wellness foods A to Z

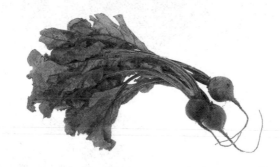

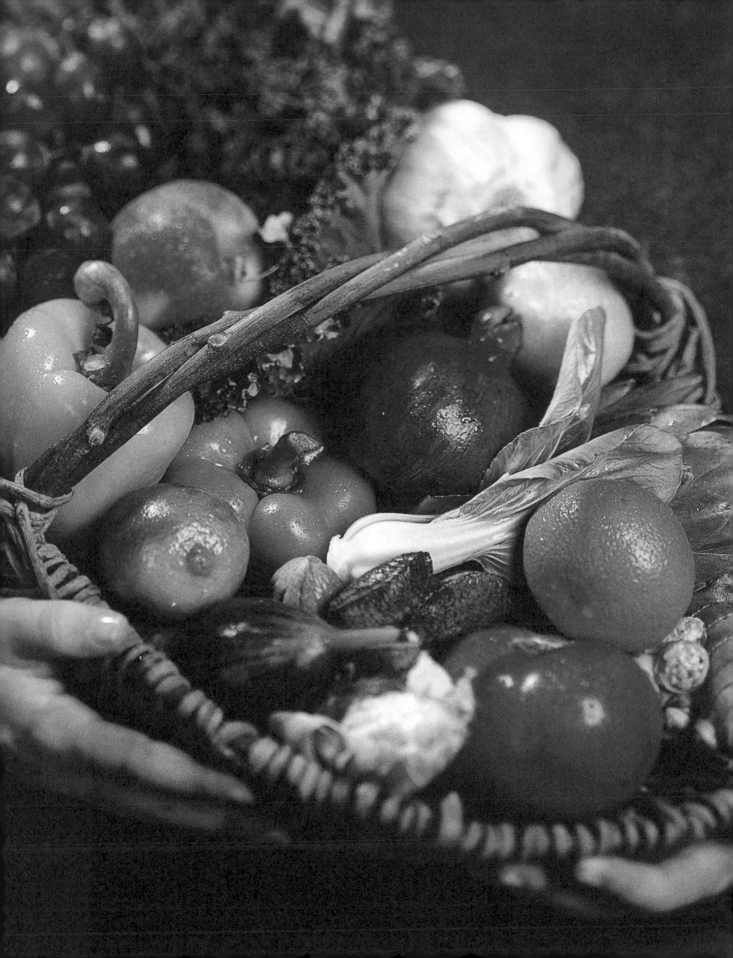

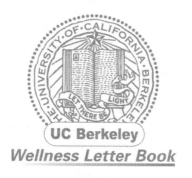

UC Berkeley
Wellness Letter Book

wellness foods A to Z

An indispensable guide for health-conscious food lovers

Sheldon Margen, M.D., and the editors of the
UC Berkeley Wellness Letter

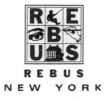

REBUS
NEW YORK

THE UNIVERSITY OF CALIFORNIA, BERKELEY
WELLNESS LETTER

www.WellnessLetter.com

The Wellness Letter is a monthly eight-page newsletter that draws on the expertise of the world-famous School of Public Health at the University of California, Berkeley to cover health, nutrition, and exercise topics in language that is clear, engaging, and nontechnical. It's a unique resource that tells you about fundamental ways to prevent illness. *The Wellness Letter* has been rated #1 among all health newsletters by *U.S. News & World Report*.

To view sample articles from the current issue and see information on our other publications, visit us online at **www.WellnessLetter.com**.

You can also order a trial subscription of this award-winning newsletter by calling 386-447-6328 or by writing to Wellness Letter, P.O. Box 420148, Palm Coast, FL 32142.

This book was created and produced by Rebus, Inc.
New York, NY 10012

COVER PHOTOGRAPHS: Lisa Koenig
HAND MODEL: Bree Rock
ILLUSTRATION: Rob Duckwall

For information about permission to reproduce selections from this book, write to Permissions, Health Letter Associates, 632 Broadway, New York, NY 10012

Library of Congress Cataloging-in-Publication Data

Margen, Sheldon.
    Wellness foods A to Z : an indispensable guide for health-conscious food lovers /
    p. cm.
    Includes index.
    ISBN 0-929661-70-2
        1. Nutrition—Encyclopedias. I. University of California, Berkeley, wellness letter. II Title.

RA784 .M2965 2002
613.2—dc21   2001058867

Printed in the United States of America
10 9 8 7 6 5 4 3

This book is not intended as a substitute for advice, diagnosis, or treatment by a physician or other health-care practitioner. Readers who suspect they may have specific health or medical problems should consult a physician about any suggestions made in this book.

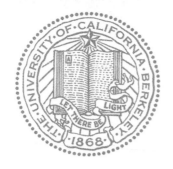

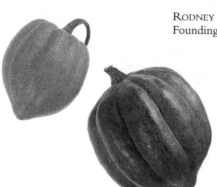

contents

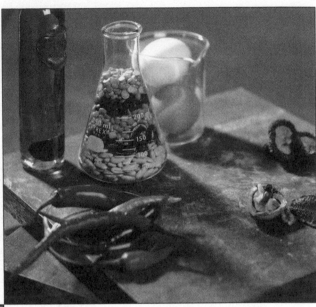
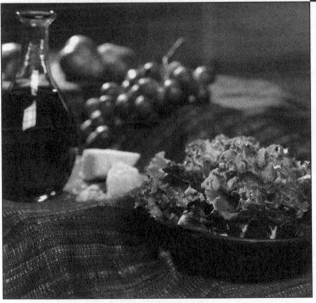

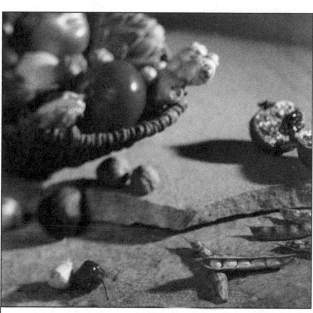

wellness foods: the basics

the nutritional bounty in vegetables,
fruits, grains, legumes, meats & poultry,
seafood, eggs, and dairy products

▼

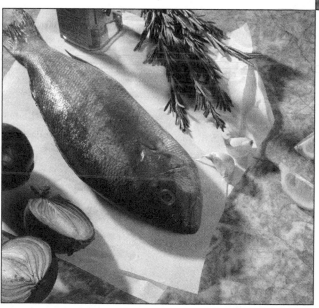

▲

foods a to z

a to z entries with nutrition profiles, key nutrient
charts, listings of different varieties, shopping
and storage information, preparation tips, and
serving suggestions

appendix

how to read a food label, facts about water,
cooking glossary, herbs & spices, salt & vinegar

index

an introduction to

wellness foods

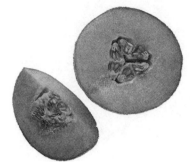

Awareness of the role that nutrition plays in maintaining health and well-being has expanded dramatically in recent years. Reporting on the latest findings connecting nutrition and disease prevention has always been a major topic in the *University of California, Berkeley Wellness Letter*. But when we launched the newsletter in 1984, it was one of a small handful of publications bringing information on that subject to a consumer audience. Today, magazine articles, television programs, and many popular books regularly describe the functions of different nutrients and the principals of sound nutrition. Terms such as "saturated fats," "cholesterol," and "antioxidants," once the province of nutritional researchers, have worked their way into everyday conversation. And it is clear from surveys that many Americans now understand the importance of a healthy diet: How choosing the right foods provides the energy and nutrients we need to function properly and maintain our overall health. Indeed, research increasingly shows that nutrients and other substances in foods can help alleviate or prevent such chronic diseases as heart disease, cancer, diabetes, and osteoporosis, once assumed to be an inevitable consequence of aging.

Despite all this nutritional advice, however, it isn't always clear to many people which dietary guidelines are important or how to apply them. Indeed, in all the talk about "good nutrition," what can get lost are the actual foods that we make choices about every day.

Certainly it is helpful to have a clear understanding of the basic facts about nutrition and the connection between nutrients and disease prevention. Indeed, the "Eating for Optimal Health" section (*page 12*) provides an excellent overview of these two topics. But the primary focus of this book is on specific foods and how you can enjoy them for both maximum taste and nutritional value. You will find answers to most questions you might have about the nutritional make-up of fresh, whole foods—from fat content (which in excessive amounts can contribute to heart disease) to antioxidant compounds (which may protect against heart disease, cancer, and age-related vision impairment, among other benefits). In addition to offering up-to-date information about a food's nutritional content and potential health benefits, we also want to emphasize the richness and variety of fresh foods, including the many culinary satisfactions they provide.

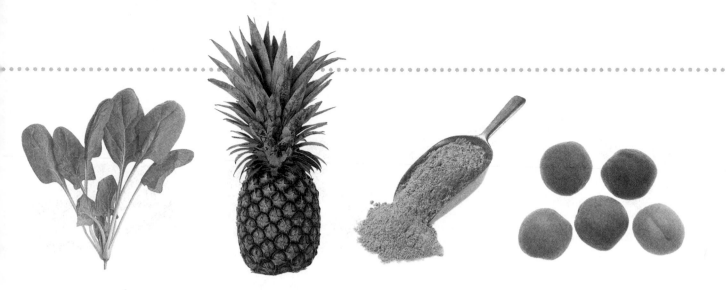

Americans today have a greater variety of foods to choose from than ever before—largely because of advances in agricultural methods and food storage and shipping. Varieties of fruits and vegetables that were once only found in gourmet or specialty food shops are now widely available in supermarkets. Produce that used to be highly seasonal is now available year round. Fresh seafood is no longer sold only to Americans who live near the seacoast, but can be purchased in most areas across the country.

One of the ironies of modern life, however, is that as the technology of food production and transportation has advanced, Americans have come to rely increasingly on processed convenience foods that are often high in fat and stripped of beneficial nutrients and fiber. In the belief that there are short-cuts to good nutrition, many people are also taking vitamin pills and other dietary supplements that contain "pure" nutrients. Some of these products may provide health benefits, but they are not adequate substitutes for foods as far as providing a healthful daily diet.

This book has a simple lesson: Eating a variety of fresh or minimally processed foods is the best way to be sure you are obtaining all of the nutritional and health benefits available from foods. These benefits, as scientists continue to discover, are plentiful, and they are linked not only to the nutrients in foods, but to non-nutrient substances that can have a profound impact on health. These substances, all of which occur naturally, are complex chemicals in plants called "phytochemicals." There are hundreds, possibly thousands, of different phytochemicals and scientists are only beginning to identify them and understand the role they play. Scientists have also realized that the substances in foods exist in an astonishingly complex balance: Some individual foods contain dozens of different compounds that very likely work together to provide a disease-protective benefit.

The array of phytochemicals in foods, and their interactions with one another and with nutrients, can't be reproduced in a dietary supplement or a heavily processed food product. Therefore, eating fresh, whole foods is the best way to be sure of obtaining all the benefits that foods offer.

As we have emphasized over the years in the *University of California, Berkeley Wellness Letter,* the most important step you can take to maintain an optimal diet is to eat a wide variety of foods, with

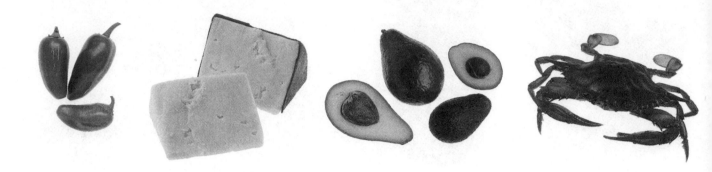

an emphasis on fruits, vegetables, and whole grains. This not only helps ensure that you get a proper balance of nutrients, but that you also benefit from the interactions that occur among foods and nutrients in your overall diet. No "special diet" that emphasizes one or two foods, or one group of foods, can do this. Achieving greater variety in the foods you consume also increases the pleasure you take in eating.

Most people aren't aware of how wide a range of foods is available to them. Did you know, for example, that you can choose from 20 or so different kinds of pastas made from roots, beans, potatoes, and many grains other than wheat? Or that there are some 500 varieties of bananas? This book will introduce you to many new foods and highlight their nutritional benefits. And in the serving suggestions provided throughout the "Foods A to Z" section, you'll find that it's possible to eat delicious foods and not abandon good nutrition; you will also have a reason to try unfamiliar foods as well as new ways of preparing those you eat every day.

how to use this book

The first section—"Eating for Optimal Health"—presents the latest information on the functions and health benefits of the different substances in food, and clarifies common misconceptions about nutrition and disease prevention. It also includes 12 "Wellness Eating Strategies" to guide you in making healthy food choices.

A comprehensive look at the protective benefits of key nutrients is in the "A Guide to Vitamins & Minerals," which also includes recently revised recommended intakes from the National Academy of Sciences and charts of leading food sources.

The third section, "Wellness Foods: The Basics" will give you a better understanding of the nutritional make-up of different food groups: vegetables, fruits, meat and poultry, seafood, eggs, and dairy products. You will also find practical information on food safety and preparation.

For information on specific foods, you can turn to the main section of the book, "Foods A to Z." Each alphabetically arranged entry supplies a "nutritional profile"; describes the different types and varieties of foods that are available; explains how to choose and store foods to retain their nutri-

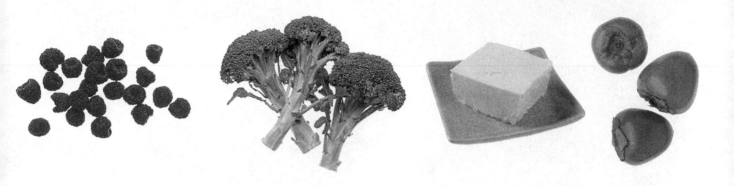

ents; and suggests the healthiest, most appetizing ways to incorporate foods into your daily menus. The entries in this section are organized under specific foods ("Salmon") as well as certain categories of food ("Fish"). If you are paging through this section and cannot locate a food, check the index.

▶ **Each entry in "Foods A to Z"** is accompanied by one or more nutrition charts (in green boxes). The charts allow you to determine and compare the nutritional value of foods at a glance. You can also use the charts to evaluate foods that don't carry nutrition labels (which are not required on fresh foods such as produce, meats, and seafood). The values are based on the United States Department of Agriculture (USDA) Nutrient Database, and they are averages: The nutritional content of any specific food item is affected by where and when it was grown; how it was shipped, stored, and displayed; and how it is prepared.

▶ **The portion sizes** used for the charts are amounts that an average person would consume at one sitting. For meat, poultry, and fish, the portion size has been standardized at 3 ounces cooked. For vegetables, it tends to be 1 cup cooked or 2 cups uncooked (salad greens, for example). Fruit portions tend to be either 1 cup of cut-up fruit or individual whole fruits. Portions of high-fat foods, such as nuts and cheese, are generally 1 ounce.

▶ **The top part of the nutrition chart** shows values for these categories: calories, protein, carbohydrate, dietary fiber, fats (total, saturated, and unsaturated), cholesterol, potassium, and sodium.

▶ **The lower section of the chart, called "Key Nutrients,"** indicates the vitamins and minerals supplied in amounts equal to or greater than 10 percent of the Recommended Dietary Allowances (RDAs) for adults. Where the RDA has not been established for a nutrient, a value called Adequate Intake (AI) is used. The RDAs and AIs were reviewed and updated between 1997 and 2002, and the values in this book reflect those updates. The RDAs are more current than the nutritional values shown on the familiar "Nutrition Facts" food labels, which make use of an older set of numbers for charting a food's nutritional content (*see pages 32 and 602 for more information*). The charts show the amount of each nutrient as well as the percent of the RDA or AI it represents. For nutrients that have different values for different age groups, the calculation uses the highest value.

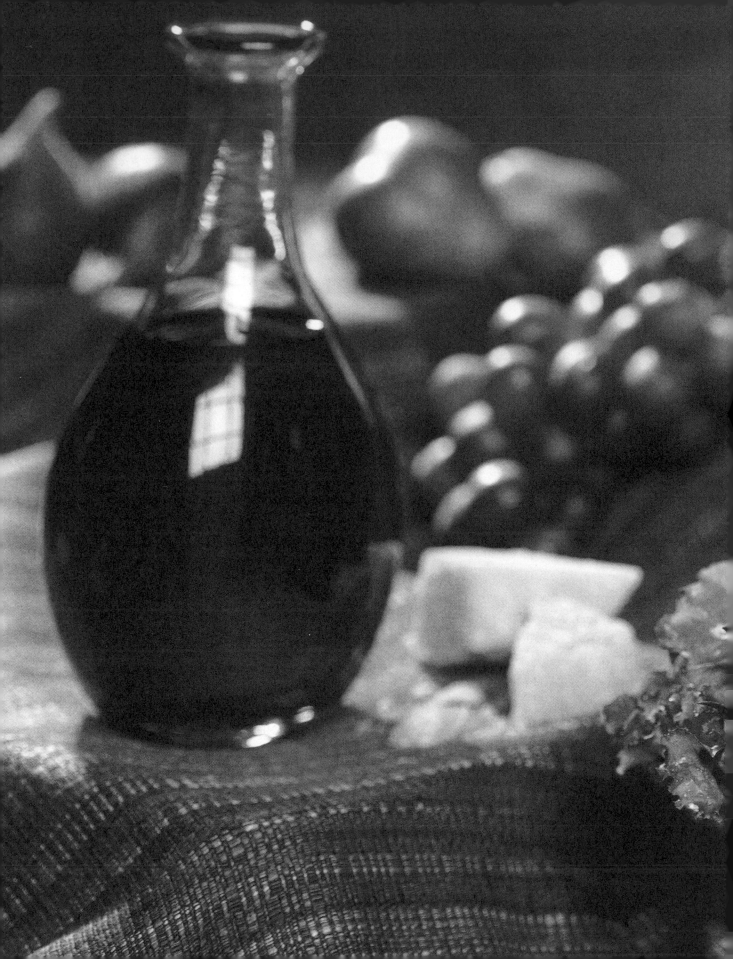

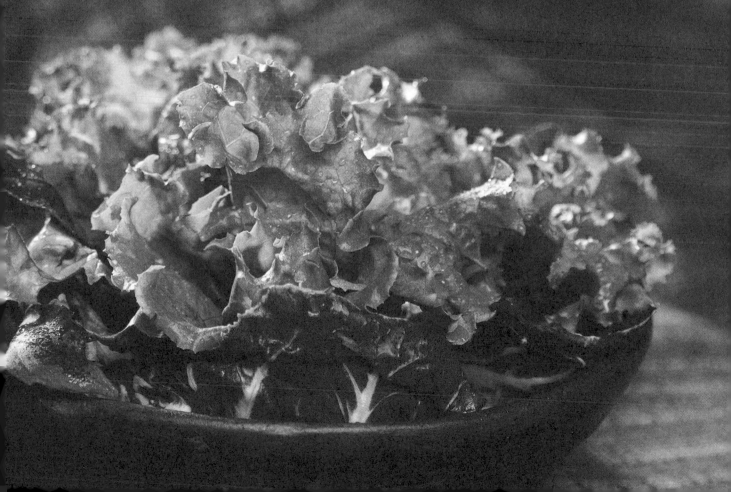

eating for
optimal health

eating for optimal health

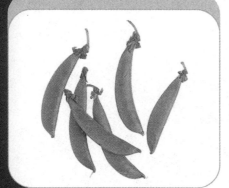

Although many Americans are aware that making some changes in their diet would benefit their health, they are often confused or misinformed on some basic nutritional concepts—believing, for example, that cholesterol is found in vegetable oils, or that foods labeled "cholesterol-free" are also free of saturated fat, which can raise blood cholesterol levels. This chapter is a handy reference of core information that highlights the components of a healthy diet and identifies the various substances in foods that affect our health, the role these substances play in our bodies, and the foods where they are found. It will also sort out some of the more common misconceptions about the nutrients in your diet. Once you understand what you should be eating and why, the rest of this book can help you immediately take advantage of all the benefits that specific foods have to offer.

a nutrition revolution

In recent years, there have been remarkable advances in what we know about the role of nutrition in disease prevention—about dietary fat and dietary fiber; carbohydrates and protein; and about vitamins and minerals. Many Americans are familiar with at least some of the benefits—and risks—associated with these nutrients. These range from the impact (both positive and negative) various types of dietary fat have on blood cholesterol levels to the bone-building benefits of calcium to the ways in which B vitamins appear to offer protection from heart disease. Americans are especially conscious about vitamins and minerals because they are available in supplement form—and millions of us take vitamin or mineral supplements every day in the belief that they will help us fight off disease.

Less familiar—and perhaps even more revolutionary—are substances in foods, especially plant foods, that are neither vitamins nor minerals, but other types of chemicals that are essential to good health. The pigments in plants, for example—the stuff that makes carrots and pumpkins orange and plums purple—may have amazing abilities to protect our health. About 2,000 pigments exist in the plants we eat, and they include over 400 known carotenoids and over 150 substances known as anthocyanins. The latter are classed as flavonoids, a large group of chemicals that includes some flavorings. Flavonoids, in turn, belong to an even larger class known as polyphenols. All of these complex substances are called phytochemicals, and scientists are discovering that some of them may have a number of possible benefits.

Some highly colored fruits and vegetables, for example, may interfere with cholesterol synthesis and thus help protect our arteries. Others act as powerful antioxidants—that is, they reduce the activity of cell-damaging free radicals—and so may help protect against cancer, diabetes, and other chronic diseases. Researchers at Cornell University, for example, found that eating fruits and vegetables rich in antioxidants helps keep lungs healthy and thus reduces the risk of asthma, emphysema, and chronic bronchitis. Phytochemicals with a high antioxidant potential may even slow down the aging process. Scientists at the USDA Human Nutrition Research Center on Aging at Tufts University can now measure the antioxidant potential in foods—and studies suggest that consuming these foods can boost the antioxidant power of human blood substantially. (*For a list of these top antioxidant foods, see page 35.*)

What's important to keep in mind is that the substances in foods interact and best carry out their functions not as individual nutrients or phytochemicals, but as part of a nutritional package—that is, when they are present in foods. That's why no single food or dietary supplement can guarantee you either a healthy life or a long one. The key to optimal health and longevity, nutritionally speaking, is a balanced and varied diet. Fortunately, there is a consensus among experts as to which dietary elements play a role in promoting or preventing disease.

the key to a healthy diet

Studies by nutritionists and epidemiologists over the past two decades have shown that healthy diets throughout the world—diets associated with lower rates of cancer, heart disease, and other chronic disorders—share certain traits. They contain plenty of fruits, whole grains, and vegetables, with modest amounts of meats and fish. In other words, a semi-vegetarian diet.

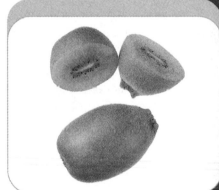

The rice-based diet in much of China is the most obvious example of this way of eating. So is the traditional Japanese diet, with its emphasis on rice or noodles accompanied by lots of vegetables, seafood, and a wide variety of soyfoods. (The Japanese have the lowest rate of heart disease in the world, and the Japanese island of Okinawa—where the average citizen consumes at least seven servings of vegetables daily and an equal number of grains—has the highest percentage of centenarians.) And the so-called "Mediterranean diet" consumed in parts of Italy, Greece, and France includes unsaturated fats such as olive oil or canola oil and wine served with meals (which can protect the heart if consumed in moderation). The pyramid recommended by the U.S. Department of Agriculture also emphasizes the semi-vegetarian approach to eating (*see "Using the Food Pyramid," page 16*). All of these diets are healthier than the typical American diet, which contains far too much saturated fat and calories from meat, dairy products, and snack foods.

12 wellness eating strategies

Here are more specific recommendations for putting together and maintaining eating habits that not only provide essential nutrients, but—in combination with other lifestyle habits such as not smoking and getting plenty of exercise—can help prevent heart disease, various types of cancer, and other chronic disorders. (The following pages spell out in greater detail the nutrients and other substances in foods that are referred to in this summary.)

using the food pyramid

Dietary advice has become more sophisticated and complicated in recent decades, so a simple diagram like the widely used pyramid developed by the U.S. Department of Agriculture (USDA) can be useful only in conveying a few general principles. The pyramid is overly simplified: It doesn't distinguish among various kinds of fat, for example, it lumps animal and vegetable protein sources together, and it doesn't distinguish between fatty and lean meats or refined grains and whole grains. Nor does it admit a difference between full-fat and fat-free or low-fat dairy products. All of these distinctions are spelled out in many of the individual food entries in this book. But the pyramid illustrates its basic point quite clearly: A variety of fruits, vegetables, and whole grains is the foundation of a healthy diet.

Portion control is also important. Serving sizes are small in the pyramid. Examples of one serving are a cup of raw leafy vegetables; one medium carrot; ½ cup of chopped, cooked, or canned fruits or vegetables; ½ cup of cooked beans; 3 ounces of cooked meat, poultry, or fish. The number of servings you need from each group on a daily basis depends on your total calorie intake. If you are a woman eating 1,600 calories per day, you should try to get at least five servings of fruits and/or vegetables—while a very active person consuming, say, 2,800 calories should aim for nine servings.

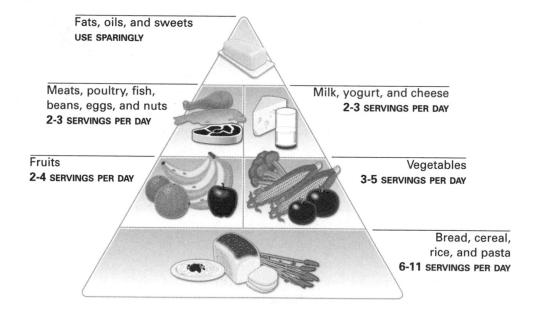

Fats, oils, and sweets
USE SPARINGLY

Meats, poultry, fish, beans, eggs, and nuts
2-3 SERVINGS PER DAY

Milk, yogurt, and cheese
2-3 SERVINGS PER DAY

Fruits
2-4 SERVINGS PER DAY

Vegetables
3-5 SERVINGS PER DAY

Bread, cereal, rice, and pasta
6-11 SERVINGS PER DAY

1. Eat a varied diet—one that emphasizes fruits, vegetable, and grains, foods that are high in complex carbohydrates. These foods should contribute most of your daily calories. Your diet should also include low-fat or fat-free dairy products, nuts, and occasional small servings of meat, poultry, and fish. This is the so-called semi-vegetarian diet. (A completely vegetarian diet can also be very healthy.)

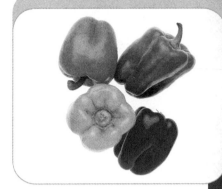

Eat five or more servings of vegetables and fruits, and six or more servings of grains or legumes, daily. Whole grains are especially nutritious. Compared to refined grains such as white rice or products made from white flour, whole-grain foods are high in fiber, contain most of the important vitamins and minerals you need, and have a moderating effect on blood glucose and insulin levels—all properties that seem to offer protection against a variety of chronic diseases.

2. Keep fat intake moderate. Your consumption of calories derived from fat should be at or below 30 percent of your total daily calories. Some experts put the fat figure even lower—25 percent of your total daily calories. You can reduce your intake by choosing the leanest meats, poultry breast without the skin, fish, and low-fat or fat-free dairy products. Cut back on butter and margarine—or foods made with these products—as well as on mayonnaise, salad dressings, fried foods, and chips. Packaged foods (cookies, cakes, crackers, TV dinners) and fast foods (hamburgers, pizza) are often sources of hidden fats and excess calories.

3. Limit your intake of saturated fat to less than 10 percent of total calories. The types of fat you consume are almost as significant as your total fat intake. Choose oils high in monounsaturated and polyunsaturated fats (canola, olive, corn, or peanut oil), but use even these in moderation. Saturated fats, which come chiefly from animal products like fatty meats, whole milk, butter, and cheese, stimulate cholesterol production in the body, as do trans fats, found in the hydrogenated fats in margarine and other processed foods (*see "Trans Fats," page 298*). Keep your intake of saturated and hydrogenated fats to a minimum.

4. Keep your cholesterol intake at 300 milligrams or less per day. Cholesterol is found only in animal products, such as meats, poultry, dairy products, and egg yolks. One large egg yolk contains about 215 milligrams of cholesterol, or about two-thirds of your daily allowance. A 3-ounce serving of meat, poultry, or fish contains about 60 milligrams (20 to 25 milligrams per ounce). Foods high in cholesterol are not necessarily high in fat.

5. Maintain a moderate protein intake—about 10 to 12 percent of your total daily calories. Choose nonfat sources of protein, such as fat-free milk and yogurt, which are also high in calcium and other nutrients. Legumes are an excellent plant source of protein. The typical American diet is overly rich in protein, particularly from animal sources.

6. Be sure to include green, orange, red, and yellow fruits and vegetables. Foods such as broccoli, carrots, tomatoes, cantaloupe, and citrus fruits are high in antioxidant nutrients such as vitamins C and E and carotenoids. Acting at the molecular level, these antioxidants inactivate a class of particles known as free radicals, highly reactive molecules in the body that can cause damage to cells. A high intake of antioxidants may be protective against cancer, heart disease, and other disorders. Researchers are only beginning to understand their importance. (*See Antioxidants, page 34.*)

7. Consume sugary foods only in moderation. For most healthy people, the only harm that sugar does, in itself, is to contribute to tooth decay. However, sugary foods are often high in calories and little else. Many foods (like cakes, pies, and cookies) that are high in sugar are also high in fat. Such foods can also trigger sudden high levels of blood sugar, which are especially bad for people with diabetes or at high risk for diabetes.

8. Limit your sodium intake to no more than 2,400 milligrams per day. This is equivalent to the amount of sodium in a little more than a teaspoon of salt. In some people, sodium may contribute to high blood pressure (about 10 percent of the population is salt-sensitive in this respect). A high salt intake can also promote water retention. Moreover, if you are consuming more than 2,400 milligrams a day, chances are you are getting much of your sodium from processed foods that don't contribute to a healthy diet. Check food labels for ingredients containing sodium; cut back on salty foods, particularly canned soups, cheeses, and pickles; and moderate your use of salt in cooking and at the table.

9. Consume enough calcium. It builds strong bones and helps maintain bone density and strength through a lifetime. This is especially important for women, whose bone density dramatically declines at menopause. The habit of eating calcium-rich foods should begin in childhood, when bone density is on the increase. The more bone you build early in life, the better you can withstand bone loss later. (*For good sources of calcium, see page 67.*)

10. Get your vitamins and minerals chiefly from foods, not from supplements. Supplements cannot substitute for a healthy diet, which supplies nutrients and other healthful compounds. Indeed, the cancer-protective elements in foods have only begun to be discovered, and these elements can't be found in pills. Scientists also believe that many compounds in food work together in ways that can't be replicated in supplements.

While supplements cannot compensate for poor eating habits, in the context of a healthy diet, certain vitamins and minerals, taken in recommended amounts, may be beneficial in many instances (*see page 31*).

11. Drink enough fluids. The body, under average conditions, loses about 2 to 3 quarts of fluid daily through perspiration, exhaled moisture, and excretion. You must replace this fluid—hence the rule-of-thumb about consuming the equivalent of at least eight 8-ounce glasses of water daily. Some of the water you need comes from solid foods, especially fruits and vegetables, which can be 80 to 90 percent water. You get the balance from liquids you consume (milk, soups, juices, and other beverages), which can be just as good as water.

12. If you drink alcohol, do so in moderation. Experts recommend that men not exceed more than two alcoholic drinks per day, and that women consume less than one drink per day. (A drink is defined as 12 ounces of beer, 4 ounces of wine, or 1.5 ounces of 80-proof liquor or spirits.) Studies have consistently found that consuming alcohol at these levels is protective against heart attacks. However, few medical experts suggest that nondrinkers start drinking for health reasons. Keep in mind that excessive consumption of alcohol can lead to a variety of health problems, counteracting any protective benefit. And alcoholic beverages can add many calories to your diet (7 calories per gram) without supplying any vitamins or minerals.

food and energy

The nutrients in food are broken down into two types. *Macronutrients*—which include carbohydrates, protein, and fats—are those that are present, and needed, in large amounts. *Micronutrients*—the vitamins and minerals—are present in much smaller amounts. (Water is a basic component of all foods, and is essential to life, but is not normally thought of as a nutrient.)

Each type of nutrient has specific functions, though every nutrient interacts with others to carry out those functions. The macronutrients provide energy and help maintain and repair the body. As micronutrients, vitamins regulate the chemical processes that take place in the body. Minerals assist with this, and play a role in body maintenance as well, notably in the formation of new tissue, including bones, teeth, and blood.

Your body is always burning a mixture of macronutrients for energy. The production of energy—and the potential for a food to supply energy—is measured in calories. (The caloric content of a food is determined by measuring the amount of heat produced when the food is burned in a laboratory device called a calorimeter. The heat that is generated is analogous to the energy produced in the human body.) At rest and at low levels of activity, carbohydrates provide 40 to 50 percent of the body's energy needs.

Carbohydrates are the most efficient fuel for the body because they can be broken down to produce energy almost instantly. Fat—either from food or from body fat stores—also provides energy, but not as readily as carbohydrates. Only after 20 to 30 minutes of continuous activity does your body begin to rely more on fat than on carbohydrates. The longer the activity and/or the longer you go without food, the more your body uses fat for fuel. And any dietary fat that is not burned is converted to body fat (as are any unused carbohydrates or proteins).

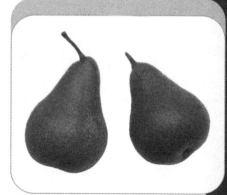

carbohydrates

Carbohydrates have become a battleground in debates about healthy eating, and these days you can meet both carbohydrate boosters and carbohydrate haters. Carbohydrates are what you are supposed to fill up on when you cut down on fat, says one side of the table. Or they are what's making Americans fat, according to the other side. Yet most people don't really know what carbohydrates are. Many of the boosters and haters talk as if all carbohydrates were the same—which is not true.

Carbohydrates include all the sugars and starches we eat—and they are found in a great variety of foods. All of the following, for example, are rich sources of carbohydrates: orange juice, table sugar, nonfat milk, pears, strawberries, whole-wheat bread, apple pie, popcorn, biscuits, green peas, muffins, honey, and sweet potatoes.

Carbohydrates are the main energy source for the body: They are transformed by the body into blood sugar (mostly glucose), the body's basic fuel. They supply 4 calories per gram, the same as protein. Fat has more than twice as many calories (9 per gram)—one reason for its bad reputation. Carbohydrates form the main source of calories in virtually every diet worldwide.

the advantages of complex carbohydrates

Since most carbohydrates are broken down into glucose, why does it matter which carbohydrates you consume? Why is the carbohydrate in a teaspoonful of sugar any better or worse than the equivalent amount of carbohydrate in lima beans or whole-wheat bread or, for that matter, in a chocolate bar?

Most carbohydrates come from plant-based foods—fruits, vegetables, grains, and legumes (beans, peas, and lentils). Dairy products are the only animal-derived foods with lots of carbohydrates. There are two general types of carbohydrates:

• *Simple carbohydrates* are sugars—glucose and fructose from fruits and some vegetables, lactose from milk, sucrose from cane or beet sugar, and others. Table sugar is pure sucrose. Most of the simple carbohydrates Americans actually consume are sugars added to processed foods such as sodas and cookies. These added sugars are the main reason why sugar now accounts for 16 percent of all calories consumed by Americans; 20 years ago, it supplied 11 percent. Soda alone supplies about one-third of this added sugar.

• *Complex carbohydrates,* which are chains of simple sugars, consist primarily of starches as well as the indigestible fiber that occurs in all plant foods. Starch is the storage form of carbohydrates in plants. Foods rich in complex carbohydrates include grains and grain products (such as bread and pasta), beans, potatoes, corn, and some other vegetables.

Many foods high in sugar (especially sucrose and other added sugars) supply "empty calories"—that is, they have few nutrients but plenty of calories. By contrast, foods rich in complex carbohydrates usually bring nutritional extras with them. *However, you need to be selective.* White bread made from refined flour contains complex carbohydrates, for instance, but whole grains (such as oats, whole wheat, brown rice) are more nutritious, since they retain the bran and the germ, which are rich in vitamins, minerals, fiber, and beneficial phytochemicals. Some experts now think that refined grains and other complex carbohydrates that are low in dietary fiber (such as pasta and white rice) cause spikes in blood sugar because they are quickly converted into glucose. Some studies suggest that a diet with too many of these foods increases the risk of diabetes, at least in those predisposed to it.

Whole grains, by contrast, are digested more slowly, and thus have a more modest effect on blood sugar than refined carbohydrates or sugars. The same is true of vegetables and beans. The fiber in these foods has many health benefits. In particular, soluble fiber (found in oats, barley, and beans) may help lower LDL ("bad") cholesterol, and regulate blood sugar (*see below*).

wellness recommendation

Include as many whole grains as you can in your daily diet—at least three servings a day, according to the government's new dietary guidelines. Limit your intake of highly refined, low-fiber grain products such as white bread.

It's much better to get simple carbohydrates (sugars) from fruit, milk, and juice—because these contain other nutrients—than from cake, cookies (even if low-fat), or soda. There's nothing wrong with small amounts of foods and beverages high in added sugar, but many Americans eat too many of them, adding lots of calories, leaving little room for more nutritious foods, and increasing the risk of chronic disease.

fiber

Dietary fiber is not one substance, but an impressive variety of compounds with varied effects in the body. Fiber compounds are found only in plant foods, and unlike macronutrients and vitamins and minerals, fiber is not broken down as it passes through the small intestine. (Though fiber is sometimes thought of as passing undigested through the entire intestinal tract, some types of fiber undergo digestion by bacterial enzymes in the large intestine, or colon.)

For simplicity, fiber can be divided into two broad categories: those that are soluble in water and those that are insoluble. Most plant foods contain both types in varying amounts, but certain foods are particularly rich in one or the other.

LEADING SOURCES	
SOURCE	**DIETARY FIBER (G)**
Raspberries, 1 cup	8.4
Bulgur, cooked, 1 cup	8.2
Kidney beans, cooked, ½ cup	8.2
Lentils, cooked, ½ cup	7.8
Rye wafers, 3 crackers	7.6
Artichoke, fresh, boiled	6.5
Potato, baked with skin, 1 medium	4.9
Figs, dried, ¼ cup	4.6
Acorn squash, baked, cubed, ½ cup	4.5
Blueberries, fresh, 1 cup	3.9
Wheat bran, crude, 2 tbsp	3.1

strong links to disease prevention

Evidence suggests that soluble fiber helps lower blood cholesterol levels and therefore reduces the risk of heart disease. It also helps keep blood glucose (sugar) levels in check, and so is beneficial in the management of diabetes. Both types of fiber can help promote weight loss because high-fiber foods are filling (so you eat less of them) and tend to be low in fat.

Insoluble fiber helps prevent constipation (when consumed with adequate fluid intake) by adding bulk to the stool and stimulating peristalsis (the involuntary contractions that move food through the intestinal tract). By reducing constipation and strained bowel movements, insoluble fiber may also help prevent diverticulosis, a condition in which tiny asymptomatic pouches, called diverticula, form within the wall of the colon. When the pouches trap food, they may become painfully inflamed (diverticulitis). About one in three Americans over age 50 suffers from diverticulosis.

In addition, dozens of studies have supported the idea that this type of fiber plays a role in preventing colon cancer, either by speeding food through the intestinal tract (thus reducing the time potential carcinogens come into contact with the colon wall) or by diluting or inactivating the carcinogens.

Some recent research, however, has cast doubt that a high-fiber intake protects against colon cancer. As reported in the *New England Journal of Medicine* in 1999, a segment of the ongoing Nurses' Health Study—which tracks the diets and health risks of more than 88,000 nurses—found that women who had the highest fiber intake (more than 25 grams daily), as opposed to the lowest (less than 10 grams), gained no protection against colon cancer. There have been other studies besides this one that have also found no protective effect against colon cancer. But other important research is under way, and the tables may be turned once more. We have barely begun to understand the connections between diet and colon cancer.

In the meantime, don't give up on "roughage," as fiber was once referred to. Indeed, according to a recent 10-year study of the dietary habits of nearly 3,000 young adults, those who had a high-fiber diet were more likely to be healthy than those who merely kept their fat consumption low. This study was reported in the *Journal of the American Medical Association*. A high-fiber intake turned out to be an independent factor (not tied to exercise or other dietary habits) in controlling weight gain and high insulin levels, which can promote heart disease and diabetes. People in the study who ate more than 10.5 grams of fiber for every 1,000 daily calories were less likely to be overweight or to have gained weight in the 10-year period. They also had fewer risk factors for cardiovascular disease—that is, they were less likely to have high blood pressure, high triglycerides, and high blood cholesterol.

The researchers emphasized that their study did not tell the whole story. But there is plenty of other evidence that a high-fiber diet—one based on fruits, whole grains, and vegetables—protects against heart disease, diabetes, and other chronic diseases.

wellness recommendation

Experts recommend that you try to get 20 to 30 grams of fiber a day from a variety of foods. Insoluble fiber is found primarily in wheat, especially in wheat bran, and in other whole grains. Soluble fiber is found mainly in vegetables, fruits, legumes, barley, brown rice, oats, and oat bran. While it's true that large intakes of fiber can decrease the absorption of some minerals, since high-fiber foods are generally quite nutritious, this is not a problem.

Be sure to drink plenty of liquids; otherwise, fiber can slow down or even block proper bowel function. And don't try to get all of your fiber at one sitting, which can cut the benefits and increase the chances of unpleasant side effects. As a rule of thumb, try to eat foods high in both insoluble and soluble fiber at every meal.

protein

Muscles, organs, antibodies, some hormones, and all enzymes (the compounds that direct cell chemical reactions) are largely composed of protein. Yet protein is not a single, simple substance, but a multitude of chemical combinations. The basic units of proteins are amino acids. Just 22 amino acids are combined in a variety of ways to create the thousands of different types of proteins. The body can manufacture 13 amino acids on its own; these are called "nonessential" amino acids.

The other nine amino acids are called "essential" because they must come from foods. Foods that contain all of the essential amino acids in sufficient amounts are called complete proteins; those that are missing one or more amino acid are called incomplete. All animal proteins—meats, poultry, fish, dairy products, and eggs—are complete proteins.

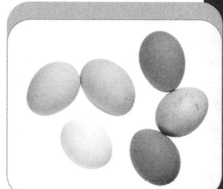

Plant proteins are incomplete proteins, with the exception of soybeans and soyfoods like tofu, which are complete. Foods that provide incomplete proteins can be made complete by eating (either at the same meal or within the same day) a complementary protein that provides the amino acids that the other food lacks. Rice and beans, peanut butter and bread, and macaroni and cheese are traditional combinations that provide complementary proteins.

wellness recommendation

In general, experts recommend that everyone get 10 to 12 percent of their calories from protein. Most Americans consume more than that. Basically, if you eat a normal, balanced diet, it is hard not to get enough protein. Even strict vegetarians get enough if they eat grains, vegetables, and nuts in the proper quantities and combinations to ensure that their protein is complete.

protein supplements don't build muscle

Some sports physiologists and coaches believe that athletes and body builders need more protein because their bodies break down and rebuild body tissue at a higher rate, and because they have more muscle mass. But even if you exercise a lot, you don't need high-protein powders, drinks, tablets, capsules, or bars. Studies suggest that endurance athletes or weight lifters do indeed need more protein than other people, but because of their greater food intake, they get extra protein with little trouble. Consuming protein supplements or isolated amino acids won't stimulate muscle growth—only exercise, specifically strength training, does. Excess protein is simply broken down in the body and burned for energy or turned into fat.

fats

In news reports and magazine articles, fat is usually portrayed as a nutritional villain. A high-fat diet has been linked in study after study with heart disease, cancer, and other health problems, including those linked to obesity. What most people forget, however, is that fats are essential to the proper functioning of the human body, and we need to consume some fat to remain healthy.

Technically fats belong to a class of substances called lipids. Unlike carbohydrates, fats are insoluble in water. Most of the fats in foods are triglycerides, which consist of three fatty acids attached to a glycerol molecule. Some of the fatty acids are called "essential" fatty acids, so named because the body cannot make them and must get them from foods (like the essential amino acids that help make up proteins).

Fats perform many other important functions. Fatty acids are the raw materials for several hormonelike compounds, including prostaglandins, that help control blood pressure, blood clotting, inflammation, and other bodily functions. Fats also serve as the storage substance for the body's excess calories, filling the balloonlike adipose cells that insulate the body. Extra calories from carbohydrates and proteins, as well as from fats, are stored as adipose tissue, or body fat. After about 20 to 30 minutes of continual activity (such as brisk walking or cycling), your body begins breaking down adipose tissue for energy, relying less and less on carbohydrates. In addition, fats help maintain healthy skin and hair, transport the fat-soluble vitamins (A, D, E, and K) through the gastrointestinal tract and bloodstream, and regulate blood cholesterol levels. Dietary fats also promote a sensation of feeling full when consumed in food, probably because they slow the emptying of the stomach.

different fats, different effects

Fatty acids vary in the length of their molecular chains and in the degree of saturation by hydrogen atoms—and these variations determine the properties of different fats. All fats are combinations of saturated and unsaturated fatty acids, which is why fats are described with terms such as "highly saturated" or "highly unsaturated." For instance, about half the fatty acids in beef are saturated, which is a high proportion.

Saturated fatty acids are loaded with all the hydrogen atoms they can carry. Fats that are largely saturated are usually solid at room temperature. Such fats come chiefly from animal sources—meats, poultry, and whole-milk dairy products. Three vegetable oils—coconut, palm, and palm kernel—are also highly saturated. And "trans fats"—fats that are transformed by hydrogenating the oils used in margarines and many packaged snack foods—act much like saturated fats (*see "Trans Fats," page 298*).

Unsaturated fatty acids do not have all the hydrogen atoms they can carry. Depending on the number of missing hydrogen atoms, these fatty acids are called either *monounsaturated* (olive, canola, peanut, and avocado oils are largely monounsaturated) or *polyunsaturated* (corn, safflower, and sesame oils are primarily polyunsaturated). These important dietary fats come from plants and fish. They are generally liquid at room temperature.

A diet high in saturated fat can raise blood cholesterol levels, which increases the risk of heart disease (*see "Cholesterol," page 26*). Unsaturated fats, by contrast, appear to have a beneficial effect on cholesterol levels—and some experts say that oils rich in monounsaturated fats, such as olive and canola, are probably more protective than polyunsaturated fats. However, the polyunsaturated oils known as omega-3 fatty acids, found mainly in fish, may be especially protective against heart disease.

This does not mean, however, that it is healthy to have a diet high in unsaturated fats: Since all fats contain 9 calories per gram (versus 4 calories per gram in carbohydrates and protein), too much of any kind of fat increases your chance of becoming overweight or obese, which is another risk factor for cardiovascular disease.

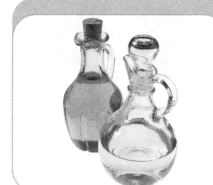

wellness recommendation

Most experts recommend that you get no more than 30 percent of your daily calories from fat—and aiming for 25 percent is preferable. It's also important to be careful about the type of fat you consume. The American Heart Association (AHA), which has recommended that less than 10 percent of fat calories come from saturated fats, now places even more emphasis on limiting saturated fats and replacing them with monounsaturated fats. New guidelines issued by the government's National Cholesterol Education Program in 2001 urge that healthy Americans with elevated cholesterol levels lower their saturated fat intake to less than 7 percent of fat calories. (The new guidelines allow up to 35 percent of total calories from fat, provided that most of those calories are from unsaturated fats. However, the Editorial Board for the *University of California, Berkeley Wellness Letter* continues to recommend the "less than 30 percent, preferably 25 percent" figures for daily fat calories.)

Some doctors believe that you should lower your fat intake to less than 20 or even 15 percent of calories. Other factors may influence your decision about how high—or how low—to maintain your fat intake. These include your weight, your personal and family risk for heart disease, your blood cholesterol levels, and medical history. But for most people, such a reduction in fat intake is probably not necessary; a diet with 25 to 30 percent of total calories from fat can be both healthy and practical.

In real life, of course, exact calculations of fat percentages are difficult if not impossible. But you can move in the right direction, for instance, by replacing butter with a highly monounsaturated oil such as canola or olive oil (or peanut, walnut, or almond oil). Replacing just 2 tablespoons of butter with the same amount of olive oil may be enough to shift your daily fat balance to meet the AHA recommendation. Small amounts of peanuts, almonds, or peanut butter are also healthy choices. Just don't go overboard: Upping your percentage of monounsaturated fats doesn't mean simply ladling on teaspoonfuls of olive oil over a salad. The oil has to replace other less-healthy fats.

Two other recommendations: Eat fish once or twice a week for its heart-protective omega-3 fatty acids. And limit your intake of the "trans fats" found in margarines and shortenings labeled "hydrogenated" (which are used in many packaged crackers, cookies, and chips). If you eat lots of margarine, cut back on or switch to a tub or liquid "squeeze" margarine or to one of the "diet" margarines that contain more water and only half the fat of other margarines. And moderate your intake of processed snack foods; instead of packaged snack foods, try a variety of fruits and vegetables.

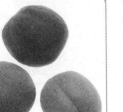

cholesterol

Cholesterol is a fatlike substance that is present in all tissues in humans and animals, and in all foods from animal sources. (There is no cholesterol in plants.)

Although cholesterol performs many essential functions in the body, the cholesterol that we get from foods is not an essential nutrient. The human body can make all the cholesterol it needs from dietary fats.

It is cholesterol circulating in the bloodstream—referred to as "serum cholesterol"—that is so often discussed and measured. And it is this cholesterol, transported through the blood by chemical packages called lipoproteins, that accumulates on the walls of blood vessels. Too much cholesterol in the bloodstream increases the risk of developing atherosclerosis—clogged arteries that can lead to heart attack or stroke.

wellness recommendation

As noted above, dietary fats can have a significant effect on blood cholesterol levels. But, surprisingly, there does not seem to be a simple relationship between dietary cholesterol and blood cholesterol. It is recommended that, regardless of their dietary habits, most people have their blood cholesterol measured periodically by their physicians. Healthy people whose blood cholesterol is at desirable levels should limit cholesterol from food to an average of no more than 300 milligrams per day. For people with elevated cholesterol levels, the government's National Cholesterol Education Program now recommends that daily cholesterol intake be less than 200 milligrams.

foods that help control cholesterol

A low-fat, low-cholesterol diet has been the tried-and-true way for anyone attempting to lower elevated blood cholesterol without medication. Besides this "negative" approach—cut back on this, eliminate that—there are also foods you can add to your diet that may help lower your cholesterol. Some of the foods listed below are proven to be effective. Others, despite media hype, have little or no effect, remain unproven, or require that you eat unrealistic amounts to get a significant effect.

Bear in mind: None of these foods, even the best, is a "magic bullet" against cholesterol that will cancel out the adverse effects of an otherwise unhealthy diet. Context is crucial. Add these foods to a low-fat diet, and you'll get the greatest effect. Even better, eat them instead of animal products high in saturated fat. And all these foods have other potential health benefits as well.

Fruits and vegetables. Some are rich in soluble fiber, notably pectin, which helps lower total and LDL ("bad") cholesterol. These include apples, citrus fruit, berries, carrots, apricots, prunes, cabbage, sweet potatoes, and Brussels sprouts. If you eat a lot of these, at least five servings a day, you'll see an extra drop in cholesterol beyond the effect of a low-fat diet.

Beans (legumes). Lima, kidney, black, and other beans, as well as lentils and chick-peas, are some of the best sources of cholesterol-lowering soluble fiber. Studies have found that eating even 4 ounces of beans a day can significantly reduce total and LDL cholesterol.

Cholesterol-lowering margarines. Benecol brand margarine can lower total and LDL blood cholesterol by an average of 10 percent, when eaten in the recommended quantities, without lowering HDL ("good") cholesterol. Benecol's "medicinal" ingredients are patented stanol esters, which are forms of plant sterols derived from pine trees. There are also other similar products, such as Take Control margarine and dressings, which contain sterols derived from soybeans. These plant chemicals act to help prevent dietary cholesterol in your digestive system from being absorbed and passing into your bloodstream.

There are also dietary supplements on the market that contain stanol esters and related compounds. However, the ingredients in the supplements are not identical to those in the margarines. Moreover, the doses are too small to have a significant cholesterol-lowering effect.

Nuts. The monounsaturated and polyunsaturated fats in nuts help lower cholesterol, especially when substituted for sources of saturated fat, such as meat or cheese. Moreover, certain phytochemicals in nuts, such as sterols, may inhibit cholesterol absorption. Studies have found that eating 2 to 4 ounces of nuts a day has a significant effect; one found that a mere 8 to 11 walnuts a day reduced cholesterol levels by 4 percent. Just remember that nuts are calorie-dense.

Oats. Oats are one of the best sources (along with barley) of a type of soluble fiber called beta glucan, which helps lower total and LDL cholesterol. Thus, oat products are allowed to bear a heart-healthy claim. But it takes a fair amount of oat fiber—the amount found in about 1½ cups of oatmeal or 3 cups of dry oat cereals—to have a significant effect.

Soyfoods. Recently the FDA allowed soyfoods to carry a heart-healthy claim if they contain a fair amount of soy protein and are eaten as part of a diet low in saturated fat and cholesterol. But no one knows whether it's the protein or other substances in soy (notably fiber, unsaturated fat, or compounds called isoflavones) that help lower cholesterol. As with oats, you have to eat a fair amount of soy—say, 2 cups of soymilk or 4 ounces of tofu—to get an effect. The benefit is usually modest, and may be significant only when soy protein replaces animal protein.

Flaxseed. This is the best source of lignans, which provide fiber. Flaxseed also contains alpha-linolenic acid (a type of omega-3 fatty acid), as well as other compounds that may have heart-healthy effects. Some researchers and marketers claim that flaxseed and its oil have greater health effects than those of other seeds and oils, but other experts dispute this. Studies on flaxseed have had inconsistent results regarding the effects on cholesterol. (Whole seeds are useless in this respect, since they pass through the intestines undigested.)

Olive oil. This oil may help lower blood cholesterol, but it is not the only oil to do so. Some studies give the edge to such highly monounsaturated fats as olive oil, but other studies have found that highly polyunsaturated oils

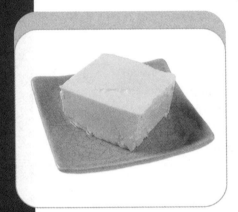

(such as corn or soybean) also lower total blood cholesterol impressively. One thing is clear: Any oil that replaces saturated fat is good. If your chief concern is lowering blood cholesterol, you have nothing to gain by choosing olive oil over other highly monounsaturated oils (such as canola or peanut) or over highly polyunsaturated oils.

Fish. Some early studies did find that fatty fish lowers cholesterol, but later ones have disputed this. If you substitute fish for meat (or for other sources of saturated fat), you'll lower your cholesterol. But the same would happen if you replaced the meat with beans or other foods low in saturated fat. When researchers control for saturated fat intake, the effect of fish on cholesterol often turns out to be minimal, at best. Fish can, however, lower triglycerides, the major type of fat that circulates in the blood. And there are other ways that fish helps keep your heart healthy.

omega-3 fatty acids

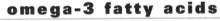

The fat in fish is rich in polyunsaturated fatty acids called omega-3s, the major marine types being eicosapentaenoic acid (EPA) and docosahexaenoic acid (DHA). Fatty fish (such as salmon) are the richest sources. Like aspirin, these omega-3s make platelets in the blood less likely to stick together and may reduce inflammatory processes in blood vessels. Thus they reduce blood clotting, thereby lessening the chance of a heart attack.

Studies on other specific heart-related benefits of omega-3s—such as the extent to which they reduce cholesterol levels or high blood pressure—have had contradictory results, however. Moreover, when there is an effect, it often appears to require large doses of fish oil—and the effect can turn out to be small in any case.

Most population studies find some beneficial effect of omega-3s on the risk of heart disease, especially against heart attacks, but again the results have been surprisingly inconsistent. Some important studies have found that fish consumption doesn't reduce the risk of heart disease, but may reduce the risk of dying from it. A 1997 study that followed 1,800 men from the Chicago area for 30 years found that those who ate at least 8 ounces of fish a week had a 40 percent lower risk of fatal heart attack than those who ate no fish (the study didn't look at nonfatal heart attacks).

Perhaps if fish oil does protect the heart, it may not be by obvious means such as lowering blood cholesterol, triglycerides, or blood pressure. For instance, some studies suggest that omega-3s may be beneficial because they modulate electrical activity in the heart, thus making the heart less susceptible to dangerous, sometimes fatal, rhythm abnormalities.

LEADING SOURCES	
SOURCE (3 oz cooked)	OMEGA-3s (G)
Boston (Atlantic) mackerel	2.2
Lake trout	1.7
Atlantic salmon, farmed	1.6
Whitefish, lake	1.5
Herring	1.4
Bluefin tuna	1.4
Chinook salmon	1.3
Sturgeon	1.3
Albacore tuna	1.3
Sardines, canned	1.2

In addition, in population studies that compare fish eaters to those who eat no fish, it's possible that the people who eat no fish have a less healthy lifestyle. Researchers adjust the data for such "confounding factors," but can't control for everything.

The area where fish holds some promise is treating rheumatoid arthritis and other inflammatory disorders, though research is preliminary. Fish oil may help relieve inflammatory symptoms of these autoimmune diseases by suppressing the immune response. More than a dozen studies have suggested that high doses of fish oil supplements taken long term and with pain medication can reduce joint swelling, ease stiffness, and lessen fatigue in people with rheumatoid arthritis. There is also some preliminary evidence that fish oil may help reduce the itching and redness of psoriasis, another autoimmune disease.

wellness recommendation

Fish is one of the best foods around. Besides its oil, it is rich in protein, iron, B vitamins, and other nutrients, and it can take the place of meats that are high in saturated fat. Studies finding that fish enhances cardiovascular health suggest that two servings a week are enough. In fact, a higher intake of fish isn't necessarily better for your health.

There are no United States government recommendations for omega-3 intake, but Health Canada, the Canadian counterpart of the Food and Drug Administration (FDA), recommends 1 to 1.5 grams a day. (*See "Comparing Fish," page 311, for more good sources of omega-3s.*)

Don't substitute fish oil supplements for fish. Not only do supplements lack some of the nutrients found in whole fish, but the supplements can cause unpleasant side effects and have some serious health concerns associated with them (*see "Fish Oil Capsules," page 309*).

vitamins

A vitamin is an organic substance (meaning it contains carbon) that your body requires to help regulate functions within cells. For the most part, vitamins must be obtained from foods, except for vitamins D and K, which can be synthesized in other ways. Only very small amounts of vitamins are

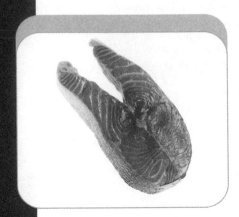

needed to carry out their functions, but these small amounts are absolutely essential. Without vitamins, higher animal organisms—like humans—could not exist. Vitamins affect all functions in the body. Among the myriad tasks vitamins perform are promoting good vision, forming normal blood cells, creating strong bones and teeth, and ensuring the proper functioning of the heart and nervous system. While vitamins themselves do not supply energy, some of them do aid in the efficient conversion of foods to energy.

Thirteen vitamins are needed by humans: A, C, D, E, K, and eight B vitamins—thiamin, riboflavin, niacin, pantothenic acid, B_6, B_{12}, folate, and biotin. In addition, vitamin A, which comes from animal sources such as meat and eggs, is present in the form of a precursor, beta carotene, in many plant foods. Carrots, for example, are rich in beta carotene, and the body converts this nutrient to vitamin A. It appears that beta carotene, apart from its role in vitamin A formation, may also act as an antioxidant.

Vitamins can all be categorized as either fat-soluble (A, D, E, and K) or water-soluble (the B vitamins and vitamin C). The distinction is important because the body stores fat-soluble vitamins for relatively long periods (usually in the liver and in fat tissue), whereas water-soluble vitamins (with the exception of B_{12}), which are stored in various tissues, remain in the body for only a short time and so need to be replenished frequently. Otherwise, symptoms associated with a deficiency of water-soluble vitamins can occur within weeks to several months.

Most vitamins are sensitive in varying degrees to heat and light, and there is always some loss of vitamins when food is being stored, handled, and cooked. These losses can be accelerated when food isn't stored away from light or properly refrigerated. Fat-soluble vitamins are more stable during cooking than water-soluble ones, which can easily be leached from foods that are cooked in boiling water. Short cooking times, and the practice of cooking foods in minimal amounts of water (*see "Cooking Glossary," page 608*), can help conserve nutrients.

minerals

The minerals that act as nutrients are absolutely essential to a host of vital processes in the body, from bone formation to the functioning of the heart and digestive system. Many are necessary for the activity of enzymes (proteins that serve as catalysts in the body's chemical reactions). In recent years, scientists have been paying great attention to minerals, looking for links between them and the major chronic diseases—high blood pressure, osteoporosis, cardiovascular disease, and even cancer. This research has been very promising.

Minerals are basic elements of the earth's crust (in contrast to vitamins, they are inorganic matter—they contain no carbon). Carried into the soil, groundwater, and sea by erosion, they are taken up by plants and consumed by animals and humans. Heating foods doesn't destroy minerals—even if you burn your food to a cinder, it will retain all its original minerals. However, when food is boiled, some of its minerals may dissolve into the water and be discarded. Minerals can also be processed out of foods, as when grains are refined to make flour.

There are more than 60 minerals in the body (making up about 4 percent of its weight), but only about 22 are considered essential. Of these, seven—calcium, chlorine, magnesium, phosphorus, potassium, sodium, and sulfur—are called macrominerals because they are present in the body in relatively large quantities. The other essential minerals are termed trace or even ultratrace nutrients because they are present in such minute quantities.

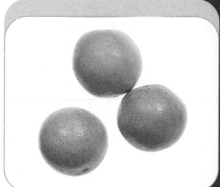

should you take supplements?

If you eat a healthy diet, you probably don't need a daily multivitamin/mineral supplement. And if you are eating an unhealthy diet, supplements cannot completely make up for it. For example, they will not offset the effects of a diet too high in fat or too low in fiber.

In certain cases, however, vitamin and mineral supplements can enhance a healthy diet. Even if you eat the right balance of foods, you may not obtain the high levels of certain nutrients (above adequate recommended levels) that many authorities now think you need. In addition, certain groups of people with special needs may benefit from taking supplements.

wellness recommendation

Consider two antioxidant supplements—250 to 500 milligrams of vitamin C and 200 to 400 international units (IU) of vitamin E daily. A large body of basic laboratory research has shown that, as antioxidants, these vitamins help inactivate free radicals—unstable molecules that can damage cells and thereby theoretically lead to chronic diseases. There have been many studies on C and E, and scientists are only beginning to understand how these and other antioxidants work. The evidence is accumulating bit by bit.

That said, some (though not all) members of the Editorial Board for the *University of California, Berkeley Wellness Letter* have concluded—based on the evidence currently available—that supplemental C and E pose little risk at the levels recommended here, and have substantial potential benefits, including protection against heart disease, certain types of cancer, cataracts, and perhaps other disorders.

If you eat lots of citrus fruits and vegetables and their juices, you may be getting that much vitamin C (1 cup of orange juice contains about 100 milligrams), and then you may not need supplemental C. If you do take a supplement, don't pay extra for "natural" forms of vitamin C; natural and synthetic forms are equivalent.

It's difficult, however, to get the recommended amount of vitamin E from foods—and most foods that are good sources of vitamin E are high in fat. Vit-

the RDA evolution

How much of a particular vitamin or mineral do you need to consume to maintain good health?

Since 1941, the Food and Nutrition Board of the National Academy of Sciences—a committee funded by the federal government—has reviewed nutrition research and established nutrition requirements. Until recently, their principal recommendations, which were updated periodically, were the Recommended Dietary Allowances, or RDAs. The primary goal behind the first set of RDAs, created in 1941, was to construct an adequate diet that could maintain good health, with a focus on preventing diseases caused by nutrient deficiencies—an example being scurvy, which results from a vitamin C deficiency.

This focus on establishing an adequate diet persisted for many years. But as deficiency diseases virtually disappeared in industrialized countries, and as evidence accumulated on the links between diet and chronic diseases such as cancer, diabetes, and heart disease, scientists began demanding modification of the RDAs to reflect current research.

Most recently, panels of experts reviewed and revised the RDAs for the first time since 1989. They issued other guidelines as well. The goal of the new guidelines has been broadened, so they are aimed not only at preventing deficiency diseases but also at reducing the risk of chronic diseases. The Canadian government helped develop the new guidelines, which will also be used in Canada.

The new guidelines, however, are not any easier to understand. The old RDAs were confusing enough, since there were different RDAs for men and women, old and young people, as well as a related set of numbers for food labels. But now, besides the RDAs, you may also read about other sets of official guidelines—DRIs, AIs, EARs, ULs—that have left even many nutrition experts scratching their heads. Also complicating matters is the fact that food labels were not revised at the same time to reflect the new guidelines; information about vitamins and minerals on food labels—expressed as a percentage of "Daily Values"—is derived from older RDA values incorporated into legal requirements for food labeling. (*See "How to Read a Food Label," page 602.*)

New Definitions

Here is a summary of the new guidelines:

DRI (dietary reference intake): The umbrella term for the guidelines, it includes the items that follow. DRIs have been devised for 17 vitamins and minerals, plus beta carotene and other carotenoids (those that the body converts into vitamin A).

RDA (recommended dietary allowance): The level of intake for a nutrient set as a goal for healthy individuals. There are often different RDAs for men and women, various age groups, and pregnant women.

AI (adequate intake): A value set when researchers decided that there wasn't enough data to calculate an RDA. An AI is a rougher estimate than an RDA.

UL (tolerable upper intake level): The highest level of daily intake likely to pose no risk of adverse effects.

EAR (estimated average requirement): The level of a nutrient that meets the requirements for half of various groups, such as women over age 50. Researchers use this to calculate the RDA.

What Counts for You

There is really no need to try to keep all these different values straight, unless you are a nutritionist. The recently revised RDAs are the main numbers to go by—or an AI when an RDA isn't available. (The values used to arrive at the "Key Nutrients" profiled in all the food entries in this book are generally RDAs or AIs.) Don't exceed the ULs. The RDAs, AIs, and ULs are summarized in the chart on pages 88–89.

It is important to note that RDAs are recommendations, not requirements. Individual dietary needs vary greatly, and the RDAs are set at a level that is assumed to cover the nutrient needs of most people, plus a generous margin of safety. If your diet follows the wellness eating strategies outlined on pages 16–19, you should have no trouble meeting the RDAs.

amin E supplements come in synthetic and natural forms. Most studies show-ing possible health benefits have used the synthetic form, which is the cheap-est and most widely available. However, if you have a choice, buy the natural form, preferably a brand that includes "mixed tocopherols" on the ingredients list. It may be easier for the body to use than the synthetic form.

You may need to supplement your calcium intake. Most nutrition-ists recommend that calcium should come from food sources. But many women, especially older women who tend not to eat dairy products, don't get enough calcium. This applies to older men as well. In that case, taking a supplement is better than ignoring calcium altogether; research has clearly demonstrated that supplements can help reduce bone loss, even in older peo-ple. (*For more information on calcium supplementation, see page 68.*)

Premenopausal women should be sure to get enough folate. According to the U.S. Public Health Service, all women capable of becoming pregnant should consume 400 micrograms of folate daily. Folate (also called folacin or, when used in a supplement or to fortify foods, folic acid) helps protect against spina bifida and other birth defects. It may also help protect against cervical cancer, particularly in women at high risk for the disease; it helps protect against heart disease; and it may have other benefits as well (*see Folate, page 45*).

If your diet is rich in leafy greens, beans, and whole grains, and particularly if you eat breakfast cereals or other grains fortified with folic acid, you may already be getting enough. But if you can possi-bly become pregnant, and yet can't be sure that you're obtaining at least 400 micrograms daily from fortified foods, you should take a multivitamin/mineral supplement containing 400 micrograms or more of folic acid or a simple 400 microgram folic acid pill.

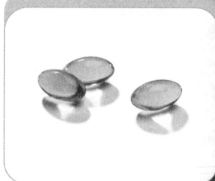

For many people, and especially those over the age of 60, taking a basic multivitamin/mineral supplement makes sense. Surveys consistently show that large groups of Americans tend to fall short in cerain key vitamins and minerals. Aging itself may make it more difficult to absorb and utilize certain nutrients. The major "problem nutrients" for older people are vitamins C, D, B_6, B_{12}, and folate, as well as minerals such as zinc, magnesium, and calcium.

Other people who can benefit from a multivitamin/mineral supplement include premenopausal women (many of whom don't consume enough iron); vegans (who consume no animal products and so may not get enough B_{12}); people on low-calorie diets, as well as heavy drinkers (who are likely to have a shortfall of vitamins and minerals); and anyone else not eating a bal-anced diet (who may not be getting enough folate, B_6, and B_{12}). Women who are pregnant should probably take a multivitamin, but should first discuss this with their doctors.

Avoid megadoses. Taking huge doses of most vitamins and minerals isn't wise. Certain vitamins—A and D—are toxic in large doses. Others, like niacin and vitamin B$_6$, produce serious side effects when taken in large doses. In fact, there's no benefit in taking high doses of most water-soluble vitamins (the B vitamins and C); excess amounts are simply eliminated by the body.

In planning your diet and in taking supplements, stick with the amounts recommended in the vitamin and mineral profiles on pages 40–89.

antioxidants

Until a few years ago, not many people had heard of antioxidants. Now ads for dozens of supplements—including cocktails of vitamins, minerals, and amino acids, as well as single compounds such as pine bark or green tea

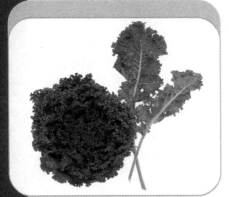

extract—make fantastic claims for antioxidants. Testimonials in glossy brochures say antioxidants have cured arthritis, restored youth, improved sex drive ("twice a night"), and generally worked miracles. Look upon all this with skepticism. But antioxidants, especially when consumed in foods, do play a crucial role in safeguarding your body's cells and may help prevent chronic diseases such as heart disease and cancer.

how antioxidants help protect life

Antioxidants are chemical substances that help protect the body from the adverse effects of oxygen. For virtually all living things the processing of oxygen is the basic source of energy and thus the basis of life. Without oxygen our cells die rapidly—within minutes. Oxidation goes on incessantly and at a tremendous rate. But oxygen can also be toxic and dangerous. The chemical changes that take place when the body uses oxygen create unstable oxygen molecules called free radicals. Free radicals may be formed in response to external factors such as heat, radiation (such as ultraviolet light and X-rays), alcohol, cigarette smoke, and certain pollutants. In addition, the cells themselves, without any aggravating environmental factors, produce their own free radicals.

Free radicals can cause varying degrees of damage to cells and structures within the cells, including protein, DNA, and other compounds. This damage can disrupt a cell's normal ability to replicate healthy cells or do other chemical work—and so may contribute to the development of chronic diseases, notably cancer and heart disease. The genetic damage to cells from free radicals can also accelerate the aging process.

However, just as our cells have methods of fighting infectious agents, they also have orderly systems for battling free radicals and repairing molecular damage—systems that quench or inactivate dangerous molecular by-products and mend the molecular defects. The free-radical fighters are called antioxidants. Some antioxidants are enzymes and other compounds manufactured by the cells themselves. Others are vitamins that we eat—namely vitamin C and vitamin E. Carotenoids (the yellow/orange/red pigments in fruits and vegetables) may also have antioxidant activity, as may other substances in foods.

Antioxidants don't just work in our bodies—they work in plants, providing protection against oxidation. In most vegetable oils, for example, vitamin E protects against rancidity, a form of oxidation. The most interesting of the antioxidants are two vitamins, C and E, as well as a class of substances called carotenoids, including beta carotene, alpha carotene, lycopene, and hundreds of others. Selenium, a mineral, is another antioxidant.

Vitamins, carotenoids, and selenium are all essential to good health and are, to some extent, under our control. We get them from food, so we can choose to consume a little or a lot of them. Once digested and absorbed by our bodies, vitamin C is present in blood and all other extracellular fluids. Vitamin E and many carotenoids are present in fats (or lipids) in the blood and in fat deposits; vitamin E is also found in cell membranes. These molecules are thus readily available to each cell. More information about the antioxidant activity of specific nutrients is provided in the vitamin and mineral profiles on pages 40–89.

unpredictable effects of antioxidants

Antioxidants come in many forms and do different kinds of work. What the supplement marketers never tell you is that not all of it is good work. For example, compounds known as polyphenols (found in tea, soybeans and other legumes, and other foods) act as antioxidants. Indeed, one of these, found in green tea and known as EGCG, is a particularly powerful antioxidant. Yet studies of these and other antioxidants have yielded contradictory results. These substances can certainly protect against oxidation in a test tube,

the top antioxidant sources

Scientists at the USDA Human Nutrition Research Center on Aging at Tufts University have been able to identify foods—and the phytochemicals in foods—with a high antioxidant potential, or what the scientists term ORAC (oxygen radical absorbance capacity). Studies suggest that high-ORAC foods boost the antioxidant power of human blood substantially. If you want to boost your antioxidant levels with phytochemicals, the foods listed below are your best sources.

ORAC Scores for 3.5 Ounces			
Fruit		**Vegetables**	
Prunes	5770	Kale	1770
Raisins	2830	Spinach	1260
Blueberries	2400	Brussels sprouts	980
Strawberries	1540	Broccoli florets	890
Raspberries	1220	Beets	840
Plums	949	Red bell peppers	710
Oranges	750	Yellow corn	400
Red grapes	739	Eggplant	390
Cherries	670	Carrots	210

Note: Juices (grape, vegetable, and citrus) are also good antioxidant sources.

but in the human body they may have the opposite effect—acting as *pro*-oxidants to encourage free radical activity. Or they may have no effect.

Another example is beta carotene, which has produced disquieting results when taken as a supplement in some studies. Sometimes it has shown no benefit against cancer. But in two studies of smokers, supplemental beta carotene actually seemed to increase the risk of lung cancer, rather than protect against it. Several theories have been proposed to explain this, but it seems clear that nutrients and other healthful compounds work in a fine balance, which scientists are only beginning to understand—and that there is also a delicate balance between free radicals and antioxidants in the body.

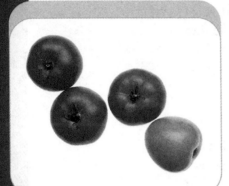

wellness recommendation

Whatever else all this new research means, it does provide the strongest possible evidence for consuming plenty of nutritious plant-derived foods. Five servings of fruits and vegetables a day should be the minimum—especially yellow, orange, and leafy green vegetables, citrus fruits, tomatoes, and berries, which are high in vitamin C and other vitamins, as well as carotenoids. Whole grains, wheat germ, and nuts supply vitamin E.

As we've mentioned, vitamins and other antioxidants work synergistically, and they may work best in their own natural settings. New compounds in food that may contribute to health are discovered every year. No individual supplements or combination of supplements can replace a varied diet. The two supplements we highly recommend—vitamin C and vitamin E—may provide some additional health benefits. But they are not meant to be a substitute for foods.

Until more is known about other recently discovered antioxidants, don't buy supplements claiming to contain them.

phytochemicals

Like vitamins and minerals—which also come from plants (as well as from animal-derived foods)—phytochemicals (meaning "plant chemicals") are essential to good health. But no one knows how many and how much of them we need.

An amazing 4,000 phytochemicals have been identified so far, and many more remain to be discovered. Only about 150 have been intensively studied. One huge class of phytochemicals is the polyphenols, which include the much-discussed flavonoids. These come in many varieties, such as flavonols, flavones, flavanones, and isoflavonoids. True to their name, flavonoids are sometimes flavorants, such as the allylic sulfides that give garlic, shallots, and onions their pungent taste and smell. Flavonoids can also be pigments, such as the anthocyanidins that make cherries red and blueberries blue.

Another large phytochemical category is the carotenoids, which are also pigments, adding color to red peppers, pink grapefruit, tomatoes, carrots, and watermelon, among other foods.

benefits for plants and for humans

Phytochemicals do big favors for plants—some protect plants from solar radiation, for instance, while others repel insects. They do big favors for humans, too, because they make foods attractive, tasty, and fragrant. Of course, if you dislike their flavor, they can keep you away from certain foods. Fortunately, the enormous range of tastes and smells means that wide choices are available. But not all phytochemicals are beneficial. Of the 4,000 known, some have effects in the human body, and some have no effect. Some are actually toxic (those in poisonous mushrooms, for example).

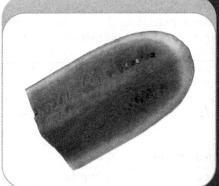

The other favor they do for us is to keep our cell chemistry stable in various ways. Most phytochemicals appear to act as antioxidants: They dispose of cell-damaging free radicals, which are by-products of the processing of oxygen in the body. Free-radical formation is boosted by various environmental factors, such as smoking, air pollution, and too much sunlight.

Phytochemicals help prevent cancer in a number of ways, some of them related to their antioxidant abilities. They can prevent potentially cancer-causing substances from forming. They may block the action of carcinogens on their target organs or tissue. Still others act on cells to suppress cancer development. They may also help protect against other diseases, notably heart disease. They may influence blood pressure and blood clotting or reduce the synthesis and absorption of cholesterol. Certain pigments (carotenoids) in plant foods may protect the eye from free-radical damage and thus prevent or postpone macular degeneration, which can lead to blindness.

wellness recommendation

All plant foods contain phytochemicals, in varying amounts. The chart that follows (*page 38*) lists categories of phytochemicals and a number of representative foods or food groups they occur in. This does not mean that any single food or any single group of foods is going to work miracles. Nor does it mean that you should concentrate on any one category or food and forget the rest. Nor should you try to include all of them in a day's diet.

Scientists are not sure which phytochemicals are responsible for the protective effects of this or that food. These substances almost surely act synergistically—that is, in conjunction with other phytochemicals—as well as with vitamins, minerals, fiber, hormones, and other compounds in foods. So while vitamin and mineral supplements make sense in some cases, phytochemical supplements do not. No one knows what the dosage should be, and there has been no demonstration of effectiveness or safety of these supplements.

If you follow our advice and base your diet on fruits and vegetables (a minimum of 5 servings a day) and grains (6 to 10 servings a day, preferably whole grains), you'll get the phytochemicals you need. Be sure that you include some servings of green leafy vegetables—ideally, at least 3 to 5 servings daily.

A GUIDE TO PHYTOCHEMICALS

The chart below shows categories of phytochemicals that have been found in certain foods in significant amounts. Keep in mind that some of the "possible benefits" listed are more theoretical than others. Much of the research has been done only in test tubes or with animals. Other theories about the benefits of some phytochemicals are based on anecdotal reports on diet—not experiments with actual phytochemicals. For example, a study that showed a link between a high intake of tomatoes and a reduced risk of prostate cancer was a study of tomato consumption. Lycopene, plentiful in tomatoes, may be the protective element, but nobody knows for sure. This is nutrition on the cutting edge.

You will find additional information on these disease-fighting compounds in many of the food entries in the Foods A to Z section of this book.

Phytochemical	Foods	Possible Benefits
Anthocyanins	Apples Berries Cherries Plums Pomegranates Red cabbage	In the test tube, and perhaps in the body, anthocyanins mop up free radicals, particles that can harm our cells and contribute to the onset of cancer and heart disease.
Capsaicin	Chili peppers	Little is known about the potential benefits of capsaicin; it may be an antioxidant or otherwise interfere with cancer development and may also prevent blood clotting. Applied topically, it can be effective at relieving the pain of arthritis.
Catechins	Apples Dark chocolate Grapes Pomegranates Raspberries Red wine Tea	Catechins may reduce the risk of certain cancers, according to research. EGCG, a particular type of catechin, appears to be a more powerful antioxidant than vitamin E; both disarm cell-damaging free radicals. Catechins may help to protect arteries against harmful plaque buildup as well.

Citrus Flavonoids
  Hesperitin
  Naringin
  Nobiletin
  Tangeritin
	Citrus fruit	The antioxidant actions of citrus flavonoids may counter unhealthy free radicals that contribute to disease. Flavonoids may also impede blood clotting.

Coumarins	Citrus fruit	Preliminary research indicates these plant chemicals may have anticancer and cardioprotective properties.
Ellagic acid	Berries Grapes Nuts Pomegranates	This robust plant substance has been shown to have numerous potent anticancer effects in lab animals.

Glucosinolates
  Indoles
  Isothiocyanates
  Sulforaphane
	Cruciferous vegetables such as broccoli, Brussels sprouts, cabbage, cauliflower, kale, watercress	Long classified as anticancer compounds, glucosinolates appear to thwart cancer by inactivating carcinogens, interfering with cancer cell replication, and mobilizing protective cancer-fighting enzymes in the body.

Phytochemical	Foods	Possible Benefits
Isoflavonoids	Soyfoods	Isoflaovnoids are converted to a kind of estrogen in the body and are thought to have some protective effect against cancer. In addition, isoflavonoids are under review for their potential beneficial effects on blood vessels, the heart, cholesterol levels, the brain, and bone health.
Lignans	Beans Flaxseed Wheat	These estrogenlike compounds are being studied for their potential to help guard against cancer and heart disease.
Limonene	Citrus fruit	According to laboratory studies, limonene may help to block abnormal cell growth and to detoxify cancer promoters.
Oleuropein & Hydroxytyrosol	Olive oil	Initial findings suggest these polyphenol phytochemicals may have disease-fighting antioxidant properties.
Phytosterols (plant sterols)	Beans Figs Nuts Seeds	Phytosterols are believed to behave as antioxidants, and they may have the potential to help reduce cholesterol levels and hinder cancer cell growth.
Quercetin	Apples Berries Cherries Red onions Red & purple grapes Tea Tomatoes	The antioxidant and additional healthful properties of quercetin may have cancer-preventing potential. Quercetin may also benefit the heart by exerting anticlotting actions and fostering healthy levels of blood cholesterol.
Resveratrol	Peanuts Red & purple grapes Red wine	Resveratrol may help promote healthy cholesterol levels, according to preliminary research. This potent phytochemical may also shield our cells from damage and curb tumor growth.
Sulfur compounds Allicin Ajoene Allyl sulfide	Chives Garlic Leeks Onions Scallions Shallots	Though evidence is far from certain, sulfur compounds may work against carcinogens and tumors, lowering the risk of colon, stomach, and other cancers. These substances may have heart-healthy properties as well. Garlic supplements are unproven and are not recommended.
Saponins	Legumes Nuts Oats Whole grains	Preliminary findings suggest saponins may help to reduce blood cholesterol and may also neutralize carcinogens in the digestive tract.
Tannins	Blackberries Blueberries Cranberries Grape juice Tea Wine	Research on the tannins isolated from cranberries (and blueberries) demonstrates their ability to inhibit the binding of *E. coli* bacteria to cells on the lining of the urinary tract. Presumably, that would allow the bacteria to be flushed from the bladder with the urine, protecting against a urinary tract infection.

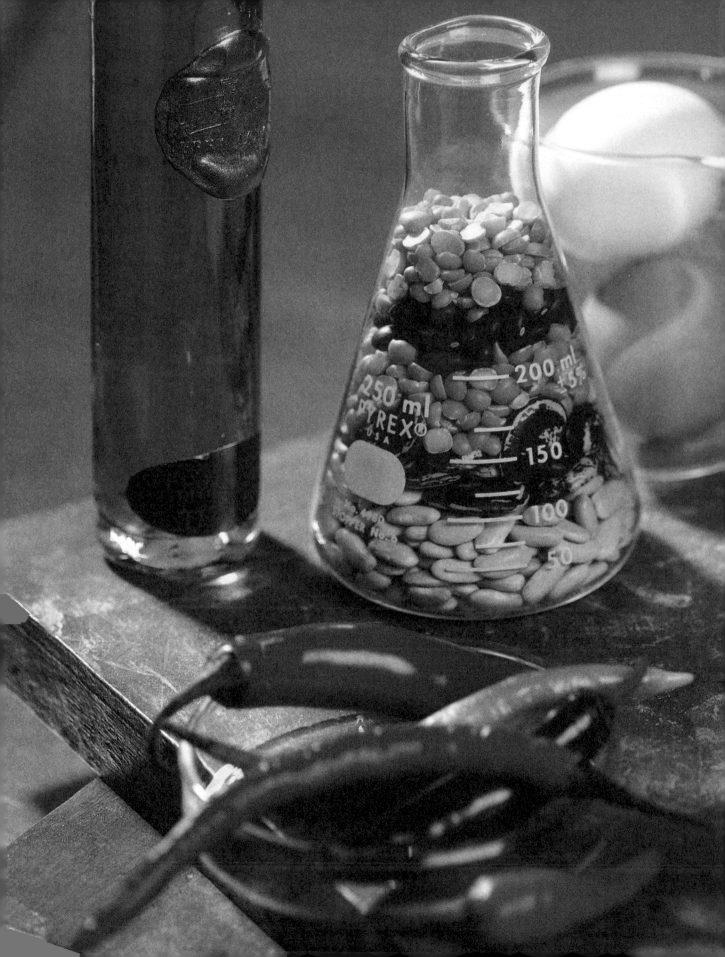

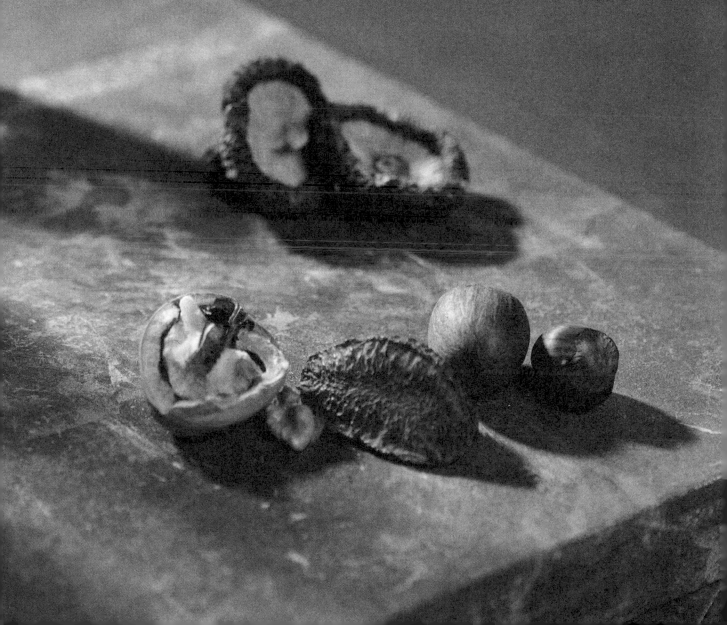

a guide to
vitamins &
minerals

biotin

Biotin, a B vitamin, is essential to growth and development. In fact, its name comes from the Greek word *bios* meaning "life." Despite its importance, biotin is of little dietary concern to most people because deficiencies are practically unheard of.

what it does

Biotin is necessary for the transfer of carbon dioxide from one compound to another in a variety of metabolic functions. It is important for the formation and oxidation of fatty acids and helps metabolize amino acids (the building blocks of protein) and carbohydrates.

This vitamin is also involved in the production of digestive enzymes and in antibody formation. It also helps the body use niacin, another B vitamin.

Biotin deficiency is rare, but when it occurs can result in weight loss, nausea, depression, dermatitis, hair loss, and elevated cholesterol.

recommended levels

For all adults, the Adequate Intake (AI) is 30 micrograms. Because deficiency is so rare, the RDA for biotin has never been established.

Supplementation: Supplementation isn't necessary or recommended.

tips & facts

• Some biotin is synthesized by bacteria in the intestines, but it is unclear whether this biotin is in a form that contributes much to the body's needs. However, large doses of antibiotics can decrease biotin levels, especially in older people.

• A protein in raw egg binds biotin and makes it unavailable to the body—though raw egg whites would have to supply 30 percent of your daily calories before absorption would be impaired. In any case, eating raw eggs or egg whites is not a good idea, since they can lead to food poisoning from *salmonella* bacteria. Cooking eggs inactivates the protein.

• People who take anticonvulsant medications, such as phenytoin and carbamazepine, may be at risk for biotin deficiency because the drugs interfere with the absorption of the vitamin. Talk to your doctor if you are on one of these medications.

• Although one of the symptoms of biotin deficiency is hair loss, it is a myth that biotin supplements or lotions containing biotin can prevent or reverse baldness.

• Wheat has a high biotin content, but most of the vitamin in this grain is bound and unavailable to the body.

where you can find it

Small amounts of biotin are found in a number of foods. Yeast, corn, soybeans, egg yolks, liver, cauliflower, peanut butter, and mushrooms are among the best sources.

carotenoids

Carotenoids are the yellow-orange pigments in fruits and vegetables. There are more than 600 carotenoids, of which over 450 that exist in food have been identified; these include beta carotene, lycopene, beta cryptoxanthin, and lutein. Some 50 carotenoids are converted to vitamin A in the intestine, and until recently scientists thought that the others were simply pigments that played no role in health. In recent years, however, research has shown that many of the carotenoids may have disease-preventing potential.

what they do

The conversion of certain carotenoids into vitamin A takes place in the intestine, and is regulated by the body, with more or less of the carotenoids being converted as the body requires. After the conversion, the carotenoids perform all of the functions of vitamin A—so there is no need to consume foods rich in preformed vitamin A (such as beef or chicken livers) to meet the RDA for that vitamin. (*See Vitamin A, page 52.*)

Potential health benefits: Carotenoids are thought to help protect against heart disease and certain forms of cancer. At least 70 studies involving humans have found that those who don't eat enough fruits and vegetables have a higher risk of cancer.

Lycopene, the carotenoid prominent in tomatoes, also appears to protect against certain cancers. One study of lycopene found that men who consumed, on a weekly basis, four to seven servings of tomato products—one of the richest sources of lycopene—reduced their risk of prostate cancer by 22 percent. According to data from two studies of lung cancer risk in 125,000 people, lycopene seemed to be most beneficial, in both smokers and nonsmokers. (Another carotenoid, alpha carotene, was associated with a lower risk only in nonsmokers.) Some studies suggest that lutein and zeaxanthin (another carotenoid) may protect against cataracts

LEADING SOURCES

This listing includes beta carotene along with some of the other known carotenoids.

BETA CAROTENE	MG
Sweet potato, cooked, ½ cup	11.5
Carrots, cooked, ½ cup	10.7
Carrot, raw, 1 medium	4.8
Cantaloupe, diced, 1 cup	4.7
Spinach, cooked, ½ cup	3.9
Apricots, fresh, 3	3.7
Kale, cooked, ½ cup	2.3
Mango, fresh, sliced, 1 cup	2.2
Acorn squash, cooked, ½ cup	2.0
Beet greens, fresh, cooked, ½ cup	1.9
ALPHA CAROTENE	**MG**
Pumpkin puree, ½ cup	4.4
Carrot, fresh, raw, 1 medium	2.2
Yellow pepper, fresh, ½ medium	0.2
BETA CRYPTOXANTHIN	**MG**
Tangerine, fresh, 1 medium	2.07
Papaya, fresh, 1 cup	0.66
Orange, naval, 1 medium	0.21
Mango, sliced, 1 cup	0.10
Peach, fresh, 1 medium	0.09
LYCOPENE	**MG**
Tomato juice, canned, 1 cup	20
Tomato sauce, canned, ½ cup	17
Tomato paste, canned, 2 tbsp	8.0
Watermelon, fresh, diced, ¾ cup	6.2
Tomato, fresh, 1 large	5.6
Guava, fresh, 1 medium	4.9
Grapefruit, pink, ½ medium	4.1
LUTEIN	**MG**
Kale, fresh, chopped, 1 cup	14.7
Red pepper, fresh, chopped, 1 cup	10.1
Spinach, fresh, chopped, 1 cup	4.2
Endive, fresh, chopped, 1 cup	2.0
Broccoli, fresh, chopped, 1 cup	1.9
Romaine lettuce, fresh, chopped, 1 cup	1.1

and another vision disorder, macular degeneration, the leading cause of blindness in Americans over age 60. And beta carotene, the best known member of the carotenoid family, is also thought to help guard against cataracts.

Some of the benefits from carotenoids come from their antioxidant potential, and they may work in other, as yet unidentified, ways as well.

recommended levels

There is no established recommended daily intake for carotenoids. You can meet the RDA for vitamin A by consuming 11 milligrams of beta carotene a day. Experts vary in their recommendations for the amount needed to obtain the disease-protective potential—and the truth is, no one really knows, since it's still unclear how carotenoids work individually or in combination with each other and with other nutrients.

You can easily get the 11 milligrams of beta carotene a day from foods with a little planning. In addition, make an effort to include foods that supply other carotenoids in your diet (see "Leading Sources" chart, page 43).

Supplementation: Supplemental beta carotene was once thought to be harmless, but some studies found that it may increase risk of lung cancer in those at high risk for the disease (smokers and asbestos workers, for example).

Exactly why the supplements would have this effect is unclear. One theory is that beta carotene's antioxidant capacity is "used up" in smokers as it inactivates the free radicals from cigarette smoke. In the process, it can turn into a "pro-oxidant" that enhances free radical formation. Also, supplemental beta carotene may need vitamin C to help produce its antioxidant effect, and smokers have low levels of vitamin C. This scenario would put smokers at increased risk for the oxidative damage that is believed to contribute to cancer.

For now, experts recommend that smokers not take beta carotene supplements. For nonsmokers, there is no harm—but also no proven benefit—to beta carotene supplements, and so we don't recommend them. If you choose to take them, take no more than 6 to 15 milligrams per day. But it's better to get beta carotene and other carotenoids from foods. (There has never been any evidence that beta carotene in foods poses any danger to smokers.)

tips & facts

• You can still meet your vitamin A needs by eating foods that contain preformed vitamin A (eggs or fortified milk, for example), and this will prevent a vitamin A deficiency. However, preformed vitamin A does not act in the body in the same way as carotenoids. If you do not eat many yellow, orange, or dark-green vegetables and fruits, you are not getting enough carotenoids, and you may be increasing your risk of developing cancer or heart disease.

• There are no adverse effects in consuming too great a quantity of carotenoids from foods. If you consume a lot of certain carotenoids, your skin may turn yellowish, especially on the palms of your hands and the soles of your feet. This discoloration is harmless, and will gradually disappear if you cut back on carotenoids.

• Spinach and other dark leafy green vegetables are good sources of beta carotene and other carotenoids. The darker the green color of the vegetable, the more beta carotene it contains. For example, romaine lettuce has 10 times more beta carotene than iceberg lettuce, and arugula has three times more than romaine lettuce.

• Broccoli that is dark-green, purple, or purplish-blue has the most carotenoids.

• The beta carotene in carrots is more available if the vegetable is cooked slightly, since raw carrots have tough cellular walls that the body cannot easily break down. The same is true for tomatoes: Ounce for ounce, processed tomato products, such as sauce or paste, contain 2 to 10 times as much available lycopene as fresh tomatoes—not only because cooking breaks down the cell walls, but also because the contents become concentrated due to loss of water during processing.

where you can find them

The most colorful foods—yellow, orange, and red fruits and vegetables—supply carotenoids. Dark-green vegetables such as watercress and Swiss chard are also good sources; the yellow/orange color of the carotenoids that are present in these vegetables is masked by the presence of chlorophyll, the green pigment produced by photosynthesis.

folate

This B vitamin, also called folacin and folic acid (in its synthetic form), is not a household word, but it should be: It has been found to have a powerful preventive effect against a variety of disorders, from birth defects to cancer to heart disease.

what it does

Folate is involved in the production of coenzymes used to form DNA and RNA, the genetic material of cells, and so is important for cell reproduction. It is also essential for the formation of hemoglobin, the oxygen-carrying component of red blood cells.

Aside from these basic metabolic functions, folate helps prevent neural tube birth defects, including spina bifida, a potentially crippling birth defect in which the spinal cord is not completely encased in bone, and anencephaly, a fatal defect in which a major part of the brain never develops. It also helps prevent oral and facial birth defects such as cleft palate.

LEADING SOURCES	
SOURCE	FOLATE (MCG)
Chicken livers, simmered, 3 oz	660
Asparagus, fresh, cooked, 1 cup	263
Oatmeal, fortified, cooked, 1 cup	199
Chicory greens, fresh, 1 cup	197
Lentils, cooked, ½ cup	179
Chick-peas, cooked, ½ cup	141
Kidney beans, cooked, ½ cup	115
Orange juice, from concentrate, 1 cup	109
Brussels sprouts, frozen, boiled, 1 cup	94
Avocado, Florida, ½ medium	81
Wheat germ, 2 tbsp	40

Potential health benefits: Folate may prevent cervical cancer, and preliminary evidence shows that it may also help protect against other cancers, such as colorectal cancer or lung cancer.

An adequate blood level of folic acid can also lower levels of homocysteine in the blood, which may help prevent heart disease. High levels of this amino acid-like substance have been linked to an increased risk of heart attack and stroke (though the research evidence on this link is not consistent).

It has long been known that people with homocystinuria—a rare genetic disorder that results in extremely high levels of homocysteine—often develop atherosclerosis at a early age. More recently it was discovered that people who do not get enough folate, vitamin B_6, and vitamin B_{12} in their diets also have elevated homocysteine levels, and therefore an increased risk of cardiovascular disease. In normal metabolic processes, these B vitamins help convert homocysteine into amino acids that the body can use, and thus homocysteine does not rise to potentially harmful levels. It remains to be proven that lowering high homocysteine levels will actually reduce the risk of heart attack in anyone except people with homocystinuria (for whom it clearly does reduce the risk). But in the meantime, it's certainly a good idea to increase your consumption of folate and other B vitamins.

recommended levels

For all adults, the RDA is 400 micrograms. Because neural tube birth defects occur well before a woman knows she is pregnant, *it's important that all women who might become pregnant be sure they consume 400 micrograms of folate a day.*

Supplementation: Women who don't eat at least five servings of fruits and vegetables a day, as well as fortified cereals and grains, should take a daily multivitamin/mineral supplement providing at least 400 micrograms of folic acid (the term used for folate in supplement form or in fortified foods). *To obtain the benefit of preventing birth defects, women should start building up folic acid stores at least one to two months before becoming pregnant.*

tips & facts

• Fortification of grain products with folic acid, in effect since 1998, has helped raise Americans' blood levels of the vitamin, such that the incidence of very low folate levels is less than 2 percent. But levels are still not high enough to prevent birth defects altogether. The government estimates that fewer than one-third of American women of childbearing age take daily supplements of folic acid.

• Two ounces of dried pasta (1 cup cooked) contains about 100 micrograms of folate, which is 25 percent of the recommended daily intake.

• The level of fortification approved by the FDA (140 micrograms per 3 ounces of grain product) is estimated to reduce the risk of heart disease by 5 percent and of severe blockage of the carotid artery by 3 percent, according to a recent study.

• Folate, along with vitamin B_{12}, may also help keep your hearing keen as you grow older. A study in the *Clinical Journal of Nutrition* found that women in their 60s with normal hearing ability had higher blood levels of folic acid and B_{12} (from diet or supplements) than those with hearing dysfunction. (The study was small, but provides an interesting new avenue of research.)

• The folic acid and B_{12} in supplements and fortified foods are much better absorbed by the body than the same vitamins found naturally in food. Thus, recent studies have shown that people who take folic acid supplements decrease their homocysteine levels more than those who get folate from food.

where you can find it

Good sources of folate include: beef and chicken livers, dried beans and peas, leafy greens, oranges, wheat germ, whole grains, and fortified grain products.

niacin

Niacin, a B vitamin, is unusual in that the human body not only can get it preformed in foods, but can also synthesize the vitamin from tryptophan, an amino acid (protein component). This means that you don't have to eat foods high in niacin to meet the niacin requirement. Most people, in fact, get about half of the niacin they need from foods containing tryptophan. For example, milk and eggs contain very little preformed niacin, but they end up being ample niacin sources because they are rich in tryptophan.

LEADING SOURCES	
SOURCE	NIACIN (MG)
Chicken breast, skinless, roasted, 3 oz	12
Yellowfin tuna, cooked, 3 oz	10
Swordfish, cooked, 3 oz	10
Turkey breast, skinless, roasted, 3 oz	6.4
White rice, cooked, 1 cup	3.4
Bagel, 1	3.2
Pita bread, white, 1	2.8
Sweet corn, 1 cup	2.6
Spaghetti, cooked, 1 cup	2.3
Peas, cooked, ½ cup	1.6
Cream of wheat, cooked, 1 cup	1.5

what it does

Niacin—also called nicotinic acid or vitamin B_3—aids in converting the macronutrients in foods into energy. It helps to synthesize glycogen (a form of carbohydrate stored in muscles and the liver). At the cellular level, niacin is an essential part of coenzymes involved in processes such as metabolizing fatty acids and mobilizing calcium stored in cells. By contributing to these functions, niacin also maintains the health of the skin, nerves, and digestive system.

The principal consequence of niacin deficiency is pellagra, a disease characterized by dry, scaly skin at any areas exposed to sunlight. The disease was common in the southern United States and parts of Europe in the early 1900s, mainly in areas where diets were based on cornmeal (which contains a form of niacin unavailable to the body). Pellagra is no longer a problem in industrialized countries—it disappeared as more varied protein sources became part of the diet—but it still occurs in parts of Asia and Africa.

Potential health benefits: Large doses of niacin in supplement form can help lower elevated levels of blood cholesterol. Studies have shown that it reduces both heart attacks and heart attack deaths—in part because it raises levels of HDL ("good") cholesterol. But at these levels—usually 1.5 to 6 grams per day—the vitamin acts as a drug, not a dietary supplement (*see Supplementation, below*).

recommended levels

The RDA for women is 14 milligrams; for men, 16 milligrams. These levels can easily be reached with your daily diet.

Supplementation: Niacin in supplement form is an effective means of lowering high blood cholesterol levels that can't be reduced by diet and other lifestyle changes. It is also used for people who have high levels of triglycerides (fats in the blood that, when elevated, can also pose a risk for heart attack)—and is much less expensive than other prescription drugs for controlling cholesterol. But don't assume that it's safe to take high-dose niacin on your own because it's a vitamin, it's "natural," and available without a prescription. There are adverse effects that range from flushing, nausea, and headache to potentially serious problems such as liver damage. *When taken in therapeutic doses, niacin should be prescribed by your doctor and used only under medical supervision.*

tips & facts

• Most of the niacin in corn is unavailable to the body. But when corn is mixed with an alkaline substance—for example, when it is ground with lime to make corn tortillas—much of the niacin becomes available.

• Grains are ordinarily poor sources of niacin, but enrichment makes them good sources. In fact, much of the niacin in the American diet comes from grain products to which niacin has been added.

where you can find it

Good sources of protein are generally good sources of niacin. Enriched cereals and breads are also good sources. Meats, poultry, and fish are rich in both preformed niacin and tryptophan. Milk and eggs are excellent sources of tryptophan. Niacin and tryptophan also occur in smaller amounts in peas and other legumes.

pantothenic acid

This B vitamin (B_5) is found in a wide variety of foods and is involved in many of the body's processes. In fact, its name comes from the Greek word *pantos*, which means "everywhere." It does not participate in biological reactions on its own; instead, it combines with other substances in the body to form two coenzymes: coenzyme A (CoA) and phosphopantetheine attached to a protein known as acyl carrier protein (ACP).

what it does

As part of CoA, pantothenic acid stimulates the release of energy from carbohydrates, fats, and protein. It also provides the basis for the formation of acetylcholine, which is used in the transmission of nerve impulses. As part of ACP, it is involved in the synthesis of fatty acids, cholesterol, and the lipids (fats) that are part of cell membranes.

A diet lacking in this vitamin results in headaches, fatigue, tingling and numbness in the hands and feet, and intestinal problems. Because pantothenic acid is found in so many foods, deficiencies are extremely rare except in severe malnutrition.

recommended levels

The Adequate Intake (AI) for all adults is 5 milligrams. Because deficiency is so rare, the RDA for pantothenic acid has never been established.

Supplementation: Supplementation isn't necessary or recommended.

tips & facts

• Some vitamin supplements supply pantothenic acid in the form of calcium pantothenate. Despite its name, this compound actually contains little calcium, and therefore makes no contribution to daily calcium needs.

• There's no truth to the claim that pantothenic acid supplements can prevent gray hair. The myth probably arose from animal studies that showed that a deficiency of the vitamin caused gray hair in rats. However, studies exploring the possibility that pantothenic acid could prevent gray hair or restore hair color in people showed no effect.

where you can find it

The richest sources of pantothenic acid are organ meats, fish, poultry, whole grains, yogurt, and legumes.

riboflavin

Riboflavin, also known as vitamin B_2, might be described as a helper vitamin. Although it has no direct function on its own, riboflavin is used to produce coenzymes that are needed to initiate many chemical reactions throughout the body. Riboflavin was first observed in 1879 as a yellow fluorescent pigment in milk, but it was not identified as a vitamin until 1933. (The word riboflavin is a combination of ribose, a sugar found in the vitamin, and *flavin*, the Latin word for yellow.)

LEADING SOURCES	
SOURCE	RIBOFLAVIN (MG)
Beef liver, fried, 3 oz	3.50
Yogurt, fat-free plain, 8 oz	0.53
Milk, fat-free, protein-fortified, 1 cup	0.48
Oatmeal, instant, fortified, cooked, 1 cup	0.37
Egg, 1 extra large	0.29

what it does

Like thiamin (vitamin B_1), riboflavin helps cells convert carbohydrates into energy, and it also aids in the metabolism of fats and proteins. More specifically, riboflavin acts as a precursor to two coenzymes that are needed to catalyze a variety of enzymes in the body. (Enzymes initiate and accelerate chemical reactions that must take place within the cells in order for life to continue.)

Riboflavin is also essential for the proper use of vitamin B_6, niacin, folate, and vitamin K. And it helps the body distribute and use medications and clear them from the body.

Potential health benefits: Riboflavin has an antioxidant effect. It is needed to produce a coenzyme that catalyzes glutathione reductase, an enzyme that is important in preventing the oxidation of the lipid (fat) in cell membranes. This helps to keep cells healthy. Some evidence suggests that an adequate intake of riboflavin may help prevent esophageal cancer in malnourished populations. But it's unknown whether riboflavin has any disease-prevention benefits for people who are healthy.

recommended levels

The RDA for women is 1.1 milligrams; for men, 1.3 milligrams.

Supplementation: Supplements are not necessary and not recommended. Riboflavin is present in a wide variety of foods, so it would be difficult not to get enough of this vitamin naturally. Deficiencies of riboflavin are rare, and when they do occur, it is usually because a diet is also lacking in other B vitamins (such as niacin and vitamin B_6); some of the signs of deficiency are actually due to an imbalance in these other vitamins.

tips & facts

• A high intake of riboflavin can turn urine bright fluorescent yellow, since any excess of the vitamin is excreted in urine.

• Milk and dairy products provide about half the riboflavin intake in the United States.

• Riboflavin is not as easily destroyed by heat as other B vitamins, but it is extremely sensitive to light. This is one reason why milk is packaged in opaque bottles or cardboard cartons—milk sold in clear glass bottles loses a significant amount of riboflavin.

• The milling of grains removes much of the riboflavin, but enriched grains have the riboflavin restored.

where you can find it

Riboflavin is found in liver, milk and other dairy products, poultry, fish, and eggs. In the United States, grain products are usually enriched or fortified with riboflavin.

thiamin

Thiamin (vitamin B$_1$) is not a vitamin that has miraculous claims attached to it, so chances are you've never wondered whether or not you're getting enough thiamin in your diet. But a lack of this B vitamin can cause beriberi—a disease that leads to mental impairment, muscle paralysis, nerve damage, and eventually death. Beriberi was once rampant in parts of Asia because of diets that consisted mostly of white rice from which rice bran, containing thiamin, had been removed. Today, deficiencies are rare, especially in Western countries, since thiamin is one of the nutrients added to grains and flours during the enrichment process.

LEADING SOURCES	
SOURCE	THIAMIN (MG)
Pork loin, roasted, 3 oz	1.5
Florida pompano, cooked, 3 oz	1.2
Sunflower seeds, 1 oz	0.7
Oatmeal, instant, fortified, cooked, 1 cup	0.7
Brazil nuts, 1 oz	0.3
Rice, white enriched, cooked, 1 cup	0.3
Baked potato with skin	0.2
Pink beans, cooked, ½ cup	0.2

what it does

Thiamin is necessary for the release of energy from food. It helps the body convert glucose and other sugars to compounds that can then be broken down to yield energy. It is also essential for healthy brain and nerve cells as well as heart function. Potential benefits for disease prevention are unknown.

recommended levels

The RDA for women is 1.1 milligrams; for men, 1.2 milligrams. Since the primary function of thiamin is to extract energy from food, the amount you need depends on your overall calorie intake. Athletes and other very active people who consume large amounts of calories may need more thiamin, but the extra food they consume should cover their extra thiamin needs.

Supplementation: Supplements are not necessary and not recommended.

tips & facts

• Thiamin is one vitamin that you should make sure you get enough of on a regular basis.

• The importance of thiamin in the diet, combined with the fact that it is plentiful in few foods, led to the requirement that food processors enrich refined grain products, such as white flour and white rice, with thiamin.

• Make sure your thiamin intake is adequate if you drink a lot of decaffeinated or regular tea or coffee. These beverages contain a substance that can deplete the body's stores of this vitamin.

• Raw fish, shellfish, beets, Brussels sprouts, and red cabbage contain an antithiamin factor that destroys the vitamin. Cooking inactivates this substance.

• Thiamin is best absorbed in an acid medium. If you regularly take antacids or medications to reduce stomach acid production, ask your doctor how this might affect your thiamin absorption.

where you can find it

Few foods contain abundant amounts of thiamin. Lean pork is one of the best sources. Whole grains, dried beans, nuts, seeds, fish, and enriched breads and cereals are also good sources.

vitamin A

LEADING SOURCES	
SOURCE*	VITAMIN A (MCG)
Beef liver, cooked, 3 oz	9,098
Chicken liver, cooked, 3 oz	4,176
Egg substitute, fortified, ¼ cup	407
Milk, fat-free, fortified, 1 cup	150
Milk, whole, 1 cup	92
Cheddar cheese, 1 oz	90
Egg, medium	84
Swiss cheese, 1 oz	72
Yogurt, low-fat, fruit-flavored, 1 cup	36

*Vitamin A is obtained from both retinol and carotenoids. The food sources in this chart supply preformed vitamin A from retinol. For a list of foods high in carotenoids, see page 43.

Vitamin A was the first fat-soluble vitamin to be discovered. The various forms of vitamin A are called retinoids because of their importance to the health of the retina of the eye. The majority of the vitamin A in our diets is supplied by precursors—various carotenoids in plants, especially beta carotene (*see Carotenoids, page 43*)—some of which may be converted to vitamin A in the intestines. Some animal foods, such as those shown in the chart at left, supply preformed vitamin A.

what it does

The most commonly known function of vitamin A is its role in promoting good vision, especially night vision. The vitamin is needed in order for the eye to adapt from bright light to darkness—for example, when you encounter headlights from an oncoming car while driving at night.

Vitamin A helps to maintain epithelial tissues—those that make up the skin surface and the linings of systems like the respiratory and gastrointestinal tracts. These tissues are rich in immune cells and are the body's first line of defense against disease. Therefore, vitamin A is important in maintaining immunity. Vitamin A is also important in the development of immune cells, and in bone growth. In addition, it is needed for normal reproduction and lactation.

A deficiency of vitamin A (which is a problem only in less-industrialized areas of the world) can cause night blindness and total blindness as well as a reduced resistance to infection and growth retardation.

Potential health benefits: Some research indicates that vitamin A may inhibit the development of certain tumors. Another possible benefit suggested by research is that it increases resistance to infection in children.

recommended levels

The RDA for women is 700 micrograms; for men, 900 micrograms. Formerly expressed in either International Units (IU) or Retinol Equivalents (RE), the latest RDA for vitamin A is stated in micrograms.

Supplementation: Supplements of vitamin A are not recommended, since an excessive intake of preformed vitamin A can be quite toxic. A single dose of 130 milligrams in adults or 40 milligrams in children can cause nausea, vomiting, fatigue, and weakness. (A milligram equals 1,000 micrograms.) Lower doses—10 milligrams in adults, 4 milligrams in children—taken daily over time can still be harmful, resulting in headaches, hair loss, drying of mucous membranes, itchy, scaly skin, and liver damage. As little as 10 milligrams of vitamin A taken daily can also cause birth defects in pregnant women. The upper safe daily limit now set by the National Academy of Sciences (which establishes the RDAs for nutrients) is only 3 milligrams, equivalent to 10,000 IUs.

Unless you eat a lot of liver or fish oil, it is practically impossible to get too much vitamin A from your diet, however. Carotenoids won't lead to toxicity, since their conversion to vitamin A is regulated by the body's need for vitamin A.

tips & facts

• Only 50 of the more than 600 carotenoids can be converted to vitamin A.

• Some acne drugs are derivatives of vitamin A, but vitamin A supplements found in health-food stores will not cure acne, and may be toxic.

where you can find it

Preformed vitamin A is found in organ meats, fish, and egg yolks. Milk is often fortified with the vitamin. Dark-green, orange, and red fruits and vegetables are good sources of carotenoids, which are converted to vitamin A.

vitamin B6

Vitamin B6 is a collective term used to describe three B vitamins: pyridoxine, pyridoxal, and pyridoxamine. These three substances are involved in over 100 chemical reactions in the body. Probably because of the varied nature of this vitamin, claims have been made for its role in the prevention or treatment of a wide variety of diseases.

LEADING SOURCES	
SOURCE	VITAMIN B6 (MG)
Tuna, yellowfin, cooked, 3 oz	0.89
Potato, baked, with skin, 1	0.70
Banana, 1 medium	0.68
Chick-peas, canned, ½ cup	0.57
Prune juice, 1 cup	0.56
Chicken, light meat, skinless, roasted, 3 oz	0.51
Avocado, Florida, ½ medium	0.43
Pepper, green or red, 1 large	0.40
Tuna, canned in water, 3 oz	0.32

what it does

The 13 nonessential amino acids (the building blocks of protein the body can produce on its own) could not be manufactured without vitamin B6. In addition, vitamin B6 helps each cell to assemble the protein it needs by facilitating the breakdown and recombination of all the amino acids.

Vitamin B6 is needed to produce the chemical changes that must take place to convert amino acids to glucose in the event that the body needs to rely on protein, rather than carbohydrates, for energy. When blood glucose levels are low, B_6 helps convert glycogen stored in the liver into glucose. In addition, it is important in maintaining a healthy immune system, facilitates the conversion of the amino acid tryptophan to niacin (*page 47*), and helps produce serotonin, dopamine, and other neurotransmitters (chemical messengers in the brain and nervous system).

Potential health benefits: Recently, vitamin B_6 was found to be a possible protector against heart disease. It works with folate and vitamin B_{12} to prevent the excess buildup of the amino acid–like substance homocysteine, which can lead to atherosclerosis. More specifically, marginal deficiencies of vitamin B_6 can contribute to the buildup of homocysteine in the body, which may increase the risk of heart disease. Vitamin B_6 may also improve the functioning of the immune system in older people.

recommended levels

For women and men through age 50, the RDA is 1.3 milligrams; for women age 51 and older, 1.5 milligrams; for men age 51 and older, 1.7 milligrams.

Supplementation: Anyone not eating a balanced diet should consider a daily multivitamin with 100 percent of the RDA. Very high doses of B_6 are toxic and can cause nerve damage if taken for months or years. Doses of less than 250 milligrams per day are considered safe.

tips & facts

• Women taking oral contraceptives also need to pay special attention to their vitamin B_6 intake. About 15 to 20 percent of these women have low levels of vitamin B_6, probably because birth control pills increase the body's production of enzymes that use up the vitamin.

• Megadoses of vitamin B_6 are not necessary to keep homocysteine levels low. Meeting the RDA for the vitamin is all that is needed.

• Vitamin B_6 supplements—50 to 200 milligrams daily—have been reported to help ease the symptoms of premenstrual syndrome (PMS), although the results from well-controlled studies have been inconclusive.

• Supplements of vitamin B_6 have also been reported to alleviate morning sickness in some pregnant women. However, if you are pregnant, do not take supplements without discussing it with your doctor first.

• Vitamin B_6 is easily destroyed by heat and other food-processing methods.

• Whole-wheat products contain vitamin B_6, but refined grain products (white flour or products made with it) do not. Much of the vitamin is removed during milling of the grains (when the bran and germ are removed) and it is not required to be replaced. Some breakfast cereals are fortified with vitamin B_6, however.

where you can find it

Fish, poultry, meats, organ meats, bananas, and avocados are all good sources of vitamin B_6.

vitamin B12

The last vitamin to be discovered, vitamin B_{12} is unique among the water-soluble vitamins. In general, water-soluble vitamins are found in a wide variety of foods (especially plant foods); are well absorbed by the body; and are not stored in large quantities. Vitamin B_{12}, by contrast, is found only in animal products and its absorption by the body is complicated. The liver is able to store large amounts of the vitamin, so that even if you stopped consuming it altogether, you would not become deficient for months or years. However, certain changes in the digestive tract that occur in older people can affect the ability to absorb vitamin B_{12}.

LEADING SOURCES	
SOURCE	VITAMIN B12 (MCG)
Clams, cooked, 3 oz	85
Chicken liver, cooked, 3 oz	16.6
Tuna, bluefin, cooked, 3 oz	9.32
Sardines, canned, 3 oz	8.22
Salmon, canned, 3 oz	3.77
Lamb shoulder, broiled, trimmed, 3 oz	2.67
Yogurt, fat-free, plain, 8 oz	1.39
Tuna, canned in water, 3 oz	1.00
Milk, fat-free, 1 cup	0.93
Swiss cheese, 1 oz	0.54

what it does

Vitamin B_{12} is important to almost every cell and system in the body, including the blood and the nervous system. It works closely with folate and is involved in many of the same metabolic functions, such as the development of healthy red blood cells, the formation of DNA, and the production of amino acids. Vitamin B_{12} is also essential for transforming stored folic acid into a metabolically active form and for the formation of myelin, the fatty sheath that surrounds nerves.

Potential health benefits: Like other B vitamins such as folate and B_6, vitamin B_{12} may be crucial in preventing heart disease. Studies show that low levels of B_{12} (as well as folic acid and B_6) are associated with high levels of homocysteine, an amino acid–like substance that may be an independent risk factor for heart disease. Increasing your intake of these vitamins can lower homocysteine—though whether that will also reduce your risk of heart disease is unknown. Evidence is mounting, but it will take time to come up with the answer.

Reduced absorption: one form of B_{12} deficiency. Because of the body's ability to store this vitamin, B_{12} deficiencies are rare. However, in order for B_{12} to be separated from food and utilized, the stomach must secrete adequate amounts of acids along with the digestive enzyme pepsin, and then the free vitamin must combine with a protein known as "intrinsic factor," secreted by the stomach lining, in order to be absorbed.

Deficiencies do affect some people over age 50 who do not secrete enough stomach acids and pepsin, so that less of the vitamin is extracted from food and thus less is absorbed. The presence of *H. pylori,* the bacterium that causes most ulcers, can also adversely affect vitamin B_{12} absorption.

In some cases, the diet may be deficient. Vegans (who eat no animal products, which are the best source of this vitamin) can be deficient, and so can heavy drinkers. Deficiency can also affect people with diseases of the intestinal tract, those who have had extensive intestinal surgery, and those taking certain drugs for gout or seizures.

The National Academy of Sciences estimates that up to 30 percent of people over age 50 produce insufficient stomach acid, and thus their B_{12} absorption is reduced. There is a great deal of controversy over this, as well as over how to test for a deficiency. But it's important to have the condition properly diagnosed (*see Tips & Facts, opposite page*).

Pernicious anemia. A much rarer but far more serious type of vitamin B_{12} deficiency is pernicious anemia, a disease where red blood cells fail to reproduce normally. It can occur at any age. What happens is that the stomach stops producing acids and intrinsic factor, and thus virtually no vitamin B_{12} can be absorbed. Because the vitamin is stored so efficiently, it may take up to five years before stores are used up and symptoms develop. These may include extreme fatigue, dementia, disorientation, and weakness in the limbs. One consequence of this condition may be irreversible neurological damage, so it's important to see a physician early. If it turns out you have pernicious anemia, it can be successfully treated with vitamin injections. Extremely high doses of vitamin B_{12} taken orally may also be effective, but anyone diagnosed with this condition should treat it under the care of a doctor.

recommended levels

The RDA for all adults is 2.4 micrograms. Some studies have shown that blood levels of B_{12} tend to decrease with age, possibly because absorption of B_{12} is less efficient as we grow older. Therefore, it's recommended that adults over age 50 try to obtain 6 to 12 mcg of vitamin B_{12} daily.

Supplementation: To prevent B_{12} deficiency, you only have to consume moderate amounts of foods containing the vitamin. But in recent years, experts have become increasingly concerned about deficiency, especially among people over age 50. Fortified foods, such as breakfast cereals, can help, since the B_{12} they contain is much better absorbed by the body. So is the B_{12} in supplements. In a supplement the vitamin is not bound, as it is in foods, and thus is more easily absorbed. Fortified foods also release the vitamin more easily, because it is simply added to the foods.

Therefore, the National Academy of Sciences now advises either consuming food fortified with B_{12} or taking a multivitamin/mineral supplement that contains B_{12}—advice that is especially important for older people to follow. If you are 50 or older, consider taking a multivitamin/mineral supplement. Most have at least 6 micrograms of vitamin B_{12}. A few multivitamins contain up to 25 micrograms, but doses that high aren't a problem. Don't waste your money on injections "for extra energy" unless you have a deficiency.

tips & facts

• One danger posed by B_{12} deficiency is misdiagnosis. Severe deficiency may cause such symptoms as tingling and weakness in the arms and legs, confusion, memory loss, hallucinations, listlessness, and stomach pain. The cause may appear to be Alzheimer's disease or some other condition. If you or someone in your family is being tested for symptoms like these, especially if dementia is suspected, make sure the doctor also tests for vitamin B_{12} deficiency. (There are blood tests for elevated levels of compounds associated with B_{12} deficiency along with low levels of the vitamin itself.)

• It has been claimed that vitamin B_{12} shots help increase energy and cure a wide array of ills. But such injections are usually a waste of time and money, since there is no benefit to them. The only legitimate use of vitamin B_{12} shots is to correct a vitamin B_{12} deficiency. Injections of the vitamin are preferred over supplements because in most cases the deficiency results from an inability to absorb the vitamin, not because of a lack of B_{12} in the diet.

• Breast-fed babies of strict vegetarian women may suffer vitamin B_{12} deficiency (infants do not have reserves of the vitamin). Lactating women who eat no animal products should be sure to take a vitamin supplement that supplies the RDA for vitamin B_{12}.

• About 4 percent of vitamin B_{12} by weight is actually the mineral cobalt. Thus vitamin B_{12} is also known as cobalamin.

• A high intake of folate, which works in tandem with vitamin B_{12}, can mask some signs of pernicious anemia because it can correct the blood-related consequences of a lack of vitamin B_{12}. However, the neurological damage caused can continue, and often goes unnoticed until it is too late to correct it.

where you can find it

Egg yolks, liver, beef, poultry, fish, shellfish, dairy products, fortified cereals, and fortified soy products are all reliable sources of vitamin B_{12}.

vitamin C

No vitamin has been touted to the extent that vitamin C has as a virtual cure-all. Many people take vitamin C regularly because they believe it keeps them healthy; others take megadoses in the winter in hopes of preventing a cold; and still others believe it can help prevent cancer. Vitamin C is one of the most versatile vitamins, performing a wide range of functions in the body. And of course, vitamin C prevents scurvy, a debilitating disease that until this century killed many people. (Vitamin C is also called ascorbic acid because of its anti-scorbutic—or anti-scurvy—properties.) Recent research has found that while vitamin C is a powerful immune protector, many of the claims for its healing properties have been overblown.

LEADING SOURCES	
SOURCE	VITAMIN C (MG)
Pepper, red, 3 oz	163
Pepper, green, 3 oz	110
Currants, black, ½ cup	101
Broccoli, chopped, cooked, 1 cup	98
Orange juice, 1 cup, from frozen	98
Brussels sprouts, cooked, 1 cup	97
Papaya, ½ medium	95
Cranberry juice cocktail, 1 cup	90
Strawberries, 1 cup	85
Grapefruit juice, 1 cup, from frozen	83
Orange, navel, 1 medium	80
Kiwifruit, 1 medium	75

what it does

Vitamin C plays many roles in the body. It provides structure to capillary and cell walls, and is crucial to the production of collagen, the connective tissue that stabilizes bone, muscle, and other tissues in the body. In addition, it helps form hemoglobin, the protein in red blood cells, and enhances iron absorption. It is important for wound healing and helps prevent bruising. And it is involved in the production of the neurotransmitters serotonin and norepinephrine. The proper functioning of the immune system is also dependent on vitamin C.

Potential health benefits: The vitamin plays a role in defending against disease. It is an antioxidant, and in this capacity can help prevent and possibly reverse the cell damage caused by free radicals (*see page 34*). Many well-designed studies show that vitamin C may reduce the risk of certain cancers as well as coronary artery disease, and may prevent or delay the onset of cataracts. Eye fluids, for example, are normally rich in vitamin C and other antioxidant compounds—thus C may protect against sunlight-induced free-radical formation in the eye.

It may also be beneficial for lowering high blood pressure. For example, a study from the Linus Pauling Institute at Oregon State University found that people with high-normal or Stage 1 hypertension (which covers a range from 130/85 to 159/99 mm Hg) who took 500 milligrams of vitamin C a day had an average drop in systolic pressure (the first of the two numbers used to express blood pressure) of 9 percent after a month. The drop in diastolic pressure was smaller. Those given a placebo pill had no significant drop in either number.

The evidence for its effectiveness as a cold-fighter is mixed. In one review of studies investigating the effect of vitamin C on colds, some researchers concluded that doses of 1,000 to 6,000 milligrams a day reduced the severity of cold symptoms by about 21 percent, and shortened the duration of the cold by one day, on average. Since there is no evidence that vitamin C prevents colds, such high doses cannot be recommended on a daily basis, but if you feel a cold coming on, it can't hurt to increase your intake for a few days.

recommended levels

The RDA for women is 75 milligrams; for men, 90 milligrams. These amounts are enough to prevent deficiency diseases, but probably not enough to produce a highly significant antioxidant effect.

Supplementation: Based on an evaluation of research to date, members of the Editorial Board for the *University of California, Berkeley Wellness Letter* recommend a daily intake of 250 to 500 milligrams of vitamin C a day. If you consume five servings of fruits and vegetables a day, you will probably have no trouble meeting the low end of this recommendation. Many studies have shown the potential for disease-prevention benefits from taking vitamin C supplements, and long-term studies have never demonstrated serious harm from vitamin C supplements. Because many people may not be able to obtain the upper end from diet alone, however, we recommend a daily supplement of 250 to 500 milligrams daily in addition to a diet rich in vitamin C.

Precautions: Most people can take high doses of vitamin C (as much as 3,000 milligrams a day) with no apparent serious ill effects—but possibly no benefit, either. However, several grams of vitamin C a day can cause diarrhea, and there are unresolved questions about the effect of such high levels on iron metabolism and nutrient balance in the body, as well as about the possibility of kidney stones.

High doses may also mask blood in the stool (a warning sign of colon cancer), causing a false negative result in a stool sample test even if blood is present. In people with diabetes, high doses may cause a false positive result for glucose in the urine.

tips & facts

• Many people take doses of 1,000 milligrams (1 gram) or more of vitamin C. Such high doses are relatively safe—your body simply excretes any excess of this water-soluble vitamin in urine and feces.. For that very reason, taking more than 400 to 500 milligrams has only a negligible effect on levels in the body, according to an analysis published in the *American Journal of Clinical Nutrition.*

• If you take vitamin C supplements, divide your dose and take half in the morning and half in the evening. The body eliminates vitamin C in about 12 hours, so doing this will keep blood levels high throughout the day and also reduce the risk of diarrhea from too high a dose.

• If you have heart disease or risk factors for it, taking a vitamin C supplement every day can help tiny blood vessels dilate, which may reduce the risk of a heart attack. This is based on a 1998 study published in *Circulation* of 46 people with heart disease; after long-term vitamin C use, their very small blood vessels were able to expand 25 percent more.

• Generally, the darker green a vegetable is, the more vitamin C it contains. Therefore romaine lettuce has more of the vitamin than iceberg, and broccoli that is bluish-green has more than green broccoli.

where you can find it

Vitamin C is present in many fruits and vegetables. Citrus fruits, peppers, and broccoli are especially good sources of the vitamin. Some foods, especially fruit drinks and juices, are fortified with vitamin C.

vitamin D

Vitamin D is unique among vitamins. Although it is classified as a nutrient—that is, it comes from foods—it is actually a hormone, and like other hormones it is manufactured in the body. All that's required is minimal exposure to sunlight, which causes skin cells to manufacture the vitamin. In fact, for many people, sunlight is the primary source of vitamin D, since it is found naturally in only a few foods.

what it does

Vitamin D helps maintain blood levels of calcium and phosphorus and helps the body utilize these two minerals. Hence, it plays a key role in building bones and teeth. Like many other nutrients, it probably has a beneficial effect on the immune system. A deficiency of vitamin D causes abnormalities in calcium bone metabolism. In children, this can result in rickets, a condition in which the bones fail to knit properly (and which is very rare in Western countries). In adults, vitamin D deficiency can contribute to osteoporosis and, more rarely, ostoemalacia (softening of the bones).

Potential health benefits: Because of its involvement in calcium absorption, vitamin D may reduce the risk of osteoporosis. Several studies have shown that vitamin D in supplement form can help reduce the risk of fractures associated with osteoporosis.

Some evidence also points to a link between vitamin D and a reduced risk of colon cancer. And some test tube studies have shown that vitamin D inhibits the growth of cancer cells, including those in the breast and prostate. But all of the research on vitamin D and cancer prevention is very preliminary.

recommended levels

The RDA for women and men through age 50 is 200 IU; for ages 51-70, 400 IU; for ages 70 and older, 600 IU. If you get even 10 or 15 minutes of sunlight on your arms and face two or three times a week, you will probably manufacture enough vitamin D to meet your needs. And because it is a fat-soluble vitamin, you can store enough to supply you in the days, or even months, when you don't get any sun exposure. Still, it's a good idea to get some vitamin D from fortified foods such as milk products and breakfast cereals. (A cup of milk in the United States contains 100 IU.) And some people, depending on their age, where they live, and on their diet, have to get some vitamin D from foods and/or supplements to meet the requirement.

Supplementation: The ability to manufacture D in the body declines with age, and simply increasing the exposure to sunlight won't necessarily help. By age 70, the body's vitamin D production is only 30 percent of what it was at age 25. Anyone over 60 who doesn't get adequate amounts of vitamin D from foods and also lacks sun exposure should take supplements. Those at highest risk are people who are homebound or institutionalized, as well as those living in the northern third of the United States and in Canada. Vegans and others who don't drink milk may also need to take a supplement. Supplemental vitamin D is recommended for everyone over age 70.

A daily multivitamin with 400 IU of vitamin D is usually the best way to get extra vitamin D. But if you fall into one of the categories above, it makes sense to discuss your risk of vitamin D deficiency with a health professional.

Precautions: Even small overdoses of vitamin D can be toxic, leading to kidney stones, kidney failure, muscle and bone weakness, and other problems. It's nearly impossible to get too much vitamin D from food and absolutely impossible to get too much from sunlight. *Nearly all documented cases of vitamin D toxicity have been caused by supplements.* Danger starts at 2,000 IU a day; to be safe, don't consume more than 1,000 IU of vitamin D daily.

tips & facts

• Your ability to make vitamin D from sunlight varies according to your location and the time of year. Generally, those who live at a latitude of 42° (a line that runs through Boston, Detroit, Chicago, the middle of Iowa, and southern Oregon) can manufacture sufficient vitamin D from a minimal amount of sun exposure between April and October. This is generally sufficient, because you will store enough vitamin D for the winter.

• People who live below 42° latitude in the United States have an even longer period—from March to November in Washington, D.C., for example—to manufacture and build up stores of vitamin D. Those living in the northern United States and in Canada have less time, but for most people it's not a problem, particularly if they get some dietary vitamin D.

• Dark-skinned people may need longer exposure to sunlight—perhaps up to twice as much as light-skinned people—since skin pigmentation screens sunlight and reduces vitamin D production.

• Sunscreen can reduce or even shut down the synthesis of vitamin D. This is a problem chiefly for older people, who are often more conscientious about using sunscreen than the young, and who also produce less vitamin D. Try to get 15 minutes of exposure without sunscreen in the early morning or late afternoon, when the sun is less damaging to the skin. Apply sunscreen the rest of the time you are in the sun, especially if you are fair-skinned.

where you can find it

The vitamin D content found naturally in unfortified foods is generally low. The exception is fatty fish (such as salmon), many of which contain 200 to 600 IU of vitamin D. Milk sold commercially is fortified with vitamin D in the United States and Canada. Some cereals, breads, and flours are also fortified with vitamin D.

vitamin E

Vitamin E, a fat-soluble vitamin, was discovered at the University of California, Berkeley, about 80 years ago. Since the early 1990s, it has been one of the most publicized nutrients, chiefly because of research findings concerning its protective effect against heart disease. In recent years, the claims made for vitamin E as a dietary supplement border on the miraculous—it's been promoted for everything from delaying aging to healing sunburn. Many of these claims should be met with skepticism, but there is good evidence to suggest that everyone should get extra amounts of vitamin E for its potential cardiovascular and other preventive benefits.

what it does

Vitamin E is actually a generic term for a group of related compounds. It occurs naturally in two groups of related forms known as tocopherols and tocotrienols. Alpha-tocopherol is by far the main type in the body, while gamma is the main tocopherol in foods. No specific metabolic function for vitamin E has been discovered, in contrast to most nutrients. The vitamin plays a role in the formation of red blood cells, reproduction and growth, and in the body's utilization of vitamin K. But its principal function appears to be as an antioxidant, helping to protect tissue against the damage of oxidation by destroying or neutralizing free radicals, which can damage the basic structure of cells and thus may lead to disease (*see page 34*). The tocotrienols have been less studied than tocopherols, and although some are potent antioxidants, their function is still unclear.

Potential health benefits: Of all its benefits, the strongest and most consistent evidence so far is related to vitamin E lowering the risk of coronary artery disease (which leads to angina and heart attacks). Many laboratory and animal studies suggest that vitamin E helps protect LDL ("bad") cholesterol from oxidation—and oxidation makes LDL more likely to promote the buildup of fatty plaque in coronary artery walls (the condition known as atherosclerosis). Vitamin E may also reduce the blood's ability to clot, thus decreasing the risk of heart attacks. Finally, it may help reduce inflammatory processes (inflammation has been linked with coronary artery disease).

The results of clinical trials, using human subjects, have been inconclusive. Some studies have shown that taking vitamin E supplements reduced deaths from heart disease, but others have found no significant reduction. Most of the studies have been done on patients with heart disease, and it is possible that there would be a more consistently protective effect in people who had not yet developed heart disease.

LEADING SOURCES	
SOURCE	VITAMIN E (MG)
Corn or soybean oil, 1 tbsp	12
Canola or sunflower oil, 1 tbsp	8
Kale, cooked, 1 cup	7
Sweet potato, 5 oz	5
Wheat germ, 1 oz	4
Almonds or hazelnuts, 1 oz	4
Sunflower seeds, 1 oz	4
Spinach, cooked, 1 cup	4
Asparagus, cooked, 4 oz	3
Blueberries, 1 cup	3
Avocado, 5 oz	2
Broccoli, chopped, cooked, 1 cup	2
Margarine, 1 tbsp	2

Other research suggests that vitamin E may lower the risk of some types of cancer as well as arthritis, Parkinson's disease, one type of stroke, Alzheimer's disease, and diabetes (*see below*). But the evidence is inconsistent or preliminary.

recommended levels

The RDA for all adults is 15 milligrams. This amount—equivalent to about 23 International Units (IU), another measure of vitamin E—is enough to prevent deficiency of the vitamin (an extremely rare occurrence). However, it is not sufficient to obtain the vitamin's potential disease-prevention benefits.

Supplementation: Consider taking 200 to 400 IU of vitamin E per day from a supplement. (That's the equivalent of 133 to 217 milligrams.) You can't get that much from food unless you eat huge amounts of nuts, seeds, or vegetable oil, all high in fat. Not all members of the Editorial Board for the *University of California, Berkeley Wellness Letter* agree that vitamin E supplements are advisable for everyone. But the majority believe that such levels are safe and potentially beneficial.

Precautions: Even very large doses of vitamin E appear to produce few serious side effects, though diarrhea, blurred vision, dizziness, and headaches have occasionally been reported at intakes of 1,200 IU or more daily.

At high doses, however, vitamin E may interfere with the clotting ability of the blood. There have been a few reports about clotting problems (leading to excessive bleeding and other problems) associated with vitamin E, especially in people taking anticoagulant medications such as warfarin (Coumadin). If you are taking an anticoagulant or any other medication that affects blood clotting, you probably shouldn't take vitamin E supplements—be sure to check with your doctor first. Also check with your doctor if you regularly take daily doses of nonsteroidal anti-inflammatory drugs (NSAIDs) such as aspirin, ibuprofen (Advil), or naproxen (Aleve), since at high doses these can also affect blood clotting.

tips & facts

• When choosing a supplement, look for "natural" vitamin E, preferably a brand containing some "mixed tocopherols" (which contain various amounts of three tocopherols). Synthetic vitamin E (often denoted as dl-alpha-tocopherol) is cheaper, but largely contains forms that are foreign to the body and are probably poorly utilized by the body. In effect, about twice as much of the vitamin ends up in the blood of people taking natural E as in those taking the same amount of synthetic E.

• Studies suggest that vitamin E may help improve control of blood sugar, notably by enhancing the action of insulin and by affecting cell membranes. Hence, if you have Type 2 diabetes, (non-insulin dependent) or are at high risk for developing it, this is added reason to take a daily vitamin E supplement. In addition, people with diabetes seem to be particularly prone to the "oxidative stress" caused by free radicals, which contributes to their increased risk for heart disease as well as diabetic complications.

• Olive oil is one vegetable oil that is not high in vitamin E. While vitamin E is abundant in polyunsaturated fats—the predominant fat in corn, safflower, and sunflower oils—olive oil is predominantly monounsaturated.

where you can find it

Vegetable oils, margarine, seeds, nuts, green leafy vegetables, and whole grains contain significant amounts of vitamin E.

vitamin K

Vitamin K is synthesized by bacteria that normally inhabit the intestinal tract. About 60 to 80 percent of our vitamin K needs are met through this process. It is fortunate that we have the ability to produce vitamin K, since unlike other fat-soluble vitamins, it is not stored by the body in appreciable amounts.

what it does

Without vitamin K, blood would not clot. Most of the factors involved in blood clotting are present in a "precursor" form in the bloodstream to prevent clot formation within the blood vessels. Vitamin K is the catalyst that changes these precursor proteins into their active form when there is a cut or wound. At the early stages of blood clotting, vitamin K transforms prothrombin into the clotting protein thrombin. Later in the process, it helps change fibrinogen into fibrin, a protein that forms the essential portions of a blood clot.

Deficiencies of vitamin K are practically unheard of in healthy children and adults. However, deficiencies can occur in people who have malabsorption syndromes or liver disease or who are on long-term or broad-spectrum antibiotic therapy. Also, some drugs used to reduce blood clotting in people with circulatory or cardiovascular diseases interfere with the body's production of vitamin K, and so require careful monitoring by a physician.

Newborns are deficient in vitamin K and so are given an injection of the vitamin to prevent excessive bleeding, which can be life-threatening in a baby.

Potential health benefits: Vitamin K is needed to make a protein that is essential for bone formation and so may be helpful in maintaining strong bones in older people. Research that tracked 72,000 middle-aged women for 10 years in the ongoing Nurses' Health Study found that those who consumed moderate or high amounts of vitamin K (nearly all from vegetables) had a 30 percent lower risk of hip fractures than women consuming little or no vitamin K. This held true even when other factors affecting bone health, such as calcium and vitamin D, were taken into account.

recommended levels

The AI (Adequate Intake) for women is 90 micrograms; for men, 120 micrograms. Some experts suggest that a higher range of vitamin K intake—100 to 150 mcg per day—may be necessary to help keep bones strong as you age. This protective effect can easily be supplied by the foods noted below.

Supplementation: For healthy people, supplements are not necessary and not recommended.

Precautions: People who take anticoagulant drugs such as warfarin (Coumadin), which decrease blood clotting by inhibiting the action of vitamin K, should avoid large servings of foods high in vitamin K, especially green vegetables. Consuming high amounts of the vitamin can defeat the anticlotting action of the drugs.

tips & facts

• High doses of vitamin E may impair the absorption of vitamin K somewhat. So people who are taking vitamin E supplements should be sure to eat some foods rich in vitamin K.

where you can find it

Spinach, lettuce, watercress, and other leafy green vegetables are good sources of vitamin K, as are broccoli and Brussels sprouts. Vegetable oils, and soybean oil in particular, also contain some vitamin K.

boron

In the late 19th century, boron was used to preserve foods such as meat, shell-fish, and butter—a function that was prized in times of poor refrigeration and food shortages. Thus, people consumed large amounts of boron with no apparent ill effects, until one study suggested that a high intake over a period of a few weeks could cause appetite loss and digestive problems. As a result, the addition of boron to foods was banned, and the mineral was pretty much forgotten. But in recent years, interest in boron was revived to such an extent that exaggerated claims were being made for its health benefits. The truth is that boron is essential to human health, though nutritionists still have much to learn about its functions and its degree of importance.

what it does

Although the role boron plays in human health is still under investigation, research has shown that the mineral helps to maintain the structure of cell membranes. It is also involved in the metabolism of several minerals—especially calcium—and may enhance the effects of estrogen. Thus, boron helps build and preserve bone mass. It may also help regulate brain function.

recommended levels

Because research into boron is in its early stages, the RDA has never been established. Any symptoms related to a deficiency of boron have yet to be discovered

Supplementation: Supplementation is not necessary and not recommended. In fact, while up to 10 milligrams per day appear to be safe, the government's Food and Nutrition Board has recommended that, based on animal studies, daily doses above 20 milligrams may have adverse consequences. Getting too much boron (which is unlikely from foods alone) can cause gastrointestinal upset, skin problems, and seizures.

tips & facts

Boron has been touted as a miracle mineral. Some people believe that it cures arthritis, improves memory, prevents the hot flashes that occur in menopause, and builds muscle mass. These claims have been exaggerated from the results of small, preliminary studies involving people whose intake of boron was extremely low. There's absolutely no evidence that a high intake of boron can produce any of these benefits.

where you can find it

Nuts, legumes, leafy green vegetables, and dried beans are good sources of boron, as are beer and wine. Animal products tend to be low in this mineral.

calcium

Calcium is essential at every stage of life. An adequate calcium intake during childhood, adolescence, and early adulthood helps ensure that a person can achieve maximum bone mass (which depends on several factors besides calcium intake, such as genetics and exercise). In addition to producing strong bones, achieving maximum bone mass makes enough calcium available to the body to perform other essential functions. Although the buildup of bone mass slows with age, and eventually calcium depletion will outpace calcium accumulation, the amount of bone lost can be significantly reduced if calcium intake remains adequate throughout life.

LEADING SOURCES	
SOURCE	CALCIUM (MG)
Yogurt, low-fat plain, 8 oz	448
Ricotta cheese, part-skim, ½ cup	337
Sardines, canned with bones, 3 oz	325
Milk, fat-free, 1 cup	302
Orange juice, fortified, 1 cup	300
Swiss cheese, 1 oz	272
Cereal, fortified, 1 cup	250
Oatmeal, instant fortified, cooked, 1 cup	215
Salmon, canned with bones, 3 oz	205
Turnip greens, cooked, 1 cup	200
Cheddar cheese, low-fat, 1 oz	118
White beans, canned, ½ cup	96

what it does

Most of the calcium in the body is used in the formation and maintenance of bone. In fact, bones and teeth contain 99 percent of the body's calcium. The remaining 1 percent is found in the cells and in the fluid that surrounds them. This amount, though small, is involved in several vital functions. Calcium helps regulate muscle contraction (and so helps control heartbeat). It is needed for the transmission of nerve impulses, signaling the release of messages from one nerve cell to another. It controls cell membrane permeability, so that substances can flow in and out of cells as needed.

Calcium is also involved in several enzymatic reactions, especially those that release energy for use by cells, and it is an important factor in blood clotting.

Potential health benefits: By building and maintaining bone density and strength, long-term calcium intake is one of the keys to preventing or delaying osteoporosis, the bone-thinning disease that makes bones fragile and brittle so that they fracture easily. About 1.3 million older Americans suffer fractures due to osteoporosis.

Calcium, along with potassium and magnesium, helps control blood pressure, and a diet containing adequate amounts of these minerals may help prevent hypertension. There is also evidence, based on a study of more than 85,000 nurses, suggesting that a calcium-rich diet may reduce the risk of ischemic stroke, the most common type of stroke. Studies have found that calcium intake helps prevent dangerous blood clots, and that it may actually lower blood cholesterol somewhat.

Another benefit: According to a review article in the *Journal of the American College of Nutrition,* calcium in supplement form may help reduce symptoms of premenstrual syndrome (PMS), such as breast tenderness, bloating, headaches, and mood disorders.

recommended levels

For adults through age 50, the Adequate Intake (AI) is 1,000 milligrams; for adults age 51 and older, 1,200 milligrams. This recent recommendation is higher than an earlier RDA for calcium. And some authorities think that women over age 50, and men over age 65, should try for 1,200 to 1,500 milligrams per day.

Supplementation: Although it is possible to meet your calcium requirements from food sources, the average American woman consumes only 625 milligrams; the average man, 865. You should get as much calcium as you can from foods. But people, and especially women, who consume less than the recommended levels should make up the shortfall by taking supplements.

Up to 2,500 milligrams from food and supplements is considered safe. However, don't take more than 500 milligrams of supplemental calcium at a time—preferably with food. If you take 1,000 milligrams or more a day, take it in two or more doses over the course of the day.

tips & facts

• Dairy products are the best sources of calcium, but, surprisingly, Americans get about half their calcium from such nondairy foods as sardines, calcium-fortified orange juice, salmon, broccoli, and fortified cereals.

• Compared to other cheeses, cottage cheese is a minor source of calcium, and cream cheese has virtually none. Fat-free and low-fat milk are slightly higher in calcium than whole milk.

• Although caffeine may enhance calcium excretion, you can compensate for this by adding a tablespoon of milk to your coffee. Specialty coffee drinks, such as cafe latte (*see "Love that Latte," page 401*) or cappuccino, can significantly contribute to your calcium intake. A 12-ounce cafe latte supplies 400 milligrams of calcium, for example. (Opt for fat-free or low-fat milk.)

• Antacid pills made from calcium carbonate (such as Tums) can serve as inexpensive calcium supplements. Each tablet contains 500 milligrams of calcium carbonate, which supplies 200 milligrams of pure calcium.

• People with recurring kidney stones were once told to avoid calcium. Research now suggests that getting recommended amounts of calcium may help prevent stones in many people. But some stone-formers may reduce their chances of recurrence by cutting down on calcium. It depends on what kind of stones you get. If you are prone to stones, discuss dietary and other measures with your doctor.

• Very high protein diets (130 grams or more of protein daily) may lead to increased calcium loss, but the long-term consequences of such a diet are unknown.

where you can find it

Milk, yogurt, and cheese are all excellent sources of calcium. Kale, Swiss chard, turnip greens, broccoli, almonds, canned sardines and salmon eaten with their soft bones, and firm tofu are all good nondairy sources, as is calcium-fortified orange juice.

chromium

Chromium is an essential trace mineral that the body requires in very small amounts. Deficiency is rare in Western countries. Yet claims have been made for extra amounts of chromium in supplement form: that it helps burn fat and build muscle, that it is a cure for diabetes, and that it will help lower blood cholesterol levels. However, there are doubts not only about the benefits, but about the safety of taking chromium supplements.

what it does

Chromium is important in the burning of carbohydrates and fats, and in some aspects of protein metabolism. It is needed for the body to use insulin properly. Without chromium, insulin cannot make blood sugar (glucose, our basic fuel) available to cells—though the exact role chromium plays in this process isn't clear.

Potential health benefits: Some very preliminary research suggests that chromium picolinate—the form of the mineral most commonly sold as a supplement—can reduce blood sugar in people with Type 2 diabetes, the most common form of the disease. But this does not mean that supplements are a reliable treatment for diabetes, which is not linked to chromium deficiency. There is some evidence that a lack of chromium can cause high blood cholesterol levels and low HDL ("good") cholesterol levels, but the studies have been inconsistent—and there is no evidence that taking supplements will help control cholesterol levels.

recommended levels

The AI (Adequate Intake) is 25 micrograms for women through age 50; 20 micrograms for women age 51 and older; 35 micrograms for men through age 50; 30 micrograms for men age 51 and older.

Supplementation: There is little evidence that chromium deficiency is widespread or that supplements of chromium picolinate have any benefit. Therefore, supplements are not necessary and not recommended. Moreover, the evidence is mounting that supplements of chromium picolinate—which millions of people have taken—can do more harm than good. A study conducted at the University of Alabama at Tuscaloosa showed that chromium picolinate enters the body's cells directly and stays there, where it can cause problems. The chromium picolinate reacts with vitamin C and other antioxidants in the cells to produce a "reduced" form of chromium capable of causing mutations in DNA, the genetic material. It's the combination of chromium and picolinate (particularly the reduced form) that can produce dangerous compounds—not the chromium alone. Moreover, the picolinate eventually breaks off and itself has adverse effects.

tips & facts

• Vitamin C enhances chromium absorption.

• Calorie for calorie, diets that are high in fat tend to contain less chromium than low-fat diets.

• Cooking acidic foods in stainless steel pots may boost the food's chromium content, since the mineral will leach from stainless steel.

• There is no good evidence backing chromium picolinate as a weight-loss or body-building aid. Another claim—that it can reduce blood cholesterol levels—is also lacking evidence.

where you can find it

Whole grains, brewer's yeast, prunes, nuts, peanut butter, potatoes, and seafood are high in chromium.

copper

Copper is part of at least 15 proteins in the body, including many enzymes, yet the human body contains only about ½₂₅₀ of an ounce of copper. But that tiny amount makes possible a number of essential functions.

what it does

Along with iron, copper helps in the formation of red blood cells. Copper also oxidizes stored forms of iron so that iron can be transported to sites in the body where it is needed. Copper is also used to construct healthy blood vessels and connective tissue, such as collagen, and it plays a role in producing hair and skin pigments and several neurotransmitters (chemicals that carry nerve signals throughout the body). Copper is also involved in fertility and the immune system.

Potential health benefits: Scientists have investigated a possible connection between copper and heart disease. Induced copper deficiencies in humans and animals seem to accelerate atherosclerosis. But other minerals, including zinc and selenium, may be involved, and some studies show that very high levels of copper in the blood may make atherosclerosis worse.

recommended levels

The RDA for all adults is 900 micrograms.

Supplementation: For healthy people, copper supplements are not necessary or recommended. Despite claims of supplement manufacturers, there is no evidence that a low copper intake can contribute to arthritis or high blood cholesterol levels.

Precautions: High doses of copper may be dangerous, especially in view of unknown interactions with other trace minerals. As little as 10 milligrams (10,000 micrograms) of copper can cause nausea—and large amounts (3.5 grams or more) can be fatal. Taking megadoses of zinc supplements—for example, taking zinc lozenges to try and prevent a cold—can interfere with copper absorption.

where you can find it

Shellfish, organ meats (such as liver), legumes, nuts, and seeds are good sources of copper.

iodine

Iodine is closely associated with proper functioning of the thyroid gland. This small butterfly-shaped gland that surrounds the trachea (windpipe), regulates metabolism and growth. Despite its small size—less than an ounce—the thyroid gland of a healthy adult has a remarkable ability to store iodine. The body typically contains 20 to 30 milligrams of the mineral, and 75 percent of it is stored in the thyroid gland.

what it does

Iodine is essential for the formation of the thyroid hormone thyroxin, which governs metabolism and physical and mental development. There is also some evidence that thyroxin is involved in the conversion of beta carotene to vitamin A, in the synthesis of protein and cholesterol, and in the absorption of carbohydrates. In addition, it is essential for reproduction.

If your diet is lacking in iodine, the thyroid gland will enlarge in an attempt to trap as much iodine from the blood as possible. Once the enlargement becomes visible, it is called a goiter. (However, not all goiters are caused by an iodine deficiency.)

A low iodine intake also causes insufficient production of thyroid hormones, which can result in fatigue, skin changes, an increase in blood fats, hoarseness, delayed reflex reactions, and reduced mental functioning. A lack of iodine in the diets of pregnant women can cause a severe form of mental retardation called cretinism in babies. In children, an iodine deficiency can adversely effect intellectual ability.

Iodine was once lacking in the American diet, but the introduction of iodized salt in 1922 did much to correct this. In fact, there have been no cases of iodine deficiency reported in the United States since the 1970s, although it still may be a problem in developing countries.

recommended levels

The RDA for all adults is 150 micrograms. Americans easily get about twice this amount from the average 2,000 calorie diet.

Supplementation: Because iodine is so plentiful in the diet, supplemental iodine is not necessary. Taking high levels of iodine has no benefit, but at the same time, it also doesn't have adverse effects for most people. The body is remarkably tolerant of high levels. There is one exception: In those who have been iodine-deficient, especially the elderly, very high intakes can cause thyroid disease. But it's hard to say how much is too much. A healthy person can probably consume up to 2,000 micrograms of iodine a day without harm, though some researchers believe 1,000 micrograms should be the limit. Extremely high doses can also cause goiters.

tips & facts

• Your salt intake should be limited to 2,400 milligrams of sodium a day. The salt you use should be iodized—a quarter teaspoon (containing 580 milligrams of sodium) has about 100 micrograms of iodine.

• Sea salt is not a good source of iodine. This type of salt, often sold in health-food stores, is made by evaporating sea water, but the iodine it contains is lost during the drying process.

• Although many processed foods contain added salt, iodized salt is not typically used. However, dough conditioners used in some baked goods are high in iodine, and so these foods contribute significant amounts of iodine to the diet.

• A government survey has shown that Americans have decreased their iodine intake over the last 20 years—though no one is sure why this is happening. Levels are still within the desirable range, but researchers plan to monitor the trend.

where you can find it

Iodized table salt is obviously a good source of iodine. Seafood is an excellent source (iodine is present in salt water), and dairy products also supply some iodine. The amount of iodine in fruits and vegetables depends on the soil in which they grow.

iron

Iron deficiency is one of the more common nutritional shortfalls in the United States. The problem mainly affects women and it's likely to occur during only a few stages of life, when the body's demand for iron increases.

what it does

About 70 percent of the iron in the body is found in the red blood cells. Iron is an essential component of hemoglobin, the protein that gives blood its red color and carries oxygen to all the cells. Iron is also essential to the formation of myoglobin, which stores oxygen in muscles to provide energy for muscle contraction. Several enzymes and proteins in the body also rely on iron.

LEADING SOURCES	
SOURCE	IRON (MG)
Clams, cooked, 3 oz	24
Tofu, 4 oz	11.9
Cream of wheat, cooked, 1 cup	9.2
Oatmeal, instant, fortified, cooked, 1 cup	8.3
Quinoa, dry, ½ cup	7.9
White beans, canned, ½ cup	3.9
Beef tenderloin, broiled, 3 oz	3.6
Lentils, cooked, ½ cup	3.3
Bagel, 1	2.8
Rice, white, cooked, 1 cup	2.8
Tuna, canned in water, 3 oz	2.7

The body carefully monitors its iron status, absorbing more iron when stores of the mineral are low and less iron when stores are adequate. The iron contained in red blood cells is re-utilized as those blood cells are broken down by the body. Very little iron is excreted; the only way significant amounts of iron leave the body is through blood loss or blood transfer to a fetus. This means that it can take a long time before a deficiency develops. However, the body's controls cannot override an iron-poor diet in the long term.

Iron deficiency. The initial stage of iron deficiency usually produces no symptoms. However, even mild iron deficiency can cause irritability in infants and hinder learning and problem-solving capacity in children. Anemia, with its accompanying fatigue and weakness, is the ultimate consequence of iron deficiency. In this disorder, there is a decrease in the number of red blood cells circulating in the body, or a below normal hemoglobin content. Either condition reduces the amount of oxygen delivered to the cells.

Who is at risk? An iron deficit isn't necessarily due to poor eating habits. An otherwise balanced diet may not supply adequate iron. The following people may need supplemental iron, but should ask their doctor to check for iron deficiency before taking iron pills.

Menstruating women, especially those who bleed heavily, since blood losses increase the need for iron.

Pregnant women, whose iron needs increase because of the demands of the fetus and placenta.

Dieters, especially women, since the less they eat, the more likely it is that they will not get enough iron.

Endurance athletes, particularly women or vegetarians, tend to have a higher incidence of iron depletion, which may impair top performance. This iron shortfall has been attributed to a variety of reasons, including the increased elimination of iron during prolonged exercise.

Strict vegetarians, since the animal products they don't eat are the best sources of iron. These vegetarians have to make a special effort to eat other foods that contain fair amounts of iron, such as legumes, dried fruits, leafy greens, and fortified cereals and grains.

Infants and children, because of their rapid growth; deficiencies may adversely affect their learning capacity.

recommended levels

The RDA is 18 milligrams for women through age 50; 8 milligrams for women age 51 and older; 8 milligrams for all adult men.

Supplementation: The average diet supplies plenty of iron—from both natural food sources such as meat and fish as well as fortified foods (most cereals, pastas, and breads are fortified with iron). For most people, there is no reason to load up on iron. In particular, men and postmenopausal women do not need iron supplements and probably don't even need the iron in a multivitamin/mineral supplement. Iron in vegetarian foods is less well absorbed than the iron in meat, but even vegetarians can get enough iron from food. Moreover, if the body already has sufficient iron, additional iron won't be absorbed, unless you have hemochromatosis (an inherited disorder in which the body overloads on iron).

People at possible risk for iron deficiency may need an iron supplement (*see "Who is at Risk?" page 73*). But that should be determined by a doctor. No one should take a separate iron pill unless a physician advises it.

Because the body reduces absorption when iron stores are high, in most cases large amounts of iron are not toxic for adults. There are some exceptions, however. An estimated 1 million or more Americans with hemochromatosis are at risk for iron overload because their bodies overabsorb the mineral. And children are especially susceptible to ill effects from excessive doses of iron. Iron-containing supplements are the leading cause of childhood poisoning death. As few as five high-potency over-the-counter pills could be fatal for a child.

A 1992 Finnish study suggested that even normal iron stores increased risk for heart disease in men. However, further study has not supported the idea.

tips & facts

• Heme iron, which is found in meat and other animal products, is much better absorbed than nonheme iron, which makes up some of the iron in animal tissues and all of the iron in dairy products, eggs, vegetables, fruits, and grains, and in the supplemental iron used to fortify flour and cereals.

• Vitamin C helps the body absorb nonheme iron. For example, you could triple the amount of iron absorbed from a vegetarian meal of navy beans, rice, corn bread, and an apple by adding 75 milligrams of vitamin C—the amount in 1 cup of steamed broccoli or 5 ounces of orange juice.

• An iron pot can add lots of iron to your food. The iron leaches into the food, boosting its iron content. Acidic foods such as tomato sauce or applesauce, which cook for a long time, absorb the most iron. Stainless steel cookware also releases some iron.

• Don't start taking iron supplements to treat anemia. Anemia is a condition caused by a decrease in hemoglobin, a protein-iron compound in the blood. Fatigue is one of the chief symptoms of anemia. But fatigue, weakness, and other symptoms associated with anemia have many causes, and anemia itself can result from other dietary deficiencies, such as a lack of folate, or from some form of internal bleeding. If you think you're anemic, you need to consult a physician.

where you can find it

Liver, beef, and lamb are excellent sources of iron. Pork, poultry, and fish have less. (Dark-meat poultry is higher in iron than white meat.) Dried beans and peas, tofu, and dried fruit are also good sources of nonheme iron.

magnesium

Magnesium is one of the major minerals, but has received far less attention than superstar nutrients such as calcium or vitamin C. However, recent research has uncovered new aspects of its crucial roles in health. This has led many people to make claims about the health benefits of magnesium—from food or supplements. There certainly are many good reasons to get it from foods.

LEADING SOURCES	
SOURCE	MAGNESIUM (MG)
Amaranth, dry, ½ cup	260
Sunflower seed kernels, ½ cup	255
Quinoa, dry, ½ cup	179
Spinach, boiled, 1 cup	156
Wild rice, raw, ½ cup	142
Tofu, 4 oz	118
Halibut, cooked, 3 oz	92
Almonds, 1 oz	86
Brown rice, cooked, 1 cup	86
White beans, canned, ½ cup	67
Avocado, Florida, ½ medium	51
Chocolate chips, ¼ cup	48

what it does

Magnesium performs hundreds of important functions in the body, including those that help convert carbohydrates, fats, and protein into energy. It is a major component of bones and teeth and works closely with calcium. It is also involved in the proper functioning of nerves and muscles—for example, magnesium is needed to relax muscles after contraction—and helps regulate heart rhythm.

Potential health benefits: Adequate magnesium levels may help prevent several chronic diseases in a variety of ways.

Coronary artery disease (CAD). Magnesium is important for the activity of the heart muscle and the nerves that initiate the heartbeat. It may help prevent heart arrhythmias, as well as keep blood vessels healthy and prevent spasms of coronary arteries that cause angina. And it helps regulate blood pressure.

A magnesium deficiency can thus lead to cardiovascular abnormalities that increase the risk of heart attack and stroke. Some studies have found that people with several types of heart problems benefit from increased magnesium (in some studies the magnesium comes from food, in others from supplements or injections). However, other studies have found no coronary benefits for people with heart disease from supplemental magnesium.

Many population studies have found that people with a diet rich in magnesium have a lower risk of heart disease and stroke. In addition, people who live in areas with hard water, which is high in magnesium, have a lower death rate from CAD. Magnesium-rich foods are a big part of the government-endorsed antihypertension diet known as DASH (Dietary Approaches to Stop Hypertension). None of this proves that magnesium is the key, however. Foods that are rich in magnesium are also rich in other protective nutrients (such as potassium) and fiber, so it is hard to separate out the effect of this single mineral. And studies using magnesium supplements to lower blood pressure have had mixed results.

Diabetes. Several important studies have found that getting insufficient amounts of magnesium increases the risk of both types of diabetes as well as insulin resistance (which often leads to diabetes). In fact, some researchers believe that the potential link between hypertension and diabetes may be a magnesium deficiency. Magnesium is known to be essential in the body's use of insulin and burning of carbohydrates. But more research is needed into its practical effects on the prevention and treatment of diabetes.

Bone health. Working closely with calcium and vitamin D, magnesium helps with the formation and maintenance of bones and teeth. By helping to keep bones strong, an adequate magnesium intake may help prevent osteoporosis. Indeed, studies have found that women with this bone-thinning disease tend to have low magnesium levels, and that people with high magnesium intakes have greater bone density. Indeed, most dietary supplements marketed for bone health contain magnesium along with calcium and vitamin D.

recommended levels

The RDA is 310 milligrams for women age 19 to 30; 320 milligrams for women age 31 and older; 400 milligrams for men age 19 to 30; 420 milligrams for men 31 and older. Few Americans are truly deficient in magnesium, but many consume less than the recommended levels. The elderly, in particular, may have low magnesium levels, because they tend to consume less of it and because, with age, the body absorbs and retains less of it. People taking certain medications, such as diuretics or certain antibiotics, and heavy drinkers, are also at risk for magnesium deficiency.

Supplementation: There is no need to take individual magnesium supplements. If you have heart disease, don't take supplements without talking to your doctor. For older people, or anyone not eating a balanced diet, a basic multivitamin/mineral is a good way to get supplemental magnesium.

Precautions: The kidneys are very efficient at maintaining magnesium balance, excreting less of the mineral through urine when intake is low and more of it when intake is high. Thus people with healthy kidneys rarely have to worry about overloading on magnesium. Those with kidney disease, however, should be careful to monitor their magnesium intake.

tips & facts

• Though magnesium qualifies as a major mineral, the body contains far less magnesium than it does of the other major minerals. On average, a 150-pound body contains about 1 ounce of magnesium—compared to nearly 3 pounds of calcium, for example. About 60 percent of the body's magnesium is stored in the bones; the rest is found in the cells.

• About 80 percent of the magnesium in grains is found in the bran and germ, which are removed in the milling of white rice and white flour. The mineral is not replaced when these grains are enriched. Therefore enriched grain products—white bread, pasta, and white rice, for example—are not good sources of magnesium.

• Thiazide diuretics prescribed for hypertension or congestive heart failure may cause magnesium deficiency, since these drugs increase urine output. If you take these drugs, be sure to eat foods high in magnesium, and ask your doctor if you need supplements.

• When used in high doses over long periods, over-the-counter antacids that contain magnesium (such as Mylanta, Maalox, and Di-Gel) or laxatives (milk of magnesia) can cause magnesium poisoning. This can seriously depress the cardiac and central nervous systems. When using these products, do not exceed the maximum dose listed on the label. If gastrointestinal symptoms persist, see your doctor.

where you can find it

Whole grains, nuts, seeds, legumes, chocolate, and green leafy vegetables are high in magnesium. If your drinking water is hard, you'll get a fair amount of magnesium from it.

manganese

Manganese has been recognized as an essential dietary element since 1931, when deficiency of the mineral was found to hinder growth and adversely affect reproductive function in animal studies. Even today, most of our understanding of the functions of manganese comes from animal studies, because researchers have not been able to fully unravel the mechanisms that control its absorption, transport, and storage in the human body.

what it does

Manganese is important for the formation and maintenance of bone and connective tissue, and for proper brain formation. It is involved in a wide variety of enzymatic functions, including those that form urea (a chief component of urine), produce fats and cholesterol, and metabolize carbohydrates for energy. It also is important for the development of superoxide dismutase, an antioxidant enzyme produced by the body.

Outside of the laboratory, there has never been a report of manganese deficiency in people. This is probably because this mineral is plentiful in the diets of most cultures, and also because magnesium can substitute for manganese in many of the body's functions. Animal studies show that a lack of manganese causes poor growth, skeletal abnormalities, and problems in carbohydrate and fat metabolism.

recommended levels

The AI (Adequate Intake) for women is 1.8 milligrams; for men, 2.3 milligrams.

Supplementation: Because these levels can easily be obtained from foods, supplementation is not necessary or recommended. Manganese toxicity does occur, but is almost always the result of inhalation of the mineral in an industrial setting. Oral toxicity is possible, but extremely rare. Too much manganese can cause central nervous system complications, iron deficiency, and reproductive problems.

where you can find it

Nuts, shellfish, whole grains, pineapple, and berries are good sources of manganese. It is also found in coffee and tea.

molybdenum

Molybdenum is needed in amounts far below those of other trace elements, and because deficiencies are unknown, there has been little research into the effects of molybdenum on health. We do know that molybdenum is required, though even a poor diet seems to supply enough to meet the body's needs.

what it does

Molybdenum is needed to produce enzymes that aid in various chemical reactions in the body, notably those that form uric acid, a waste product that is excreted by the body through urine. It may help the body retain fluoride and aid in the release of iron from iron stores in the liver when the body requires it. It is also involved in interactions involving copper and sulfur.

recommended levels

The RDA for women and men is 45 micrograms.

Supplementation: Because these levels are easily obtained from foods, supplementation isn't necessary or recommended. There's never been a report of a molybdenum deficiency in people with normal diets, and surveys indicate that the daily intake of this trace mineral is well above recommended guidelines.

where you can find it

Milk, legumes, grains, and cereals are good sources of molybdenum. The molybdenum content of plant foods depends on the soil they are grown in.

phosphorus

Phosphorus and calcium are often called "twin nutrients," since about 85 percent of the phosphorus in the body is combined with calcium in bones and teeth. Yet nutritionally, phosphorus doesn't command the same attention as calcium, probably because phosphorus, unlike calcium, is found in such a wide variety of foods that it is relatively easy to consume the required intake.

what it does

Phosphorus helps build bone and maintain the integrity of the skeleton. In fact, the bones and teeth will not harden without phosphorus. But phosphorus does much more than that. It also regulates the release of energy. A compound called adenosine triphosphate, or ATP, which requires phosphorus, plays a major role in controlling energy flow in the body.

Phosphorus also helps transport fats, in the form of phospholipids, throughout the bloodstream by making the fats water-soluble. In addition, phosphorus attaches to many nutrients to help transport them into and out of cells, and is needed to produce DNA and RNA.

A diet lacking in phosphorus can cause fragile bones, fatigue and weakness, loss of appetite, stiff joints, and an increased susceptibility to infection. Premature infants, and people who regularly take large amounts of aluminum-containing antacids, may be susceptible to phosphorus deficiency (the aluminium found in some types of antacids can bind with phosphorus and make it unavailable to the body). Premature infants require more phosphorus than is found in human milk, and without supplementation, are at risk of developing rickets.

recommended levels

The RDA for women and men is 700 milligrams.

Supplementation: Because these levels can easily be obtained from foods, supplementation is not necessary or recommended.

where you can find it

Phosphorus is found in most foods. High-protein foods—meat, seafood, poultry, seeds, and dairy products—are excellent sources. It is also part of an additive that is used in a wide variety of processed foods. Grains contain some phosphorus, but about 85 percent of it is chemically bound and unavailable to the body.

potassium

LEADING SOURCES	
SOURCE	POTASSIUM (MG)
Baked potato, with skin, 1 medium	844
Avocado, Florida, ½ medium	742
White beans, canned, ½ cup	595
Yogurt, fat-free plain, 8 oz	579
Pompano, broiled, 3 oz	545
Tomato juice, 1 cup	535
Orange juice, fresh, 1 cup	496
Tuna, yellowfin, broiled, 3 oz	488
Cantaloupe, diced, 1 cup	482
Banana, 1 medium	467
Water chestnuts, raw, sliced, ½ cup	362

Like sodium and chloride, potassium is an electrolyte—a mineral that, when dissolved in body fluids, becomes an electrically charged particle called an ion. Positive and negatively charged ions work together to distribute fluids throughout the body and to maintain proper fluid balance. Foods that are good sources of potassium may also reduce the risk of high blood pressure and stroke.

what it does

As an electrolyte, potassium helps balance the acidity/alkalinity of the body's fluids. It is also vital for normal muscle contraction, nerve impulses, the functioning of the heart and kidneys, and the regulation of blood pressure.

Potential health benefits: There is good evidence that an adequate amount of potassium helps prevent or lower elevated blood pressure and reduces the risk of stroke and other forms of cardiovascular disease. Among people in the developing world whose diet is rich in potassium and low in sodium, high blood pressure is nonexistent. When these people move to industrialized countries, their blood pressure rises, and the change in diet may be a factor in this.

However, studies show that even a large increase in potassium consumption by itself has only a modest effect on blood pressure. Hence, diet alone is seldom an adequate treatment for hypertension. But for people who are hypertensive, eating more fruits, vegetables, whole grains, and dairy products will supply beneficial amounts of potassium as well as calcium and magnesium, two other minerals that regulate blood pressure.

The benefit of potassium helping to prevent hypertension is such that the Food and Drug Administration (FDA), which allows only a handful of health claims on foods, recently approved a claim for potassium: "Diets containing foods that are good sources of potassium and low in sodium may reduce the risk of high blood pressure and stroke."

Scientists are also discovering new benefits of potassium. For instance, it may act as an antioxidant and may help reduce the tendency of the blood to clot.

recommended levels

There is no RDA for potassium, but nutritionists generally recommend that adults consume 3,000 milligrams of potassium per day. The government's Daily Value for potassium (used on food labels) is 3,500 milligrams.

Supplementation: Because potassium is widely available from foods, supplements are not necessary or recommended. While you can't get an overdose of potassium from foods, potassium pills can supply dangerous amounts. Megadoses can cause muscle paralysis and abnormal heart rhythms, even in healthy people.

For those with kidney disease, diabetes, or heart problems, and those on certain antihypertensive drugs, a few extra grams of potassium can be especially dangerous. *Take supplements only if your doctor has recommended them.*

tips & facts

• More potassium is found in lean cuts of meat than in fatty cuts, since potassium is concentrated in muscle tissue.

• Ounce for ounce, avocados and bananas have more potassium than any other fresh fruit.

• To qualify for the new health claim concerning potassium, a food must have at least 350 milligrams of potassium and less than 140 milligrams of sodium per serving (and must also be low in fat and cholesterol).

• Endurance exercise can deplete your body of electrolytes, but except under the most extreme circumstances, you don't need special sports drinks to replace them—your normal diet should suffice. In any case, sports drinks actually contain only small amounts of potassium.

• People who take diuretic medications used in treating heart disease or high blood pressure should have their blood levels of potassium monitored, since the use of diuretics can cause a loss of potassium.

where you can find it

Fruits and vegetables are excellent sources of potassium. Fish, beans, and nuts are also good sources.

selenium

Selenium is a trace mineral found in many foods. It was not demonstrated to be a necessary part of the human diet until 1979, but it has since became a "hot" mineral, with many claims made for its disease-fighting potential. As a result, many people now take it as part of an "antioxidant cocktail" along with vitamins C and E. Though none of selenium's purported benefits have been proven, scientists have been studying its possible protective effects—against cancer and heart disease and perhaps even rheumatoid arthritis and AIDS.

what it does

Selenium is used in an array of important compounds in the body. It is an integral part of glutathione peroxidase, an antioxidant enzyme present in all cells, works synergistically with vitamin E, and also helps regulate the body's use of vitamin C. In addition, selenium is needed for the proper functioning of the thyroid gland. A lack of

LEADING SOURCES	
SOURCE	**SELENIUM (MCG)**
Brazil nuts, 1 oz	839
Tuna, canned in water, 3 oz	69
Flounder, broiled, 3 oz	50
Shrimp, steamed, 3 oz	29
Turkey, light meat, roasted, 3 oz	27
Chicken breast, roasted, 3 oz	23
Rice, brown, cooked, 1 cup	19
Egg, 1 large	15
Wheat germ, 2 tbsp	11
Tortillas, flour, 1 medium	7
Milk, fat-free, 1 cup	5

selenium impairs the immune system, but high doses don't seem to improve immunity in healthy people.

Selenium deficiency is rare, except in regions of the world (notably China) where the selenium content of the soil is five to ten times lower than the lowest levels in the United States, and locally grown foods are the only ones consumed. Too little selenium may impair the immune system and reduce the ability of the body to neutralize toxic substances it is exposed to, such as certain drugs or chemicals in the environment.

Potential health benefits: As an antioxidant, selenium appears to play a key role in reducing the risk of some cancers—but the role is unclear.

A 1996 study showed that selenium supplements (200 micrograms per day) reduced the risk of three cancers—lung, colorectal, and prostate—by 45 to 63 percent. Another study, in the *Journal of the National Cancer Institute*, found that men who had consumed about 160 micrograms of selenium daily cut their risk of prostate cancer by about 65 percent, compared with those consuming about 85 micrograms a day.

There is also evidence that people living in areas of the world where the selenium content of the soil is high have lower risks of cancer of the lung, breast, and digestive tract. And benefits against all cancers were found when, in a clinical trial, people consumed selenium-enriched yeast fortified with vitamin E and beta carotene.

However, other studies have found no protective effect—and a few studies found that the mineral can increase the risk of some cancers. In addition, though the benefits of selenium supplements have been shown in people who are deficient, nobody is sure that supplemental selenium will do you any good if your diet is supplying adequate selenium. Yet it's difficult, if not impossible, to calculate how much selenium is in a given food—in part because selenium levels vary from one geographical region to another.

recommended levels

The RDA for women and men is 55 micrograms. A number of foods offer good sources of selenium.

Supplementation: Selenium supplements are not recommended. If you do take them, don't take more than 200 micrograms a day. Multivitamins offer anywhere from 20 to 200 micrograms.

Precautions: Selenium can be toxic at high doses. The highest daily intake considered safe is 400 micrograms. High levels of selenium can cause nausea, vomiting, hair loss, and tooth loss. Rather than protecting cells, too much selenium can damage them.

tips & facts

• Make whole grains part of your daily fare. They contain selenium as well as fiber, vitamins, and other minerals. Fish is an excellent source of selenium, so eat two or three servings weekly.

• Selenium comes in organic forms (such as that from yeast) and inorganic forms (including sodium selenite or selenate). The organic forms are better absorbed by the body, so if you want to take a supplement and can find a multivitamin/mineral pill containing organic selenium, that's preferable. There is no harm in taking inorganic selenium, however; it's certainly better than no selenium at all. But get as much selenium as you can from food.

• Vitamin E works with selenium and increases its effectiveness in the body. Since it's difficult to get the recommended levels of vitamin E from food, we advise taking a daily supplement of 200 to 400 IU (*see page 63*).

where you can find it

Selenium is found in Brazil nuts, meats, poultry, seafood, grains, and grain products. The amount of selenium in plant foods depends on the selenium content of the soil. The values in the "Leading Sources" chart (*page 81*) are provisional data from the United States Department of Agriculture.

sodium

Most people are familiar with sodium in the form of table salt—sodium chloride—which is about 40 percent sodium. Sodium is necessary for life, playing an essential role in the regulation of body fluids and blood pressure. But most Americans eat more salt than they need, largely because much of the sodium we consume—about 75 percent—doesn't come from the salt shaker, but has been added to processed foods, snacks, and fast foods to enhance their taste. Being aware of this "hidden sodium" is often the key to keeping your sodium consumption within recommended guidelines.

what it does

All cells in the body are bathed in a fluid that maintains cell function; the minerals in this fluid are 90 to 95 percent sodium salts. The quantity of sodium in these particles determines the fluid balance of the entire body. If the body is retaining more sodium, it must also retain more water to maintain the proper electrolyte ratio.

Many organs interact to regulate the amount of sodium in the body. The chief monitors are the kidneys, adrenal glands, heart, and brain. This regulatory system will conserve sodium if you need it and excrete it if you have an excess. Although your sodium intake may vary from day to day, the amount of sodium in your body generally does not vary by more than 2 percent. Eating too much salt triggers the body's thirst mechanism and encourages you to drink more fluids, and the regulatory system in the body will then increase urine production to help excrete the excess sodium.

Sodium and high blood pressure. Researchers aren't sure how, but a high sodium intake promotes high blood pressure (hypertension). In countries where salt intake is low, so is the rate of hypertension. A good deal of sound research has found that a diet containing more than 6 grams of salt a day—2,400 milligrams of sodium, a little more than 1 teaspoon of salt—is associated with high blood pressure. Some people who overuse salt won't end up with high blood pressure, but it's impossible to identify in advance the people who are sodium-sensitive—meaning that sodium raises their blood pressure. That's why recommendations for keeping sodium intake in check apply to everyone. In addition, even though you may not be sodium-sensitive at age 30 or 40, your sensitivity may increase as you get older. (Sodium sensitivity increases with age.)

Some evidence suggests that excessive sodium intake can also accelerate calcium excretion in the urine, thus contributing to osteoporosis. This loss could affect your bones even if you consume lots of calcium.

recommended levels

There is no RDA for sodium. The minimum amount you need for good health is only about 115 milligrams a day. To ensure an adequate intake, the National Academy of Sciences recommends consuming at least 500 milligrams daily—the amount in a scant quarter teaspoon. Considering that a single serving of many processed foods supplies twice that amount, meeting the minimum intake is hardly a problem for most people. Instead, focus on limiting sodium intake. People with high blood pressure or kidney disease may be advised to consume even less than 500 milligrams.

Because sodium is so abundant in the diet, and because the body's regulatory system is so efficient, sodium deficiencies are practically unheard of. However, severe vomiting or diarrhea, or profuse sweating may dramatically lower sodium levels. In such circumstances, the body can release a hormone called angiotensin, which promotes sodium retention in the body. But sodium levels can rapidly fall dangerously low under conditions of extreme sweating if fluid is not adequately replaced.

tips & facts

• It's not all that difficult to reduce your daily sodium intake. Read food labels. Ask for less salt when eating out. Avoid or at least limit fast foods, canned soups, chips, salted nuts, and other salty snacks—most of which are high in fat as well as salt. And you don't have to throw out the salt shaker: A light shake of salt on a ripe tomato or other favorite food supplies only a tiny amount of sodium.

LEADING SOURCES

SOURCE	SODIUM (MG)
LOW SODIUM	
Coffee, 8 fl oz	1
Fruit juice, 8 fl oz	2-10
Fruit, 1 fruit or 1 cup	1-5
Tea, 8 fl oz	5
Broccoli, ½ cup	8
Tomato, fresh, 1	14
Soft drink, 8 fl oz	10-60
Egg, 1	69
Beef, pork, lamb, poultry, fish (fresh), cooked, 3 oz	60-100
MEDIUM SODIUM	
Clams, steamed, 3 oz	95
Butter, salted, 1 tsp	115
Margarine, 1 tsp	115
Milk, whole, 8 fl oz	120
Cake, 2 oz	150-400
Ketchup, 1 tsp	180
Bread, 2 slices	200-600
HIGH SODIUM	
Yellow mustard, 1 tsp	188
Potato chips, 1 oz	250
Cheese, cheddar, 1½ oz	300
Tuna, canned, 3 oz	250-500
Lobster, steamed, 3 oz	326
Olives, black, 2 oz	385
Ham, cured, 2 oz	400-800
Cheese, cottage, ½ cup	425
Pancakes, 3 prepared	400-800
Soy sauce, 1 tsp	420
Parmesan, 1 oz	528
Frankfurter, 1	450
Chicken broth, ½ cup	500
Roll, crescent, 2 oz	500
Tomato juice, canned, 6 oz	500
Pizza, 1 slice	500-1,000
Cheese, American, 1½ oz	600
Pickle, dill, 2 oz	700
Hamburger, 1 prepared (Big Mac, Whopper)	1,000
Spaghetti and meatballs, canned, 7½ oz	1,000
Soup, canned, 10 oz	1,000-1,500
TV dinner, 11 oz	1,000-2,000

• Cravings for salt are not primarily based on a physiological need for more sodium. Instead, people who eat a lot of salty foods crave salt because their systems are used to it. The cycle can be broken with relative ease. If you gradually cut back on salt, in a few weeks you'll be surprised at how good food can taste when it isn't oversalted—and also surprised at how quickly heavily salted foods lose their appeal.

• Sodium comes in forms other than table salt. A few of the common sources of sodium found in foods include: baking powder, baking soda, monosodium glutamate (MSG), sodium citrate, sodium nitrate, sodium phosphate, sodium saccharin. In addition, the following flavorings are high in sodium: brine (as for pickles), soy sauce, ketchup, garlic and onion salt, kelp, and sea salt.

• On packaged foods, note that unsalted does not mean sodium-free, but that no salt was added to the product. Such foods may still be naturally high in sodium. The lowest-sodium foods will be labeled "very low sodium" (35 milligrams or less per serving) or "sodium-free" (less than 5 milligrams per serving). Those labeled "low sodium" have 140 milligrams or less per serving; "reduced- sodium" on a label indicates the product has at least 25 percent less sodium than the regular version.

• Reduce the sodium content of canned vegetables, beans, and water-pack tuna by draining the liquid and rinsing the food under cold running water before using.

• Bottled water may be high in sodium, especially mineral water, sparkling water, and club soda. Seltzer is generally sodium-free. Check nutrition labels.

where you can find it

Fresh or unprocessed fruit, vegetables, meats, and eggs are generally low in sodium. Many packaged and canned foods are high in sodium, since it is added during processing, as are condiments, cheese, and fast foods. The chart (*oppostie page*) shows the sodium content of common food products.

zinc

Zinc is essential for proper sexual maturation and the manufacture of testosterone, and since it is plentiful in oysters, this might be why oysters have a reputation as an aphrodisiac. But megadoses of zinc (or of oysters, for that matter) do not actually have any effect on libido or sexual prowess. Still, zinc is a remarkable nutrient. It is present in all the body's tissues and is involved in over 100 enzymatic reactions.

LEADING SOURCES	
SOURCE	**ZINC (MG)**
Oysters, steamed, 3 oz	30
Crab, Alaska king, steamed, 3 oz	6.5
Turkey, dark meat, roasted, 3 oz	3.9
Pork loin, roasted and trimmed, 3 oz	2.1
Wheat germ, 2 tbsp	1.8
Tofu, 4 oz	1.7
Cashews, dry-roasted, 1 oz	1.6
Swordfish, broiled, 3 oz	1.3
Sardines, cooked, 3 oz	1.2
Rice, brown, cooked, 1 cup	1.1

what it does

It's been known for over a century that zinc is essential for health in both animals and plants. In humans, zinc is a fundamental part of the enzymes that are used to regulate cell division, growth, wound healing, and proper functioning of the immune system. Male children severely deficient in zinc will not develop sexually, though no such cases have ever been reported in the United States. The mineral also plays a role in acuity of taste and smell. It is also involved in protein metabolism, particularly in the synthesis of collagen, and helps the body utilize vitamin A and insulin.

Severe zinc deficiency is most often found in the developing world, but mild deficiencies may also occur elsewhere in undernourished people and in those on strict vegan diets, which may not contain much zinc.

Because zinc is so widely dispersed in the body's tissues, a diagnosis of mild deficiency is difficult. Some experts suggest that it is more common than most people think, especially in children, adults on special diets, and the elderly. (Zinc absorption is not impaired by aging, but many older people may not consume enough zinc.) In infants and children, a zinc deficiency will inhibit growth and sexual maturation. Even mild deficiencies in children will dull the sense of taste, cause poor appetite, and result in suboptimal growth.

In both children and adults, a low intake can also contribute to an impaired sense of taste and smell, delayed wound healing, weakened immune function (particularly in the elderly), and skin problems (especially acne). In pregnant women, a zinc deficiency can result in low-birth-weight babies.

Potential health benefits: There are a number of benefits attributed to zinc, in particular that it can prevent prostate problems, prevent or cure colds, and help prevent eye disease.

Some evidence exists to support the last claim. Zinc may protect against age-related macular degeneration (a major cause of blindness in older adults), which is thought to result from damage to the retina by compounds known as free radicals. Zinc helps guard retinal tissue, and at least one study has suggested that people with high intakes of zinc from food have a lower risk for age-related macular degeneration. More studies are needed, but at this point it is too soon to recommend taking zinc supplements in the hope of preventing macular degeneration.

On the other hand, there is no evidence that zinc can prevent prostate problems or boost sexual performance. The prostate gland normally contains high concentrations of zinc, and it's true that a zinc deficiency can cause a drop in testosterone levels. But that doesn't mean that extra zinc will have any effect on your prostate or your potency.

As for colds, zinc lozenges are a popular alternative weapon against colds, but the evidence for them is mixed. A few studies have indicated that taking zinc soon after the onset of symptoms can help shorten the duration of a cold. But other studies have failed to show that zinc has any more effect than a placebo. There is no evidence that zinc will actually prevent a cold.

recommended levels

The RDA for women is 8 milligrams; for men, 11 milligrams. These levels can easily be reached on the semi-vegetarian diet recommended in this book—a diet that emphasizes fruits, vegetables, whole grains, and low-fat dairy products, plus small amounts of meat and fish.

Supplementation: Most people don't need zinc pills or lozenges, and there are drawbacks and dangers in zinc supplementation. As little as 18 to 25 milligrams of zinc per day, if taken for long periods, interferes with the absorption of copper. In addition, large doses can impair blood-cell formation and depress the immune system. Just 50 to 75 milligrams of zinc per day can reduce levels of HDL ("good") cholesterol. Nausea, vomiting, and diarrhea may also result from doses of 200 milligrams of zinc per day.

tips & facts

• Small amounts of zinc taken frequently are better absorbed than a single dose of the same total amount, so try to include good sources of zinc in every meal.

• Fiber and phytates (chemicals present in some grains, such as wheat) can interfere with zinc absorption. It is possible that people on a high-fiber diet might not get enough zinc, especially if they eat little or no meat.

• Taking calcium pills may interfere with zinc absorption, though there is no evidence this can lead to actual deficiency. If you take calcium supplements to help keep your bones strong, but consume little or no dietary zinc, you might need to take a multivitamin/mineral supplement containing zinc. Most multivitamin/mineral pills contain 100 percent of the RDA for zinc.

• Zinc may be able to ease cold symptoms for some people, but zinc takers in studies have reported nausea, mouth irritation, and a bad taste in the mouth among the adverse effects. You will have to decide for yourself whether it is worth risking these side effects to possibly shorten the duration of a cold. If you do try supplements, don't take them for more than five days.

where you can find it

Turkey, pork, shellfish (especially oysters), and some nuts are good sources of zinc. Whole grains also contain zinc, but the mineral is not as readily absorbed from them.

RECOMMENDED INTAKES FOR VITAMINS & MINERALS

The chart on this page features two sets of figures recently issued by the Food and Nutrition Board of the National Academy of Sciences to help people improve the nutritional quality of their diets.

Recommended Dietary Allowances (RDAs) are optimum levels of nutrients sufficient to prevent deficiency diseases and also promote good health in most of the population (*see page 32*). When too little data exists for a particular nutrient to set an RDA, the Food and Nutrition Board has set an Adequate Intake (AI).

Upper Levels (ULs), also called Tolerable Upper Intake Levels, are the highest amount of a vitamin or mineral that can be taken without any risk of an adverse effect to healthy individuals. For most nutrients, exceeding the ULs is possible only by taking dietary supplements or fortified foods. Some nutrients do not have a UL because no data exists to set a specific figure.

The figures listed are for adults only. Recommended intakes for pregnant and lactating women can differ and are not included here.

Vitamins	Recommended Dietary Allowance (RDA)**	Upper Level (UL)**
Biotin	30 mcg*	None established
Folate (Folic acid)	400 mcg	1,000 mcg (from supplements and fortified foods)
Niacin	Women: 14 mg Men: 16 mg	35 mg (from supplements and fortified foods)
Pantothenic acid	5 mg*	None established
Riboflavin	Women: 1.1 mg Men: 1.3 mg	None established
Thiamin	Women: 1.1 mg Men: 1.2 mg	None established
Vitamin A	Women: 700 mcg Men: 900 mcg	10,000 IU (3,000 mcg)
Vitamin B_6	Women to age 50: 1.3 mg Women over 50: 1.5 mg Men to age 50: 1.3 mg Men over 50: 1.7 mg	100 mg
Vitamin B_{12}	2.4 mcg	None established
Vitamin C	Women: 75 mg Men: 90 mg	2,000 mg
Vitamin D	To age 50: 200 IU Ages 51-70: 400 IU Over 70: 600 IU	2,000 IU
Vitamin E	15 mg	1,000 mg (1,000 IU synthetic, 1,500 IU natural)
Vitamin K	Women: 90 mcg* Men: 120 mcg*	None established
Minerals		
Calcium	To age 50: 1,000 mg* Over 50: 1,200 mg*	2,500 mg

*Adequate Intake (AI) **RDA and UL values are for adults only

Minerals	RDA**	UL**
Chromium	Women to age 50: 25 mcg* Women over 50: 20 mcg* Men to age 50: 35 mcg* Men over 50: 30 mcg*	None established
Copper	900 mcg	10 mg
Iodine	150 mcg	1.1 mg
Iron	Women to age 50: 18 mg Women over 50: 8 mg Men: 8 mg	45 mg
Magnesium	Women to age 30: 310 mg Women over 30: 320 mg Men to age 30: 400 mg Men over 30: 420 mg	350 mg
Manganese	Women: 1.8 mg* Men: 2.3 mg*	11 mg
Molybdenum	45 mcg	2 mg
Phosphorus	700 mg	Up to age 70: 4,000 mg After age 70: 3,000 mg
Selenium	55 mcg	400 mcg
Zinc	Women: 8 mg Men: 11 mg	40 mg

Other Recommended Intakes

For a few nutrients, existing evidence isn't sufficient to establish a requirement. The guidelines listed below are based on guidelines established by various health organizations and experts, including the Food and Nutrition Board.

Carotenoids

There is no established daily intake for carotenoids. Some carotenoids are converted by the body into vitamin A; you can meet the RDA for vitamin A by consuming 11 milligrams of beta carotene a day. No specific group of carotenoids can be singled out for providing disease prevention benefits. The Food and Nutrition Board advises eating more carotenoid-rich fruits and vegetables. Don't take beta carotene supplements. Smokers in particular should avoid high doses of beta carotene, which are associated with an increased risk of lung cancer.

Potassium

Nutritionists generally recommend that adults consume 3,000 milligrams of potassium per day.

Sodium

Try to limit daily intake to 2,400 milligrams.

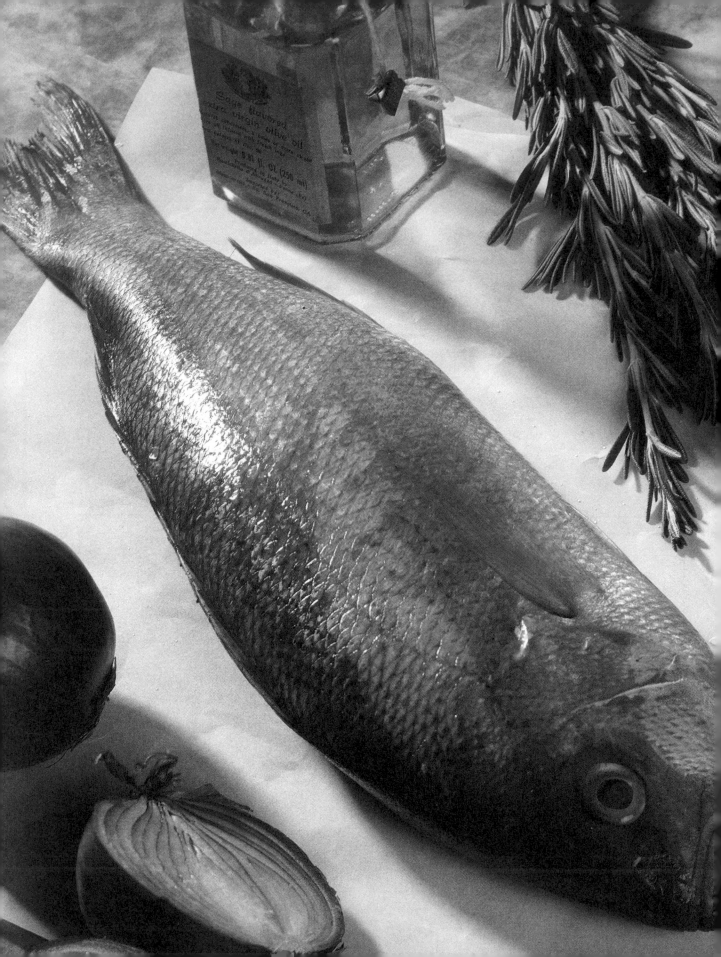

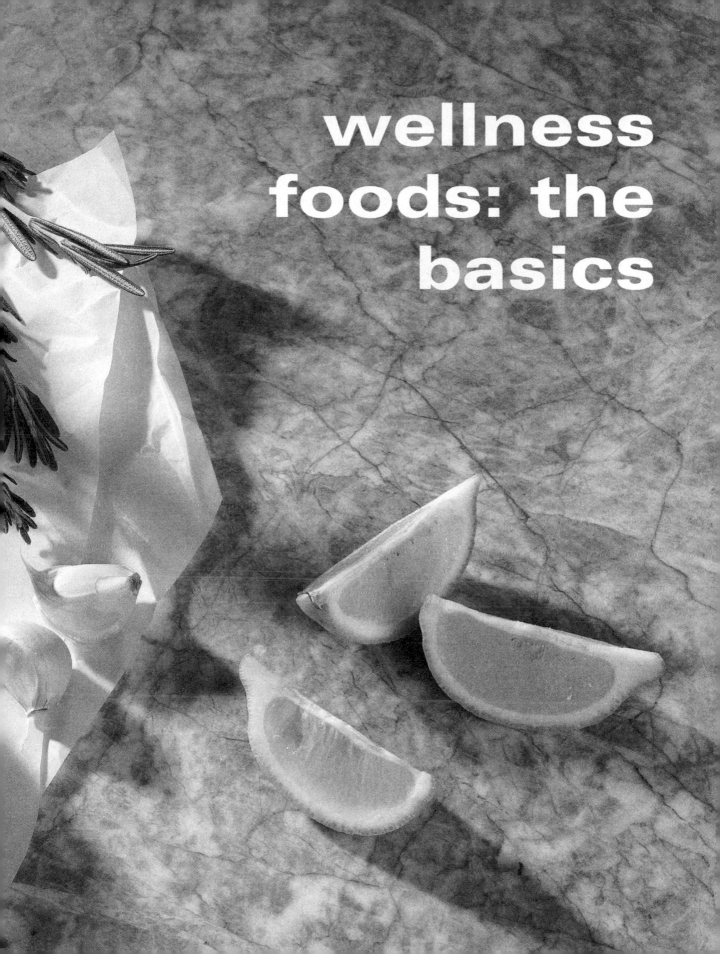

wellness foods: the basics

vegetables

If the key to good nutrition is consuming a variety of foods, then vegetables can truly stand as the cornerstone of a healthy diet. Of all foods, they offer the most diversity: There are literally hundreds of varieties available to us, and because of careful plant breeding, today's vegetable harvest is continually being expanded and improved. In addition, vegetables are replete with nutrients. They supply nearly all of the vitamins and minerals required for good health, and many of them—especially starchy vegetables like potatoes and winter squash—contain complex carbohydrates, which furnish us with energy. Most also provide dietary fiber, and a few, such as legumes (dried beans, peas, and lentils) can also contribute to your protein intake. At the same time, vegetables contain no cholesterol, have little or no fat, and are low in calories. (Even half a cup of boiled potatoes or squash contains fewer calories than a tablespoon of butter.) In nutritional parlance, vegetables are "nutrient dense"—that is, their store of nutrients is relatively high for the number of calories they supply. When you consider how inexpensive most vegetables are compared to meats and other animal foods, you really are getting the most out of the calories you consume when you emphasize vegetables in your diet.

out of favor, in favor

With such diversity of choice, it's nearly impossible for anyone to say categorically, "I don't like vegetables." Along with an impressive range of sizes and shapes, vegetables offer a rich mix of colors—among them green, yellow, orange, red, white, and purple in dozens of shades—and a correspondingly wide array of flavors and textures. Moreover, most vegetables are easy to prepare, and can be eaten raw or cooked. Yet in the United States, vegetables have typically been served as accompaniments to meat or fish, rather than as equal partners or as the main course (as they are in Asian and Middle Eastern cuisine, for example). According to the U.S. Department of Agriculture, the average American eats about 4.4 servings of fruits and vegetables a day, which reflects a steady improvement in Americans' food choices compared with 3.9 servings of fruit and vegetables per day in 1991. While food consumption surveys coordinated by the U.S. Department of Agriculture (USDA) and National Cancer Institute (NCI) show that Americans are motivated by the health benefits of eating fruits and vegetables, not everyone is eating even five servings a day.

Furthermore, the vegetables that Americans favor are, as often as not, among the lowest in vitamins and minerals: The top six most popular vegetables include iceberg lettuce, cucumbers, and celery, which are very low in nutrients.

Per capita vegetable consumption statistics include vegetables in all forms, including processed foods, such as frozen French fries. So even if vegetable consumption is at 4.4 servings, this does not translate to consumption of fresh vegetables. Following several decades during which per capita consumption of fresh vegetables declined, there has been a steady increase, though not a dramatic one. Excluding potatoes, which are in significantly greater demand than any other vegetable, consumption of fresh vegetables has increased modestly from 1970 to 1995. The biggest gains were for broccoli, bell peppers, carrots, and tomatoes.

There has also been increased interest in new or unusual vegetables. Some are familiar foods in different guises—white eggplants or baby squash, for example. Other "new" vegetables have been around for some time and are simply being rediscovered by imaginative cooks—beet greens and kale, to mention two traditional Southern favorites, or bok choy and daikon radish, which were once found only in Asian markets and are now available at corner greengrocers and in many supermarkets.

types of vegetables & their nutrients

Most of the vegetables that we eat today are descended from ancient wild plants that were domesticated centuries ago and have been widely cultivated over the last few hundred years. There are several ways to classify vegetables, but two of the most basic are by their botanical families, or by which part of the plant is eaten—the root, stalk, or leaves, for example. Although the botanical designation of a vegetable is sometimes useful, it doesn't determine the vegetable's nutrient content. That depends largely on what part of the plant it comes from.

Leafy vegetables—including spinach, salad greens, collards, kale, radicchio, and watercress—may grow in tight or loose heads or individually on stems; a few leafy greens, like turnips and beets, are actually the tops of root vegetables. Lettuces and other salad greens are nearly always served raw, while sturdier, more flavorful greens, like kale, are generally cooked. Some greens can be eaten either way. All leaves contain lots of water and few carbohydrates (or calories). Most green leaves are rich in beta carotene and other carotenoids and vitamin C, and are good sources of fiber and folate (a B vitamin). They also supply varying quantities of iron and calcium.

Flowers, buds, and stalks range from the ordinary, such as celery, broccoli, and cauliflower, to some of the aristocrats of the vegetable kingdom—asparagus and artichokes, for example. These plants tend to be rich in vitamin C, calcium, and potassium, as well as dietary fiber. Cauliflower and broccoli also offer cancer-fighting compounds. Their mild to slightly sweet flavors are appealing alone, or with a range of sauces or other accompaniments.

Seeds and pods are the parts of plants that store energy. Snap beans, lima beans, peas, and sweet corn have more protein than other vegetables, and also contain more carbohydrates than do leafy, stalk, or flower vegetables. When the vegetables are immature (and freshly picked), the carbohydrates are in the form of sugars; with time—on the plant or after harvesting—these sugars turn to starch. The B vitamins and the minerals zinc, potassium, magnesium, calcium, and iron are also nutritional bonuses for these foods.

Roots, bulbs, and tubers grow underground and act as nutrient storehouses. Onions, turnips, potatoes, beets, carrots, radishes, and parsnips are sturdy and dense, making them satisfying foods. Interestingly, however, in some cases—such as beets and onions—the tops of the plant (beet greens and scallions) are richer in vitamins and minerals than the roots or bulbs. Because of their high starch content, some of these vegetables are higher in calories than most of their aboveground counterparts. And some of them can also act more like simple sugars, which means that they can trigger rapid rises in blood sugar and insulin. But the foods in this group make various valuable nutritional contributions: Potatoes are good sources of vitamin C and potassium; both sweet potatoes and carrots contain abundant amounts of beta carotene; radishes and turnips are good sources of fiber and vitamin C; and a number of studies suggest that onions and garlic may lower blood pressure and cholesterol levels.

Fruit vegetables, which include eggplants, squash, peppers, and tomatoes, are the pulpy, seed-bearing bodies of the plants on which they grow. Technically speaking, these are fruits rather than vegetables (because the fleshy part of the plant contains seeds), but we use them like vegetables and refer to them as such. Generally higher in calories than leafy vegetables, stalks, or flowers, they tend to be good sources of vitamin C. These vegetables also offer myriad flavors and textures, and so are useful as seasonings and accents (think of tomato paste or chili sauce), as well as staple foods.

Color is a good clue to nutrient content. Most yellow and orange vegetables, such as carrots, winter squash, or sweet potatoes, get their color from beta carotene and other carotenoids, which are precursors to vitamin A. Dark-green leafy vegetables also contain carotenoids (as well as the pigment chlorophyll, which gives them their green color). The more intense a vegetable's green or orange color, the more beta carotene it contains.

cruciferae—the disease fighters

One group of vegetables has received a great deal of attention from researchers for its role in disease prevention. Named after the Latin word for "cross," because they bear cross-shaped flowers, cruciferous vegetables include cabbage and close relatives such as broccoli, Brussels sprouts, cauliflower, kale, and collards, as well as mustard greens, rutabagas, and turnips. All are part of a botanical genus known as *Brassica*. Studies of cruciferous vegetables have shown that they contain nitrogen compounds called indoles, which appear to be effective in protecting against certain forms of cancer, particularly cancers of the stomach and large intestine. More recent research has revealed other promising anticancer compounds in these vegetables: Some of them seem to stimulate the release of anticancer enzymes, while antioxidant nutrients—such as carotenoids and vitamin C—help to sweep up cancer-promoting unstable oxygen molecules known as free radicals. In addition, most cruciferous vegetables are good sources of dietary fiber. A few—chiefly kale, collard greens, and turnip greens—also supply calcium, while others such as Brussels sprouts provide iron.

available year round

At one time the vegetables consumers bought were grown on local farms (or came from the family garden), but today the major vegetable crops are part of the vast American industry called "agribusiness," which began developing after World War II. Advances in agricultural and food-handling technology created a movement toward large-volume production. Small farmers expanded their land holdings if they could, or entered into cooperative marketing ventures with other farms. As a result, farm acreage increased tremendously in warm-weather states, such as California, New Mexico, Arizona, Texas, and Florida, which now produce the bulk of the domestic vegetable crop. Growers in these states, aided by machinery at nearly every stage of cultivation, can harvest a steady, year-round stream of vegetables, which are then dispatched in refrigerated train cars and trucks to food brokers and wholesalers nationwide. Consequently, consumers are never limited to seasonal foods from their own locality. These domestic supplies are supplemented by crops grown in the southern hemisphere, to fill in where North American crops leave off.

Greater availability, however, has come at a price. Mechanized growing and handling methods, combined with the rigors of long-distance shipping, have prompted large-scale commercial growers to emphasize hardiness over flavor and texture in developing many vegetable varieties. Vegetables displayed in supermarkets often appear fresh and sturdy, and are of a uniform size, but they probably don't equal the taste of produce grown locally. An appreciation for flavor and freshness on the part of consumers has prompted a resurgence of small farms that send their harvests to greenmarkets in nearby cities, allowing urbanites to take advantage of local crops. Residents of suburbs and small towns can often buy local vegetables at roadside farmstands, directly at the farms, or in urban farmers' markets. And, more and more, Americans are growing their own vegetables, which offers greater opportunity to cultivate flavorful varieties, pick vegetables as soon as they're ripe, and cook them almost immediately.

If you have access to local sources of produce, by all means take advantage of them. But remember that most vegetables sold in supermarkets have perfectly adequate flavor and nutritional quality, and will probably be very good if they have been properly shipped and handled. Even vegetables transported a thousand miles and left in bins for a day or two are full of nutrients. It's important, however, to be able to distinguish between such vegetables and those that may have lost half of their vitamins and their flavor because of careless storage and display. The shopping and storage guidelines in the Foods A to Z section should help you in your selection.

fresh, frozen, or canned

If vegetables are truly farm fresh—harvested the same day you serve them—they will offer maximum nutritional value. To get the most from fresh vegetables, shop frequently and use them as soon as possible. Some types of vegetables, however, if stored incorrectly (or for too long), will lose a significant amount of their nutrients. If produce looks or feels wilted and pallid, or if you have inadvertently allowed the green beans to sit in the refrigerator for a week, you'll be better off purchasing and eating the frozen or even the canned version.

In general, frozen vegetables are preferable to canned. Once vegetables are harvested, a loss of nutrients starts to occur. But if the vegetables are flash-frozen soon after picking, they retain most of their nutrients, except for small amounts of vitamin C and other water-soluble vitamins. However, their texture probably won't be equal to that of well-prepared fresh vegetables, and they may suffer further nutrient loss if improperly stored or overcooked.

Canned vegetables, on the other hand, undergo a heating process that can destroy some of the vitamin C and B vitamins. Minerals aren't destroyed, but they may be lost if the canning liquid is not saved and used. In addition, large amounts of sodium are often added during processing. Though they have enough nutrients to be worth eating if nothing else is available, most canned vegetables lack the flavor and texture of produce that is fresh or frozen.

pesticides & waxes

Pesticides and other "agrichemicals" kill insects that can damage crops, thus helping to ensure the huge volume and variety of vegetables in the market today. These chemicals have been accepted for years as a necessity of modern farming, but now they are being perceived as, perhaps, an unnecessary evil—a health risk that might not outweigh the advantages gained from eating fresh vegetables. The residues of scores of these compounds remain on the food we eat, while their toxic effects remain in question.

While the Environmental Protection Agency registers pesticides for food use and sets tolerance levels—the upper permitted limit for pesticide residues in individual foods—the Food and Drug Administration (FDA) enforces these limits for all foods except for meat and poultry, which fall under the USDA's jurisdiction. The FDA collects and analyzes thousands of samples of fruits and vegetables yearly for pesticide residues. Most of the domestic and imported fruits and vegetables in the United States are found to be free of illegal pesticide residues or have low-level residues that fall within established tolerances. Though some scientists believe that the FDA's acceptable levels are, in fact, too high, the FDA believes the benefits of eating fresh produce far exceed any risk from low levels of residues.

Associated with the use of pesticides is the practice of waxing certain vegetables before sending them to market. Wax coatings keep food fresh and bright looking; they also slow moisture loss and thus extend shelf life. But waxes also seal in pesticide and fungicide residues (sometimes the chemicals are combined with the wax). Washing or scrubbing removes some, but not all, of these surface chemicals; the only way to completely remove them is by peeling the skin, which means discarding the portion richest in fiber and some nutrients. Vegetables that are commonly waxed include rutabagas, cucumbers, squash, and tomatoes. Sometimes, as with rutabagas and cucumbers, the layer of wax is visible on the surface—you can scrape some off with your thumbnail. The FDA requires retailers to post signs identifying waxed produce (and the type of wax used), but few comply with the regulation.

protective steps

Despite the gaps in current research, enough evidence of toxicity in these residues has been gathered to justify concern. Fortunately, there are a number of sensible measures you can adopt.

• Try to buy fresh vegetables in season. When prolonged storage and long-distance shipping are not required, there's less need for antispoilage chemicals.

• Wash vegetables carefully. Many water-soluble residues rinse away with thorough washing. Peel vegetables with wax coatings, which washing does not remove. If you're not sure whether a vegetable has been waxed or not, check with the produce manager.

• Trim away tops and the very outer leaves from celery, lettuces, cabbages, and other leafy vegetables, which may contain the bulk of a vegetable's toxic residues. Be sure to wash the inner leaves.

• To avoid chemical residues in vegetables as much as possible, you can buy organic produce, which is available not only in health-food stores, but also in some farmers' markets and big-city supermarkets. "Organic" means that the food has been grown without chemical fertilizers or pesticides. Though there is a new federal definition for organic, and foods whose labels claim to be organic must be certified as such by the USDA, small-scale purveyors and farmers are exempt from this stricture. Check with produce sellers to ascertain that you are actually getting organically grown vegetables; be aware, though, that they may not really know for certain.

fruits

Most people like fruit—contrary to the nutritional myth that says anything fun to eat can't be good for you. There are two traits shared by most fruits that make them so appealing: They taste sweet, yet are relatively low in calories. Not only do fruits make excellent snack foods and desserts, they also add sweetness (along with vitamins and minerals) to prepared dishes. A combination of sugars—fructose, glucose, and sucrose—are present in fruits in varying proportions. Fructose is often considered the principal fruit sugar, and it is the sweetest; but sucrose is the main sugar in some fruit, such as oranges, melons, and peaches. What keeps the calorie content of fruit low is water, which makes up 80 to 95 percent of most fruits and gives them their refreshing juiciness.

Fiber is another benefit that fruits provide. The characteristic textures of different fruits—the crispness of apples, the graininess of certain pears, the chewiness of dates and figs—are partly due to insoluble fibers. In most fruits, particularly apples and citrus fruits, some of the fiber takes the form of pectin, the soluble fiber that may help lower cholesterol levels and stabilize blood sugar. With few exceptions—most notably avocados—fruits are nearly free of fat, and they contain no cholesterol.

Fruits supply some minerals—among them potassium (in bananas, pears, and oranges, three of the most popular fruits), iron (in various berries and dried fruits), and even small amounts of calcium and magnesium. But the chief contribution fruits make to our diet is vitamins, particularly vitamin C and beta carotene, the precursor of vitamin A. Citrus fruits, berries, and melons are all good sources of vitamin C, as are a number of tropical fruits, such as kiwifruit and papaya. Yellow and orange fruits like apricots, cantaloupes, peaches, nectarines, and mangoes are the best sources of beta carotene.

Modern methods for harvesting, shipping, and storing fruit have made these fresh foods more widely available than ever. At the same time, fruits are often picked before they are ripe, and may be offered for sale when they are not at their best. Some fruits are bred more for appearance and their ability to ship and store well than for flavor.

types of fruits

All fruits develop from a plant's flower—actually from the ovary, the flower's female tissue. Most fruits are simply the matured and thickened ovary, including its seeds, though in many instances the ovary is surrounded by a fleshy layer of adjacent tissue—the fruit's pulp—and enclosed by a protective skin. Beyond this basic arrangement, of course, there are enormous differences in the structure of various fruits: Just think of a pineapple compared to a raspberry. Moreover, some plants—such as tomatoes and peppers—are technically fruits that we treat as vegetables, while others—rhubarb, for example—are botanically classified as vegetables but used as fruits. Indeed, fruits are so diverse that they don't all fit neatly into categories, botanical or otherwise. However, it is possible to loosely organize the most familiar fruits based on some of their shared characteristics.

Apples and pears, which are known botanically as pomes, have firm, moist flesh surrounding a central seedy core. Though not especially high in vitamins, they rank as some of the best sources of dietary fiber.

Apricots, peaches, nectarines, and **plums** are drupes, or fruits with a single stone or pit. Sweet, juicy, and comparatively fragile, they supply both beta carotene and vitamin C, along with some potassium and fiber. Cherries are also drupes, but with fewer nutrients per ounce than their larger cousins.

Berries have seeds embedded in succulent layers of flesh. As a botanical group, they embrace a wide range of fruits, from dates to grapes (as well as eggplants, peppers, and tomatoes). But the plants we conventionally think of as berries are small, juicy rounded fruits that range in taste from sweet to sour. Berries supply varying amounts of vitamin C, and many are a surprisingly good source of fiber.

Citrus fruits—oranges, tangerines, grapefruit, lemons, and limes—are multisectioned, warm-weather fruits best known for their vitamin C content. Oranges and grapefruit also provide fair amounts of dietary fiber.

Melons are usually divided into two classes, watermelons and muskmelons (which include cantaloupe, honeydew, casaba, and many others). Vitamin C is the principal nutrient supplied by these exceptionally juicy fruits, though orange-fleshed melons provide beta carotene as well.

Many other fruits don't lend themselves to simple classification. Bananas, for example, are botanically lumped with berries, but are distinct in shape and texture. A papaya, too, is a berry, though it can weigh up to 10 pounds. Pineapples are multiple fruits; each one develops from dozens of separate flowers that are discernible as "eyes" on the rough skin and yellow flesh. And many tropical fruits, from mangoes and avocados to some of the truly exotic examples, are singular varieties that boast unique flavors and textures.

ripening & freshness

With many vegetables, "ripeness" often means they are beyond the point of freshness (summer squash, lettuce, and cucumbers, for example, are not palatable if truly ripe). With fruits, on the other hand, ripeness is the key to enjoying them. As most fruits reach the final stage of maturity, several important changes occur that make them delectable as well as nutritious. The fruit softens, its color changes, the vitamin content increases, acidic content decreases, and the starch changes to sugar, giving the fruit a mild, sweet flavor and aroma. These changes are brought about by various enzymes that can continue to act on the fruit even after harvesting—though the degree of ripening depends on the particular fruit. Melons and citrus fruits, for example, won't get any sweeter after they are picked, while bananas and peaches ripen very nicely after picking. Still other fruits, such as avocados and pears, must be picked before they can begin to ripen. If the ripening action of the enzymes continues for too long, however, the fruit decays: Flavor and texture deteriorate, the flesh turns brown, and the vitamin content drops.

In order to withstand the rigors of shipping and distribution, many fruits are harvested while still in a firm, underripe stage. Some fruits are then allowed to ripen on their own in storage, but others are treated with ethylene gas. Fruits give off this gas during normal ripening, and for many years growers and distributors have introduced ethylene gas into storage rooms to speed up the ripening of certain fruits, reducing the time by as much as 50 percent. Ethylene can stimulate pigment change in a fruit—bringing out the yellow in bananas or the golden-brown in pineapples—and will help soften and sweeten firm tropical fruits as well as certain varieties of apples and pears that need to be ripened quickly to meet market demand. Ethylene is completely safe, and it does not affect a fruit's vitamin content. By the time you buy the fruit, all traces of the gas are gone.

Cold temperatures can slow the ripening process and also stave off the growth of microbes, the other principal cause of fruit spoilage. Some fruits are held after harvesting in controlled atmosphere (CA) storage, in which oxygen levels are significantly reduced, a change that greatly prolongs the life of the fruit. CA storage, combined with modern shipping methods, makes apples, pears, and citrus fruits available all year. Other fresh fruits, particularly berries and many tropical fruits, are seasonal and cannot extend their seasons with CA storage. However, between staggered plantings and imports, almost all fruits are available year round.

canned & frozen

Canning is the most common way to preserve whole fruits, making them reliably available out of season. A few fruits, most notably berries and cherries, are frozen. Most frozen fruits are processed without cooking, and so there is little if any nutrient loss. Canned fruits, on the other hand, lose varying amounts of vitamin C and beta carotene. However, the vitamin loss is not as substantial as it is with vegetables (because fruits are processed at lower temperatures). In addition, people usually consume the juices that are canned along with the fruit, so the nutrients dissolved in them aren't really lost. It is true that canned fruits are often packed in heavy syrup, which can more than double the calories. (For example, a cup of raw sliced peaches has 75 calories, as compared to 190 when the slices are canned and packed in syrup.) Fortunately, canned fruits are also available packed in unsweetened juice, where the nutrients are retained, and the caloric increase is far smaller (a cup of juice-packed peaches has only 110 calories).

dried fruits

Another way to preserve fruit is by drying, either in the sun or with heated air. This process turns such fruits as apples, apricots, bananas, dates, figs, grapes (raisins), peaches, pineapples, and plums (prunes) into concentrated packages of nutrients. Drying reduces the fruit's water content, usually from about 80 percent to between 15 and 25 percent. Consequently, the proportion of minerals and vitamins is substantially increased—especially iron, copper, potassium, and beta carotene (though vitamin C is sometimes lost). Dried fruit is also a compact source of dietary fiber. The catch is that drying also concentrates the sugars and calories, so that, in return for the high vitamin and mineral content, you are getting a snack food that can sometimes be as as calorie-laden as many kinds of cookies.

Some light-colored dried fruits—apples, peaches, pears, apricots, and golden raisins—have sulfite preservatives added to them to keep them from turning brown; this treatment also helps minimize any loss of vitamin C and beta carotene. But these preservatives can produce allergic reactions, sometimes severe ones, in certain people, especially asthmatics. Manufacturers are required to list the preservatives—usually sulfur dioxide—clearly on packages, shipping containers, and bulk bins. Sulfite-sensitive people should be sure to check labels. Fortunately, there are some sulfite-free, light-colored fruits available, usually labeled as such.

juices

The next best thing to whole fruits is their juice, in which most of their nutrients are retained, though not the fiber. All citrus juices are high in vitamin C, containing almost 100 percent of the RDA in an 8-ounce glass. Potassium is also abundant in nearly all fruit juices. Fresh-squeezed juice usually has the highest vitamin C content, followed by canned or frozen (which retain their vitamin C for months). Since vitamin C deteriorates when in contact with oxygen, chilled cartons and refrigerated mini-boxes, which are permeable to air, retain the least vitamin C. If the "sell by" date on a juice carton is close or has passed, there may be significant loss of vitamin C— and of flavor. To protect the vitamin C from air, keep all juices refrigerated in tightly closed glass containers.

When buying juice, watch the wording on labels. Beverages labeled "juice" must be 100 percent juice, but "juice blends," fruit "punches" or "drinks," and "juice cocktails" usually contain little fruit juice—the rest being water and sugar. In some cases, these products cost more than real juice, so you're paying a lot for water. If you want diluted fruit juice, you're better off mixing real juice with water or seltzer. And remember to buy only pasteurized cider and juices. There have been outbreaks of food poisoning from unpasteurized juices.

legumes, nuts & seeds

D ried beans, peas, and lentils are collectively called legumes, and the dried fruits that constitute nuts, are all storehouses of concentrated nutrients, especially protein—in fact, they have more protein than any other vegetable food. Although the protein is incomplete (being deficient in one or more amino acids), this problem is easily overcome when they are served with complementary foods, such as grains. Their rich nutritional endowment can be attributed to the fact that legumes and nuts are seeds; that is, they contain within their small pods or shells the means to reproduce themselves, along with enough nutrients to sustain the new plants until they can draw nutrients from the soil.

These three foods, however, have very different roles to play in a healthful diet. Nuts are a nourishing snack food with one significant drawback—they are very high in fat, as are most other seeds. Hence, their contribution to a diet should be a modest one. Legumes, on the other hand, are low in fat, inexpensive, and versatile (they can be used in a variety of interesting dishes). Consequently, they deserve to be a culinary mainstay. For years, many Americans have shied away from legumes, in the belief that they have no value other than as starchy "fillers," or that they cause gas, or that they take too long to prepare. But more and more people have begun to sample these pod-borne vegetables, and they are discovering that any problems associated with legumes are either untrue or exaggerated—and that this food, which was once looked down upon as "poor man's meat," is actually an ideal alternative to meat and other fatty sources of protein.

Although nuts and legumes are technically seeds, there is also a category of foodstuffs actually called seeds. These, too, are the storehouses of energy for future plants, and as such are nutrient-rich and high in fat. The difference with these seeds, is that we tend to eat them in smaller amounts, though they bring with them some outstanding health benefits. Examples of these so-called edible seeds are flaxseeds, pumpkin seeds, sunflower seeds, sesame seeds, and poppy seeds. There are also quite a few seeds we eat in even smaller quantities; these are the flavorful seeds we use as spices.

grains

In most countries of the world, grains and grain products—flour, bread, cereal, and pasta—are the chief forms of sustenance. They provide about 50 percent of the world's calories and indirectly contribute much of the other half, since grains are also fed to the animals from which we get meat, eggs, and dairy products. Any number of national dishes—for example, the polenta and pasta of Italy, the kasha of Russia, the couscous of North Africa, the tabbouleh of Lebanon—are made from local grains that have been cooked and then served as a main dish, either on their own or in combination with seasonings or other foods.

Grains are among the best sources of complex carbohydrates, and health professionals and nutritionists recommend that 55 to 60 percent of our calorie intake should come from carbohydrates, which is why grain foods, such as bread, cereal, pasta, and rice, make up the largest part of the food guide pyramid. Yet despite the advice to increase complex carbohydrates in the diet, Americans still fall two servings shy of the USDA's recommended six to 11 daily servings of grains or grain products. The USDA's Healthy Eating Index reports that fewer than one in 10 Americans eats the recommended number of grain food servings a day. Studies also show a yearly increase in the consumption of highly refined, low-fiber grain products such as bagels and pretzels.

While the United States is one of the largest producers of grains, more than half of it is used for animal feed. By comparison, in countries such as Japan, India, and China, grains (mainly rice) provide about 65 percent of the calories eaten, and in less-developed countries, 80 to 85 percent.

grains in the american diet

Economic conditions are primarily responsible for differences in levels of grain consumption. As a country becomes wealthier, its population can afford to use more of its grain for feeding livestock to provide meat; poorer countries, on the other hand, are almost totally dependent upon their crops to feed people. (The amount of land required for raising enough beef to feed one person can yield enough wheat to feed 15 people or enough rice to nourish 24.) This inverse relationship is evident in our own recent past. In 1910, when the average American had fewer material resources, per capita consumption of wheat flour was about 210 pounds. The rate steadily declined as the nation grew wealthier, reaching a low in the early 1970s of about 110 pounds of wheat flour per person. During that same period, meat consumption increased to 170 pounds per person.

Affluent countries also rely more and more on convenience foods. In the case of grain products, many of these are now heavily refined—that is, they have been processed to remove their outer layers, making them easier to chew and quicker to cook. The parts that are discarded, however, contain most of the fiber, B vitamins, and trace minerals found in the whole grain, along with a fair amount of protein. Today, most refined grains are "enriched" with the addition of key nutrients, but this process does not replace all of what has been lost. Moreover, many grain-based convenience foods, from doughnuts and crackers to packaged, frozen side dishes, have fat, sugar, and sodium added to them, further compromising their nutritional wholesomeness. The appeal of convenience foods is that they are either ready to eat or quick to prepare. Whole grains, by contrast, have a reputation for being time-consuming to cook.

Another reason Americans have not embraced whole grains and grain products is that they have a reputation for being fattening. For years, weight-loss diets typically excluded or minimized foods like pasta and bread. Actually, though, grain products are less fattening than the foods emphasized in some of the most popular diets. For example, a 3-ounce cooked hamburger patty made from lean ground beef has 225 calories and over 13 grams of fat—or 54 percent of its calories from fat. The same amount, by weight, of cooked pasta (about ⅔ cup) has just 132 calories—and virtually no fat. If a grain dish is high in calories, it's usually because of the fat added to it in the form of butter, cheese, or a sauce made with whole milk or cream. Grains eaten without these fatty ingredients are generally less fattening than most meats and dairy products, which are inherently high in fat.

Even though Americans still don't eat enough grains to supply them with the recommended amounts of complex carbohydrates and dietary fiber, overall grain consumption has risen. According to USDA's 1994-96 food intake surveys, U.S. adults consume an average of 6.7 servings of grain products per day, but of these products only one serving was whole grain.

grain benefits

Between 65 and 90 percent of the calories in grains come from carbohydrates (mostly complex), which should comprise about two-thirds of the calories you consume each day. Grains are also rich in both soluble fiber (the kind that lowers blood cholesterol levels) and insoluble (the kind that helps to prevent constipation. People living in areas where unrefined whole grains make up a significant part of the diet are alleged to have a lower incidence of cancer, heart disease, and type 2 diabetes than those who live in the industrialized countries of Europe and North America. Whole grains also help alleviate constipation and provide assistance in maintaining a healthful weight. Moreover, grains—especially whole grains—and grain products offer significant amounts of B vitamins (riboflavin, thiamin, and niacin), vitamin E, iron, zinc, calcium, selenium, and magnesium.

In addition, grains are an excellent low-fat source of protein. The protein, however, is incomplete—that is, it is deficient in some essential amino acids that act as "building blocks" for protein in the body. But it's possible to complete the protein by eating grains with foods that contain complementary proteins, such as legumes, small amounts of meat, poultry, dairy products, eggs, or, in some cases, other grains. A classic example of a dish with complementary proteins is rice and beans. The beans provide the amino acid lysine missing from the rice, while the rice contributes methionine, an amino acid missing from the beans. Peanut butter sandwiches, macaroni and cheese, breakfast cereal with milk, and rice and buckwheat in a pilaf (buckwheat is not deficient in lysine) are other examples of food combinations that provide complementary proteins.

what's in a grain

Not all grains are botanically related—true grains, such as wheat, rice, oats, rye, millet, corn, triticale, and barley, are members of the grass family, *Gramineae*; other so-called grains, such as amaranth, quinoa, and buckwheat, belong to different botanical families. But the kernels of the different grains all have a similar composition. A kernel is an edible seed composed of three parts—the bran, the endosperm, and the germ, or embryo. Some grains, notably rice, oats, and some varieties of barley, are also covered by an inedible papery sheath called the hull, which must be removed before the grain can be processed or consumed. Within each kernel are the nutrients needed for the embryo to grow until the plant can take root and get nourishment from outside sources.

The bran is the outer covering of the kernel. It makes up only a small portion of the grain but consists of several layers—including the nutrient-rich aleurone—and contains a disproportionate share of nutrients. The bran layers supply 86 percent of the niacin, 43 percent of the riboflavin, and 66 percent of all the minerals in the grain, as well as practically all of the grain's dietary fiber. In some grains—wheat and corn, for example—the fiber is primarily insoluble, while in other grains, such as oats and barley, it is mainly soluble. Whole grains almost always contain the bran, but it is usually stripped away during milling and so is missing from most refined grain products.

The starchy endosperm accounts for about 83 percent of the grain's weight. Most of the protein and carbohydrates are stored in the endosperm, as are some minerals and B vitamins (though less than are in the bran). This layer also has some dietary fiber; for example, about 25 percent of the fiber in wheat is found in the endosperm. In wheat, the endosperm is the part of the grain used to make white flour.

The smallest part of the grain is the germ; it constitutes about 2 percent of the kernel's weight. Located at the base of the kernel, the germ is the part of the seed that if planted would sprout to form a new plant. It contains a good amount of polyunsaturated fat, and, as a consequence, is often removed during milling to prevent grain products from turning rancid. The germ is also relatively rich in vitamin E and the B vitamins (though it has fewer of the latter than are found in the bran or endosperm), and some minerals.

milling & enrichment

Grains have been milled since they were first cultivated, to make them easier to cook and digest. During milling, the inedible hull and varying amounts of the bran are removed from the grain, and then the grain is ground into smaller granules. For example, barley is milled into three types—hulled, Scotch or pot, and pearled—each with progressively less bran. Similarly, wheat can be milled into cracked wheat (most bran), finely ground cracked wheat, or wheat flour (least bran).

To turn wheat kernels into flour, the seeds are put through an alternating series of high-speed steel rollers and sifters of increasingly finer mesh in order to separate the three parts of the seed.

White, or refined, flour consists almost entirely of the ground endosperm, while whole-wheat flour retains the three constituents, which are recombined after milling. (Stone-ground flour, however, does not go through the separating process.)

In the United States, it is the refined grains that are most popular. Most of the bread and rolls we eat are made from white flour, and the pasta we cook is usually made from refined wheat. In addition, the rice is most often white, rather than brown. Admittedly, these are all nourishing foods, but they lack some of the dietary fiber and some of the nutrients found in the whole grain. White flour, for example, can lose up to 80 percent of the vitamins and minerals present in the whole-wheat kernel, and it retains only 25 percent of the fiber.

Today, most of the refined grain products are enriched—that is, certain nutrients lost during processing are added in amounts that approach their original levels. Some grain products—bread, flour (except whole-wheat flour), and pasta, for example—must meet federal standards for how much of each nutrient must be added to the product. After milling, white flour, cornmeal, white rice, and semolina (the flourlike product used for pasta) are enriched with thiamin, niacin, and riboflavin, and fortified with iron. Some white wheat flours may also be fortified with calcium. (To fortify means adding nutrients to a food that you would not usually find in that food, especially at those levels. For example, the addition of potassium iodide to salt was one of the earliest successful fortification programs.) Because white flour is enriched, it has just slightly less of the B vitamins than whole-wheat flour, but more iron.

Enriched grains are more nutritious than unenriched ones, and they also supply the same amount of complex carbohydrates as whole grains. Moreover, refined grains store longer because the natural oils in the bran and germ have been removed, and these oils tend to spoil quickly, especially in warm environments. But from a nutritional vantage point, high-quality whole grains are still superior to refined grains; they contain more dietary fiber as well as a host of trace nutrients, such as zinc and copper, that are removed during milling.

shopping & storage

Shopping and storage guidelines for whole grains are similar. Most grains are sold in boxes or cellophane bags: Be sure the package is tightly sealed and check for a freshness date. If you buy grains in bulk from bins, try to be sure the store has a good turnover and that the bins are emptied before adding new stock. Grains should be clean and dry, free from chaff or other debris, and smell pleasantly fresh.

Though they have a long shelf-life compared to fruits and vegetables, whole grains are subject to spoilage. They contain natural oils that can turn rancid, and they can also fall prey to insect infestation and mold. Therefore, keep grains in tightly closed containers or plastic bags. You can store them at room temperature (except in hot weather) in a dark, dry place for about 1 month. However, they will keep considerably longer in the refrigerator—at least 4 to 5 months. Use moisture-proof containers to prevent them from drying out or getting soggy.

If you freeze grains, they will keep almost indefinitely. The exceptions are oats and oat bran, which are higher in fat than other grains and so can turn rancid after only 2 or 3 months in the freezer. Therefore, buy only as much of them as you will need in that period of time.

meat & poultry

Americans have always appreciated meat. In colonial days, they hunted game animals for it, and by the early 1800s, as more people left farms to settle in towns, they brought it with them preserved with salt. In the 1870s, the growth of the cattle industry, and new methods of feeding and transporting domestic animals, introduced fresh meat into the average person's daily diet. Meat and poultry became the central focus of meals, and they have remained so, to a striking degree: Americans, who make up only 7 percent of the world's population, eat one-third of the world's meat supply.

In the past several decades, however, the role of meat and poultry in the American diet has come under greater scrutiny than that of any other food. Nutritionists have recommended that we eat less meat—particularly red meat—because of the total fat, saturated fat, and cholesterol it contains. Vegetarian and semi-vegetarian diets are in vogue, and many consumers now regard red meats as "bad" foods. Poultry, on the other hand, has come into favor because it is lower in fat. While we are eating more meat and poultry than ever before, the kinds of meat we choose has changed. Beef and pork consumption have declined somewhat since the 1970s, while that of chicken and turkey has risen. Consumption of poultry in the United States continues to increase, while beef consumption falls; in fact, surveys show that we eat more poultry than we do beef.

two concerns: fat & cholesterol

Red meat is one of the major sources of fat and cholesterol in the American diet; these substances have long been implicated in various illnesses. Studies have shown that too much dietary fat and cholesterol can increase the risk for heart disease. A high-fat diet may also lead to an increased risk for some types of cancers. For instance, the rate of breast cancer in Japanese women is far less than that of Western women. This has been attributed in part to many lifestyle, dietary, and environmental factors. These include the fact that the Japanese eat much less saturated fat and more of the protective omega-3 fatty acids as well as a diet rich in plant foods, such as soybeans and soyfoods, which may protect against disease. And it is important to note that when Asian women immigrate to the United States, their risk of breast cancer rises considerably—a six-fold increase compared with the women in their native countries—with incidence rates approaching those of Caucasian women. In addition, a diet high in total fat promotes obesity, which itself is a risk factor for heart disease, cancer, and diabetes.

The amount of saturated fat in some meats can also pose a threat to health. A diet high in saturated fat can lead to elevated blood cholesterol levels, which, in turn, may result in the coronary arteries becoming clogged, setting the stage for a heart attack. Studies have found that vegetarians have, on average, blood cholesterol levels that are lower than people who eat meat regularly. And vegans (those who shun all animal foods, including cheese and eggs) have diets even lower in saturated fat. Vegetarians consume less saturated fat because their diets are based on whole plant foods that are naturally lower in total and saturated fat.

A high intake of saturated fat may also increase the risk of colon cancer. Studies show that colorectal cancer is most common in countries where the diet is typically "Western": high in fat (particularly saturated fat), meats (especially red and processed meats), calories, sugar, and refined grains, and low in fruits, vegetables, and whole grains. Eating large amounts of fat may be unhealthy for the colon because some fat passes into the colon undigested, and the bacteria there act upon the fat, producing potentially carcinogenic substances that may damage the colon lining. In addition, a diet high in saturated fat typically promotes constipation, and chronic constipation may be linked to colon cancer. A healthy diet, on the other hand, is high in vegetables, fruits, and whole grains, and low in animal fats. It can include small amounts of low-fat meats and poultry as well as fish and low-fat or fat-free dairy products.

The amount of cholesterol in meat is also a concern. Fat and saturated fat content vary according to the species of animal, the cut, whether the fat is trimmed or the skin is removed (on poultry), and in some cases, the grade of meat. (The individual entries will tell you which are the leanest types of meat or poultry.) But the cholesterol content of all types of meat, whether it is lean or fatty, is roughly the same—20 to 25 milligrams per ounce. This amount does not fluctuate because cholesterol is found in lean tissue as well as in the fat. However, saturated fat has a far greater effect on blood cholesterol levels than does dietary cholesterol.

the nutrients in meat

You don't need to eat meat and poultry to survive; it's possible to get all the nutrients you need from a vegetarian diet, especially if you also include low-fat dairy products and/or fish. But meat and poultry are exceptionally rich in iron, zinc, and vitamins B_6 and B_{12}—nutrients that are difficult to obtain in a meatless diet.

Iron, for example, is essential for the production of hemoglobin in our bodies. But, according to the National Academy of Sciences, about 14 percent of women between the ages of 15 and 44 have some degree of iron deficiency. Meat and poultry contain heme iron, the type that is best absorbed by the body; the iron in plant foods, by contrast, is nonheme iron, and is not as well absorbed. For example, about 15 percent of the iron in beef, lamb, chicken, and pork is absorbed by the body, compared to 4 percent in navy beans.

About 70 percent of the zinc in the American diet comes from animal products, mostly meat. Chicken and pork contain impressive levels of vitamin B_6. As for vitamin B_{12}, it is not easy to find sources other than animal products, unless you consume fortified soy milk, some nutritional yeasts, or supplements. And of course, meat and poultry are known for their high protein content. Animal foods are the major sources of protein in the American diet, with meat, fish, and poultry combined accounting for 42 percent of all animal protein consumed. Moreover, the protein in meat, unlike that in vegetables and grains, is complete, meaning that it provides all of the amino acids needed by the body.

balancing the meat in your diet

Moderation, not abstinence, is the key: It is overconsumption of meat that puts health in jeopardy; small servings will provide significant amounts of nutrients without adding excess fat to your diet. Just 3 ounces—about the size of a deck of cards— of trimmed, cooked sirloin steak or skinless chicken breast yields more than half of the protein you need daily. The steak also furnishes well over 10 percent of the RDA for riboflavin, niacin, vitamin B_6, and iron, about half the RDA for zinc, and 100 percent of the RDA for vitamin B_{12}. The chicken breast offers about 15 percent of the RDA for vitamin B_{12}, about 30 percent of the vitamin B_6, and about 75 percent for niacin. Removing the skin from chicken cuts the fat content by three-quarters and the total calories by half. Still, dark-meat chicken (such as thighs or wings) without the skin has two to three times as much fat as skinless breast—and 25 percent more calories. In fact, some well-trimmed, lean cuts of beef or pork (look for the word "loin" or "round") have no more fat, ounce for ounce, than skinless dark-meat chicken.

Few experts recommend eliminating all meat, or even all red meat, from our diets, because of its nutritional value. In fact, all types can be part of a low-fat diet, if you follow some simple guidelines.

• Eat small portions—3 to 4 ounces.

• Choose lean cuts of beef, pork, or lamb—those that have less than 10 grams of fat in a 3-ounce serving.

• Substitute poultry for some of the red meat in your diet.

• Treat meat as a side dish that complements a meal of vegetables, grains, or legumes.

• Limit fattier cuts of meat, such as prime beef, bacon, and sausage, to special occasions.

• Trim all of the external fat from red meats and remove the skin from poultry.

• Choose low-fat cooking methods—such as roasting, grilling, broiling, and poaching—over frying. Stir-frying and sautéing can be acceptable if you use little additional fat.

tough or tender

Meat is muscle, made up mostly of water and protein, with some fat. Beef, without external fat, for example, is, on average, 72 percent water, 21 percent protein, and 6 percent fat by weight. Chicken, without skin, is 75 percent water, 21 percent protein, and 3 percent fat. If you looked at a cut of meat or poultry under a microscope, you would see that it is composed of individual, cylindrical muscle fibers. These are held together by thin bands of connective tissue, of which there are two main types: collagen and elastin. Connective tissues are more abundant in those parts of the animal that do a lot of work, because exercise builds connective tissue; this partially accounts for the toughness of cuts from these areas. (Cuts of meat high in connective tissue also tend to be fattier than more tender cuts, because fat is deposited around connective tissue first.) Collagen turns to gelatin when it is heated in liquid—this transformation explains why stewing tenderizes tough cuts of meat. Marinating in an acidic liquid also softens collagen. Elastin is not affected by cooking and can be broken down only by pounding or cutting.

Muscle fibers generally run in only one direction, called the grain. Cutting tough meat across the grain helps to tenderize it by shortening the muscle fibers.

the color of meat

Hemoglobin, the pigment that makes blood red, is not responsible for the red color of beef and lamb and the dark color of chicken or turkey drumsticks. When an animal is slaughtered, most of the hemoglobin is removed as the animal is bled. The color of meat comes instead from myoglobin, another red pigment present in the muscles, which stores oxygen. The parts of an animal containing well-exercised muscles—which require more oxygen—are darker than underused areas. For example, the legs of chickens and turkeys are dark because these animals stand or walk a lot, but their wing and breast meat is white because they hardly fly. On the other hand, goose, duck, and game birds use many of their muscles for flying, and consequently all their meat is dark. As for cattle, a cut of beef from the shoulder, which is involved in walking, is darker than a cut from the loin, which is minimally active. In addition, the type of animal dictates the color of the meat. Beef muscles contain more myoglobin than those of pork or veal.

are meat & poultry safe?

All meat sold in the United States is inspected for wholesomeness by the Food Safety and Inspection Service (FSIS) of the United States Department of Agriculture (USDA), which includes a team of veterinarians. Animals are examined before slaughter for signs of disease, and unhealthy animals are not slaughtered for food.

Every so often, reports appear in the media about excessive hormone, antibiotic, or chemical residues in meat and poultry, and such stories cause great concern among consumers. It's true that hormones—the natural sex steroids estradiol (estrogen), progesterone, and testosterone, as well as two synthetic ones—are used in the raising of livestock, particularly cattle; 60 to 90 percent of the cattle in the United States are given hormones to make them gain weight faster. These growth stimulants are popular among cattlemen because they save money—savings that are passed on to the consumer. Hormone-treated cattle eat less and reach market sooner, yet gain approximately 50 pounds more lean muscle tissue than an untreated animal. So not only do we save money and resources, but we also get leaner meat.

The FDA says that hormone-treated beef is safe to eat and, at the prescribed dosages used in feedlots, these hormones have been certified safe. Currently, there is very little definitive evidence to the contrary.

Antibiotics are not a part of regular raising practices, but they are prescribed for sick animals. Numerous studies have shown that their minuscule residues are not a risk to human health. When excessive levels of drugs, chemicals, or hormones are found, they usually occur in the animal's liver, kidneys, or fat—not in the lean tissue. By avoiding organ meats (which are very high in cholesterol), choosing lean cuts, and trimming excess fat, not only do you reduce the amount of fat in your diet, but you significantly reduce the risk of contamination from these substances should they be present.

food poisoning: reducing the risk

An important safety concern is the risk of bacterial contamination in meats and poultry. Every year, an estimated 76 million people become sick from foodborne illness. Of these, 300,000 people are hospitalized and approximately 5,000 die, according to estimates by the Centers for Disease Control. Beef, pork, and chicken, as well as eggs and other meats, can harbor salmonella, while *Escherichia coli* (*E. coli*) bacteria and campylobacter organisms are common culprits of foodborne illness from meat and poultry. Poultry is more prone to spoilage than other meats, in part because it is sold with its skin, which carries more bacteria than its flesh. Poultry that has been improperly handled is probably the main source of foodborne illness.

The way almost all poultry is raised and processed also contributes to its increased levels of contamination. Chicken production is a highly—but not completely—automated industry that strives for efficiency: A high-speed production line can slaughter and gut as many as 90 chickens a minute, and generate a great deal of filth. Mechanical eviscerating and other processing methods increase the bacteria count. Recently the industry has come under fire from the press, consumers, and Congress. According to a variety of estimates, a high percentage of all raw chicken marketed harbors salmonella, campylobacter, or both. (Newer methods of maintaining safe poultry are in development, however.)

The USDA is responsible for meat and poultry inspection, but its performance in the past has reportedly been less than thorough. Although the poultry industry grew, the number of USDA inspectors declined. The USDA seal, according to industry critics, is no longer a guarantee of a clean, wholesome product.

The risks of getting food poisoning from poultry and other foods are eliminated through proper handling and cooking. To prevent food poisoning from meat and poultry, follow the general guidelines below. Other safety tips are included in each entry as they pertain to the particular meat.

• Keep your refrigerator below 40° and the freezer at, or below, 0°.

• Wash your hands thoroughly before and after handling raw meats. Use soap and warm water, and wash for at least 20 seconds, working soap into the hands, including the fingernail area and between the fingers.

• Use a fresh dish towel every time you cook meat.

• Defrost frozen meats only in the refrigerator, in the microwave, or, in some cases, in cold water. Never thaw foods at room temperature. The outside surface thaws before the inside, leaving the outside prone to bacterial contamination and growth.

• After preparing raw meat or poultry, wash the utensils, counter, cutting board—anything that came into contact with the meat—thoroughly in hot, soapy water before preparing other foods.

• Marinate meats and poultry only in the refrigerator. Don't put cooked meat back into an uncooked marinade, and don't serve the marinade as a sauce unless you heat it to a rolling boil and then boil it for several minutes.

• Don't serve barbecued meat or poultry on the plate that previously held the raw meat or poultry, and don't use the cooking utensils for serving.

• Never eat meat raw. Steak tartare may be considered a delicacy by some people, but it is dangerous to eat.

• Keep meats and poultry at room temperature for no more than an hour before or after cooking, and promptly refrigerate leftovers.

• Cook meats and poultry to the internal temperature recommended by the recipe you are following.

fish & shellfish

Though Americans have traditionally favored meat far above fish and shellfish, in the past decade these water-borne foods—which have long been appreciated by creative cooks—have become increasingly popular among the public at large. In part, this is due to the fact that fish and shellfish are no longer limited to a few familiar choices such as swordfish, fillet of sole, and shrimp. Today, many supermarkets display a surprising array of fish and shellfish from local waters and, increasingly, from other regions and even other countries. But certainly another reason behind the growing enthusiasm for these foods is their nutritional value. Like meat and poultry, fish and shellfish offer an excellent source of protein, yet unlike these animal foods, they are relatively low in calories, fat, and cholesterol. They contain some cholesterol, as do all animal products, but most fish or shellfish is no higher in cholesterol than skinless chicken breast or lean beef. Shrimp is the exception, with 166 milligrams per 3-ounce serving, as compared with 61 milligrams in a similar serving of lobster and about 72 milligrams in white meat chicken (without the skin). The good part is that all fish and shellfish are low in saturated fat. Whitefish such as flounder, cod, and haddock, as well as shellfish, are very low in total fat. They're also a good source of vitamin B_{12}, iodine, phosphorus, selenium, and zinc.

In addition, some of the fat in fish, unlike the fat in meat and poultry, appears to promote health. Fish fat, which takes the form of oils, contains certain types of polyunsaturated fatty acids—known as omega-3s—that have anticlotting properties and thus may be protective against heart attack and perhaps high blood pressure. Like other unsaturated fats, fish oils can help lower blood cholesterol levels when they replace saturated fats in the diet. They may also help control inflammatory responses in the body that cause such conditions as arthritis and psoriasis (a chronic skin condition characterized by redness and scaling). Omega-3s are distributed throughout the fish's flesh, so you should still trim and discard any visible fat as well as the liver and skin, since contaminants, if present, are most likely to settle in these three areas.

Experts have concluded that fish and shellfish—if cooked—are safe and wholesome and Americans should be eating them. The American Heart Association recently revised its dietary guidelines to advise eating at least two servings of fish a week. It emphasized fatty fish such as salmon and herring, since this is one instance where fat may help protect the heart. Research suggests that the higher the fat content of fish, the greater the cardiovascular benefits. Fish with a moderate fat content are barracuda, striped bass, and swordfish and whiting. The high-fat fish include some of the more popular fish such as herring, mackerel, salmon, and tuna. Most canned fish also retains most of its omega-3s.

Fish oil supplements are another story. You should avoid cod liver oil and other fish oil supplements, which may contain toxic levels of vitamins A and D, as well as environmental contaminants that often concentrate in the fish's liver. Large doses of fish oil may also thin the blood excessively and may increase your risk for certain kinds of stroke. And there is no evidence that taking fish oil supplements provides the same protection against heart attacks as eating fish.

how safe is seafood?

Not so long ago, food poisoning from eating raw fish or shellfish was considered the only possible hazard associated with enjoying these foods. But in recent years, frequent headlines about pollutants in both fresh and salt water, coupled with reports about contamination due to improper shipping and handling within the seafood industry, have led increasing numbers of people to wonder if many varieties of fish, whether cooked or raw, are hazardous. It is true that fish and shellfish are among the most perishable of commodities—even when properly refrigerated, they don't last as long as chicken or beef. Even fish from the purest water has to be handled carefully. Complicating matters is the fact that lakes, rivers, and oceans here and all over the world are polluted with sewage, industrial waste, and heavy metals such as mercury and lead, as well as other contaminants. There are U.S. government agencies that inspect fish (fresh and canned) and make rules about where food fish may be harvested. But fish and shellfish are not subject to mandatory federal inspection; enforcement is largely the responsibility of each state, and the quality and effectiveness of state programs vary greatly. Funds to finance these programs are always short, and consumer groups have long complained that more vigilance and more funding are needed.

Any fish or shellfish may carry some bacteria and viruses—and animals from sewage-polluted waters may carry large doses of them. Many varieties of fish commonly carry the larvae of tapeworms and roundworms. Cooking will kill all such parasites and microorganisms. (Of course, if bacteria reach a certain level, the fish will be unfit for consumption no matter how much you cook it.) But heat won't eliminate mercury, lead, or such industrial pollutants as polychlorinated biphenyls (PCBs). These compounds were once widely used in electrical insulation, pesticides, plastics, inks and dyes, and other industrial products, and they seeped into the food chain in various ways. Banned by the U.S. government in 1979, PCBs persist in the environment. When they accumulate in the body they can cause birth defects, and are classified as probable carcinogens. PCBs are not the only possible contaminant: Chlordane, dioxin, DDT (which is also banned but still present), and the heavy metals are also of concern.

Although fish and shellfish—if cooked—are safe and wholesome, these animals nonetheless are more subject to chemical contamination than food animals raised on land, because they feed not just on plants but on other animals, and they filter gallons of water through their bodies daily. Chemicals that may be present have "an opportunity to become more concentrated through bioaccumulation." Another problem is that the potential ill effects from consumption of these chemicals are not obvious and dramatic (like food poisoning from eating bad clams, for example). Indeed, the effects are very hard to detect. Maybe the consumption of small amounts of PCBs or mercury might slightly raise the risk of cancer or of birth defects. Clearly, consumers as well as scientists would like a lot more information about fish—where they were caught or harvested, how they've been handled, what pollutants they may contain, and what the long-term effects of such pollutants may be on human health.

Many fish and shellfish, including catfish, salmon, tilapia, trout, oysters, and mussels, are now raised by aquaculture, or fish farming. The quality of the fish and shellfish depends on conditions at the fish farm. Contrary to what many people imagine, farm-raised fish don't necessarily live in clean tanks. The water the fish are raised in may be polluted with agricultural runoff, pesticides, or river water. The fish farmers may also add drugs (including antibiotics and sulfa drugs) to prevent or treat disease, or put hormones into the water. As with other fish and shellfish, proper handling in processing and transporting is important, too. The FDA inspects fish farms, but some critics believe the inspection system is inadequate.

safety guidelines

Following some basic rules can help minimize the risk from contamination. Eat fish and shellfish in reasonable amounts—that is, in modest portions no more than three times a week—and choose different varieties, so you aren't likely to always be eating fish from the same area. In addition, follow the suggestions in the individual entries for purchasing, storing, and handling fresh fish and shellfish. Before you eat freshwater fish caught locally, check with the local health department to make sure the waters are safe.

Finally, it's best to simply avoid eating raw fish or shellfish, including sushi—the risk of illness is too high. Even the freshest fish may harbor various kinds of bacteria and other potentially harmful organisms. Certain shellfish—clams, oysters, mussels—live by filtering 15 to 20 gallons of water a day. If the water they inhabit is polluted, they'll retain bacteria and viruses along with the microscopic foodstuffs they absorb. Raw shellfish can thus be a source of hepatitis, gastroenteritis, and other diseases. Raw fish, as used in sushi, sashimi, ceviche, and other dishes, may be a source of parasites, such as tapeworms and roundworms, as well as bacteria and viruses. (Marinating raw fish in lemon or lime juice is not the equivalent of cooking—it won't kill all bacteria and parasites.) It's true that a well-trained sushi chef may know how to purchase and handle fish so as to minimize the risk of illness and parasitic infection. But while sushi chefs are licensed in Japan, there's no way to check their credentials in this country. Preparing and eating raw fish at home is definitely not recommended, since this practice has proved the most common source of parasitic infection from fish in this country. If you make gefilte fish or other dishes that use raw, ground fish, remember not to sample it until it's cooked.

Inadequately cooked shellfish, too, can be a source of infection. Steamed clams, for example, are typically cooked just to the instant of opening, about a minute or two, so the clam never gets hot enough inside to kill bacteria or inactivate any virus that may be present. If it is health certainty you want, learn to enjoy your shell-fish on the well-done side.

In January 2001, the FDA warned pregnant women—and those who might become pregnant or who are nursing—not to eat shark, swordfish, king mackerel, or tilefish because these may contain mercury, which can damage the brain and nervous system of the fetus. It also advised pregnant women to eat no more than 12 ounces of fish a week, and to vary the types of fish they eat. And, of course, in addition to pregnant and nursing women, the very old and very young, and anyone coping with a serious illness should be cautious and not take any chances with raw fish and shellfish.

The surest way of getting untainted seafood is to buy it from a reputable source, whether it's a fish seller or a supermarket with a well-stocked fish department. Not only is the seafood likely to be properly handled and displayed, but the people who work there can answer questions you might have about storing and preparing your purchase once you get it home.

milk & eggs

Milk and eggs are basic, nutrient-rich foods. Milk is the sole nourishment for infant mammals; eggs contain the nutritional material to sustain unborn birds and reptiles. Human beings have been consuming eggs and the milk of other animals for thousands of years, and both foods are still among the most nutritious available to us. Milk and milk products—including cheese and yogurt—are the most important dietary sources of calcium, providing about 75 percent of this mineral in the American diet. And both milk and eggs provide a roster of other vitamins and minerals, along with ample supplies of protein. Because the protein is complete, dairy foods complement the protein in legumes and grains, by supplying the amino acids present in low amounts in some non-animal protein sources.

From a culinary standpoint, these foods are widely enjoyed and remarkably versatile. Eggs and milk (and its derivative dairy products) can be eaten alone, but they are also used to enhance innumerable other foods: They can lighten cakes or thicken sauces and soups, and they serve as accompaniments, flavorings, or sauces in hundreds of different dishes, from breakfast cereals to vegetables. In many others—from the omelet to the ice cream sundae—they are the central ingredient. But despite the universal appreciation for milk and eggs, they have several drawbacks when it comes to health concerns. With dairy products, the most serious shortcoming is that the fat in milk is mainly saturated. In addition, some dairy products are also quite high in sodium. The downside to eggs is their cholesterol content: One egg contains about two-thirds of the total suggested daily maximum intake. Whole eggs are high in fat, too, containing about 5 grams per large egg.

avoiding the fat

Should you give these foods up entirely in order to limit your fat and cholesterol intake? Not really. Eggs do no harm if eaten occasionally. They may be high in cholesterol, but the fat they contain is primarily unsaturated. The whites are fat-free and an excellent source of protein. And during the past decade or two manufacturers have created an astonishing variety of low-fat or fat-free dairy products that preserve the taste, texture, and nutritional value of whole milk products. As a result, consumers have a wider choice than they have ever had before when it comes to buying milk, sour cream, yogurt, ice cream, and cheese.

In low-fat or fat-free forms, these products have an important role to play in the American diet, given their rich supply of calcium—a mineral that as many as two-thirds of American women, and one-half of American men, should be consuming in greater quantities. Calcium intake is the primary factor in building strong bones. It's vital to start consuming adequate amounts of calcium when young—especially between the ages of 11 and 24—and continue to do so through adulthood. Calcium plays a role in preventing osteoporosis—a loss of bone mass and subsequent weakening of bones that often occurs in postmenopausal women and occasionally in older men. The link between calcium and osteoporosis is not clear-cut, but getting enough calcium is one way a woman can help reduce her risk of getting the disease. One of the reasons that milk and dairy products are reliable sources of well-utilized calcium is that they contain lactose (or milk sugar) and vitamin D, which enhance calcium's absorption. It's also easy to remember that 4 to 5 cups of milk or 4 to 5 servings of other calcium-rich dairy products will supply the 1,200 milligrams of calcium you need each day.

dairy & egg safety

Most milk comes from large dairy cooperatives, where milk from many farms is pooled and then processed to a uniform standard. The milk is pumped directly from the cows' udders—via milking machines—to steel tanks, and from there to refrigerated trucks. These modern practices contribute to our safe, reliable milk supply—a far cry from the days when raw milk, sold from open pails or cans, was a common vehicle for the spread of disease. That's why pasteurization—a mild heating process that kills dangerous microorganisms—is considered one of the greatest advances in food sanitation. Today, raw milk (unpasteurized)and products made from it are still legally sold in some states, but that doesn't mean that they are safe to consume. While less than 1 percent of milk consumed by Americans daily is raw, this small percentage of raw milk has gotten increased attention in recent years as the source of serious and sometimes fatal occurrences of food poisoning.

Unpasteurized milk products contain a salmonella strain that is resistant to five antibiotics used to treat most salmonella infections. Health officials attest that raw milk and raw milk products can pose a risk of infection, not only because of salmonella, but because of many other pathogens as well. Unpasteurized cheeses have been implicated in multiple outbreaks and their consumption poses an important health threat. Everyone, but especially infants, pregnant women, and those with weakened immune systems, should avoid unpasteurized milk products.

Some proponents of raw milk contend that it is more nutritious, because the heat of pasteurization destroys some nutrients. In fact, the nutrient loss is so minimal as to be almost undetectable, and there is no evidence that raw milk enhances resistance to disease, another claim that has been made for it. Very few dairies still produce what is called certified milk, which is processed under extremely rigid sanitary standards in an attempt to preserve its cleanliness without pasteurization. However, even certification is no guarantee that milk is not contaminated. Many states have banned the sale of any raw milk, certified or not, and the Centers for Disease Control calls raw milk "unsafe"; the FDA considers it "a public health problem." These statements would seem to be enough to convince any consumer that the dubious benefits of raw milk in no way outweigh its risks.

Raw eggs should be given the same wide berth as raw milk. Eggs have also been implicated as the major cause of severe outbreaks of salmonella. The majority of cases involving this kind of salmonella have occurred in northeastern states, and over three-quarters of the outbreaks are thought to have been caused by Grade A, whole fresh eggs. Researchers suggest that the salmonella bacteria in these outbreaks can come from inside the hens, and hence are inside the eggs, rather than by the usual route of cracked or dirty eggshells. (*For more on salmonella and eggs, see page 280.*)

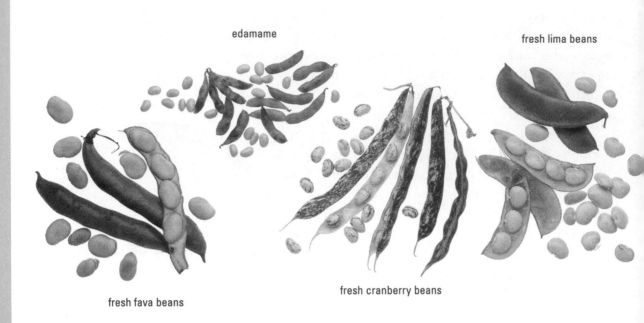

edamame

fresh lima beans

fresh fava beans

fresh cranberry beans

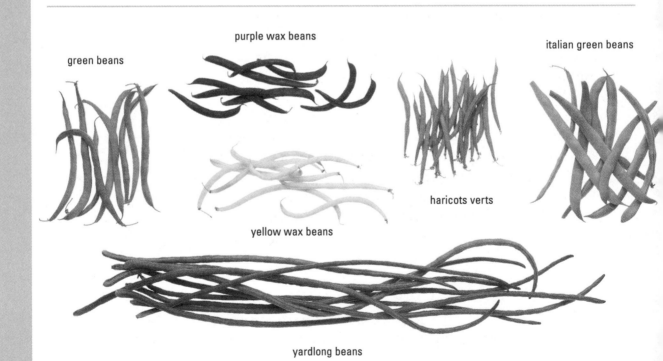

purple wax beans

green beans

italian green beans

haricots verts

yellow wax beans

yardlong beans

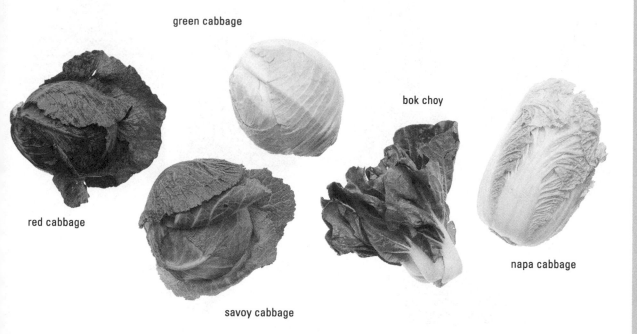

green cabbage

bok choy

red cabbage

napa cabbage

savoy cabbage

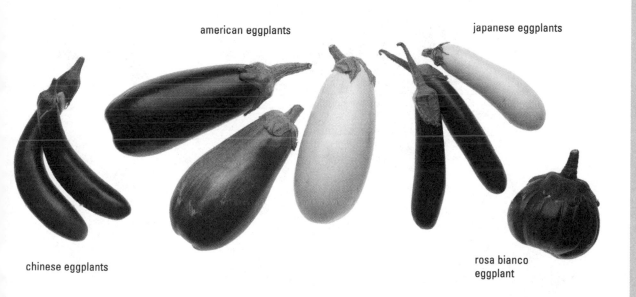

american eggplants

japanese eggplants

chinese eggplants

rosa bianco
eggplant

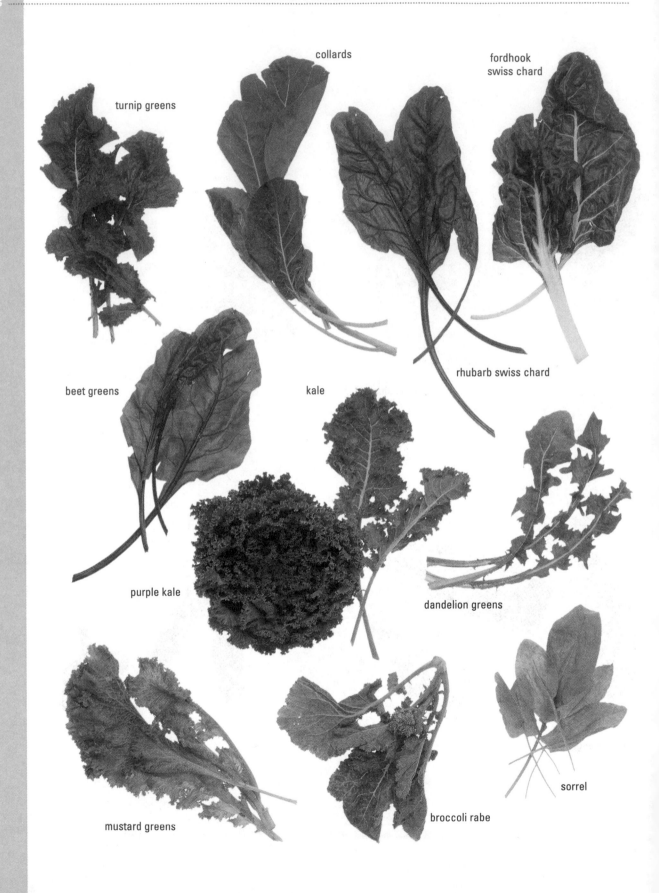

turnip greens

collards

fordhook
swiss chard

rhubarb swiss chard

beet greens

kale

purple kale

dandelion greens

mustard greens

broccoli rabe

sorrel

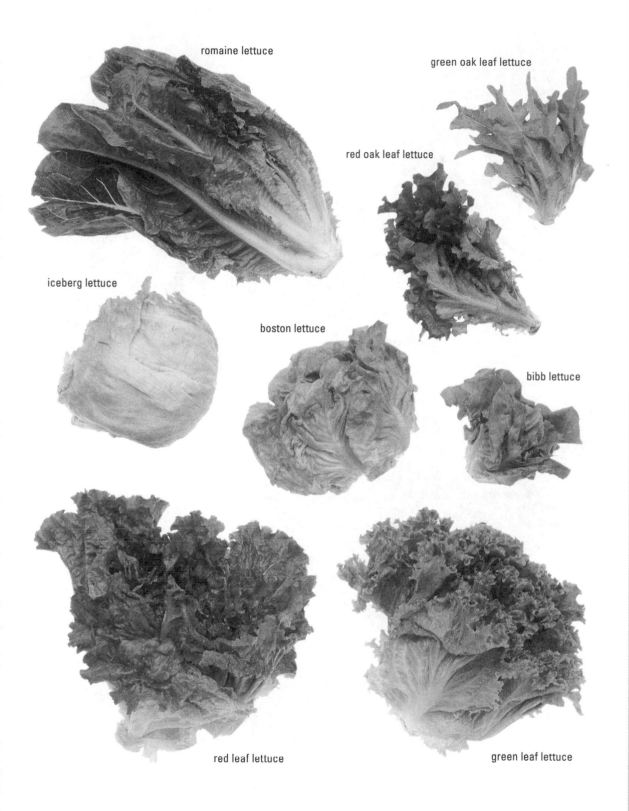

romaine lettuce

green oak leaf lettuce

red oak leaf lettuce

iceberg lettuce

boston lettuce

bibb lettuce

red leaf lettuce

green leaf lettuce

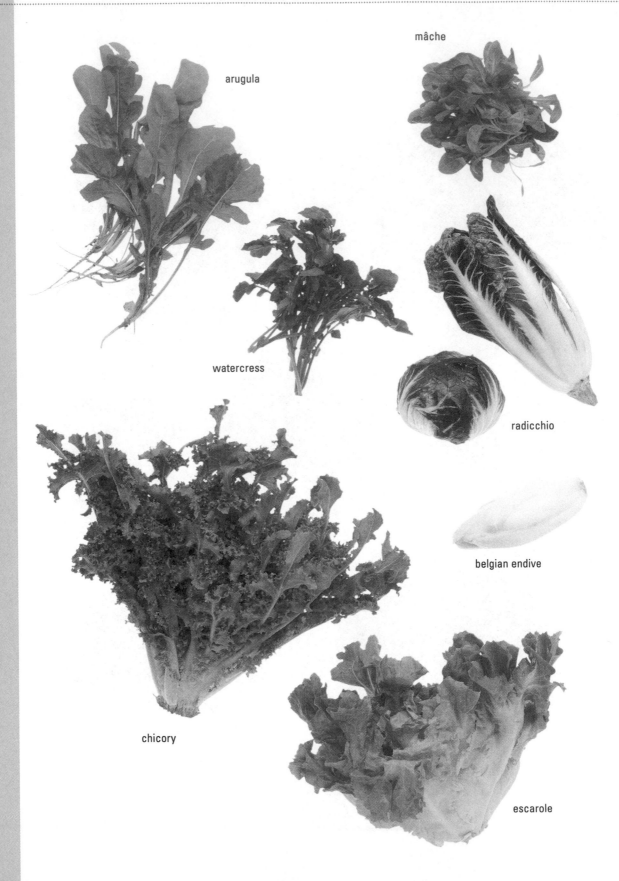

mâche

arugula

watercress

radicchio

belgian endive

chicory

escarole

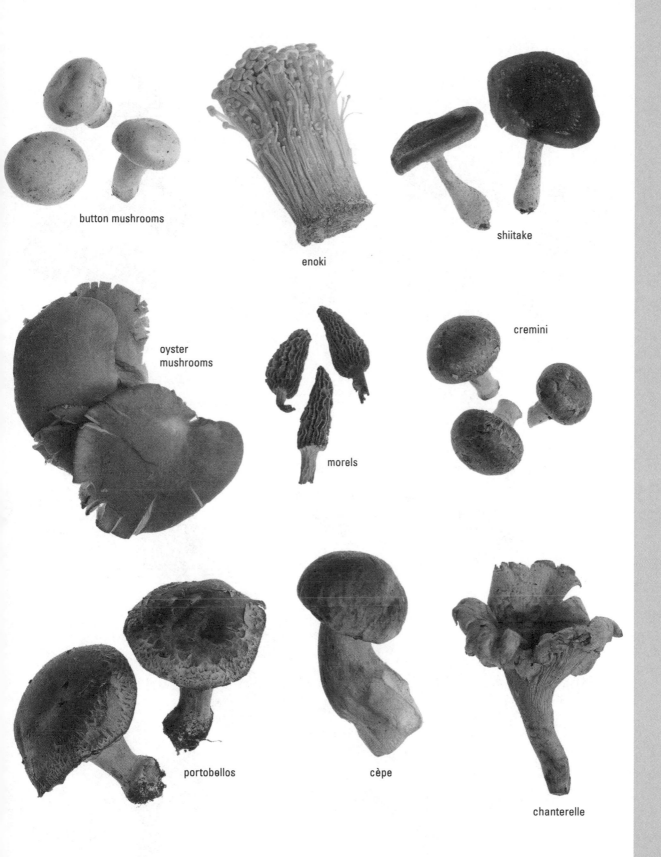

button mushrooms

enoki

shiitake

oyster mushrooms

morels

cremini

portobellos

cèpe

chanterelle

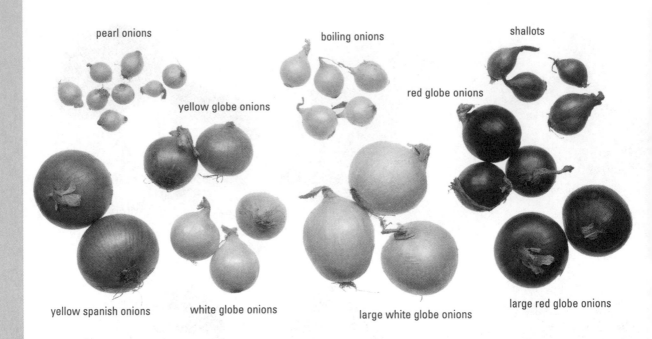

pearl onions

boiling onions

shallots

red globe onions

yellow globe onions

yellow spanish onions

white globe onions

large white globe onions

large red globe onions

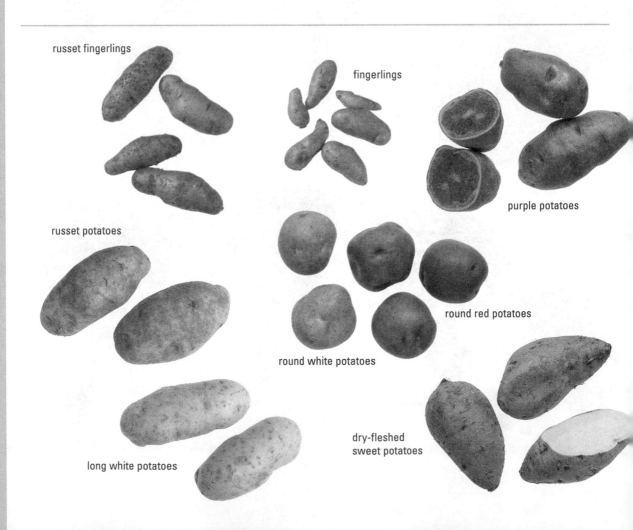

russet fingerlings

fingerlings

purple potatoes

russet potatoes

round red potatoes

round white potatoes

dry-fleshed sweet potatoes

long white potatoes

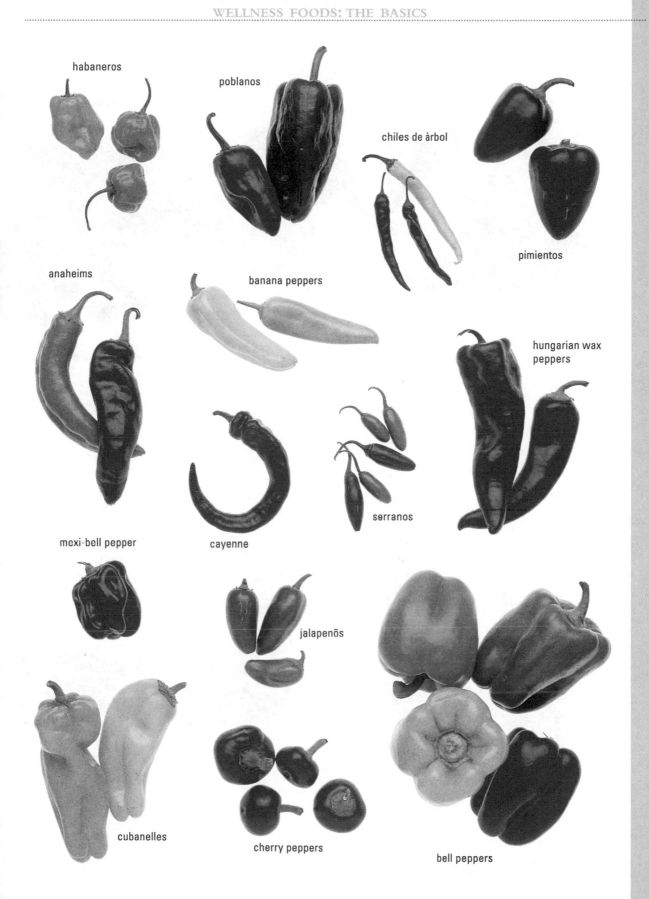

habaneros

poblanos

chiles de àrbol

pimientos

anaheims

banana peppers

hungarian wax peppers

serranos

mexi-bell pepper

cayenne

jalapenõs

cubanelles

cherry peppers

bell peppers

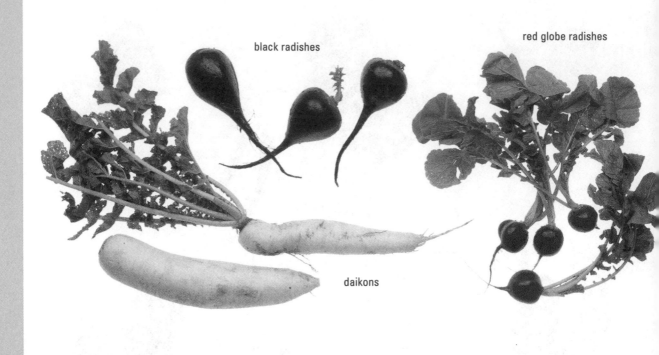

black radishes

red globe radishes

daikons

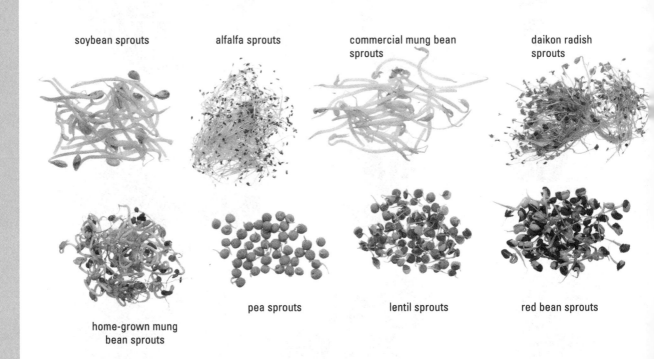

soybean sprouts

alfalfa sprouts

commercial mung bean sprouts

daikon radish sprouts

home-grown mung bean sprouts

pea sprouts

lentil sprouts

red bean sprouts

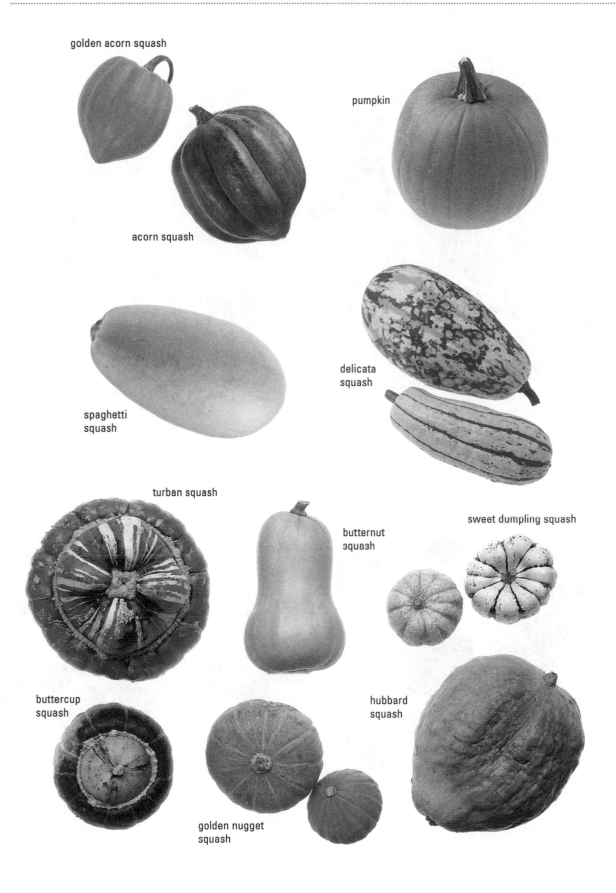

golden acorn squash

acorn squash

pumpkin

spaghetti squash

delicata squash

turban squash

butternut squash

sweet dumpling squash

buttercup squash

golden nugget squash

hubbard squash

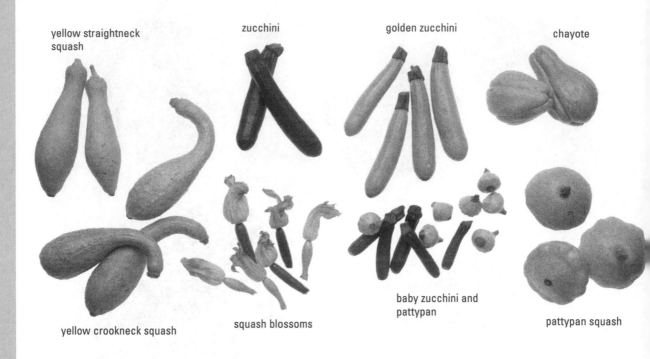

yellow straightneck squash

zucchini

golden zucchini

chayote

yellow crookneck squash

squash blossoms

baby zucchini and pattypan

pattypan squash

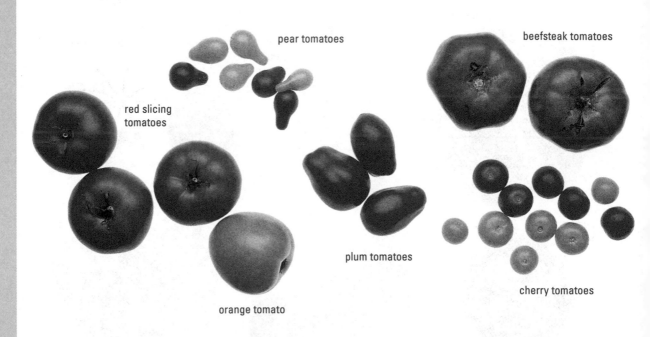

pear tomatoes

beefsteak tomatoes

red slicing tomatoes

plum tomatoes

cherry tomatoes

orange tomato

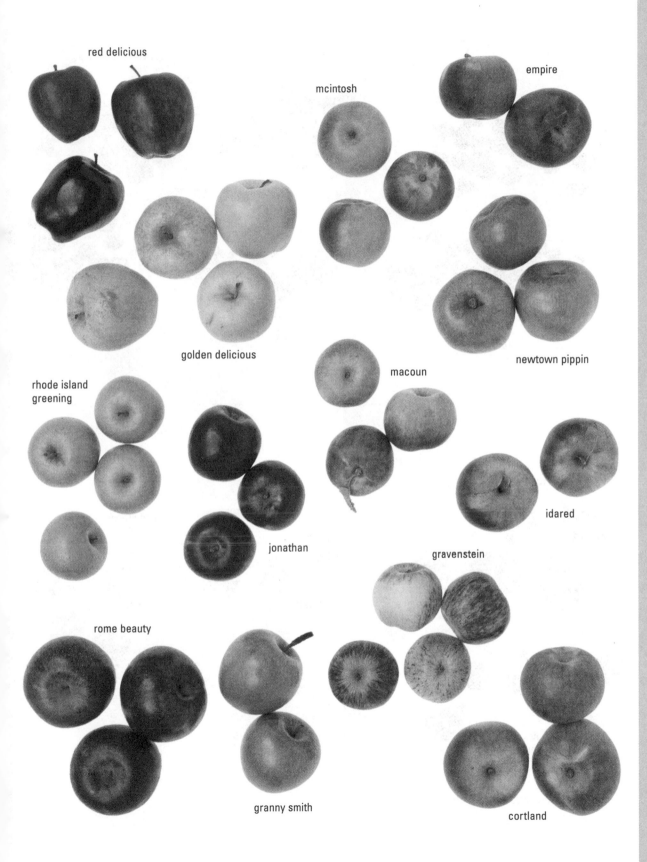

red delicious

mcintosh

empire

golden delicious

newtown pippin

rhode island greening

macoun

idared

jonathan

gravenstein

rome beauty

granny smith

cortland

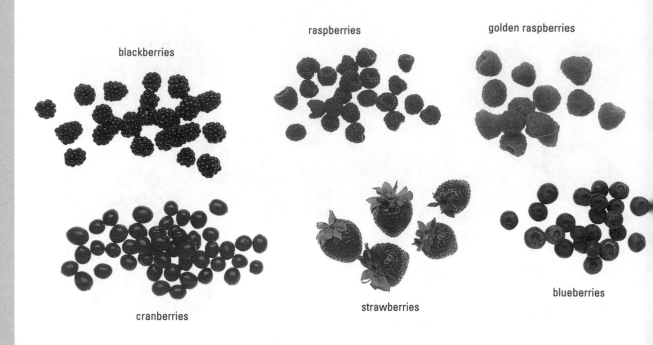

blackberries

raspberries

golden raspberries

cranberries

strawberries

blueberries

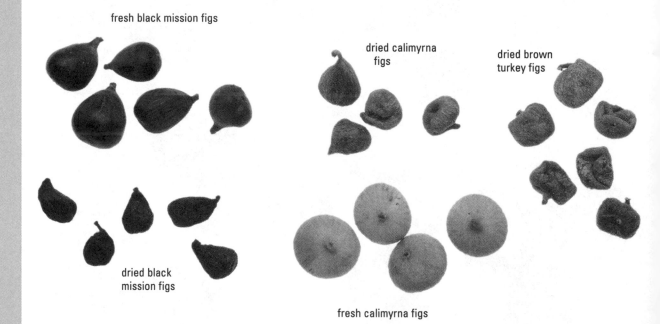

fresh black mission figs

dried calimyrna figs

dried brown turkey figs

dried black mission figs

fresh calimyrna figs

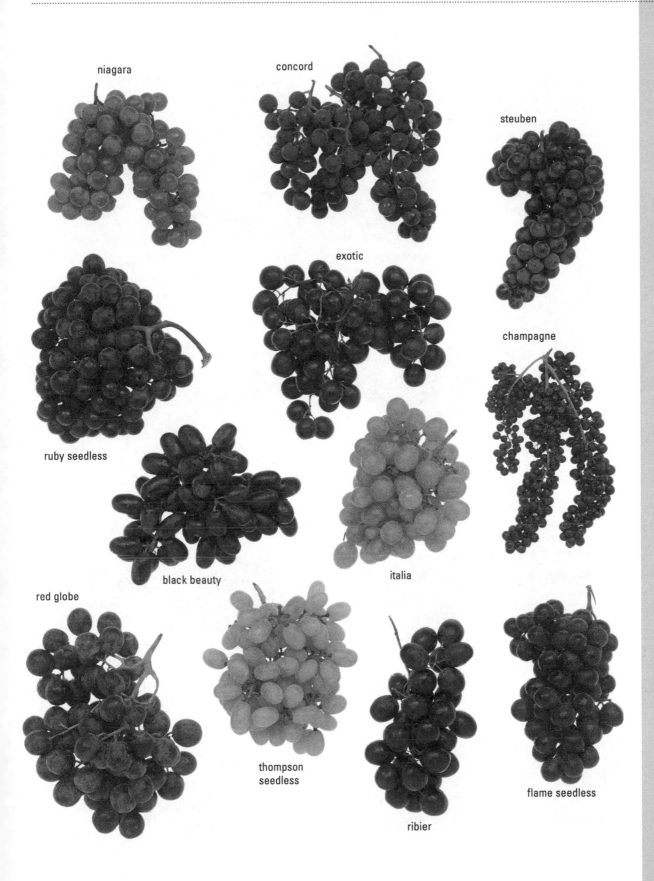

niagara

concord

steuben

exotic

champagne

ruby seedless

black beauty

italia

red globe

thompson
seedless

ribier

flame seedless

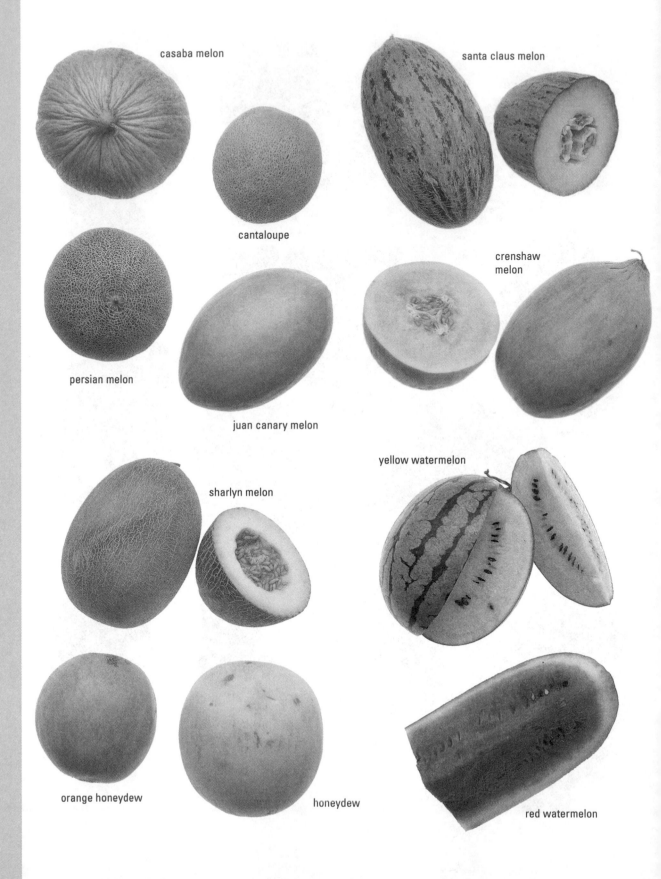

casaba melon

santa claus melon

cantaloupe

crenshaw melon

persian melon

juan canary melon

sharlyn melon

yellow watermelon

orange honeydew

honeydew

red watermelon

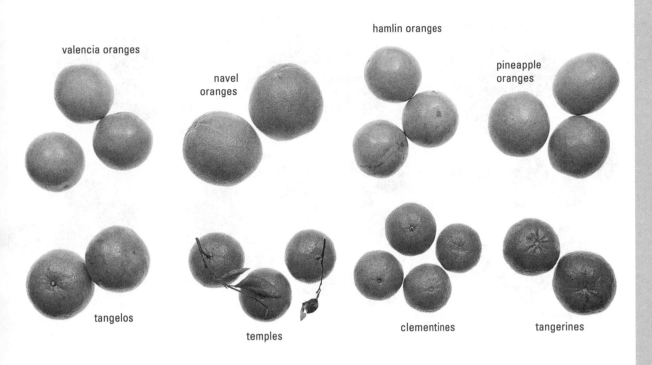

valencia oranges

navel oranges

hamlin oranges

pineapple oranges

tangelos

temples

clementines

tangerines

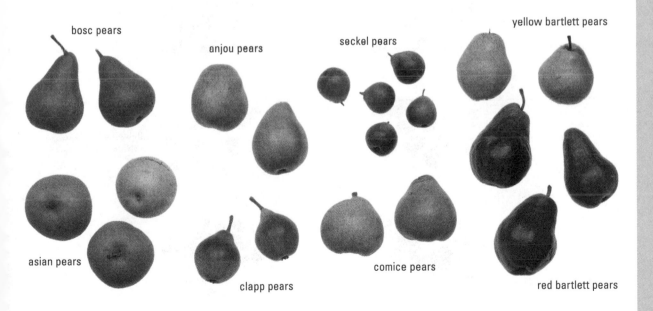

bosc pears

anjou pears

seckel pears

yellow bartlett pears

asian pears

clapp pears

comice pears

red bartlett pears

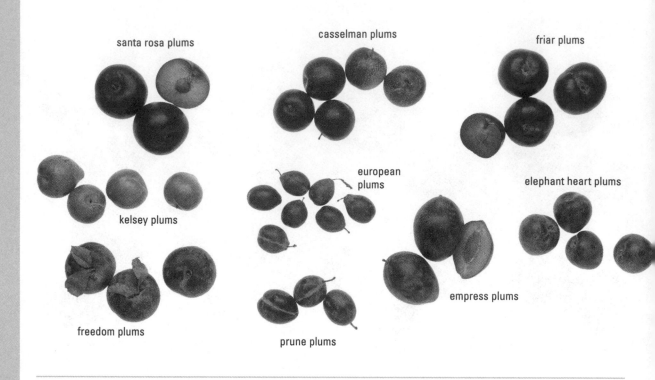

santa rosa plums

casselman plums

friar plums

kelsey plums

european plums

elephant heart plums

freedom plums

prune plums

empress plums

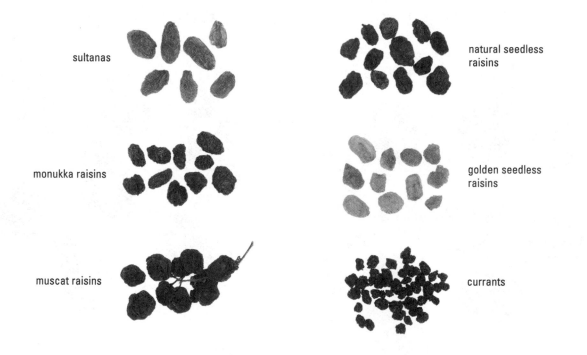

sultanas

natural seedless raisins

monukka raisins

golden seedless raisins

muscat raisins

currants

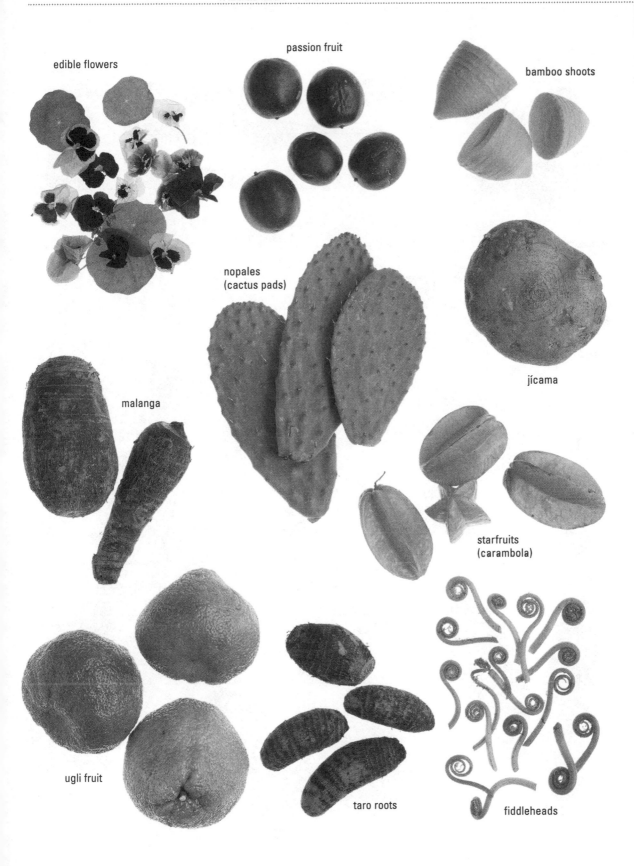

edible flowers

passion fruit

bamboo shoots

nopales
(cactus pads)

jícama

malanga

starfruits
(carambola)

ugli fruit

taro roots

fiddleheads

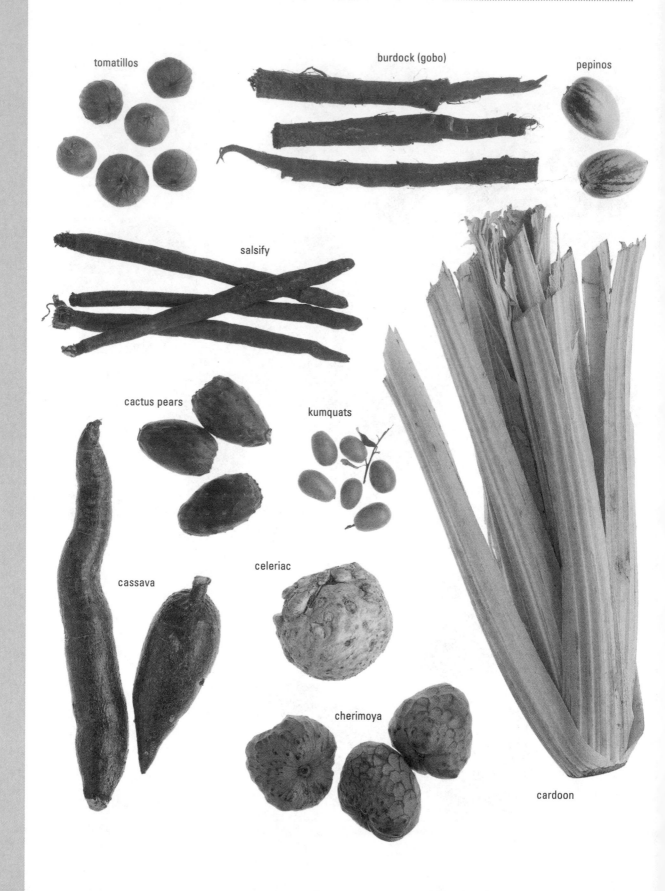

tomatillos

burdock (gobo)

pepinos

salsify

cactus pears

kumquats

cassava

celeriac

cherimoya

cardoon

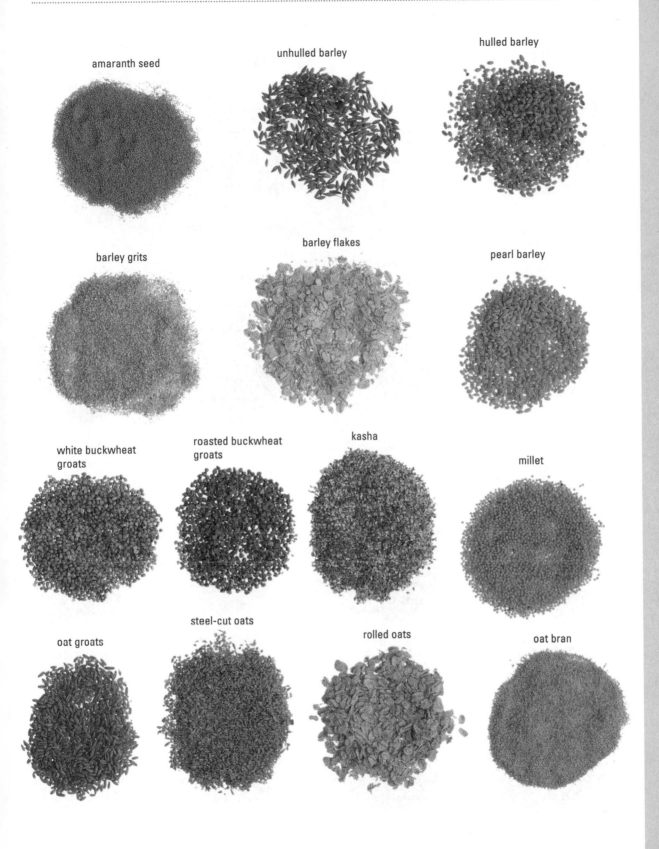

amaranth seed

unhulled barley

hulled barley

barley grits

barley flakes

pearl barley

white buckwheat groats

roasted buckwheat groats

kasha

millet

oat groats

steel-cut oats

rolled oats

oat bran

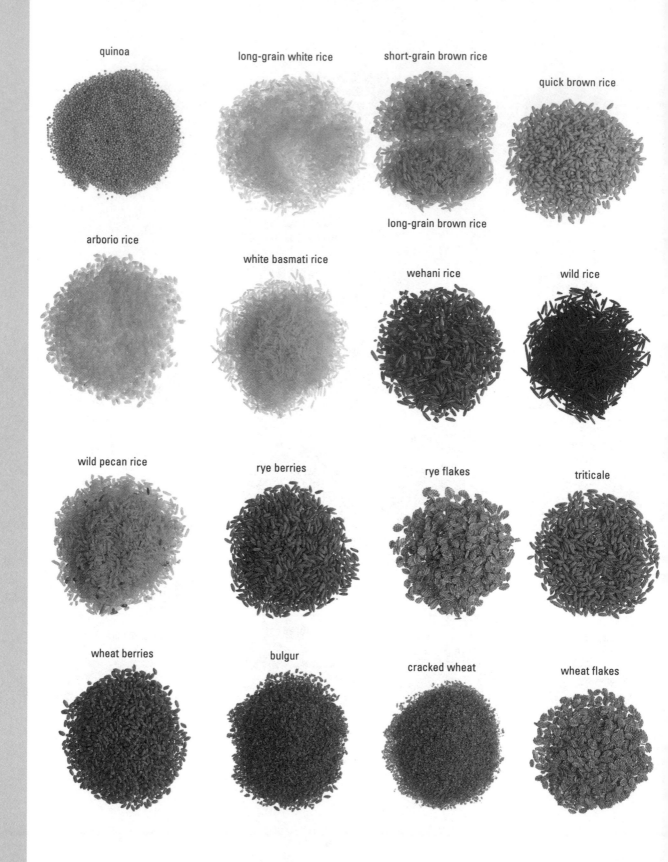

quinoa

long-grain white rice

short-grain brown rice

quick brown rice

long-grain brown rice

arborio rice

white basmati rice

wehani rice

wild rice

wild pecan rice

rye berries

rye flakes

triticale

wheat berries

bulgur

cracked wheat

wheat flakes

spaghetti

whole-wheat spaghetti

corn spaghetti

amaranth spaghetti

jerusalem artichoke spaghetti

beet spaghetti

red bell pepper and basil spaghetti

fettuccine

squid ink fettuccine

linguine

spinach linguine

vermicelli

capellini

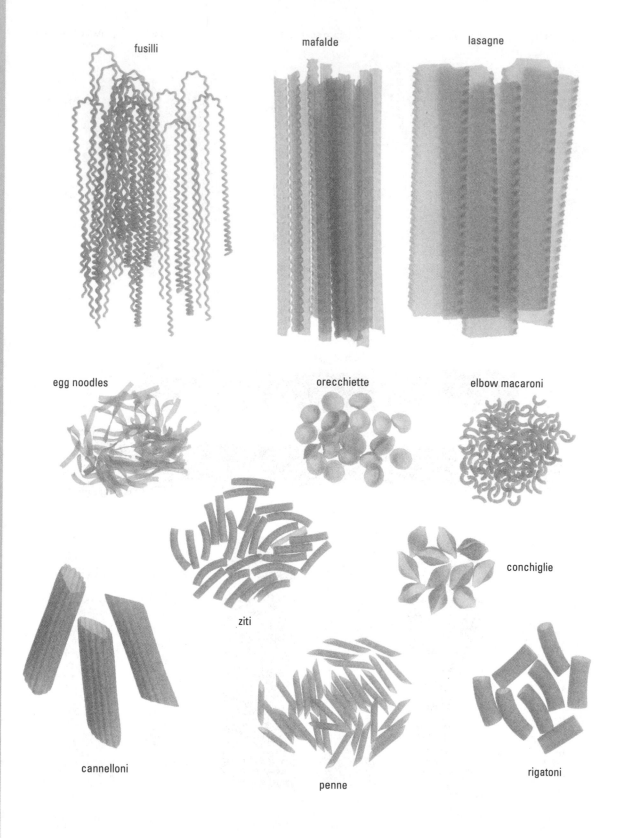

fusilli

mafalde

lasagne

egg noodles

orecchiette

elbow macaroni

conchiglie

ziti

cannelloni

penne

rigatoni

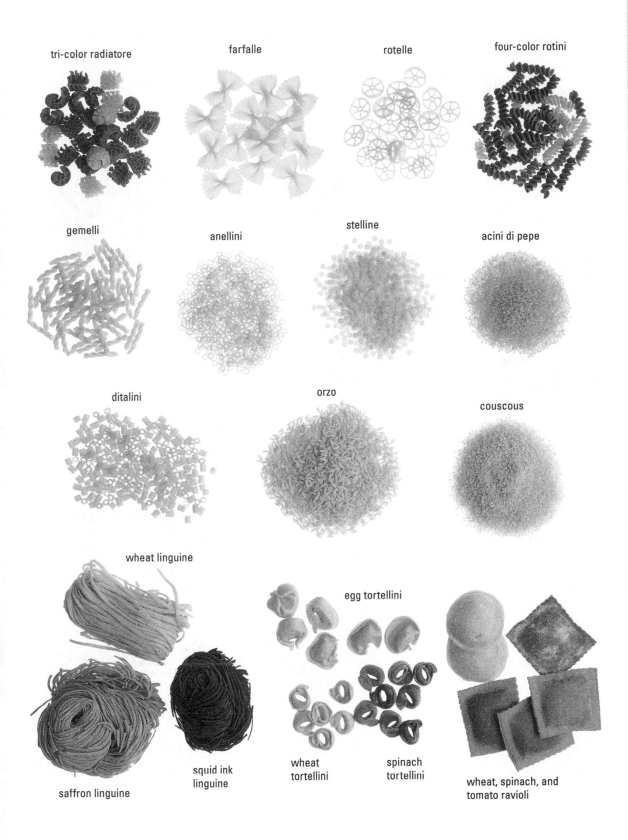

tri-color radiatore

farfalle

rotelle

four-color rotini

gemelli

anellini

stelline

acini di pepe

ditalini

orzo

couscous

wheat linguine

egg tortellini

saffron linguine

squid ink
linguine

wheat
tortellini

spinach
tortellini

wheat, spinach, and
tomato ravioli

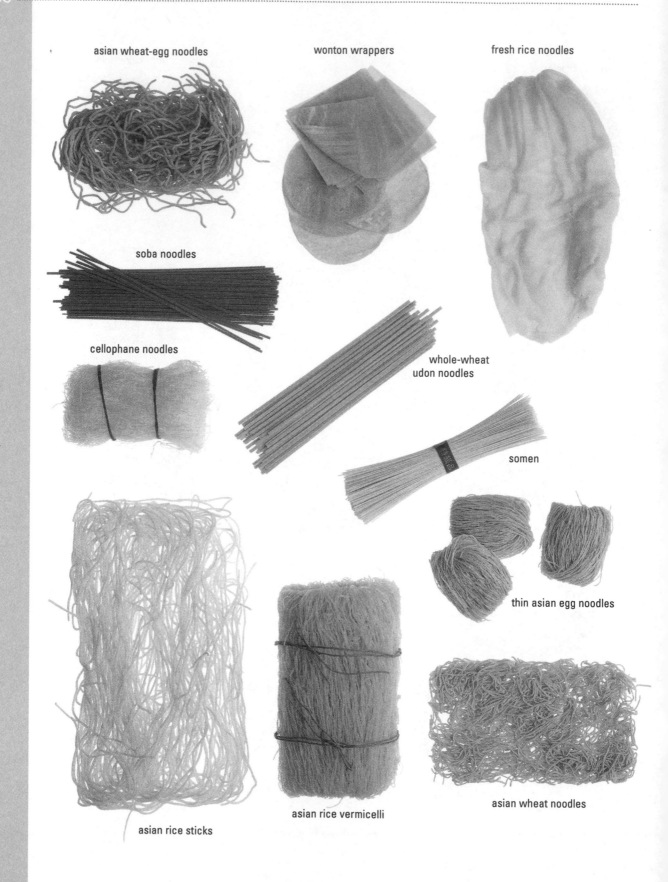

asian wheat-egg noodles

wonton wrappers

fresh rice noodles

soba noodles

cellophane noodles

whole-wheat
udon noodles

somen

thin asian egg noodles

asian rice sticks

asian rice vermicelli

asian wheat noodles

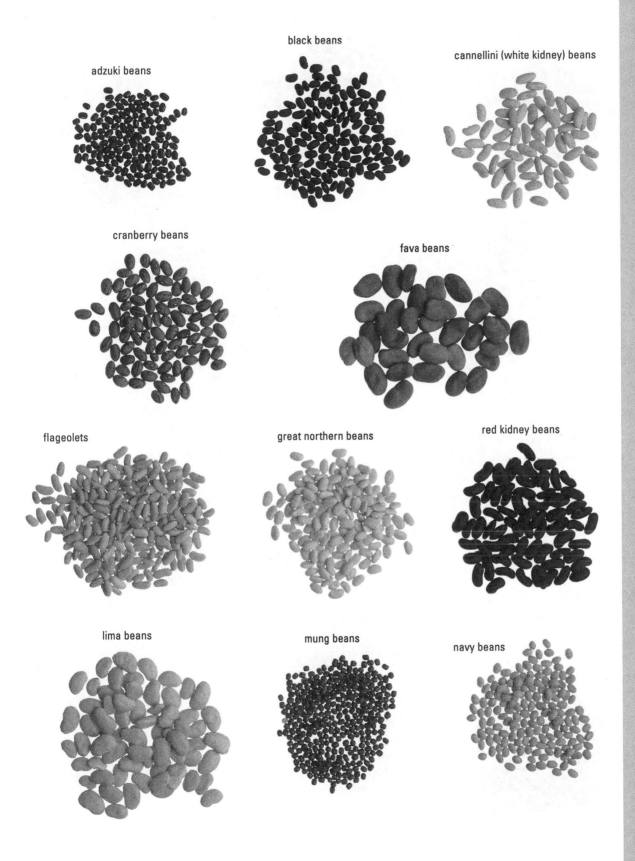

adzuki beans

black beans

cannellini (white kidney) beans

cranberry beans

fava beans

flageolets

great northern beans

red kidney beans

lima beans

mung beans

navy beans

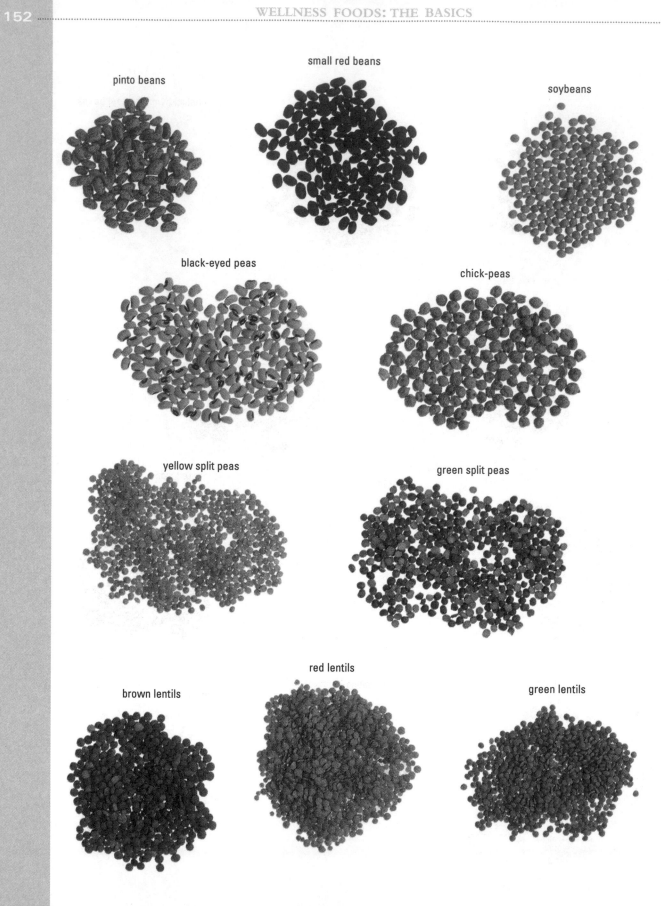

pinto beans

small red beans

soybeans

black-eyed peas

chick-peas

yellow split peas

green split peas

brown lentils

red lentils

green lentils

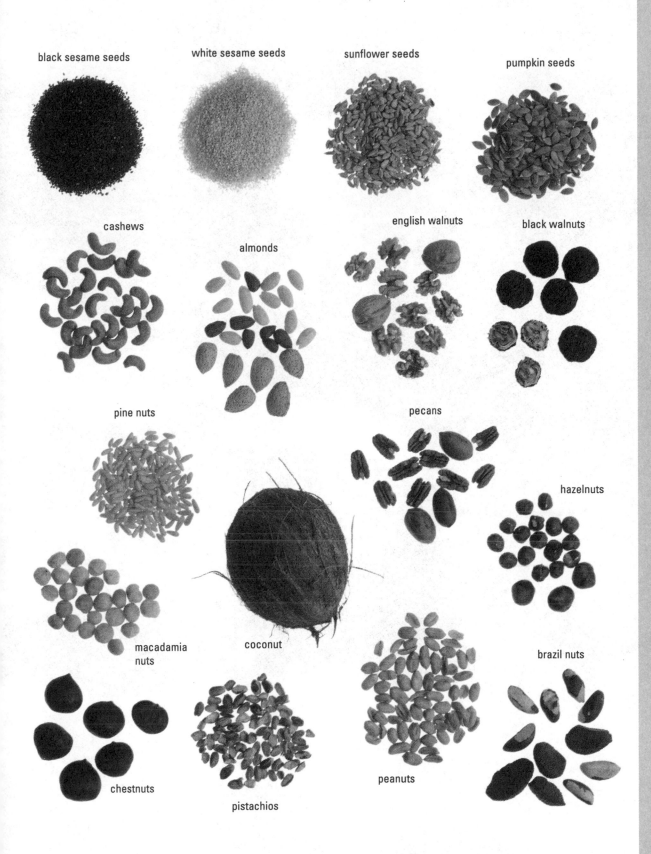

black sesame seeds

white sesame seeds

sunflower seeds

pumpkin seeds

cashews

almonds

english walnuts

black walnuts

pine nuts

pecans

hazelnuts

macadamia nuts

coconut

brazil nuts

chestnuts

pistachios

peanuts

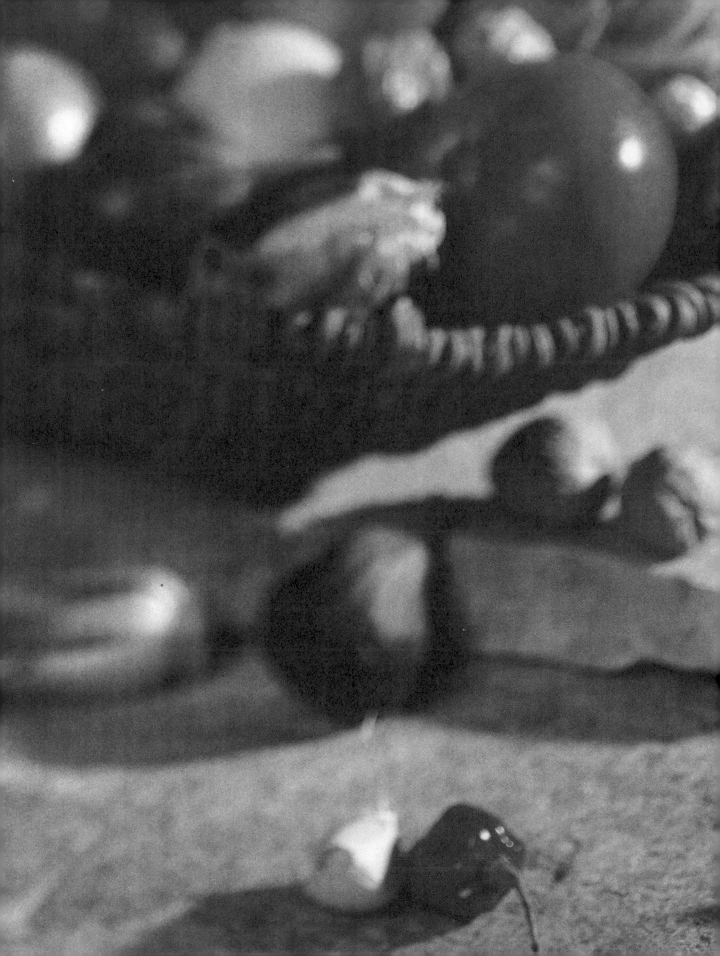

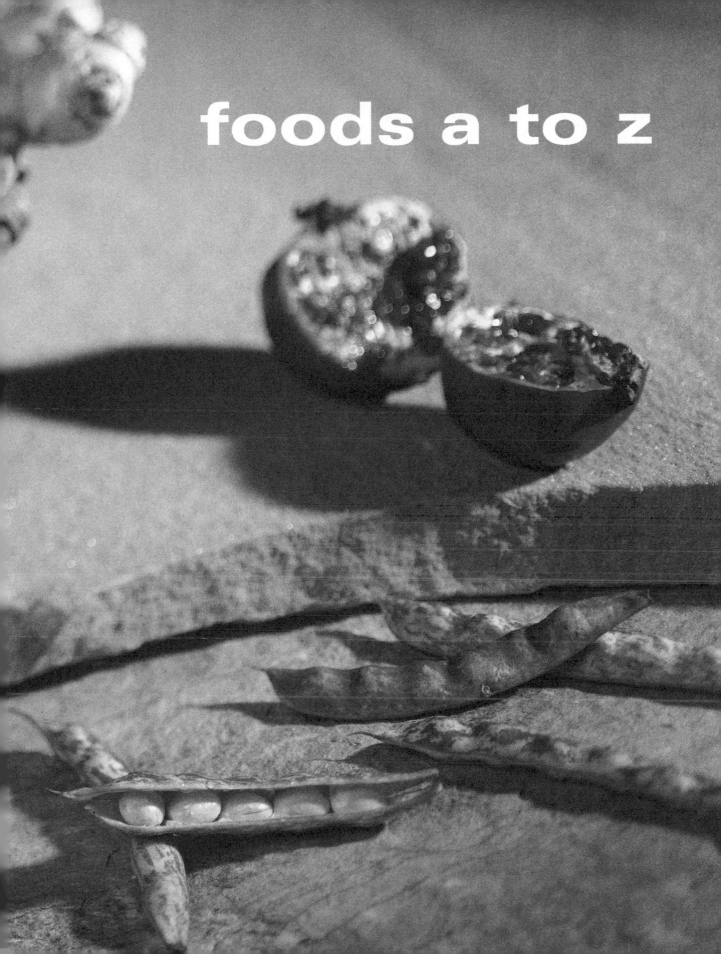

foods a to z

almonds

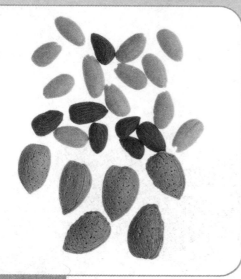

almonds

Almonds belong to the rose family and are related to stone fruits such as peaches, apricots, and plums. In fact, almonds grow inside a fruit that is covered in a peachlike fuzz. When the velvety almond "fruit" ripens, it splits open to reveal the shell that envelops the almond seed (or nut). Sweet, with a rich, smoky flavor, almonds have many culinary uses and are suitable for both savory and sweet dishes.

Native to Asia, the almond has been consumed by humans for thousands of years, and is mentioned in the Book of Genesis numerous times. In the 12th century B.C., the Phoenicians most likely introduced the nut to the Mediterranean region. Dishes calling for almonds were common throughout Europe, and almond milk (ground almonds steeped in hot water) was used in soup and as a digestive aid.

First introduced to the United States in the mid-19th century, almonds are grown commercially in California. They also are grown commercially in parts of the Mediterranean.

nutritional profile

Like some other nuts, almonds are rich in vitamin E, and they also provide protein, riboflavin, iron, and magnesium. Their fat content is mostly monounsaturated fat (about 10 grams per ounce), which may help to reduce LDL ("bad") cholesterol while preserving HDL ("good") cholesterol levels. Studies indicate that almonds and other nuts have a protective effect upon heart health, when part of a diet low in saturated fat. In addition, almonds are an excellent source of fiber: Supplying 3 grams per ounce, they have more fiber than most other nuts. Although almonds are brimming with nutritional benefits, don't go overboard with them, because, like other nuts, they are high in calories.

in the market

Almonds are sold in a number of forms, in shell and out. Whole, shelled almonds are sold "natural" (with their brown skin on) and blanched (with the skin removed). Almonds are also sold sliced (natural or blanched), slivered, or chopped. Most of the almonds sold are simply labeled almonds, but there are a number of specialty almonds:

Bitter almonds Because raw bitter almonds contain traces of a poison called prussic acid (though they are only mildly toxic), their sale is illegal in the United States. However, in their processed form, they are used to make almond extract and other almond-flavored products, such as almond liqueurs.

Chinese almonds These aren't true almonds, but the kernels of several varieties of apricot that are grown specifically for their seeds. They are similar in flavor to bitter almonds (which they are sometimes mistakenly called) and,

ALMONDS / 1 ounce	
Calories	167
Protein (g)	6
Carbohydrate (g)	6
Dietary fiber (g)	3.1
Total fat (g)	15
Saturated fat (g)	1.4
Monounsaturated fat (g)	9.6
Polyunsaturated fat (g)	3.1
Cholesterol (mg)	0
Potassium (mg)	208
Sodium (mg)	3

KEY NUTRIENTS (%RDA/AI*)	
Riboflavin	0.2 mg (17%)
Vitamin E	7 mg (46%)
Iron	1 mg (13%)
Magnesium	84 mg (20%)

*For more detailed information on RDA and AI, see page 88.

also like bitter almonds, are mildly toxic if eaten raw: They should always be blanched or roasted before eating.

Green almonds These almonds have a green furry covering, much like a fuzzy peach. The furry covering is actually the almond "fruit," and the almond is the seed within. In harvesting mature almonds, the fruit portion is discarded. But in the almond's green stage, you can eat the whole fruit. The flesh of the fruit is crunchy and tastes like an unripe peach. The almond itself, since it hasn't yet hardened into a seed, is soft and jellylike, with a faint almond flavor.

Jordan almonds This plump, round Mediterranean variety imported from Spain is rich tasting, with a sweet, almond flavor. It is often sold encased in a sugar coating, but can sometimes be found simply shelled.

▶ **Availability** Packaged almonds are widely available all year round. Almonds in the shell are easiest to find in fall and early winter. Green almonds are available in mid to late summer.

choosing the best

For the sake of freshness, buy almonds in sealed packages when possible. When buying from a bulk source, choose a store where there's a rapid turnover and where the bulk foods are kept in covered containers. Smell the almonds to be sure that they're fresh and sweet.

▶ **When you get home** Like all nuts, almonds have a high fat content, which makes them susceptible to spoilage. To keep them fresh if not using right away, freeze them in their original unopened package or in a tightly covered jar or a zip-close plastic bag. It's not necessary to thaw them before using.

preparing to use

If a recipe calls for blanched almonds, you can either substitute unblanched almonds (the result will taste the same; you just may have some brown specks from the skin) or blanch them yourself: Drop unblanched almonds into a pan of boiling water and boil 30 seconds. Drain and, with your fingers, pop the almonds out of their skins. Dry before using.

serving suggestions

- Use almond butter in place of peanut butter in your favorite cookie recipe.

- Coat fish in coarsely ground almonds and bake or sauté until golden brown and cooked through.

- Steep ground almonds in warm milk. Strain and use the milk to make a pudding.

- Add toasted almonds to pasta dishes.

- Substitute almonds for pine nuts in a traditional pesto recipe.

- Stuff dates or prunes with whole almonds.

- Stir ground almonds into chilis or stews.

other almond products

Almond butter As for peanut butter, almonds are ground until they give off their own natural oils and become pasty. Almond butter can be used in place of peanut butter.

Almond extract Used in baking, this flavoring is produced by combining bitter almond oil with ethyl alcohol. It is quite strong and a little goes a long way.

Almond flour See "Nut & Seed Flours" (*page 327*).
Almond oil See "Nut Oils" (*page 299*).

Almond paste This rich paste is a combination of blanched ground almonds, sugar, and glycerin (added to help prevent crystallization). It is primarily used in baking and candy making. Marzipan is similar and often contains egg whites.

amaranth

While amaranth is often touted as the miracle grain of the Aztecs, it is not a true grain at all. Rather, it is a tiny seed about the size of a poppy seed. In fact, there may be as many as 40,000 to 60,000 seeds generated by one plant. Amaranth seeds range in color from purple to pale yellow. The flavor of the amaranth seed is nutty, almost maltlike, but mild and sweet.

The leaves of the amaranth plant are also edible and are highly nutritious. A vigorous, hardy plant, amaranth is a relative of pigweed, the common wild plant also known as lamb's-quarter. Because amaranth leaves taste quite a bit like spinach, they are often sold in ethnic markets as Chinese spinach or Indian spinach. They are used in those cuisines much like spinach, usually steamed or stir-fried. Amaranth leaves are best eaten young and tender (before the seeds develop).

Amaranth has a rather dramatic history. An ancient grain, perhaps 8,000 years old, amaranth was a staple crop of the Aztecs in the 13th century. The grain was not only valued as a dietary necessity by the Aztecs, but it was offered as a royal tribute and used in religious rituals. After witnessing the role that amaranth played in Aztec culture (including sacrificial drinks that mixed ground amaranth seeds and human blood), the cultivation of the plant was forbidden by Cortés, who prohibited its use either as a food or as a sacred grain. As a direct result, all knowledge of amaranth was virtually lost to the Western world for hundreds of years.

Fortunately, the cultivation of amaranth continued in a few remote areas of the Andes and Mexico. It reappeared several centuries later and was brought to Asia, where it was grown on the Indian subcontinent and in China. Today, amaranth crops are cultivated in Mexico and Central America, and in recent years, the plant has been introduced to wheat-growing regions of the United States, but on a modest scale.

nutritional profile

The old adage that good things come in small packages holds true for the tiny amaranth seed. The tiny fiber-rich seeds of this weedlike plant provide admirable amounts of minerals such as iron, zinc, and magnesium. Small amounts of calcium are also found in amaranth. When compared with other grains, amaranth protein quality scores high, probably because, unlike true grains, amaranth is not deficient in the essential amino acids lysine and methionine.

Not to be overlooked are the amaranth leaves, which can range in color from deep spinach-green to burgundy-red. The leaves supply beta carotene, B vitamins, and a large amount of vitamin C. Their mineral content is also admirable, supplying good amounts of calcium, iron, and potassium.

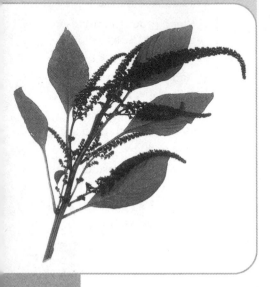

purple amaranth

AMARANTH SEEDS ¼ cup	
Calories	182
Protein (g)	7
Carbohydrate (g)	32
Dietary fiber (g)	7.4
Total fat (g)	3.2
Saturated fat (g)	0.8
Monounsaturated fat (g)	0.7
Polyunsaturated fat (g)	1.4
Cholesterol (mg)	0
Potassium (mg)	178
Sodium (mg)	10

KEY NUTRIENTS (%RDA/AI*)	
Iron	3.7 mg (46%)
Magnesium	130 mg (31%)
Zinc	1.6 mg (14%)

*For more detailed information on RDA and AI, see page 88.

in the market

Amaranth seeds Harvesting amaranth seeds is a labor-intensive process, so amaranth is a relatively expensive product. Some large supermarkets do stock amaranth alongside rice, barley, and other grains; if you don't find it there, look for the seeds at a health-food store.

Amaranth flour See Flour, Nonwheat (*page 324*).

Amaranth pasta See Pasta, Nonwheat (*page 443*).

Amaranth leaves Amaranth leaves are available as "spinach" in Chinese and Indian markets; as amaranth in farmers' markets; and as callaloo in Caribbean markets (especially in Jamaican neighborhoods). Many seed companies offer several varieties of amaranth for the home gardener (including a purple variety that some gardeners choose for decoration). Because amaranth is an extremely hardy plant (it grows like a weed) with such a wealth of nutrients, it would be well worth the trouble to grow this delicious green.

▶ Availability Amaranth seeds are available year round, but amaranth leaves are more seasonal. Local supplies are usually at their peak in the spring and early summer, but imports from Mexico are available much of the year in ethnic markets.

choosing the best

Amaranth seeds should be well wrapped in airtight packages. Amaranth leaves should be bright and unwilted; the stems should look moist and fresh, not dry and split.

▶ When you get home Like all seeds, amaranth contains fat, which means that the seeds are best stored in the refrigerator or freezer to prevent them from going rancid. Amaranth leaves should be stored in the refrigerator as you would store spinach: loosely wrapped in the crisper drawer. Do not wash the leaves until ready to use.

preparing to use

Amaranth seeds need no particular preparation. Amaranth leaves should be washed and the tougher stem ends should be trimmed off.

AMARANTH LEAVES 1 cup cooked	
Calories	28
Protein (g)	3
Carbohydrate (g)	5
Dietary fiber (g)	2.3
Total fat (g)	0.2
Saturated fat (g)	0.1
Monounsaturated fat (g)	0
Polyunsaturated fat (g)	0.1
Cholesterol (mg)	0
Potassium (mg)	846
Sodium (mg)	28

KEY NUTRIENTS (%RDA/AI*)	
Beta carotene	2 mg (18%)
Riboflavin	0.2 mg (14%)
Vitamin B$_6$	0.2 mg (14%)
Vitamin C	54 mg (60%)
Folate	75 mcg (19%)
Calcium	276 mg (23%)
Iron	3 mg (37%)
Magnesium	73 mg (17%)
Zinc	1.2 mg (11%)

For more detailed information on RDA and AI, see page 88.

apples

A member of the rose family, the apple has a compartmented core and is thus classified as a pome fruit (the Latin word *pome* means "apple"). Fossil remains have shown that apples were gathered and stored 5,000 years ago, and it is likely that they were already being cultivated in Neolithic times.

The Egyptians grew apples, and invading Roman legions introduced them to Britain. The early colonists brought apples to America from their home country, establishing orchards in Massachusetts and Virginia; these became the foundation for most of the apples grown in the United States today.

nutritional profile

An apple a day provides respectable amounts of both insoluble and soluble fiber. One large apple supplies almost 30 percent of the minimum amount of fiber experts say should be consumed daily. About 81 percent of the fiber in the apple flesh is soluble, most of it presumed to be a type called pectin. Studies indicate that pectin and other soluble fibers are effective in lowering cholesterol levels.

Fresh apples also have some vitamin C and some potassium. When apples are processed (into apple juice or applesauce), however, almost all of their vitamin C is lost (though the potassium is retained). Commercial brands of apple juice are very often fortified with vitamin C—and occasionally with calcium as well.

The fruit is fibrous, juicy, and nonsticky, making it a good tooth-cleaner and gum stimulator (although you should still brush your teeth or rinse your mouth with water after eating an apple because of the acids in the juice).

in the market

There are about 7,500 varieties of apples grown all over the world, and 2,500 in the United States alone. You won't encounter most of these, except in local farmers' markets or at pick-your-own apple farms. In fact, just 16 varieties account for 90 percent of the domestic apple production, and eight of them—Golden Delicious, Granny Smith, Jonathan, McIntosh, Red Delicious, Rome Beauty, Stayman, and York—make up 80 percent.

Braeburn The crisp, aromatic Braeburn blends sweetness and tartness and is just right for snacks and salads. Its color varies from greenish-gold with red sections to nearly solid red.

Cortland This large apple has deep purplish-red skin and snow-white flesh that resists browning. Available primarily in the East and Midwest, the Cortland is good for eating raw and also for baking in pies.

Crispin Also known as Mutsu, the Crispin is a large green apple developed from crossing a Golden Delicious with a Japanese apple called Indo. It is an all-purpose variety, with a firm texture and sweet flavor.

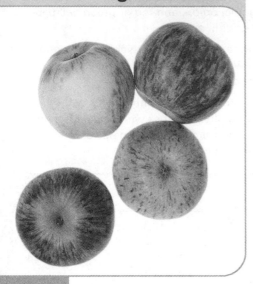

gravensteins

APPLE / 1 large with peel	
Calories	125
Protein (g)	>1
Carbohydrate (g)	32
Dietary fiber (g)	5.7
Total fat (g)	0.8
Saturated fat (g)	0.1
Monounsaturated fat (g)	0
Polyunsaturated fat (g)	0.2
Cholesterol (mg)	0
Potassium (mg)	243
Sodium (mg)	0

KEY NUTRIENTS (%RDA/AI*)	
Vitamin C	12 mg (13%)

*For more detailed information on RDA and AI, see page 88.

Empire The result of crossing the McIntosh with the Red Delicious, the Empire's deep red skin is rather thick, but the crisp texture and sweet-tart taste make it ideal for eating fresh.

Fuji Like fine wine, its flavor improves with age. Fuji's spicy, crisp sweetness makes it excellent fresh or as applesauce. Fuji varies from yellow-green with red highlights to very red.

Gala Gala is heart-shaped and has distinctive yellow-orange skin with red striping. With a crisp, sweet taste that can't be beat, Gala is great in salads.

Golden Delicious Despite its resemblance to the Red Delicious apple in shape and name, the Golden Delicious is an entirely separate variety. It is an all-purpose apple, suitable for baking, eating raw, using in pies, and making applesauce. Its freckled, golden-yellow skin makes it distinctive, as does the fact that its flesh, when sliced, doesn't darken as readily as that of other apples—a virtue that makes it a worthy ingredient in salads.

Granny Smith This pale green apple is originally from Australia, but is now widely grown in this country. It is an all-purpose variety, with a crisp texture and tart flavor.

Gravenstein This distinctive, red-striped apple is used primarily to make commercial applesauce, but it is also sold fresh. Moderately tart, it is an all-purpose apple that is perfect for homemade applesauce.

Idared This all-purpose apple, red-skinned and with a mild flavor, is a favorite in the Northeast and parts of the Midwest.

Jonagold A blend of Jonathan and Golden Delicious apples, Jonagold offers a unique, tangy-sweet flavor. With a yellow-green base and a blush stripe, it is excellent both for eating fresh and for cooking.

Jonathan Deep red with yellow undertones, this is a small- to medium-sized apple, with juicy, firm, yellow flesh. Use it for eating or baking pies, or for making applesauce. It's not a good choice for baking whole because it loses its shape.

Macoun Tart and juicy, the red-green Macoun is excellent eaten fresh, but it arrives late in the year and doesn't keep well.

McIntosh A green-red apple, the McIntosh is a parent variety of many other apples, such as Cortland and Empire. It is very juicy, with a slightly tart flavor. Although it is excellent raw or cooked, the exceptionally smooth texture of the cooked apple may not appeal to some people. McIntosh bruise more easily than other apples and should be handled with care.

Mutsu See Crispin (*opposite page*).

Newtown Pippin A tart green apple, this variety is generally used for cooking, but is also suitable for eating fresh.

Northern Spy This large red-green apple has firm yellow flesh and a tart flavor, making it suitable for pies or for snacking.

Pink Lady Pink lady apples have a sweet-tart taste and firm, crisp flesh. Their skin has a pink blush (hence the name) over yellow. They are good both fresh and for cooking.

serving suggestions

- If you love melted cheese sandwiches, cut the fat and boost the flavor by substituting thick apple slices or grated apple for some of the cheese.

- Offer apple slices or rounds with sweet or savory dips.

- Add thin apple slices to mixed green salads.

- Grate apples into meatloaf, meatball, or burger mixtures to enhance flavor and add moisture.

- Be creative the next time you make applesauce: Include fruits and nuts, such as cranberries, blueberries, chopped pecans, or almonds.

- Glaze meat or poultry with apple cider, but make it sweet and hot by mixing in some mustard, a touch of vinegar, or curry powder.

- Blend prepared horseradish into applesauce to make an unusual condiment for beef.

Red Delicious This familiar bright red apple (which may have yellow undertones) is the most popular variety in the United States, accounting for almost half the domestic crop. It has thin but tough skin, and crisp, juicy, sweet-tasting flesh. Red Delicious is best eaten fresh; when cooked, it disintegrates and loses most of its flavor.

Rhode Island Greening Though it isn't widely available, many apple fanciers consider this green apple the best choice for pies.

Rome Beauty A favorite for baking, the red or red-striped Rome Beauty holds its spherical shape well during cooking, which also brings out its flavor. Eaten fresh, however, it tastes rather bland and mealy.

Stayman This is a good all-purpose apple, with purplish-red skin and white flesh that is mildly tart and juicy.

Winesap As its name suggests, this all-purpose apple—one of the oldest varieties in the United States—has a tangy, winelike flavor. The flesh is firm and juicy, and the skin is a deep red-purple. Winesaps are often used to make apple cider.

York Also known as York Imperial, this variety has a lopsided shape and pinkish-red skin, often dotted with pale spots (which don't affect the quality of the fruit). The flesh is yellow and moderately juicy. Yorks are good baking apples, holding their shape and flavor when cooked.

▶ Availability Most apples are available year round, largely because of "controlled atmosphere" storage (*see "CA Storage," below, left*).

choosing the best

Never buy apples that have not been kept cold, since they can become overripe and mealy in as little as 2 to 3 days, and will also turn brown near the core. After January, almost any apple you buy will probably have been stored in CA after harvesting: Although CA storage slows aging, it does not stop it, and CA-stored apples, once removed from their controlled environment, begin to deteriorate just as quickly as fresh apples do.

Apples should be firm to hard—if you can dent one with your fingers, it will make disappointing eating. Large apples are more likely to be overripe than smaller ones, so pay extra attention to firmness when buying them. Apples should also be well colored for their variety. The skins should be tight, unbroken, and unblemished, although brown freckles or streaks (russeting) are characteristic of some varieties, such as Golden Delicious, and do not affect taste.

▶ When you get home Cold temperatures keep apples in "suspended animation," preventing them from ripening further after they are picked. Because most apples are picked at the peak of ripeness, additional "ripening" actually means "decaying"—and this process is speeded up tenfold when the fruit is not refrigerated. Whether an apple is freshly picked or has emerged from months of cold storage, it must be kept cold or its flesh will degenerate into mushiness.

preparing to use

Wash apples before using them peeled or unpeeled. If peeling, use a vegetable peeler or a sharp paring knife to remove the thinnest possible layer of skin.

Core apples by quartering them and cutting out the semi-circular wedge that contains the seeds; or, core whole apples with an apple corer, an inexpensive utensil consisting of a pointed metal tube affixed to a handle. Insert the tube into either end of the apple, push the corer through, then draw it out again; the core will stay in the tube.

To prevent browning, rub the cut surfaces of apples with a mixture of lemon juice and water, or drop sliced or peeled apples into cold water (with a little lemon juice added to it) as you work.

> ### ➤ phytochemicals in apples
>
> • The skin of red apples contains anthocyanins, natural food pigments that in the test tube, and perhaps in the body, mop up free radicals, particles that can damage our cells.
>
> • Apples are a major dietary source of an antioxidant phytochemical called quercetin. Claims have been made for quercetin that range from cancer protection, to allergy symptom relief, to anticlotting effects. There is no clear evidence yet for any of these benefits.

mini apples

Crab apples Crab apples are tiny (like a big cherry tomato) yellow apples with a reddish blush. They are not eaten fresh like other apples because their flesh is a bit tart and mealy, and there is too high a percentage of core and seeds to flesh. However, they are often used to make jellies and apple butter, probably because they have a high proportion of pectin, the soluble fiber that is not only heart-healthy but helps jellies to jell. They are available in some produce stores, but more often are found at farmstands.

Lady apples Lady apples are petite members of the apple family. They are light green in color, with bright red dabs over part or much of the fruit and are mildly sweet with moderate acidity. Lady apples are good to eat both fresh and cooked.

apricots

These golden, fragrant, delicate fruits originated in China about 4,000 years ago and were transplanted throughout Asia and Europe. In the late 1700s, the Spanish introduced apricots to California, where they were planted in the gardens of Spanish missions. Today, California supplies about 95 percent of the apricots grown in the United States.

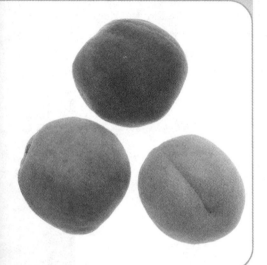

apricots

nutritional profile

The deep gold color of apricots indicates that they contain carotenes, specifically beta carotene, which is converted to vitamin A by the body. Apricots are a good source of vitamin C, fiber, and potassium, with a decent amount of iron (especially dried apricots). About half the apricot crop is canned and is consequently somewhat less nutritious than fresh: Apricots packed in light syrup have double the calories and half the beta carotene and vitamin C of fresh.

For an extra boost of beta carotene and potassium, and as a change from orange or apple juice, try apricot nectar—the juice of fresh apricots. Apricot nectar (which like all nectars has an added sweetener) is only slightly higher in calories than orange juice, and because it is not naturally high in vitamin C, it is usually fortified with this vitamin.

in the market

There are approximately a dozen varieties of apricots: All are similar in taste, but differ somewhat in size and color (which ranges from yellow to deep orange). *Blenheim, Perfection, Katy, Tilton, Patterson,* and *Castlebrite* are among the better-known varieties. There are also some interesting apricot hybrids available:

Aprium This cross between a plumcot and an apricot is more apricot than plum. It looks like a large apricot and has a scant fuzz on the skin.

Plumcot A plumcot is a cross between a plum and an apricot. It is one of several efforts that have been made to develop a fruit with the delicate flavors of the apricot but with the hardiness (and shipability) of a plum. It's shaped more like a plum, but the skin can look like apricot skin.

Pluot This is a cross between a plumcot and a plum; see Plums (*page 477*).

choosing the best

Fully ripe apricots ship poorly, so unless you live near an apricot-growing region, you may have a difficult time finding any ripe ones. (Domestic apricots are available from mid-May through mid-August.) Fruits at this stage of maturity are soft to the touch. You should eat them as soon as possible, as they will not keep. Apricots that still need a day or two of ripening at room temperature should be plump, firm, and orange-gold in color. Don't buy hard fruits that are tinged with green—they will never develop full flavor. When

FRESH APRICOTS / 3	
Calories	50
Protein (g)	2
Carbohydrate (g)	12
Dietary fiber (g)	2.5
Total fat (g)	0.4
Saturated fat (g)	0
Monounsaturated fat (g)	0.2
Polyunsaturated fat (g)	0.1
Cholesterol (mg)	0
Potassium (mg)	311
Sodium (mg)	0

KEY NUTRIENTS (%RDA/AI*)	
Beta carotene	1.6 mg (15%)
Vitamin C	11 mg (12%)

*For more detailed information on RDA and AI, see page 88.

choosing plumcots or apriums, look for firm, fragrant fruit without bruising.

▶ **When you get home** If you buy apricots that are not quite ripe, store them in a paper bag at room temperature, away from heat or direct sunlight, for 2 to 3 days. Once ripe, they may be stored in the refrigerator, where they will keep a day or two at most. Don't wash the fruits until you're ready to eat them.

preparing to use

Rinse apricots under cold running water before using them. Ripe apricots are soft and delicate, so if you need to peel them for a recipe, do so carefully. Place the fruits in boiling water for 15 to 20 seconds, then remove them and cool them under cold water. Use a knife to pull away their skin; it should slip right off. To halve apricots, cut down to the pit around the longitudinal seam and twist the two halves to separate them; discard the pit. Dip peeled or cut-up apricots into diluted lemon juice to keep them from browning.

serving suggestions

• Try sliced fresh apricots in a sandwich where you would ordinarily use tomatoes.

• For a healthful jam, cook dried apricots with apple juice until very soft and tender, then puree—no sweetening is needed.

• For a quick salsa: Combine chopped fresh or canned apricots with chili peppers, lime juice, chopped onion, and ground cumin. Serve alongside chicken or fish.

dried apricots

When fresh apricots are dried, their vitamin C content is reduced, and their calorie content (compared with the same weight of fresh) is increased. However, in their dried form, apricots turn into a nutrient-rich food, supplying a concentrated source of iron, potassium, beta carotene, and fiber.

Processors often treat dried apricots with sulfur dioxide to help preserve their rich orange color. Sulfites, however, can cause severe allergic reactions in people who are sensitive to them. When sulfites are used, government regulations stipulate that they be listed on the label or package. Unsulfured apricots can be found in health-food stores; they are brown, not orange.

The two types of dried apricots that are available are California-style, which come as dried halves; and Turkish, which are smaller and whole. The Turkish type are a bit sweeter.

¼ cup (about 9 halves)

Calories	77
Protein (g)	1
Carbohydrate (g)	20
Dietary fiber (g)	2.9
Total fat (g)	0.2
Saturated fat (g)	0
Monounsaturated fat (g)	0.1
Polyunsaturated fat (g)	0
Cholesterol (mg)	0
Potassium (mg)	448
Sodium (mg)	3

KEY NUTRIENTS (%RDA/AI*)

Beta carotene	1.4 mg	(13%)
Iron	1.5 mg	(19%)

*For more detailed information on RDA and AI, see page 88.

artichokes

The artichoke has a noble history. Pliny, the early Roman scholar and writer, noted that it garnered more esteem—and fetched a higher price—than any other garden vegetable. It was avidly cultivated in 15th-century Florence and was reputedly taken to France by Catherine de Médici, wife of Henry II. The French and Italians, along with the Spanish, continue to be the leading growers—and consumers—of artichokes. European immigrants brought artichokes to the United States in the 19th century, first to Louisiana and later to the midcoastal region of California, where the cool, foggy climate has proven ideal for their cultivation—fully 99 percent of the U.S. commercial crop is grown in this area.

A single artichoke is actually an unopened flower bud from a thistle-like plant with the Latin name of *Cynara scolymus*. Each green, cone-shaped bud consists of several parts: overlapping outer leaves that are tough and inedible at the tip, but fleshy and tender at the base; an inedible choke, or thistle, which is enclosed within a light-colored cone of immature leaves; and a round, firm-fleshed base. Although the base is often referred to as the "heart" of an artichoke, it is more accurately called the bottom. Minus the leaves and choke, it is the part that you work your way toward when eating a large artichoke. What is commercially packaged as an artichoke heart, however, is the tender central portion of a tiny artichoke that has no choke—it includes the bottom with some of the innermost leaves attached.

artichokes

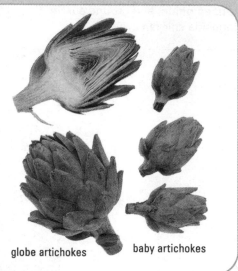

globe artichokes   baby artichokes

ARTICHOKE 1 medium, cooked	
Calories	60
Protein (g)	4
Carbohydrate (g)	13
Dietary fiber (g)	6.5
Total fat (g)	0.2
Saturated fat (g)	0
Monounsaturated fat (g)	0
Polyunsaturated fat (g)	0.1
Cholesterol (mg)	0
Potassium (mg)	425
Sodium (mg)	114

KEY NUTRIENTS (%RDA/AI*)	
Vitamin C	12 mg (13%)
Folate	61 mcg (15%)
Iron	1.6 mg (19%)
Magnesium	72 mg (17%)

For more detailed information on RDA and AI, see page 88.

nutritional profile

Low in sodium and virtually fat-free, artichokes are a good source of vitamin C, iron, potassium, magnesium, and folate. They are also an especially good source of dietary fiber. A 2-ounce serving (the bottom of one big artichoke) has only 26 calories, but 3 grams of fiber.

in the market

There are probably as many as 50 different artichoke varieties grown in warm climates around the world, but only the *Green Globe*, an Italian type, is cultivated commercially in the United States. Ideally, it has a spherical or slightly elongated bud that is solidly green (many European artichoke varieties have purplish or reddish leaves) and grows to about 4 inches in diameter.

Artichokes vary greatly in size. Differences are not related to quality or maturity, but are determined by the part of the stalk the buds grow on—large ones on the center stalk, smaller ones on side branches, and *"baby" artichokes* (weighing about 2 ounces) at the base. The largest artichokes—entree-sized specimens weighing a pound or more—are best when stuffed with a savory filling and served hot or cold; the medium-sized ones are recommended for eating with sauces as an appetizer; and the babies—which are completely edible when properly trimmed—are often marinated and served in salads and in hot or cold antipastos.

The shape of this vegetable also varies. While spherical and oval-shaped artichokes are preferred for market, a more cylindrical shape is quite common. Even conical-shaped artichokes have been produced.

choosing the best

Whatever its size or shape, an artichoke should be compact and heavy for its size, with leaves, or scales, that are fleshy, thick, firm, and tightly closed; if the leaves look dry and woody, or have begun to spread apart, the artichoke is past its prime. Check the stem end for tiny holes—these are signs of worm damage, which will probably be even more extensive inside the artichoke.

Artichokes are harvested year round. The crop peaks in the spring—March through May—and again, to a lesser extent, in October. Spring artichokes should be a soft green; those picked in the fall and winter tend to be olive green and may have bronze-tipped leaves or a slightly blistered, whitish outer surface. This "winter-kissed" effect, as it is called by the growers, is the result of exposure to a light frost in the fields; it does not affect the taste or tenderness of the artichoke. Don't, however, confuse blackened or wilted leaves, or dark bruised spots, with the normal bronzing of frost-touched artichokes.

If you're not sure about the freshness of an artichoke, squeeze it: You'll hear a squeaky sound if the leaves are still plump and crisp.

▶ When you get home Although artichokes appear hardy, they are quite perishable; store them in the refrigerator, in a plastic bag, for no more than 4 or 5 days. Do not rinse or wash the vegetables (or cut or trim them) before storing, as this could cause them to become moldy.

preparing to use

If artichokes are to be served whole with a dipping sauce, they need little preparation—it's the eating itself, of course, that is labor-intensive.

Wash each artichoke under cold running water or hold it by the stem and swish it vigorously in a basin of water. Cut off the top inch of the artichoke, which consists of inedible leaf tips, with a large, sharp knife. Clip the sharp tips off the remaining outer leaves using kitchen shears. Pull off any short, coarse leaves from the bottom and cut off about 1 inch of the tough stem. With a paring knife, peel the remaining stem. Don't cut an artichoke with a carbon-steel knife; it will turn the cut parts black. Rub the cut parts with lemon juice to keep them from darkening or drop the prepared artichoke into a bowl of cold water to which a tablespoon of lemon juice or vinegar has been added. (This is often called "acidulated water" in recipes.)

serving suggestions

• Add quartered artichoke hearts to baked pastas, chicken or tuna casseroles, potato salad, or rice pilaf.

• Puree cooked artichoke bottoms and green peas, season with garlic and lemon juice, and toss with freshly cooked pasta.

• For a dip, puree cooked artichoke bottoms with reduced-fat cream cheese, softened sun-dried tomatoes, and chopped fresh basil. Serve with crudités.

When an artichoke flowers, it produces a beautiful purple thistle.

For small or baby artichokes, cut off the stems as well as the top parts of the leaves. Remove the outer leaves by bending them back until they snap (the meaty portion will remain attached); stop when you reach the inner, pale green leaves. Pare the outer layers from the artichoke bottoms. Halve each vegetable lengthwise, scoop out the thin center petals, then slice the artichoke halves lengthwise.

Some recipes call for the choke to be removed to form an artichoke "cup" for stuffing. To make artichoke cups, prepare the vegetable as for serving whole with the following exception: Cut the stem flush with the base so the artichoke will sit upright when you serve it. Boil, steam, or microwave, then let stand until cool enough to handle. Spread the outer leaves apart with your fingers, pull out the petals covering the choke, and then use a teaspoon to scrape out the choke. The artichoke can be stuffed and served as is, or baked.

Some recipes require only artichoke bottoms (though the recipe will probably refer to them as "hearts"). To prepare artichoke bottoms, prepare and cook a whole artichoke. Remove all the leaves from the cooked artichoke (you can eat them separately or scrape off the flesh from the base of each leaf to incorporate in the dish). Discard the thin petals covering the choke, then scrape off the choke with a paring knife. Trim around the bottom with a knife to neaten it.

serving suggestions

Instead of dipping artichoke leaves in melted butter, try one of these ideas:

• *Japanese-style dip:* Combine miso (soybean paste), lemon juice, wasabi powder, and a dash of sesame oil.

• *Garlic dip:* Cook several garlic cloves along with the artichokes, then mash them to a paste with a little olive oil and lemon juice.

• *Lemon-pepper dip:* Puree silken tofu with lemon juice and lots of black pepper.

• *Balsamic-mustard dip:* Combine balsamic vinegar and Dijon mustard with a bit of olive oil (you can also make this with no oil).

how to eat an artichoke

When you are served a whole artichoke, remove the outer leaves, one at a time, beginning at the bottom. Pull off a leaf and dip its fleshy base into the sauce. Place the bottom half of the leaf, concave-side down, in your mouth and draw it between your teeth so that you scrape off the tender flesh and pull out the fibrous portion of the leaf.

Continue eating the fleshy leaves until you encounter the inner petals, which are thin (like flower petals), rose-colored, and bunched to a point at the top. The bases of these can be bitten off rather than scraped through your teeth. Underneath the petals you'll find the choke, a tuft of slender hay-colored fibers resembling corn silk. Pull or scrape off the choke to expose the artichoke bottom, which resembles the center of a daisy (the artichoke is a member of the daisy family). That is your reward—dense and velvety, the entire bottom can be cut into quarters, dipped, and eaten.

asparagus

The slender, regal asparagus plant gets it name from the Greek word (*asparagos*) for "sprout" or "shoot." Asparagus was a highly sought delicacy in ancient Rome, with emperors maintaining special asparagus fleets to gather and transport the choicest spears for the empire. Referred to as the aristocrat of vegetables and dubbed the "food of kings" by King Louis XIV of France, asparagus has enjoyed an international popularity that continues today.

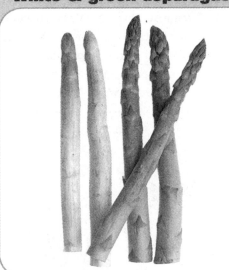

white & green asparagus

nutritional profile

A member of the lily family and thus closely related to garlic, onions, and leeks, asparagus offers an admirable variety of nutrients. Low in fat and high in fiber, asparagus is a good source of iron, vitamin C, and B vitamins—most exceptionally folate.

in the market

Green Green asparagus is the primary asparagus on the market and the only one grown on a commercial scale in this country. *Martha Washington* and *Mary Washington* are the principal varieties.

Purple A purple variety of asparagus called *Viola* contains about 20 percent more sugar than other varieties. The large burgundy spears have a creamy, white interior. Tender, with a sweet, mild, nutty flavor, purple asparagus can be used just like other asparagus.

White White (actually cream- or ivory-colored) asparagus is planted under heaps of soil, which is piled on the plants as they grow, thereby blocking the sunlight necessary for them to produce chlorophyll. The process yields spears that are more fibrous than the green ones and have a stronger, slightly bitter flavor. While you can find fresh white asparagus in the United States at gourmet food shops and local markets, it remains more popular in Europe. Some domestic asparagus growers, however, cultivate white asparagus specifically for canning.

▶ Availability There was a time when asparagus was a spring delicacy, but with vegetables available from around the world, year round, this is no longer so. Naturally when the asparagus in the market is imported, it will be more costly than locally grown, in-season vegetables.

choosing the best

After harvesting, asparagus deteriorates rapidly unless it is kept cold. In stores, therefore, asparagus should either be refrigerated or displayed on trays with the stalks standing in several inches of cold water. In outdoor markets, the trays should be shaded from the sun.

The best-quality spears are firm yet tender, with deep green or purplish tips that are closed and compact; partially open and wilted tips are the most

ASPARAGUS / 1 cup cooked	
Calories	43
Protein (g)	5
Carbohydrate (g)	8
Dietary fiber (g)	2.9
Total fat (g)	0.6
Saturated fat (g)	0.1
Monounsaturated fat (g)	0
Polyunsaturated fat (g)	0.2
Cholesterol (mg)	0
Potassium (mg)	288
Sodium (mg)	20

KEY NUTRIENTS (%RDA/AI*)	
Thiamin	0.2 mg (18%)
Riboflavin	0.2 mg (17%)
Niacin	1.9 mg (12%)
Vitamin B$_6$	0.2 mg (13%)
Vitamin C	19 mg (22%)
Folate	263 mcg (66%)
Iron	1.3 mg (16%)

For more detailed information on RDA and AI, see page 88.

obvious signs of aging. Avoid excessively sandy spears (sand grains can lodge within the tips and be difficult to wash out). Stalks should stand straight, be green for most of their length, and have a nicely rounded shape; flat or twisted stalks are often tough and stringy.

Personal preference abounds and some people prefer very thin asparagus (often called "pencil grass"), while others prefer the thicker stalks. Size is not directly related to quality, but stalks that measure at least ½ inch in diameter at the base are usually preferable. Asparagus is usually sold in bundles, but if you can buy it loose, select spears of uniform size, which will cook evenly. When deciding on quantity, remember that asparagus loses about half of its total weight once it's been trimmed and cooked. Buy at least ½ pound per person.

▶ **When you get home** Keep fresh asparagus cold to preserve its tenderness and as much of its natural sweetness and vitamin C as possible. When kept at room temperature, asparagus loses roughly half of its vitamin C content within 2 days. It also loses some of its residual sugars (which impart flavor), and the stalks become tougher and stringier.

preparing to use

Wash asparagus in cool running water. If the tips have any sand on them, dunk them in and out of water, then rinse thoroughly.

To trim asparagus before cooking, hold a spear in both hands, closer to the tough woody end than to the tip. Bend the stalk until it snaps. It will naturally snap at the place where the asparagus begins to turn woody. Be sure to save the trimmings to throw into soups, stocks, or broths.

the asparagus syndrome

Eating asparagus can cause some people to temporarily excrete urine with an odd smell. About 40 percent of the population has a gene that causes this harmless reaction, which occurs when a sulfur compound in asparagus is converted during digestion into a closely related compound that has the same distinctive sulfurous odor.

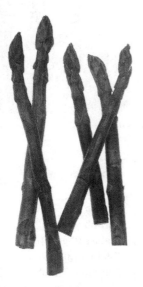

Purple asparagus turns green when cooked.

serving suggestions

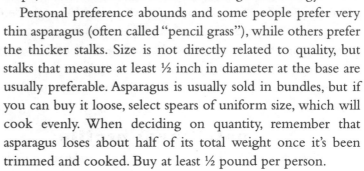

• Roast asparagus with a bit of olive oil, in a 450° oven. Serve drizzled with balsamic vinegar.

• Wrap asparagus in foil with slivered garlic, oregano, rosemary, or thyme, and a drizzle of olive oil. Bake until tender.

• Cook asparagus until tender and mash along with avocado to make an asparagus guacamole.

• Serve steamed asparagus with simple, light seasonings such as lemon juice, an herb vinaigrette, or a light mustard sauce.

• Puree leftover asparagus with some broth and cooked rice to make a low-fat "cream" of asparagus soup.

• Top a cheese pizza with cooked asparagus spears.

avocados

A smooth, creamy texture and a mild, nutty flavor are the hallmarks of the avocado, a tropical fruit that is often considered a "vegetable" because of its unique flavor and the ways in which it can be prepared. A favorite of the Aztecs, the avocado is native to Central America and has been cultivated for thousands of years. Avocados were first cultivated in the United States in the mid-1800s in Florida and California, where domestic avocado production still thrives. California produces nearly 90 percent of the domestic crop, and the two states together provide a year-round supply that adds up to the world's largest commercial production.

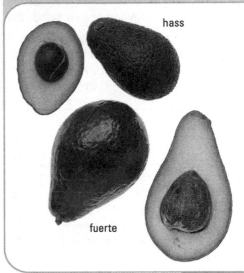

avocados

hass

fuerte

nutritional profile

Avocados provide ample amounts of folate and good amounts of fiber, potassium, niacin, and vitamin B_6. Although the avocado is exceptionally high in fat, its fat is mostly monounsaturated. The only other fruit that has comparable amounts of this beneficial fat is the olive. Research shows that when monounsaturated fat is substituted for saturated fat, it helps to lower LDL ("bad") cholesterol levels. Still, because they are high in calories, it is prudent to avoid eating large amounts of these velvety, nutrient-rich fruits.

in the market

Hass avocados are the most popular variety by far, but some two dozen avocado varieties grow in California and Florida. They range in size from a few ounces to several pounds, with skins bright green to black, some smooth, some pebbly, in texture. The Florida fruit tend to be larger and less costly, but ounce for ounce they contain two-thirds of the calories of their smaller California cousins and half the fat. (Though because they are considerably higher in water content, they are also lower in flavor.)

Bacon These medium-size, mild-flavored avocados have smooth, thin, green skin and yellow-green flesh. They range in weight from 6 to 12 ounces.

Cocktail avocados These miniature avocados are Fuerte avocados that are picked when they are only 2 to 3 inches long. They are shaped somewhat like pickles and have smooth, dark green skin.

Fuerte A popular California variety, the Fuerte can weigh up to a pound, has a more pronounced pear shape, a milder flavor (and higher water content), and a thinner, smoother skin than the Hass.

Gwen Similar in taste and texture to Hass avocados, Gwens are slightly larger with a plump, oval shape, green pebbly skin, and gold-green, creamy flesh. They range in size from 6 to 15 ounces.

Hass The most popular California variety (about 90 percent of the state's production), Hass avocados weigh about half a pound and have a thick, pebbled skin that changes from green to purplish-black as the fruits ripen.

HASS AVOCADO / ½ medium	
Calories	153
Protein (g)	2
Carbohydrate (g)	6
Dietary fiber (g)	4.2
Total fat (g)	15
Saturated fat (g)	2.2
Monounsaturated fat (g)	9.7
Polyunsaturated fat (g)	1.8
Cholesterol (mg)	0
Potassium (mg)	548
Sodium (mg)	10

KEY NUTRIENTS (%RDA/AI*)	
Niacin	1.7 mg (10%)
Vitamin B_6	0.2 mg (14%)
Folate	57 mcg (14%)
Iron	1.0 mg (13%)

*For more detailed information on RDA and AI, see page 88.

Lula (Lulu) These are large (almost a pound) and are grown in Texas.

Pinkerton This long, pear-shaped fruit has a small pit, medium-thick, slightly pebbly green skin and is easy to peel. The Pinkerton has creamy, pale green flesh and is relatively large in size, ranging from 8 to 18 ounces.

Reed Large and round in shape, the thick, green, slightly pebbly skin of this avocado covers buttery flesh. The skin on Reeds remains green even as the fruit ripens. They range in size from 8 to 18 ounces.

Zutano This pear-shaped avocado is easily recognizable by its shiny, yellow-green skin. Its flavor is mild and light. Zutanos range in size from 6 to 14 ounces.

choosing the best

Select heavy, unblemished fruit. Most markets sell hard, unripe avocados, which should be bought 3 to 6 days ahead of when they are to be used to allow time for ripening. But if an avocado yields slightly to gentle pressure, it is already ripe enough to slice. If pressing the fruit leaves a small dent, it is too ripe to slice, but is suitable for mashing. If pressing leaves a large dent, the fruit is overripe, and will have black, unusable flesh.

▶ **When you get home** If avocados need ripening, you can speed up the process by placing them in a paper bag with an apple or banana. Never put hard avocados in the refrigerator, for they will ripen very slowly.

preparing to use

To pit an avocado, cut it lengthwise or crosswise all the way around and twist the two halves apart. Use a teaspoon to pry out the large seed. To skin the fruit, place the halves face down and pull off the peel like a banana skin. (If the flesh is very soft, scoop it out of the hull with a spoon.) If the skin is too tough to peel easily, use a paring knife to score it into peelable strips. Slice the flesh thinly or chop it into chunks.

The flesh of a cut avocado, exposed to the air, turns dark within a few minutes. This process does not affect nutrition or flavor, but makes the flesh look less appetizing. To delay darkening, rub slices with lemon or lime juice, and add the juice to mashed avocado. Plastic wrap pressed down onto mashed avocado, with all the air bubbles pressed out, will deter darkening.

bananas

Bananas are readily available all year, are convenient for carrying in a lunchbag or a briefcase, have a peel that comes off easily with no mess, and can be purchased (and consumed) at several stages of ripeness. They are also highly nutritious and are easily digested by virtually everyone, including infants and the elderly. It's no wonder that Americans have made bananas their favorite fruit. In fact, Americans consume about 33 pounds per person, on average, each year.

Bananas are not grown commercially in the United States; rather, they are cultivated in tropical regions such as Central and South America, and are shipped to northern ports on a grand scale. Because of their abundance, intense competition among growers, and cheap land and labor, bananas remain moderately priced.

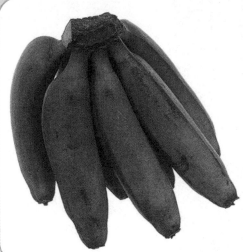

red bananas

nutritional profile

Bananas have earned the status of an ideal food. Since they contain less water than most other fruits, their carbohydrate content, by weight, is higher—which is one of the reasons that bananas have become the snack of choice for endurance athletes. Along with helping to replenish the body's store of carbohydrates, bananas provide substantial amounts of potassium, a mineral that is lost during bouts of physical activity, yet is vital for controlling the body's fluid balance. Potassium also is required to regulate heartbeat and blood pressure, and, in older people, it may help to reduce the risk of fatal stroke. An excellent source of vitamin B_6, bananas also contain a type of soluble fiber called pectin, which helps to lower LDL ("bad") cholesterol levels.

in the market

There are more than 500 varieties of bananas, although only a few make it to the market. By far the most common banana in this country is the Cavendish, though it is certainly never labeled as such. A growing number of markets also sell so-called *"finger bananas"*—an umbrella term for a variety of small bananas.

Baby (Niño) These short, chubby bananas, sometimes sold as *Lady Finger* bananas, average 3 inches in length. When ripe, the skin is bright yellow. They are very sweet and creamy.

Burro Squatty and slightly square at the edges, these bananas are slightly tangy and lemony. When ripe, the fruit is soft and the skin is yellow with black spots. Also called Horse, Hog, or Orinoco bananas.

Cavendish This is the familiar yellow banana sold in U.S. supermarkets. There are also other sizes of Cavendish, including Dwarf and Giant, though they are difficult to find.

BANANA / 1 medium	
Calories	109
Protein (g)	1
Carbohydrate (g)	28
Dietary fiber (g)	2.8
Total fat (g)	0.6
Saturated fat (g)	0.2
Monounsaturated fat (g)	0.1
Polyunsaturated fat (g)	0.1
Cholesterol (mg)	0
Potassium (mg)	467
Sodium (mg)	1

KEY NUTRIENTS (%RDA/AI*)	
Vitamin B_6	0.7 mg (40%)
Vitamin C	11 mg (12%)

*For more detailed information on RDA and AI, see page 88.

Ice Cream (Blue Java) These rather chubby bananas can grow to up to 7 inches long. The skin is a blotchy, silvery-blue and the flesh is creamy white. The flavor is somewhat like rich ice cream.

Manzano Also called apple bananas, these short chubby bananas have a mild flavor reminiscent of apples (and some say strawberries). The skin turns black when fully ripe.

Red bananas These sweet bananas have purple or maroon skin when ripe. Their flesh is creamy white tinged with pink or orange.

choosing the best

The taste and texture of a banana is directly related to its stage of ripeness. The carbohydrates in green bananas are primarily starches that convert to sugar as the fruits ripen and turn yellow. Very green bananas are hard and have an astringent taste, whereas fully ripened yellow bananas are soft, sweet, and creamy. Bananas that are yellow and lightly flecked with brown spots will be at their peak flavor, but many people prefer the texture and less-sweet taste of bananas that with green tips and no freckling. There's no harm in eating a less-than-ripe banana, except that if it is very green, it may be hard to digest.

Choose bananas according to how—and when—you'll eat them. If you prefer fully ripe, brown-flecked bananas, and the store carries only greenish ones, you'll need to shop several days in advance of the time you plan to eat the fruit. If you prefer bananas just yellow, a day or two will suffice to ripen

plantains

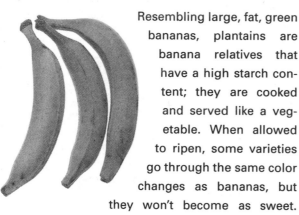

Resembling large, fat, green bananas, plantains are banana relatives that have a high starch content; they are cooked and served like a vegetable. When allowed to ripen, some varieties go through the same color changes as bananas, but they won't become as sweet. Nutritionally, they are similar to bananas. They are a good source of potassium, vitamin C, and vitamin B_6. Surprisingly, plantains also contain beta carotene (unusual in a noncolorful fruit), with ½ cup cooked containing enough to provide 5 percent of the RDA for vitamin A—compared with 1 percent in the same amount of raw bananas.

Plantains are usually available in Hispanic markets—where they may be labeled *plátanos*—or in urban supermarkets. They may appear bruised, but as long as they are firm and their skin is intact, they are fine to eat. You can use them as you would potatoes—either as a side dish or as an addition to soups and stews. Plantain skins are thick and can sometimes be difficult to peel. With a paring knife, make two lengthwise slits through the skin, but not into the flesh. Slip your thumbs under the cut skin and pull the peel apart and off.

Traditionally, plantains are fried, but this method will increase their fat content considerably. Instead, try baking green plantains in their skins—first, trim off the tips, slit the skin lengthwise, then bake in a 375° oven until a fork will easily pierce the flesh (about 40 minutes). Or, add peeled, sliced plantains to stir-fries.

greenish ones. Don't buy any that have a dull, grayish cast; these may have been stored at very cold temperatures, and will not ripen properly.

Bananas should be plump, firm, and brightly colored. Look for unblemished fruit: Occasional brown spots on the skin are normal, but sunken, moist-looking dark areas will likely show up as bruises on the fruit. Bananas should have their stem ends and skins intact: A split skin or stem may become an entry point for contamination. There's no quality difference between small and large fruit. Bananas bruise easily, so handle them with care.

▶ **When you get home** Bananas that require further ripening should be left at room temperature, but away from heat or direct sun. To speed ripening, place them in a plastic or paper bag; you can also put an apple in the bag with the bananas to hasten the process (the apple, however, will overripen to a mealy mush). Once ripened to your liking, bananas can be held at room temperature for about a day or two. Then, you can store them in the refrigerator to slow down ripening. Although the skins of refrigerated bananas will turn dark, the fruits will remain perfectly edible. (You can keep refrigerated bananas for up to 2 weeks.) You should never refrigerate unripe bananas, however: The exposure to cold interrupts their ripening cycle, and it will not resume even if the fruits are returned to room temperature.

You can salvage an overabundance of overripe bananas by peeling them, wrapping them whole or in chunks in plastic wrap, and freezing them. Eat them frozen (a sweet treat in summer) or thaw them and use in baking.

preparing to use

When peeling and slicing bananas that you won't be serving immediately, dip them into lemon, lime, or orange juice to slow browning.

serving suggestions

- Add bananas to stews, soups, and pasta sauces. They add a slight sweetness and help thicken the sauce.

- Make a banana salsa for poultry, meat, or fish: Dice bananas and combine with onion, red bell peppers, honey, and lime juice.

- Bake bananas in their skin, then peel and toss in a brown sugar–lime sauce.

- Stir mashed bananas with sautéed onion, curry spices, and yogurt to make a sweet-savory accompaniment for Indian food.

a tree that's not a tree

Despite their elongated shape and distinctive packaging, bananas are actually a type of berry, and banana "trees" are really huge plants botanically classified as herbs. The plants can grow anywhere from 15 to 30 feet high and have a slender "trunk" made up of tightly wrapped layers of leaves—making them the largest plants in the world without a woody stem. Yet some varieties of banana trees are very fragile; a strong wind can wipe out a growing field in minutes.

Each plant consists of huge leaves—so large that they are used to thatch roofs and make umbrellas in some parts of the tropics. The plant develops a single stem and bud that sustains rows of tiny flowers, each one of which becomes an individual banana, called a "finger." A cluster of 10 to 20 fingers, called "hands," grow out and upward so that they appear to be upside down. One banana plant produces 7 to 9 hands every 6 to 8 months.

barley

One of the first crops cultivated by man, barley has been used as a food, a medicine, and as a form of currency since biblical times. Today, barley ranks as one of the most important cereal crops; because it grows well in a range of climatic conditions, from the cold of Scotland to the heat of Ethiopia, it has become a major food staple in many parts of the world. But most of the barley cultivated in the United States is not eaten directly as a food; rather, it is either converted into malt for beer production or used as food for animals. More flavorful and chewy than white rice, though not as strongly flavored as brown rice, this versatile grain deserves a place in the kitchen of the health-oriented cook.

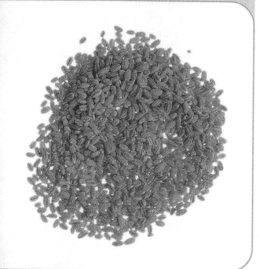

pearl barley

nutritional profile

A high-carbohydrate food, barley is rich in fiber, particularly the soluble fibers—beta glucan and pectin—that may help lower LDL ("bad") cholesterol, and possibly blood pressure. Some forms of barley in which the bran is removed (pearl barley, for example), supply fewer nutrients, while hulled barley, the form of the grain in which the bran is left intact, has retained more of its vitamins and minerals and has more nutritional value. A moderate source of protein (it lacks the essential amino acid lysine), barley is a good source of B vitamins (especially thiamin), as well as iron, zinc, and the antioxidant mineral selenium.

in the market

Most of the barley eaten in the United States has been milled to remove the bran. It is possible, however, to find less-refined forms, mostly at health-food stores.

Flakes (flaked barley) Like the rolled oats they resemble, barley flakes are grains that have been flattened. They are usually cooked and offered as a hot cereal, but they can also be mixed into muesli and baked goods.

Flour See Flour, Nonwheat (*page 324*).

Grits Most people associate the term grits with southern hominy grits, which are cracked white corn. However, other grains that are cracked to various degrees of fineness are also sold as grits (though in the case of wheat, the "grits" are known as bulgur). Barley grits are barley grains that have been toasted and then cracked. They can be cooked and served in place of rice or breakfast cereal.

Hulled This form of barley is not as widely available as the other types, but its superior nutrient content makes it worth seeking out (try a health-food store). Because only the outer, inedible husk (called the spikelet), and not the bran, is removed, hulled barley is rich in dietary fiber. It also contains more iron and trace minerals than pearl barley—and more than four times

PEARL BARLEY 1 cup cooked	
Calories	193
Protein (g)	4
Carbohydrate (g)	44
Dietary fiber (g)	6.0
Total fat (g)	0.7
Saturated fat (g)	0.2
Monounsaturated fat (g)	0.1
Polyunsaturated fat (g)	0.3
Cholesterol (mg)	0
Potassium (mg)	146
Sodium (mg)	5

KEY NUTRIENTS (%RDA/AI*)	
Thiamin	0.1 mg (11%)
Niacin	3.2 mg (20%)
Vitamin B_6	0.2 mg (11%)
Iron	2.1 mg (26%)
Selenium	14 mcg (25%)
Zinc	1.3 mg (12%)

*For more detailed information on RDA and AI, see page 88.

the thiamin. The grains are brown, and they take longer to cook than pearl barley. Hulled barley has a pronounced flavor, which makes it an appealing ingredient in hearty, country-style soups and stews.

Pasta See Pasta, Nonwheat (*page 442*).

Pearl (pearled) To produce these uniform, ivory-colored granules, the barley grains are scoured six times during milling to completely remove their double outer husk and their bran layer. Unfortunately, as with white rice, this process also removes nutrients. The thorough milling, however, shortens the grain's cooking time considerably. Pearl barley has a delicate nutlike taste that readily absorbs the flavors of its companion ingredients in soups, salads, and side dishes.

Pot barley (Scotch barley) A less-refined version than pearl, pot barley is milled just three times, so that part of the bran layer remains. It is usually added to soups and stews. Although some supermarkets carry this form, it is more likely to be found in health-food stores.

Quick-cooking Sometimes sold as instant barley, this barley has been pressed to flatten it slightly and presteamed to cut cooking time from about 45 minutes for regular pearl barley to only 10 minutes. It is as nutritious as the regular pearl barley.

Unhulled Whole barley grains in their tough outer husk can be found in some health-food stores and are good for making barley sprouts (*see Sprouts, page 543*).

choosing the best

As with any grain product, buy barley in well-wrapped packages. If buying in bulk, buy from a store with good turnover.

serving suggestions

- Use barley in place of rice in pilafs and risottos.
- Cook barley flakes, grits, or instant barley to make a hot breakfast cereal.
- Use barley as a stuffing for cabbage rolls, bell peppers, or hollowed-out winter squash.
- Try a Polish soup called krupnik, which combines barley with dried mushrooms, potatoes, and dill.
- Toss cooked barley with sliced mushrooms, chopped tomatoes, or slivered bell peppers and a little oil and vinegar. Add diced cooked turkey or tuna, if you like.
- Make a pudding by cooking barley in a mixture of milk and water sweetened with a little honey. Stir in chopped dried fruits and nuts.

malted barley

Much of the barley grown in the United States is malted; some malted barley is sold as a cereal, but generally it is used to make alcoholic beverages. Malt is made by soaking whole barley grains—including the husks—for several days under controlled conditions so that they germinate (sprout). During the soaking, the protein contained in the bran of the barley is converted into enzymes that change the starches to sugars. Then the barley is dried to prevent further sprouting. Theoretically, this process would work with any grain, but barley is well suited to malting because the bran layer is particularly rich in proteins that form many complex enzymes in the sprouting process. The conversion of starch to sugar creates the conditions necessary for fermentation by yeast, which produces alcohol.

beans, dried

Dried beans have supported human life for thousands of years, beginning with prehistoric tribes. Roman armies relied on them, because they were easy to store and transport, but the general populace in ancient Rome also admired beans. In fact, so honored were beans that prominent Roman families derived their surnames from the Latin names for legumes. For example, Cicero is from *Cicer arietinum* or chick-peas, and Fabius is from *Vicia faba*, or fava beans. Throughout the Middle Ages, these legumes were a staple food of northern European countries. In the New World, they became an important protein source when game was scarce. From this rich history, a wide range of bean-centered cuisines has arisen.

Beans are legumes (also sometimes referred to as "pulses"), an extensive family of plants distinguished by their seed-bearing pods. Both the edible pods and the seeds of these plants are called beans. There are some beans that are eaten pod and all (*see Beans, Fresh, page 183*) and some where only the inner seed is eaten. By and large, the seeds of most beans are eaten in their fully mature, dried form. In the United States and Canada, almost all the dried beans we eat (excluding the soybean) are descendants of the common bean that was first cultivated in South and Central America over 7,000 years ago.

Other legume relatives of beans include Lentils (*page 378*), Peas (*dried, page 460; fresh, page 461*), and Peanuts (*page 452*).

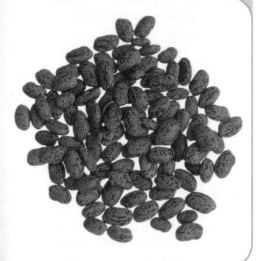

pinto beans

nutritional profile

Once considered mundane, beans have finally emerged from their status as "poor man's meat" to extraordinarily versatile and adaptable superstars in both the nutritional and culinary arenas. Robust, versatile, and full of texture, beans are rich in complex carbohydrates, low-fat protein, fiber, B vitamins, and minerals.

Beans are particularly rich in soluble fiber, which is thought to help reduce the risk of heart disease by lowering LDL ("bad") cholesterol levels. The insoluble fiber in dried beans helps speed up the passage of food through the intestine and thereby improves regularity. The ample fiber content of dried beans also supports weight-control efforts by contributing to satiety (feeling full). Even small servings can fill you up quickly.

Beans are also an excellent source of hearty, low-fat plant protein (without the harmful saturated fat and cholesterol associated with meat). To illustrate the advantage of plant-based protein in beans, compare 3 ounces of cooked kidney beans (about ½ cup) with the equivalent serving of broiled sirloin. The beans offer about 8 grams of protein (for 112 calories), yet contain no cholesterol and virtually no fat. The beef supplies about 25 grams of protein,

PINTO BEANS ½ cup cooked	
Calories	117
Protein (g)	7
Carbohydrate (g)	22
Dietary fiber (g)	7.4
Total fat (g)	0.4
Saturated fat (g)	0.1
Monounsaturated fat (g)	0.1
Polyunsaturated fat (g)	0.2
Cholesterol (mg)	0
Potassium (mg)	400
Sodium (mg)	2

KEY NUTRIENTS (%RDA/AI*)	
Thiamin	0.2 mg (13%)
Folate	147 mcg (37%)
Iron	2.2 mg (28%)
Magnesium	47 mg (11%)
Selenium	6.1 mcg (11%)

*For more detailed information on RDA and AI, see page 88.

but with it comes 8.5 grams of fat (more than one-third of which is saturated fat), 183 calories, and about 75 milligrams of cholesterol.

Though beans are rich in protein, they are nonetheless limited in the essential amino acids methionine and cystine, making their protein incomplete. A notable exception to this is soybeans, which have a full complement of essential amino acids (making their protein comparable to dairy protein). But combining other beans in a dish (or meal) with grains provides a complete set of amino acids.

The B vitamin folate is abundant in dried beans, with pinto, mung, baby lima beans, and cranberry beans supplying the most impressive amounts.

Beans are also a good source of minerals, including potassium, magnesium, selenium, and, most notably, iron. Soybeans, red kidney beans, cannellini beans, adzuki, pinto, and large lima beans are the best bean sources of iron.

in the market

In the past few years, there has been an explosion of newly available "heirloom" beans. Though most of them derive from the same legume ancestor, they have a wide variety of colors and patterns. The best chances for finding unusual beans are specialty food stores and health-food stores.

Adzuki (azuki, aduki, adsuki, asuki) These are small russet-colored beans with a thin white line on the ridge. Adzukis have a light, slightly sweet, nutty flavor and are rather thick-skinned. These are the type of bean commonly used to make Japanese red-bean ice cream.

Anasazi These heirloom beans are kidney-shaped red beans with white mottling. They cook fairly quickly and are a good substitute for cranberry or pinto beans.

Appaloosa Creamy-white with russet splotches, the marking of these heirloom beans is similar to that of Appaloosa horses. They are a good substitute for pinto beans.

Black beans (turtle beans) These matte-black beans have a thin white line on the side. The skin is black and the flesh is cream colored. Black beans have an earthy, rich flavor.

Black soybeans This soybean variety has black skin with a yellow interior. Like regular soybeans, they require long soaking and cooking.

Calypso (yin yang, orca) These white beans with a band of dark russet will keep their coloring if cooked in a plentiful amount of water. They are a good substitute for cannellini beans.

Cannellini (white kidney, fagioli, haricots blancs) These are white, kidney-shaped beans with a thick skin and a creamy, smooth texture.

Chick-peas See Chick-peas (*page 237*).

---

favism

Certain individuals with an inherited enzyme deficiency can experience a serious reaction when they eat fava beans. Most of the people who have this disorder are of Middle Eastern or southern European origin. The disorder, which is called favism, causes severe hemolytic anemia when fava beans are eaten. Symptoms of favism are flulike and commonly include fatigue, nausea, abdominal and/or back pain, fever, and chills. Fava plant pollen in the respiratory tract also can create a severe reaction in these people.

China yellow bean These greenish-yellow beans hail from Maine, not China. They have a silky texture and a mellow flavor.

Cranberry beans (Roman beans) Similar in size and shape to kidney beans, cranberry beans are a dark tan with splotches of wine coloring. Once cooked they lose their marking and become uniform in color. Cranberry beans are sweet and delicate in flavor. See also Beans, Fresh (*page 184*).

Eye of the goat Small, round, and plump, these heirloom beans are reddish brown with a band of maroon. They remain firm and richly colored after cooking and are a good choice for salads.

Fava beans (broad beans) Available whole in their skins, or peeled and split, these large, light brown beans are nutty-tasting with a slightly grainy texture. Smaller Egyptian favas, known as *ful,* are also available. See also Beans, Fresh (*page 185*). Fava beans can cause a severe reaction in certain people; see "Favism" (*page 179*).

Flageolet This small French kidney bean ranges in color from pale green to creamy white. Flageolets are thin-skinned and delicate in flavor and are traditionally used to make the French bean dish called *cassoulet.*

French navy beans (coco blancs) These small, plump heirloom beans are white with a slightly green undertone. They have a rich flavor and a smooth, silky texture.

Great Northern These large white beans are creamy and full-flavored. They are very popular in baked bean dishes.

Jacob's cattle (trout bean, coach dogs, Dalmatian beans) White with small and large maroon splotches, this heirloom bean is sweet and good in soups and salads. It can be used in place of pinto or kidney beans.

Lima beans (Madagascar beans) These beans are creamy white with the slightest hint of green. Savory and buttery in flavor and somewhat starchy in texture, limas are great in soups and stews. The most popular varieties are the small baby limas and the large Fordhooks (also called butter beans). See also Beans, Fresh (*page 185*).

Lupini These large Italian beans resemble favas and are slightly bitter.

Marrow beans These large, round white beans are often described as tasting like bacon.

Mung beans Usually eaten in the form of bean sprouts (*see Sprouts, page 542*), the dried version of these small olive-skinned, yellow-fleshed beans can be found in health-food stores. Mung beans are also skinned and split, and sold in Indian markets as *moong dal.* The Chinese grind these beans to a flour to make cellophane noodles (*see Pasta, Nonwheat, page 442*).

Navy beans (Yankee beans) These small white beans are so-named because the U. S. Navy used to carry them on ships as a standard provision. They're often used in both homemade and commercial pork and beans.

Pea beans The smallest of the white beans, these are often packed along with, or labeled as, navy beans. Like navy beans, pea beans are often the choice for Boston baked beans.

---

facts & tips

The salty black beans used in Chinese cooking are made from small black soybeans that are fermented and then preserved in salt.

Pink beans These smooth, reddish-brown beans are the beans of choice for chili con carne and refried beans.

Pinto beans (red Mexican beans) Pale pink beans with streaks of reddish-brown, these beans are meaty-tasting. Once cooked, the streaks disappear and the bean is light red, much like pink beans.

Red beans These small, roundish red beans are the color of red kidney beans, only a bit darker. They are the classic ingredient in the Louisiana dish red beans and rice.

Red kidney beans This firm, medium-sized red bean has deep red skin and cream-colored flesh. With their rich, full-bodied flavor, kidney beans are often used in chili con carne.

Runner beans These red-streaked, cream-colored beans are similar to pink and pinto beans. Runner beans can be used interchangeably for pink or pinto beans.

Scarlet runner beans Red with dark maroon mottling, these beans are similar to pinto beans.

Soldier beans (European soldier, red-eye) Kidney-shaped and chalk-white, these beans are distinguished by slashes of color that resemble the silhouette of a soldier.

Soybeans While they come in a variety of colors, the most readily available are yellow and black soybeans. The size and shape of a large pea, soybeans require lengthy soaking and cooking. See also Beans, Fresh (*page 184*) and Soyfoods (*page 533*).

Steuben yellow-eye beans (butterscotch calypso, molasses face) These somewhat flat white beans with an amber eye were probably the original bean used for Boston baked beans.

Swedish brown beans These elliptical light brown beans can be used in place of kidney beans.

Tolosana beans (Prince beans) Kidney-shaped and brown, with a thick covering of russet, these beans can be substituted for red kidney beans.

Tongues of fire Light brown with russet markings, this bean closely resembles the cranberry bean. Despite its name, it is not hot.

Winged beans (goa beans) More often found fresh (*see Beans, Fresh, page 184*), this nutritious bean can also be found in its dried form, out of its winged pod. It is the size and shape of a soybean.

choosing the best

Shop for beans in a market that has a brisk turnover. If buying beans in bags, check to see that they are whole, not broken or powdery. Some beans may only be available in ethnic, gourmet, or specialty food shops. The heirloom beans are generally only available in specialty food shops, or by mail order.

Label and date beans once they've been purchased, so that you don't mix a newer batch with an older one. Older beans require longer cooking than younger ones.

▶ **When you get home** Beans kept in airtight containers will keep for quite a long time. It is worth noting, however, that the longer beans sit, the more moisture they will lose. The importance of this lies only in the beans' cooking time (which can as much as double for older beans).

preparing to use

All dried beans should be picked over before cooking; spread them on a white kitchen towel so that you can easily see and discard any dirt, debris, or damaged specimens. Then place the beans in a strainer and rinse them under cold water.

Dried beans are normally soaked before cooking. If you don't have time to presoak beans, expect the cooking time to be lengthened by an hour or more. You can quick-soak beans in an hour, or long-soak them for 6 hours or overnight. (The longer soaking time eliminates more of their gas-producing sugars; see "The Gas Problem," at left.)

For long soaking Place the beans in a large pot or bowl (they will double in size during soaking) and add enough water to cover them by at least 2 inches (about 10 cups of water per pound of beans, or two to three times the beans' volume in water). Let the beans stand for at least 6 hours. (For longer soaking, or in warm weather, place the pot of beans in the refrigerator or they will begin to ferment.)

For quick soaking Place the beans and water in a large pot, bring to a boil, and boil for 2 minutes. Remove the pot from the heat and let stand, covered, for an hour.

For either method, drain off the soaking water and start with fresh water to cook the beans.

the gas problem

For many people, a major obstacle to eating beans is that they contain oligosaccharides, which are indigestible complex sugars that can cause flatulence, often accompanied by indigestion and bloating. These sugars pass undigested into the large intestine, where they are fermented into gas.

Rest assured that there are ways to reduce the gas-producing properties of beans. If you presoak beans (for at least 6 hours) before cooking them and then discard the soaking water, you will be eliminating some of the offensive oligosaccharides. In addition, it may be a good idea to eat beans in small amounts—as a ½-cup side-dish serving rather than as a big bowl of bean chili—along with low-fat foods (which are easier to digest than fatty foods).

beans, fresh

Of the many types of beans that we consume, only a few varieties are eaten fresh. These beans aren't a distinct species, but are simply picked at an immature stage, when the inner seed (also referred to as the bean) has just started to form; left on the plant, the seeds eventually grow to full size and dry in the pod. Though they belong to a number of plant species, fresh beans can be classified into two broad categories: edible-pod beans and shell beans. The fact that we call these beans "fresh," by the way, doesn't mean they are always marketed fresh—actually, we eat the bulk of fresh beans in canned or frozen form.

nutritional profile

Edible-pod beans are immature pods, and as such they contain the type of nutrients (such as beta carotene, lutein and zeaxanthin, and vitamin C) that are associated with fresh plants. Low in calories and rich in carbohydrates and fiber, green beans also contain folate.

Most shell beans offer some protein, B vitamins, iron, and fiber. Fresh soybeans (edamame) tend to have more fat than other beans, and they are also especially nutrient-dense. In addition to the nutrients common to other shell beans, soybeans have a highly favorable quality of protein (containing a full complement of essential amino acids), which exceeds that of other beans.

in the market

Edible-pod beans are beans that can be eaten in their entirety, pod and all. Green beans and other snap beans are the prime examples. Shell beans are beans whose pod is naturally not particularly edible and the seeds are allowed to mature, or beans that are allowed to grow past the edible-pod stage in order to have bigger seeds. Lima beans are an example of a shell bean.

edible-pod beans

Snap beans (green beans and wax beans) are the most popular beans with edible pods. There are, however, many other delicious varieties of edible-pod beans on the market.

Dragon tongue beans Dragon tongue beans are light yellow beans that are streaked with purple. They are shaped like longer, wider, flatter green beans.

Haricots verts These French green beans are much thinner than American green beans. They're also more expensive, since they're mostly imported.

Italian green beans Also called Romano beans, these are distinguished by broad, flat, bright green pods. Like snap beans, these beans also come in a yellow (wax bean) version.

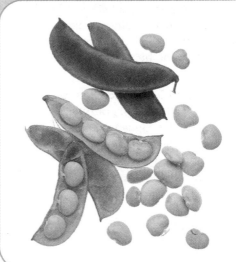

lima beans

GREEN BEANS 1 cup cooked	
Calories	44
Protein (g)	2
Carbohydrate (g)	10
Dietary fiber (g)	4
Total fat (g)	0.4
Saturated fat (g)	0.1
Monounsaturated fat (g)	0
Polyunsaturated fat (g)	0.2
Cholesterol (mg)	0
Potassium (mg)	374
Sodium (mg)	4

KEY NUTRIENTS (%RDA/AI*)	
Vitamin C	12 mg (13%)
Folate	42 mcg (10%)
Iron	1.6 mg (20%)

*For more detailed information on RDA and AI, see page 88.

serving suggestions

• Toss cooked snap beans with tomato sauce (or add them to fettuccine or other pasta and top with sauce).

• Toss snap beans with a little olive oil, salt, and pepper and roast in the oven or grill on the barbecue.

• Layer snap beans with chopped onion, diced tomatoes, bell peppers, or other vegetables. Season to taste, add some broth, cover tightly, and bake until the vegetables are tender.

BABY LIMA BEANS
½ cup cooked

Calories	105
Protein (g)	6
Carbohydrate (g)	20
Dietary fiber (g)	4.5
Total fat (g)	0.3
Saturated fat (g)	0.1
Monounsaturated fat (g)	0
Polyunsaturated fat (g)	0.1
Cholesterol (mg)	0
Potassium (mg)	485
Sodium (mg)	15

KEY NUTRIENTS (%RDA/AI*)

Thiamin	0.1 mg (10%)
Vitamin B$_6$	0.2 mg (10%)
Vitamin C	9 mg (10%)
Iron	2.1 mg (20%)
Magnesium	63 mg (15%)

*For more detailed information on RDA and AI, see page 88.

Purple wax beans These small wax beans have a dark purple pod that turns green when cooked.

Scarlet runner beans The pods are broad, flat, and green; the seeds are scarlet. These beans also have an edible blossom that may be red or white.

Snap beans A great favorite of cooks as well as home gardeners, snap beans are so called because of their tender, crisp pods that snap when bent (the ends are snapped off before cooking). The most familiar types are *green beans* and *yellow wax beans,* which are identical in taste and texture, though yellow wax beans are lower in beta carotene. Both are actually immature kidney beans, and their pods can be flat, oval, or rounded, depending on the variety. These beans were formerly known as *string beans* because the varieties developed in the 19th century had a long, tough string down the seam of the pod that had to be stripped off. However, the string has been bred out of most snap bean varieties; occasionally, though, a bean does need stringing.

Wax beans See snap beans (*above*).

Winged beans (goa beans) Not only are the pod and inner seed of these beans edible, everything else on the plant (shoots, flowers, roots, and leaves) is, too. The pods have a distinctive shape, with four sides that flare into ridges or "wings." The pods are green and shades of purple-red and the beans within are starchier than green bean seeds.

Yardlong beans (Chinese long beans, asparagus beans) Originally from Asia, these mild-tasting, thin, green beans can measure up to 18 inches long. When young and tender, long beans are good for stir-frying.

shell beans

Shell beans are mature seeds (beans) whose pods are usually no longer edible, but the beans are still fresh and have not been dried. Many of the varieties listed below are also available dried (*see Beans, Dried, page 178*), but their nutritional content differs. And though shell beans can be used interchangeably with dried beans in many recipes, keep in mind that shell beans keep the same bulk whether they're raw or cooked, whereas dried beans swell up, so you'll need to adjust recipes accordingly.

Cannellini This is the fresh form of the beloved dried white kidney bean of minestrone fame.

Cranberry beans These beans—so named because of the red markings on both the white pods and the beans themselves—are occasionally available fresh. They are usually served as a side dish or added to soups and stews.

Edamame (fresh soybeans) Edamame are a specialty soybean grown specifically to be picked and used in their immature stage so that they can be consumed fresh. Distinguished by their small, fuzzy, dark green pods, fresh soybeans have a mild flavor, along with a higher protein and fat content than other beans (but the fat is unsaturated). Moreover, the protein is complete—meaning that it provides the essential amino acids needed in one's diet—so soybeans are equivalent to animal products in terms of protein quality.

Fava beans Some people prefer the taste and texture of these beans to lima beans, which favas closely resemble. Also called broad beans, their pods are longer than those of limas—up to 18 inches—with larger beans. Young favas can be shelled and eaten raw or cooked, but more mature favas must be both shelled and skinned (the skins are much too tough to eat). Note that favas can cause a serious adverse reaction in certain individuals; see "Favism" (*page 179*).

Lima beans The most common shell bean in the United States, limas are named after the capital of Peru, where they have been cultivated since ancient times. Nearly all of the domestic crop is marketed frozen or canned, but you can sometimes find fresh limas sold in their pods. As do their dried counterparts, limas come in two varieties: *Fordhooks* (also called butter beans) and *baby limas*, which are not really young lima beans but are a smaller, milder-tasting variety.

▶ Availability Fresh shell beans are generally available for only a few months of the year—lima beans, cranberry beans, and edamame from mid-summer through early fall; fava beans from late spring though early summer.

choosing the best

The best way to choose podded beans (either shell beans or edible-pod) is at a market that sells them loose so that you can pick out pods of equal size (for uniform cooking). Snap beans, when broken, should snap crisply (although the very thin haricots verts are not as crisp). If edible-pod beans are very stiff, or the seeds are visible through the pod, the beans are overly mature and will be tough and leathery. Shell beans should bulge through a tightly close pod. If they're sold shelled, the beans should be plump and tight-skinned. Shelled limas should be grass-green (chalky-white limas will be starchy). Favas should be a light gray-green.

preparing to use

Wash edible-pod beans, then snap or trim both ends of each bean. Leave the beans whole for cooking or cut them crosswise or diagonally into 1- to 2-inch lengths. Slicing green beans lengthwise, "French style," should be necessary only with beans that are old and tough; it robs young beans of their crisp texture and allows their sweet flavor to cook out.

To remove shell beans from the pod, split the pod open and push out the beans with your thumb; rinse the shelled beans before cooking. It may be easier to open the pod if you shave the seam of the curved side with a paring knife or vegetable peeler.

Large fava beans not only need to be shelled, but their tough skins must be peeled either before or after cooking; small, young favas need not be skinned. To peel the raw beans, split the skin with your thumbnail or a sharp paring knife. The skins of cooked favas will slip off easily.

EDAMAME / ½ cup cooked	
Calories	127
Protein (g)	11
Carbohydrate (g)	10
Dietary fiber (g)	3.8
Total fat (g)	5.8
Saturated fat (g)	0.7
Monounsaturated fat (g)	1.1
Polyunsaturated fat (g)	2.7
Cholesterol (mg)	0
Potassium (mg)	485
Sodium (mg)	13

KEY NUTRIENTS (%RDA/AI*)	
Thiamin	0.2 mg (20%)
Riboflavin	0.1 mg (11%)
Vitamin C	15 mg (17%)
Folate	100 mcg (25%)
Calcium	131 mg (11%)
Iron	2.3 mg (28%)
Magnesium	54 mg (13%)

*For more detailed information on RDA and AI, see page 88.

beef & veal

The United States was once a nation of confirmed beef eaters, but no longer. In part, concern about fat, saturated fat, and cholesterol, and the role these substances play in heart disease, obesity, and cancer has steered many people away from beef.

Today's beef isn't as fatty as that of years past; fat content has dropped about 27 percent since the early 1980s. Noting the preference for low-fat protein, ranchers are crossbreeding traditional breeds with leaner, larger cattle—as well as bison (*see "Where the Beefalo & Buffalo Roam," page 188*). In addition, cattle are being fed more grass and less corn, and are being sent to market younger so that they will develop less fat. And meatpackers and retailers are trimming more external fat, leaving about ⅛ inch, down from ¾ inch a decade ago.

nutritional profile

Beef can be a part of a low-fat diet if you follow three simple steps: Choose lean cuts, eat small portions (3 to 4 ounces, cooked), and trim all visible fat before cooking. Beef is an excellent source of iron, zinc, and vitamin B_{12}—nutrients that can be hard to obtain elsewhere. You don't need to eat slabs of steak or roast to get the nutritional benefits beef has to offer. Furthermore, trimming the fat has no effect on the vitamin and mineral quality of the meat. Whether the meat is lean or fatty, the levels of these nutrients are approximately the same.

Beef's fat content is widely variable, however, and only the leanest pieces are as low in fat as broiled fish or skinless chicken. There are two factors to consider when choosing low-fat beef: grade and cut. Grading is a voluntary service established by the USDA and offered to slaughterhouses. Government inspectors evaluate beef carcasses in terms of their marbling, the white streaks or specks of fat within the flesh itself that help give meat its juiciness and distinct flavor. Ironically, the system rewards the production of fatty beef; the cuts with the most marbling are given the highest grade—Prime—followed by Choice and Select.

On average, a cut of beef graded Select has 5 to 20 percent less fat than Choice beef of the same cut, and 40 percent less fat than Prime. Since grading is not compulsory and costs the meatpacker money, much of the beef in the supermarket is ungraded. This ungraded beef is usually sold under the store's brand and is often a commercial grade, just below Select. Of the beef that is graded, Choice is the most common designation.

Perhaps more important than grade when determining fat content is cut, which refers to the part of the animal from which a piece of meat comes. It's not uncommon for Select-grade beef of one cut to have more fat than Choice beef of another cut.

SIRLOIN / 3 ounces cooked	
Calories	183
Protein (g)	25
Carbohydrate (g)	0
Dietary fiber (g)	0
Total fat (g)	8.5
Saturated fat (g)	3.4
Monounsaturated fat (g)	3.6
Polyunsaturated fat (g)	0.3
Cholesterol (mg)	76
Potassium (mg)	331
Sodium (mg)	55

KEY NUTRIENTS (%RDA/AI*)	
Riboflavin	0.2 mg (18%)
Niacin	3.5 mg (22%)
Vitamin B_6	0.4 mg (22%)
Vitamin B_{12}	2.4 mcg (99%)
Iron	2.8 mg (34%)
Zinc	5.3 mg (48%)

*For more detailed information on RDA and AI, see page 88.

veal

Delicately flavored and light-textured, veal is a highly versatile meat that comes from very young calves. It is an expensive food and has always been considered a specialty in the United States, where consumption of veal now stands at less than a pound per person each year (down from about 9 pounds per person annually in the 1940s). Italians, by contrast, eat veal as often as Americans eat beef, and a fondness for it extends throughout much of western Europe. The reason for its widespread use overseas is partly tied to economics: There is less grazing land in Europe than in the Americas, hence farmers slaughter male cattle at a young age rather than pay the expense of raising them. Not surprisingly, most of our favorite veal dishes are distinctively European: veal cutlets and scaloppine served with various sauces, stews, and braises, and stuffed veal roasts.

The finest veal comes from animals that are only 2 to 3 months old and haven't been weaned. The meat from milk-fed veal is light pink, and the texture is firm but velvety. It is generally available only at restaurants and from specialty butchers. The veal sold at supermarkets is usually from older animals—16 to 20 weeks old—so that the flesh has become darker and less tender than that of milk-fed veal.

While the cuts of veal are similar to those of beef, there are fewer of them. For the primal cuts, veal is divided up like lamb: foreshank and breast, shoulder, rib, loin, and leg (which includes the sirloin). The most popular retail cuts of veal are loin and rib chops, boneless rolled loin roast, boneless shoulder, as well as roasts, cutlets, and scallops made from the leg. The leg cutlets and scallops are the leanest cuts of veal. One good bargain, nutritionally as well as economically, is ground veal; if the meat is taken from the leg or shoulder, it has much less fat than either ground beef or lamb.

All cuts of veal are relatively tender. At the same time, veal's lack of marbling means that broiling it tends to yield meat that is dry and tough. Steaks, cutlets, scallops, and chops are best sautéed or braised; the tougher cuts from the lower leg and the shoulder benefit most from moist-heat methods—roasting, braising, and stewing.

When you shop for veal, look for light pink, fine-grained meat with little marbling; any fat should be firm and white. (Some veal may carry a USDA grade of Prime or Choice.)

Trim off any fat from the meat, including the membrane that surrounds veal scallops; this will prevent the meat from curling as it cooks. Veal scallops are also usually pounded before cooking to flatten and tenderize them.

VEAL SCALLOP / 3 ounces cooked

Calories	136
Protein (g)	24
Carbohydrate (g)	0
Dietary fiber (g)	0
Total fat (g)	4.0
Saturated fat (g)	1.6
Monounsaturated fat (g)	1.5
Polyunsaturated fat (g)	0.3
Cholesterol (mg)	88
Potassium (mg)	331
Sodium (mg)	58

KEY NUTRIENTS (%RDA/AI*)

Riboflavin	0.3 mg (21%)
Niacin	8.5 mg (53%)
Vitamin B$_6$	0.3 mg (16%)
Vitamin B$_{12}$	1.0 mcg (41%)
Iron	0.8 mg (10%)
Zinc	2.6 mg (24%)

*For more detailed information on RDA and AI, see page 88.

in the market

Primal cuts, listed below, are wholesale terms that refer to the sections of the animal. Within the primal cuts are many retail cuts, which are the names given to the steaks and roasts you find in the supermarket. According to the National Livestock and Meat Board, there are some 300 different retail cuts, and a typical meat counter may display more than 50 cuts at one time. Meat labels always give both the primal and retail cut names. The list of primal cuts below also identifies common retail cuts.

Brisket The front part of the breast is a boneless cut of beef with lots of fat. Brisket cuts—*flat half brisket, corned brisket, point half brisket,* and *whole brisket*—are best braised or cooked in liquid.

Chuck This cut encompasses meat from the shoulder, arm, and neck of the animal. One of the hardest-working areas of the animal's body, the chuck contains a lot of connective tissue, and, therefore, is not very tender. Chuck cuts include: *chuck eye roast, boneless top blade steak, arm pot roast, boneless shoulder pot roast, cross rib pot roast, blade roast, short ribs, flanken style ribs,* and *stew beef.* (Ground beef is also produced from chuck cuts, among others.) All of these should be cooked in liquid for long periods of time at moderate temperatures; that is the best way to break down the connective tissue and tenderize the meat. The exception is chuck eye roast, which may be roasted.

Flank From this section, which is just behind the belly, comes *flank steak,* also called *London broil* in some parts of the country. It is a flavorful, relatively tender, and lean cut, which is suitable for broiling—though if cooked beyond the medium-rare stage, it gets very tough. It can also be braised, pan-broiled, or stir-fried. The meat should be cut very thin on a sharp angle across the grain to make it easier to chew.

Foreshank The meat from the front legs of the steer is quite tough, and is used primarily for stew and ground beef. You may also find small steaks labeled *shank cross cuts,* which are well suited for braising or cooking in liquid.

Rib cuts Cuts from the ribs are quite tender; however, those from the section nearest the chuck are less tender than the ones from the area nearest

WHERE THE BEEFALO & BUFFALO ROAM

In recent years, there's been a growing number of ranchers who have turned to raising bison (the proper name for the American buffalo) and beefalo (a cross between bison and domestic cattle). Both types of meat have a significantly higher lean-to-fat ratio than regular beef, with very little intramuscular fat, or marbling. The following figures are for 3 ounces cooked of a composite of cuts, well trimmed of external fat.

	Calories	Fat (g)	% Calories from Fat	Saturated Fat (g)	Cholesterol (mg)
Beef	232	15	58	5.8	74
Beefalo	160	5.4	30	2.3	49
Bison	122	2.1	15	0.8	70

the loin. Most rib cuts are packaged as roasts—*rib roast, large end* (near the chuck), *rib roast, small end* (near the loin), *rib-eye roast*—but sometimes the roasts are cut into steaks, called *rib steaks* and *rib-eye steaks* (also known as *Delmonico steaks*). In general, rib cuts should be roasted, but the steaks can be broiled or grilled. *Back ribs,* another cut from this section, come with the bone intact and should be either roasted or braised.

Round This rear section of the steer is so named because it contains the round bone, or femur. Although the muscles in the round are as hardworking as those in the chuck, meat from the round is more tender because the muscles all run in one direction. The round offers three of the leanest cuts of beef available: *eye of round, top round*, and *round tip*. As roasts, these cuts can be roasted or braised; as steaks, they can be broiled or panbroiled. Other cuts from this section include: *boneless rump roast* and *bottom round roast*, which should be roasted or braised, and *round steak*, which should be braised.

Short loin The tenderest cuts come from the loin, the part between the lower ribs and the pelvis, and the muscle that does the least work. Two of the leanest cuts of beef—*top loin* and *tenderloin*—are from this section. The tenderloin muscle yields the tenderest meat; from it comes *tenderloin roast* and a number of steaks. *Filets mignons* are small steaks cut from the tenderloin. *T-bone steaks* come from the middle of the loin and include some tenderloin.

COMPARING BEEF CUTS 3 ounces cooked

As a general rule of thumb, 4 ounces of raw boneless beef will yield 3 ounces of cooked beef. For 3 ounces of cooked beef from a bone-in cut, you would start with about 8 ounces of raw. Most retail cuts of beef will be trimmed to ¼ inch or ⅛ inch of fat. Before cooking, you should trim all remaining visible fat. The values below are for beef whose external fat has been fully trimmed and are an average of Prime, Choice, and Select grades. The cuts are organized by percentage of calories from fat.

	Calories	Fat (g)	% Calories from Fat	Saturated Fat (g)	Cholesterol (mg)
Rib roast	300	24	72	9.7	72
Blade roast	284	21	67	8.2	88
Porterhouse	237	17	65	6.2	57
Brisket	247	17	62	6.4	79
T-bone	210	14	60	5.1	48
Chuck roast	238	14	53	5.6	85
Flank steak	192	11	52	4.5	58
Tenderloin	219	12	49	4.7	79
Top loin	180	8.7	44	3.4	65
Sirloin	183	8.5	42	3.3	76
Bottom round	160	6.2	35	2.1	66
Eye of round	145	4.6	29	1.7	59
Top round	178	5.4	27	1.9	77

hamburger dilemma

Hamburger lovers have it rough: If they like their burgers rare, there's the risk of food poisoning. If well-done, there's the problem of potentially carcinogenic compounds (called heterocyclic aromatic amines, or HAAs), formed when meat is cooked at high temperatures, as in panfrying, broiling, or barbecuing. But scientists at Lawrence Livermore National Laboratory in California have found two ways to reduce the risk of HAAs.

1. Flip burgers every minute while panfrying—that way they'll cook faster, and as much as 90 percent less HAAs will be produced. This also kills any bacteria, while leaving the burgers moister.

2. Precook burgers in a microwave before frying. This also reduces HAA levels greatly, compared to burgers that are simply fried, and reduces fat content by 30 percent. Microwave the patties for 1 to 3 minutes, pour off the liquid, then panfry the patties. This removes substances that form the HAAs when meat is fried.

Porterhouse steaks have the most tenderloin. *Shell steaks* or *strip loin steaks* are porterhouse or T-bone steaks without the tenderloin. (These are sometimes called New York or Kansas City steaks.) Roasts from this section can be roasted or broiled; the steaks can be broiled.

Short plate The rear of the breast, this section contains tough, fatty meat. Cuts include *skirt steak*, which is the preferred meat for fajitas, *short ribs,* and *spareribs*. Skirt steak can be braised, broiled, or panbroiled; short ribs and spareribs should be braised. Boneless cuts of beef for stew and ground beef also come from this section of the animal.

Sirloin Lying between the round and short loin, this section also contains lean, tender meat. The cuts are primarily steaks—*sirloin flat bone, sirloin round bone, sirloin pinbone,* and *top sirloin*—though you may also find *top sirloin butt roast*; some sirloin is ground. Pinbone is closest to the loin and is the most tender, but it has a lot of bone. Flat bone—the center cut—has less waste than the pinbone, but is tougher. Round bone is nearest to the round and is the toughest sirloin cut. Sirloin steaks, sold with or without the bone, can be broiled; top sirloin butt roast can be roasted.

Ground beef Most ground beef comes from the chuck, sirloin, or round. Packages are labeled by cut of beef, by fat/lean content, or both. Evaluating the fat content of packaged hamburger meat can be even more difficult than judging full cuts. While a steak or other cuts of beef labeled "lean" must have no more than 10 percent fat by weight, and "extra lean," no more than 5 percent by weight, these standards don't apply to meat that is ground. Ground beef labels use what is called compositional labeling, in which the percentage of lean meat is used to define the ground meat's fat status. For example, ground meat that is 75 percent lean, is also 25 percent fat by weight. And meat that is 25 percent fat *by weight* actually derives about 77 percent of its calories from fat when cooked; that's a lot

COMPARING GROUND BEEF **3 ounces cooked**

Ground beef is labeled according to the percentage of lean (by weight) there is in that particular mix. Here is a quick overview of the percentages you're likely to encounter in the supermarket and how they stack up.

	Calories	Fat (g)	% Calories from Fat	Saturated Fat (g)	Cholesterol (mg)
80% lean (20% fat)	248	17	62	6.5	86
84% lean (16% fat)	225	13	52	5.3	84
91% lean (9% fat)	159	7.4	42	2.9	38

of fat. To get the leanest ground beef, look for those labeled at least 90 percent lean. This will translate to meat that is closer to the official definition of "lean." Better still, buy a lean cut of sirloin or round and have the butcher trim it of all external fat and grind it for you, or you can do it yourself, using a meat grinder or food processor.

choosing the best

While cut and grade are good indicators of fat content, you still need to use your eyes when selecting beef. Look for cuts that have little marbling and external fat. Or ask the butcher to trim the external fat.

Fresh beef is easy to spot. Many stores use freshness dates on their labels, so choose the meat with the furthest "sell by" date. In addition, fresh beef has creamy-white fat, not yellow, and feels springy to the touch.

Another means of judging freshness is color. When beef is first exposed to oxygen, it develops a cherry-red color, called bloom. The inside of the beef, and any surfaces that are not exposed to oxygen (such as a cut of beef covered by another cut), are dark purple. (If the meat is vacuum packed, all of it will be dark purple, not cherry-red, because the packing seals off any oxygen.) As time goes by, exposure to oxygen will cause the meat to turn brown. This color change doesn't mean that the meat is spoiled, only that it isn't as fresh as it could be and should be used immediately.

preparing to use

Trim the fat before cooking. External fat and seam fat—the fat between individual muscles in a cut of beef—are the biggest sources of fat in beef. You can't remove the seam fat until the meat is cooked, but external fat can be taken off beforehand. Trimming external fat completely before cooking results in a 19 percent reduction in fat content, according to researchers at Texas A&M University. And pretrimming has no negative effect on flavor, tenderness, or juiciness (except in the case of beef brisket).

A marinade containing acidic ingredients, such as wine or vinegar, can add flavor to beef and help tenderize tough cuts. Make enough marinade to completely cover the meat, and place it in a covered nonreactive container in the refrigerator. Let the meat marinate for at least 6 hours, but not more than 24 hours; otherwise, the meat will turn mushy. Marinating for 15 minutes to 2 hours can add flavor, but does not tenderize the beef.

If you want to use the marinade as a sauce, cook it at a rolling boil for several minutes before serving. Uncooked marinade becomes contaminated from raw meat sitting in it and is therefore not safe to consume.

Rubs are blends of seasonings that are applied all over the surface of meat before cooking. Their purpose is to flavor, not tenderize. For a more pronounced flavor, coat the meat several hours before cooking and refrigerate.

An easy way to tenderize meat is to pound it with a mallet. This technique, which involves breaking up the connective tissue, is useful for moderately thin cuts, such as eye of round, top round, and round tip.

beets

Beets are a root vegetable with two edible parts, the root and the green leaves. In ancient civilizations, only the green part of the beet plant was eaten; the roots—which did not look like those of modern beets—were used medicinally to treat headaches and toothaches. Beets with rounded roots, like those we eat today, were probably developed in the 16th century as animal fodder, and it took another 200 years before they gained any popularity as a human food.

Beets (also called red beets, root beets, and table beets) belong to the botanical species *Beta vulgaris*, which also includes sugar beets (which are processed for sugar, and thus not eaten) and Swiss chard (grown for their greens, not their roots). Beets, sugar beets, Swiss chard, and other varieties that are used for animal fodder, are descended from a wild, slender-rooted plant that grew in southern Europe.

nutritional profile

Beets are a good source of fiber, potassium, iron, and folate, a B vitamin that helps to ward off certain birth defects. While it is more concentrated in the leaves, folate is found in both the root and the leaves of the beet. Notable for their sweet, earthy flavor, beets have the highest sugar content of any vegetable, while remaining very low in calories. And unlike many other vegetables, their full flavor is retained whether they are fresh or canned (which is the way most beets are packaged in the United States). Fresh beets, though, have a characteristic flavor and a crisp texture that you don't find in canned versions.

in the market

The vast majority of beets available in the market are the familiar red beets. But these earthy root vegetables come in other hues: purple, pink, golden, white, and even striped. The unusual beets listed below are mostly only available at farmers' markets and specialty food stores. Very small "baby" beets— radish-sized immature roots that have been pulled to thin the farmer's rows—are a delicacy. Sold (and cooked) with the tender leaves attached, they may be found in early summer at farmers' markets, roadside stands, and specialty greengrocers.

Chioggia Though these look like ordinary beets from the outside, on the inside they have distinct red-and-white-striped flesh (they are also, for this reason, called Candy Cane beets). These heirloom Italian beets are highest on the sweetness scale.

Golden Golden beets are carrot-colored and have the advantage of not bleeding once they're cooked. They are mild in flavor and not as sweet as either Chioggia or red beets.

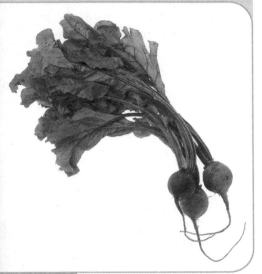

beets

BEETS / 1 cup cooked	
Calories	75
Protein (g)	3
Carbohydrate (g)	17
Dietary fiber (g)	3.4
Total fat (g)	0.3
Saturated fat (g)	0.1
Monounsaturated fat (g)	0.1
Polyunsaturated fat (g)	0.1
Cholesterol (mg)	0
Potassium (mg)	519
Sodium (mg)	131

KEY NUTRIENTS (%RDA/AI*)	
Folate	136 mcg (34%)
Iron	1.3 mg (17%)

*For more detailed information on RDA and AI, see page 88.

White White beets look much like turnips and are not quite as sweet as either the red, striped, or golden varieties.

▶ Availability Though fresh beets are always in good supply, June through October are peak months. At the start of the peak season you can find young beets with small, tender roots, which are suitable for cooking whole. But as the season goes on, the beets get larger—and tougher. In the off-peak months, you may also find clip-topped beets that have been in storage, but these are less tender than freshly harvested beets.

choosing the best

Beets are marketed in a range of sizes. Early-crop beets are usually sold in bunches with the tops attached, or as clip-topped beets in perforated plastic bags. If those you buy are bunched, choose equal-sized ones so that they will cook evenly.

Small, young beets (about 1½ inches in diameter) are pleasingly tender and cook in less time than larger ones; their fine texture is also an asset if you intend to use them raw in a salad. Medium-sized beets are fine for most cooking purposes, but very large specimens (over 2½ inches in diameter) may be tough, with unpalatable woody cores.

Look for smooth, hard, round beets. The surface should be unbruised and free of cuts; avoid beets with soft, moist spots or shriveled, flabby skin. The taproot, which extends from the bulbous part of the beet, should be slender.

If the leaves are attached—and especially if you're planning to eat them—it's preferable that they be small, crisp, and dark green. If the beets are clip-topped, at least ½ inch of the stems (and 2 inches of the taproot) should remain, or the color will bleed from the beets as they cook.

▶ When you get home To reduce moisture loss from the roots, cut off beet greens before storing, but leave at least an inch of the stem attached (tiny leaf-topped baby beets can be stored for a day or two with their tops intact). Do not wash beets before storing.

preparing to use

Generally speaking, to preserve their color and nutrients, beets should never be cut or peeled before cooking (especially if they're being cooked in a liquid); otherwise, the beets will "bleed" their rich red juices while cooking and turn an unappetizing dull brown. Scrub the beets very gently and rinse well, but be careful not to break the skin, which is quite thin. Leave at least an inch of the tops and don't trim the root. Peel them after cooking; the skins will slip right off.

---

serving suggestions

• Toss grated raw beets with apples in a lemon dressing.

• Add diced cooked beets to cooked lentils or a mixture of brown and wild rice.

• For a colorful beet salad, combine cooked red, white, golden, and striped beets in a balsamic dressing.

• Substitute grated peeled raw beets for carrots in your next carrot cake.

• Add grated raw beets to coleslaw.

• Combine cooked beets with smooth, rich avocado for a delicious salad. Toss with a citrus vinaigrette.

• Top meat or poultry sandwiches with sliced cooked beets and onions.

---

facts & tips

Betacyanin is the pigment that makes beets their deep ruby color. Interestingly, because of a genetic predisposition, some people cannot properly metabolize betacyanin, and after eating beets, the pigment passes into their urine and feces, which turn pink or red for a day or two. This is a harmless occurrence that should not cause alarm.

berries

Our appreciation of berries has deep historical roots. In fact, evidence shows that in Siberia, prehistoric peoples stored berries in icy pits to ensure a supply during the winters. Thousands of years later, Native Americans made good use of berries by not only eating fresh and cooked berries, but also by drying berries to eat over the winter. Early settlers, who learned about berry-hunting and preserving from the Native Americans, quickly developed a knowledge of the many varieties growing wild in woods and fields. Today, wild varieties are still gathered with enthusiasm, though most of the berries in markets are from cultivated acreage.

nutritional profile

Tantalizingly sweet, juicy, and compact, berries are rich in vitamin C, fiber, and, depending upon the type of berry, potassium. Most berries also provide a wide range of phytochemicals. Low in calories and high in flavor, berries are an outstanding food choice that can serve as a fresh and succulent snack or be used in a broad spectrum of recipes, from smoothies to pies.

in the market

The principal types of berries available commercially differ in size, color, season, nutrient content, and sweetness. Berry types include smooth-skinned varieties such as currants, gooseberries, and blueberries; others are called "aggregate fruits," because they are actually a cluster of many smaller fruits, such as blackberries, raspberries, and salmonberries; and the strawberry, which is known as a "false" fruit, because it grows from the base rather than from the ovary of a flower, and so is not a true berry.

Bilberries (whortleberries) A relative of the cranberry and blueberry, this European fruit resembles a blueberry but is too tart to eat as is. It is not commonly found fresh in this country, though extracts and juices are available, mostly in health-food stores.

Blackberries See Blackberries (*page 198*).

Blueberries See Blueberries (*page 200*).

Cape gooseberries (goldenberries) These berries are relatives of the tomatillo (*see Exotic Vegetables, page 295*). Like the tomatillo, the berry is enclosed in a papery husk that resembles a Japanese lantern. Fully ripe, the smooth-skinned berries range from a yellow-green to orange and their flesh looks a bit like a yellow cherry. Ripe berries smell somewhat like pineapple and have a sweet-tart flavor with undertones of tomato—you can even use them in salads, the way you would a cherry tomato. Not widely available, your best bet is a farmers' market in the spring.

Cranberries See Cranberries (*page 266*).

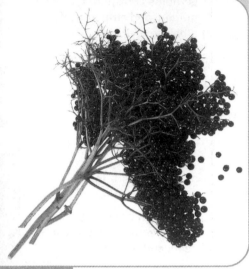

elderberries

CURRANTS / 1 cup	
Calories	63
Protein (g)	2
Carbohydrate (g)	16
Dietary fiber (g)	4.8
Total fat (g)	0.2
Saturated fat (g)	0
Monounsaturated fat (g)	0
Polyunsaturated fat (g)	0.1
Cholesterol (mg)	0
Potassium (mg)	308
Sodium (mg)	1

KEY NUTRIENTS (%RDA/AI*)	
Vitamin C	46 mg (51%)
Iron	1.1 mg (145%)

*For more detailed information on RDA and AI, see page 88.

Currants These small berries grow on vines in clusters, like grapes. Only red and white currants are grown domestically (Europeans also cultivate a black variety), and these have an intense tartness that makes them well-suited for jams and jellies. The supply of fresh currants is quite limited. The berries appear in mid to late summer.

Elderberries Elderberries are very small, dark-purple (almost black), smooth-skinned berries. They have a low percentage of flesh to seeds and are quite tart, which is why they are mostly used for making jams, jellies, and wine. Some farmers' markets carry them fresh in late summer and early fall.

Gooseberries Closely related to currants, gooseberries are very tart, grapelike fruits that turn from pale green to amber as they ripen. American-grown gooseberries are small (½ inch diameter) and round, and European varieties are twice the size and more oval in shape. Fresh gooseberries have a very short season (late May through late July), but you can occasionally find wintertime imports.

Huckleberries These shiny, purple-skinned berries are similar to blueberries. They are generally not cultivated, but wild huckleberries can be found in specialty markets in the summer.

Juneberries (serviceberries) Juneberries closely resemble blueberries, but are blander and seedier. They were a staple of the American Plains Indians, who dried the berries and combined them with dried meat and fat to make a portable food called pemmican. They are native to the north central United States and appear mostly in local farmers' markets. They are best put to use in jams, jellies, or wine.

Lingonberries These relatives of the cranberry are bright red and about the size of a blueberry. They thrive only in cold climates and are a distinctive ingredient in Scandinavian cuisine (usually as jam or preserved in a sweet syrup). You can find them fresh in some farmers' markets in northern states and the Pacific Northwest.

Mulberries Like raspberries and blackberries, mulberries are "aggregate fruits," made up of many tiny druplets. Unlike raspberries and blackberries, however, mulberries grow on trees, not vines. There are three main types of mulberry tree: white, red, and black. The color of mulberries do not necessarily match their tree name: For example, a white mulberry tree can produce berries that are white or purple (and shades in between). White mulberries have the least interesting flavor, being blandly sweet. Red and black mulberries have more interesting sweet-tart flavors. The berries, however, are extremely difficult to harvest (they tend to get crushed in the process), so it's rare to find fresh mulberries in the market.

Ohelo berries These berries—which are native to Hawaii and grow only in the lava beds of Maui and Hawaii—are small, slightly sweet, red or yellow fruits. Quantities are limited and only available in season (summer). It's very rare to find these outside Hawaii, except in the form of jams and jellies.

Raspberries See Raspberries (*page 504*).

*serving
suggestions*

• Stir sweet berries into vanilla yogurt or honey-sweetened plain yogurt.

• Add berries to savory tossed salads.

• Make a fresh lingonberry relish, using any cranberry relish recipe.

• Try a gooseberry sauce with broiled salmon.

GOOSEBERRIES / 1 cup	
Calories	66
Protein (g)	1
Carbohydrate (g)	15
Dietary fiber (g)	6.5
Total fat (g)	0.9
Saturated fat (g)	0.1
Monounsaturated fat (g)	0.1
Polyunsaturated fat (g)	0.5
Cholesterol (mg)	0
Potassium (mg)	297
Sodium (mg)	2

KEY NUTRIENTS (%RDA/AI*)

Vitamin C	42 mg (46%)

For more detailed information on RDA and AI, see page 88.

serving suggestions

Berry sauces can be made in minutes: Gently heat fresh or frozen sweet berries in a small saucepan, then crush some of the berries with a fork so that they release their juices and "melt" into a pourable sauce. (Stir in cornstarch dissolved in cold water for a thicker sauce.) Reserve some whole berries and stir them in after you take the pan off the heat. Vanilla extract, cinnamon, or grated lemon or orange zest are often used to heighten berry flavor. Add a little sugar to the sauce, if necessary, or sweeten with frozen fruit-juice concentrate, such as orange or apple. You can create interesting sauces by cooking different berries together, or with other fruits, such as the classic combination of strawberries and rhubarb.

Salmonberries Salmonberries are members of the rose family and are closely related to blackberries. The immature berry is salmon-colored, but as it ripens, the berry turns red.

Strawberries See Strawberries (*page 553*).

Thimbleberries Like the blackberry, the thimbleberry (which is so named because it resembles a small thimble) is in the rose family. It looks a bit like a red raspberry, but with a powdery bloom. It is a quite fragile berry and does not travel well, so it is mostly available from local farmers' markets in midsummer.

choosing the best

For best flavor, buy berries when they're in season where you live; they'll undoubtedly be riper, tastier, and less-expensive than berries that are flown in from distant regions "out of season." Also, the closer the berries are to the market, the less damage they're likely to suffer in transit.

Choose berries very carefully; they are often packed in opaque boxes that may conceal inferior fruit beneath a display of perfect specimens on top. If the box is cellophane wrapped, your best bet is to examine the berries you can see, and check the box for dampness or stains, which indicate that the fruit below may be decaying. If the box is not wrapped, you can remove a few of the top berries and peek beneath. Check, too, for twigs or other debris (there shouldn't be any).

All berries should be plump, dry, firm, well-shaped, and uniformly colored. Don't purchase berries that are withered or crushed. For berries that are sold on their branchlike stems—currants and elderberries—the fruit should be firmly attached to the stems.

▶ **When you get home** Berries are among the most perishable of fruits; they can turn soft, mushy, and moldy within 24 hours. When you bring home a box of berries, turn it out and check the fruit. Remove soft, overripe berries for immediate consumption; discard any smashed or moldy berries

freezing berries

Berries have a short season and are also highly perishable. Fortunately, though, some freeze beautifully, allowing you to enjoy them practically year round (though they will never resemble their plump, fresh form and are best for cooking, not eating out of hand).

Freezing berries yourself is simple. Spread them out in a single layer on a baking sheet. Place the berries in the freezer until they are solidly frozen, and then transfer them to a heavy plastic bag. They'll keep for 10 months to a year.

and gently blot the remainder dry with a paper towel. Return the berries to the box, or, better yet, spread them out in a shallow refrigerator container lined with paper towels.

Storage times vary slightly, but most berries should be kept for no longer than 2 days.

preparing to use

Sort berries again before serving, discarding any bad ones. Rinse the fruit, drain, and gently pat dry.

Frozen berries need not be thawed before using them in recipes, but extra cooking time may be necessary. Commercially frozen berries do not require washing, but home-frozen berries—which should not have been washed previously—should be quickly rinsed under cold water.

Gooseberries should have their stems and "tails" removed. Cape gooseberries need to have their husks removed. Currants and elderberries can be stripped from their stems by slipping a fork over each stem and pushing off the berries.

COMPARING BERRIES 1 cup fresh

Because the fruits we call berries cover a wide range of varieties, the nutrients in them also vary. However, most berries have certain nutrients in common. Here's how they stack up.

	Calories	Fiber (g)	Vitamin C (mg)	Potassium (mg)
Blackberries	75	7.6	30	282
Blueberries	81	3.9	19	129
Cranberries	47	4.0	13	68
Currants	63	4.8	46	308
Elderberries	106	10.2	52	406
Gooseberries	66	6.5	42	297
Mulberries	60	2.4	51	272
Ohelo berries	39	1.9	8	53
Red raspberries	60	8.4	31	187
Strawberries	46	3.5	86	252

blackberries

Plump, sweet blackberries grow wild across most of North America. The blackberry is actually an ancient fruit, prescribed by the Greeks for gout, mentioned in the Bible, and written about in British folklore. Wild blackberries are relatives of the rose, and the soft, juicy fruit grows on thorny bushes or trailing vines. Like the raspberry, the blackberry is an "aggregate fruit," so called because each berry is really a cluster of tiny fruits, or druplets. Each druplet has a seed, but, *unlike* raspberries, blackberry druplets remain attached to the core even after the berry is picked.

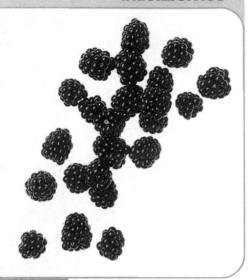

blackberries

nutritional profile

Low in calories and rich in flavor, blackberries are a good source of the antioxidant vitamin C, and they also contain folate and iron. Blackberries are a good source of pectin, a type of soluble fiber that may help to lower cholesterol levels.

in the market

True blackberries, which taste tart to relatively sweet, outwardly resemble raspberries, but they are longer, firmer, and have a black to purple-black color. (The blacker the color, the riper—and sweeter—the berry.) One type of blackberry grows on brambles, another (sometimes called a dewberry) on trailing vines. Berry growers have also developed some hybrid varieties that are cultivated mainly on the West Coast. These include:

Boysenberries This large, reddish-purple blackberry was developed in the 1920s by a farmer named Boysen. Later abandoned by Boysen, the berry was rescued from oblivion by another farmer named Knott, who ultimately founded Knott's Berry Farm and made the "Boysen" berry famous.

Loganberries These large, dark red, and very tart blackberry hybrids were created by a man named Logan in the late 19th century. The berry is actually a cross between two types of blackberry and a red raspberry. Loganberries are grown mainly for juice, pies, and wine.

Marionberries These are a large, flavorful, round blackberry hybrid.

Ollalieberries A cross between black loganberries and youngberries, the olallieberry first made an appearance in 1950.

Youngberries These are another blackberry hybrid very similar to the loganberry.

▶ Availability Blackberries are available from May through September, with the peak season occurring in June and July. For best flavor, buy local in-season berries; undoubtedly they will be riper, tastier, and less expensive than berries flown from distant regions "out of season."

BLACKBERRIES / 1 cup	
Calories	75
Protein (g)	1
Carbohydrate (g)	18
Dietary fiber (g)	7.6
Total fat (g)	0.6
Saturated fat (g)	0
Monounsaturated fat (g)	0.1
Polyunsaturated fat (g)	0.3
Cholesterol (mg)	0
Potassium (mg)	282
Sodium (mg)	0

KEY NUTRIENTS (%RDA/AI*)	
Vitamin C	30 mg (34%)
Folate	49 mcg (12%)
Iron	0.8 mg (10%)

*For more detailed information on RDA and AI, see page 88.

choosing the best

Blackberries should be deep purple to black, and should not have any green or white patches. Choose blackberries that are moderately firm, plump, and dry, with uniform color. Fresh blackberries are not always readily available in stores because quality is lost during shipping. When purchasing, be sure to check the bottom of the blackberry container for dampness and stains to ensure that there are no moldy or crushed berries.

▶ When you get home Blackberries are among the most perishable of fruits; they can turn soft, mushy, and moldy within 24 hours. Blackberries are best used the same day that they are gathered or purchased. When you bring home a box of berries, turn it out and check the fruit. Remove soft, overripe berries for immediate consumption; discard any smashed or moldy berries and gently blot the remainder dry with a paper towel. Place the berries in a shallow refrigerator container lined with paper towels.

▶phytochemicals in blackberries

Anthocyanin pigments give purplish-black color to blackberries and are under review for their potential to suppress tumor growth as well as fatty plaque buildup in arteries. Ellagic acid in blackberries is also a potent antioxidant and does not appear to deteriorate when cooked, so blackberry desserts and jams retain this phytochemical.

preparing to use

Use fresh blackberries as soon as possible because they are highly perishable. Sort berries again before serving, discarding any stems and moldy or squished berries. Gently rinse the fruit, drain, and gently pat dry.

Although blackberries have a short season and are highly perishable, they freeze quite well, allowing you to enjoy them practically year round. You can buy prepackaged frozen berries, but these may have sweetener added. Freezing berries yourself is simple. Place the berries in a single layer, slightly apart, on a cookie sheet. Place the berries in the freezer until they are solidly frozen, and then transfer them to an airtight container, label, and date.

Use fresh or frozen berries in cooked desserts. When using frozen blackberries in pies, tarts, and cobblers, there's no need to thaw.

Fresh or frozen blackberries may be used for jams. If using fresh berries, keep a few unripened berries in the mixture as they help to set the jam.

Canned blackberries may also be used in pies, tarts, and cobblers. The juice that the berries are packed in, which carries the delicious flavor and color of the blackberries, can be used for syrup or as a flavoring.

blueberries

It's all good news with blueberries. Not only are they delicious, but they contain more disease-fighting antioxidants than practically any other fruit or vegetable, even antioxidant-rich foods such as kale, broccoli, and oranges.

Though naturally quite sweet, blueberries are so low in calories that even people trying to lose weight can enjoy them. In fact, their high-fiber content makes them very satisfying. The benefits of blueberries are so powerful that many researchers are incorporating them into their own diets and recommending that you do, too.

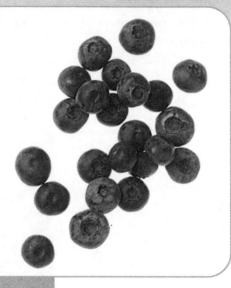

blueberries

nutritional profile

The antioxidants in blueberries can protect against the cell damage that accelerates aging, leading to wrinkled skin and increased susceptibility to disease. In laboratory tests, researchers at the USDA Human Nutrition Research Center on Aging at Tufts University found that ⅔ cup of blueberries supplied the same antioxidant protection against free radicals as 1,773 IU of vitamin E or 1,270 milligrams of vitamin C. In fact, blueberries ranked third in the list of 40 fruits and vegetables tested for their antioxidant potential.

Blueberries contain a good amount of the soluble fiber pectin that helps lower cholesterol levels. In addition, researchers believe that antioxidants in the fruit may help protect LDL ("bad") cholesterol from oxidation and slow the buildup of plaque in the coronary arteries. Pectin is also beneficial to the digestive system, adding bulk to stools without stimulating bowel movements. Keep in mind, however, that large amounts of the fresh fruit may have a laxative effect in some people.

in the market

Cultivated blueberries This is the variety you see most often in the supermarket. The marble-sizes berries are round and plump, with a deep blue color and whitish "bloom" (a dusty-looking surface).

Wild blueberries These are far rarer. You may find them sold fresh locally (they grow in cool climates such as Maine and eastern Canada), but more often they are available canned or frozen. They are much smaller than the cultivated variety—there are 1,600 wild blueberries to the pound, compared to 500 cultivated blueberries—and have a chewy, dense texture and deep flavor. Because you get more blueberries to the pound, ounce for ounce wild blueberries provide more of the skin (which is where the blueberry's color compounds live). One side effect of this is that you'll get blue lips and teeth from eating a pie made with wild blueberries, but you will also be getting a lot more anthocyanins, the substances that make blueberries blue.

▶ Availability Though cultivated blueberries are available most of the year (including imported berries), the wild blueberry season is short, and the

BLUEBERRIES / 1 cup	
Calories	81
Protein (g)	1
Carbohydrate (g)	21
Dietary fiber (g)	3.9
Total fat (g)	0.6
Saturated fat (g)	0.1
Monounsaturated fat (g)	0.1
Polyunsaturated fat (g)	0.2
Cholesterol (mg)	0
Potassium (mg)	129
Sodium (mg)	9

KEY NUTRIENTS (%RDA/AI*)	
Vitamin C	19 mg (21%)
Vitamin E	2.7 mg (18%)

*For more detailed information on RDA and AI, see page 88.

berries are not shipped much beyond their growing area. If you don't live in wild-blueberry country, look for canned or frozen berries.

choosing the best

Fresh blueberries should be deep blue and covered with a chalky white "bloom." The bloom is a sign of freshness. The berries should move freely when you shake the container; if they don't, it's a sign that they may be soft and stuck together.

Inspect the box. If it's a wooden or cardboard container, and is damp or stained, the fruit inside may be crushed, moldy, or decayed.

▶ **When you get home** Before refrigerating, empty the container of blueberries into a bowl and remove any that are crushed or moldy, then return the berries to the container. This will prevent the other berries from going bad too quickly. Do not wash the berries before storing, however.

If you've bought more berries than you can use, freeze them. Spread the unwashed berries on a cookie sheet and place it in the freezer until the berries are hard. Then transfer the berries to a heavy-duty plastic bag.

preparing to use

Before eating or cooking, rinse fresh blueberries and pat dry. Except for removing an occasional leaf, snippet of fine stem, or unripened berry (the reddish ones can be cooked, but aren't good raw), they are ready to eat.

Let frozen berries thaw at room temperature for a few minutes before adding them to uncooked dishes. When using frozen berries in cooked dishes, lengthen the cooking time by a few minutes.

When adding fresh berries to batter, dust them first with flour. The coating keeps them from dropping to the bottom of the baking pan.

▶ phytochemicals in blueberries

• Blueberries are rich in antioxidants, which are potential cancer-fighters. Though it has yet to be determined, it is suspected that anthocyanins—a group of phytochemicals that put the "blue" in blueberry—are responsible for much of the fruit's antioxidant power.

• Flavonoid phytochemicals (a class that includes anthocyanins) may make blood platelets less likely to stick together and form the type of clots that can cause heart attacks.

• Similar to cranberries, blueberries have shown promise in preventing infectious bacteria from taking hold in the urinary tract, a process that can trigger a urinary tract infection. Researchers believe that the procyanidins in the berries may be responsible.

• In a well-publicized study conducted at Tufts University, blueberries were found to reverse mental decline in elderly rats (the rats were better able to remember the correct path through a maze after having their diets supplemented with blueberry extract for 2 months). Though there are plenty of good reasons to eat blueberries whenever you can, keep in mind that what smartens up a lab rat may not have the same effect on humans.

---

other blueberry products

Blueberry juice Wild and domestic blueberry juice (sweetened with fruit juices such as grape and apple) is available in health-food stores.

Blueberry-juice concentrate This unsweetened concentrate is available in health-food stores.

Dried blueberries Dried blueberries are available in specialty food markets and can be used as you would raisins. Like all dried fruit, they provide a concentration of the whole fruit's nutrients—in this case, they are a particularly rich source of anthocyanins.

brazil nuts

Brazil nuts are the large seeds of majestic trees that grow wild in the Amazon jungle. Shaped like rough, brown-orange segments, the nuts are extremely hard and are found in clusters inside a 4- to 6-inch round fruit, called a pod, which resembles a coconut. After the pods have fallen from the trees, they are gathered and chopped open to retrieve the nuts (each pod provides about 10 to 25 nuts). Although thousands of tons of Brazil nuts are exported each year from Brazil, almost all of the Brazil nut production comes from wild forest trees. Brazil nuts taste sweet and rich, and their texture is similar to that of coconut meat.

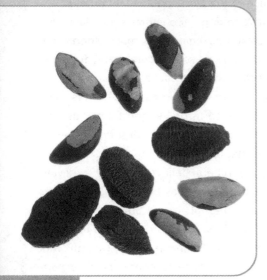

brazil nuts

nutritional profile

Brazil nuts are nutrient-dense, which means that, in relation to their size, they contain a wide variety of nutrients including protein, fiber, vitamin E, thiamin, iron, magnesium, and zinc. They also supply heart-healthy monounsaturated fatty acids.

Brazil nuts' most important nutritional claim, however, is their extraordinary selenium content. A single Brazil nut can provide more than twice the RDA for selenium (a large nut has 140 micrograms, or 254 percent of the RDA). The trace mineral selenium is an antioxidant that works synergistically with vitamin E to protect against free-radical damage to cells.

in the market

Brazil nuts are available raw (in the shell and shelled), roasted (salted and unsalted), and dry-roasted. Some stores also carry sliced Brazil nuts.

▶ Availability Brazil nuts in the shell tend to be seasonal—supplies are best in the fall and early winter.

choosing the best

When choosing Brazil nuts in the shell, look for clean, well-filled shells—shake them; they shouldn't rattle.

▶ When you get home Keep Brazil nuts in the refrigerator or freezer as they tend to spoil quickly, especially if they're shelled.

preparing to use

While it's best not to subject them to extremes of heat, Brazil nut shells are very hard, and some people find it easier to crack them open after they've been frozen, steamed, or boiled for a few minutes. Boil or steam the nuts for about 3 minutes, then run cold water over them before cracking the shells with a nutcracker.

BRAZIL NUTS 1 ounce shelled	
Calories	186
Protein (g)	4
Carbohydrate (g)	4
Dietary fiber (g)	1.5
Total fat (g)	19
Saturated fat (g)	4.6
Monounsaturated fat (g)	6.5
Polyunsaturated fat (g)	6.8
Cholesterol (mg)	0
Potassium (mg)	170
Sodium (mg)	>1

KEY NUTRIENTS (%RDA/AI*)	
Thiamin	0.3 mg (24%)
Vitamin E	2.2 mg (14%)
Iron	1 mg (12%)
Magnesium	64 mg (15%)
Selenium	839 mcg (1,526%)
Zinc	1.3 mg (12%)

*For more detailed information on RDA and AI, see page 88.

broccoli

Broccoli is the most nutritious of the cruciferous vegetables—a family of vegetables named for their cross-shaped flowers. (Other members of this esteemed family of healthful vegetables include cauliflower, cabbage, and Brussels sprouts.) The name "broccoli" comes from the Latin word *brachium*, which means "branch," or "arm"—an apt description for a vegetable with numerous thick, fleshy stalks supporting a head of compact florets. Native to the Mediterranean, broccoli was a beloved food of the ancient Romans. It was first introduced to France in the 1500s and to England in the mid-18th century, and began to be cultivated in the United States in the 1920s. Since then, it has become one of the best-selling vegetables in the United States.

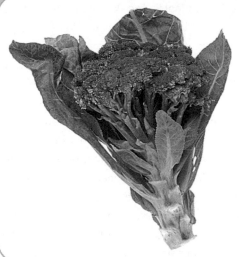

purple broccoli

nutritional profile

Supplying a mother lode of healthy compounds, broccoli is a true nutritional powerhouse. A high-fiber, nutrient-dense food, it is an excellent source of the important B vitamin, folate, as well as riboflavin, potassium, iron, and vitamin C.

Broccoli also contains the carotenoids beta carotene and lutein. Beta carotene, in addition to being used by the body to form vitamin A, is an antioxidant that may help to prevent certain types of cancer by seeking and destroying harmful free radicals. Research indicates that lutein helps to prevent the onset of cataracts and possibly macular degeneration. Lutein also functions as an antioxidant, helping to shield the eyes from free-radical damage caused by sunlight's UV rays.

The leaves and stems of broccoli are very nutritious, but the florets seem to contain a higher concentration of nutrients and phytochemicals. Raw broccoli has more vitamin C than cooked, but cooking makes the carotenoids in the vegetable more bioavailable.

in the market

Though green broccoli is the most common type of broccoli in the United States, there are a number of other broccoli relatives and derivatives:

Broccoflower A cross between broccoli and cauliflower, this looks much like a green cauliflower. Its taste is more like cauliflower than broccoli.

Broccolini A cross between Chinese broccoli and broccoli, this vegetable is also known as *baby broccoli.* Broccolini can be recognized by its deep green color and long, slender stalks ending in small buds, like broccoli florets. Sweeter and more tender than broccoli, broccolini is cooked by the same methods as its larger cousin, but will require a shorter amount of time. While some people peel broccoli stalks before using them, broccolini requires no peeling. Broccolini is somewhat more expensive than broccoli, but it is completely edible, from stem to flower.

BROCCOLI / 1 cup cooked	
Calories	44
Protein (g)	5
Carbohydrate (g)	8
Dietary fiber (g)	4.7
Total fat (g)	0.6
Saturated fat (g)	0.1
Monounsaturated fat (g)	0
Polyunsaturated fat (g)	0.3
Cholesterol (mg)	0
Potassium (mg)	505
Sodium (mg)	42

KEY NUTRIENTS (%RDA/AI*)	
Beta carotene	1.4 mg (12%)
Riboflavin	0.2 mg (14%)
Vitamin B$_6$	0.2 mg (13%)
Vitamin C	123 mg (137%)
Folate	94 mcg (23%)
Iron	1.4 mg (17%)

*For more detailed information on RDA and AI, see page 88.

Broccoli rabe (raab, rapini, rape) Similar in appearance and flavor to broccoli, but more pungent and bitter, broccoli rabe is only distantly related to broccoli: same family (it's a crucifer) but different genus. The seeds of the broccoli rabe plant are used to make rapeseed oil, also known as canola.

Broccoli sprouts See Sprouts (*page 543*).

Chinese broccoli (gai lan) Also known as Chinese kale, Chinese broccoli is longer, leafier, and more sharply flavored than common green broccoli. It is similar in flavor to broccoli rabe. It can have clusters of white flowers and be eaten in its entirety.

Green broccoli With light green stalks topped by umbrella-shaped clusters of purplish-green florets, this is the most common type of broccoli in the United States. Its technical name is sprouting broccoli or Italian green broccoli. This popular variety is also known as Calabrese, named after the Italian province of Calabria, where it was first grown.

Purple broccoli This hybrid has small purple florets that turn green once cooked. While its florets look more like purple cauliflower than broccoli, it tastes decidedly like broccoli.

choosing the best

For fresh broccoli to taste its best, it must be picked young. Left growing too long, the plant begins converting its sugar to lignin, a type of fiber that cannot be softened by cooking. (Broccoli that has been stored too long after harvesting also develops lignin.) Overly mature broccoli, no matter how it's prepared, will be tough and woody, and have an unpleasantly strong cabbagey odor.

Examine the stalks attached to the florets; they should be on the slender side and so crisp that if you broke one, it would snap clean. The florets should be tightly closed and uniformly green; yellowing florets are a sign that the broccoli is past its prime. Good color also indicates nutritional quality. Florets that are dark green or purplish- or bluish-green have more beta carotene and vitamin C than paler florets. The leaves, if any, should have good color and not appear wilted. Avoid broccoli with soft slippery spots on the florets or with stalk bottoms that are brown or slimy. Fresh broccoli has a clean smell.

Broccolini, Chinese broccoli, broccoflower, purple broccoli, and broccoli rabe should all have firm, crisp stems, without any slime. The leaves should be deep green and crisp as well. The heads should be tight.

▶ **When you get home** Refrigeration slows the conversion of sugar to lignin (a type of fiber that makes a vegetable woody) and also protects vitamin C content. Do not wash broccoli before storing it; although it needs moisture to remain fresh, any water on its surface will encourage the growth of mold.

➤ *phytochemicals in*
  broccoli

Broccoli is a rich source of cancer-fighting chemicals. After broccoli has been eaten, glucosinolates—precursors to broccoli's phytochemicals—break down into indoles and isothiocyanates.

• An indole in broccoli called indole-3-carbinol appears to be particularly beneficial in protecting against hormone-related cancers, such as breast and prostate, by interfering with the replication of cancer cells.

• Isothiocyanates, including the powerful compound sulforaphane, inhibit the damaging effects of cancer-causing substances and suppress the development of tumors.

• An additional anticancer substance in broccoli, dithiolthione, is believed to activate cancer-fighting enzymes in the body.

preparing to use

Very fresh young broccoli can be served raw as an hors d'oeuvre or in salads. Its taste and texture, however, don't agree with all palates; in general, most people prefer broccoli cooked. If you'd like to serve broccoli raw, broccolini might be a better choice. Whichever way you serve the vegetable, first rinse it thoroughly under cold running water to remove surface dirt. If you see dirt embedded in the florets, soak the broccoli in cold water for several minutes to flush it out.

Most people cut off and discard the leaves; however, they are eminently edible and contain even more beta carotene than the florets. (If you decide to remove them, consider using them in soups, purees, or stir-fries.) If you wish, peel the stalks—which get tougher the longer you keep the broccoli—but remove only a thin layer to preserve the nutrients.

Because the broccoli florets tend to cook much faster than the stalks, either split the stalks about halfway up or cut an "X" in the bottom of each stalk. Another option is to cut off the florets and add them to the pot after the stalks have cooked for 2 to 3 minutes. You can also cut both the florets and stalks into smaller pieces for fast, even cooking.

Broccolini and Chinese broccoli can be eaten from stem to flower. Broccoflower and purple broccoli should be treated like broccoli. Broccoli rabe should be trimmed at the bottom, to remove the very tough ends. Any very large or damaged leaves should be discarded as well.

serving suggestions

• Puree cooked broccoli. Add milk and seasonings for a quick soup.

• Make a raw broccoli slaw.

• Sauté broccoli or broccoli rabe in a small amount of olive oil and serve as is or tossed with pasta.

• Toss sautéed broccoli rabe with raisins or sun-dried tomatoes and a sprinkling of toasted almonds. The bitterness of broccoli rabe pairs nicely with the sweetness of dried fruit.

• Top a pizza with broccoli.

• Add broccoli, Chinese broccoli, broccolini, broccoflower, or purple broccoli, to sautés and stir-fries.

brussels sprouts

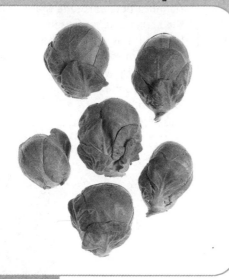

Named after the capital of Belgium, where they may have first been cultivated, Brussels sprouts look like diminutive heads of cabbage. The resemblance is not surprising, since both belong to the same botanical family. A relative newcomer to the cabbage family—standard cabbage has been around for some 3,000 years, Brussels sprouts for a mere 500—Brussels sprouts are one of the few vegetables to have originated in northern Europe. In the 19th century, They were introduced to France, then to England—where they are still highly popular—and later to America, where French settlers grew them in Louisiana. Since this plant is actually a form of cabbage, Brussels sprouts are similar to cabbage in taste, but are slightly milder in flavor and denser in texture.

nutritional profile

Brussels sprouts are nutrient-dense and offer a plentiful supply of vitamin C, fiber, folate, and other B vitamins, as well as the carotenoids lutein and zeaxanthin. With over 25 percent of their calories coming from protein, they are a healthy, low-fat plant source of this nutrient.

BRUSSELS SPROUTS
1 cup cooked

Calories	61
Protein (g)	4
Carbohydrate (g)	14
Dietary fiber (g)	4.1
Total fat (g)	0.8
Saturated fat (g)	0.2
Monounsaturated fat (g)	0.1
Polyunsaturated fat (g)	0.4
Cholesterol (mg)	0
Potassium (mg)	495
Sodium (mg)	33

KEY NUTRIENTS (%RDA/AI*)

Thiamin	0.2 mg (14%)
Riboflavin	0.1 mg (10%)
Vitamin B$_6$	0.3 mg (16%)
Vitamin C	97 mg (107%)
Folate	94 mcg (23%)
Iron	1.9 mg (23%)

For more detailed information on RDA and AI, see page 88.

how brussels sprouts grow

If you have only seen Brussels sprouts in a store, you probably don't know how unusual they look growing in the garden. Whereas other members of the cabbage family form a single large head on a short stem, a Brussels sprout plant consists of a tall, thick stem from which many tiny "cabbage" heads sprout. The heads grow closely together on the stalk from the bottom up in a circular fashion, so that on any given plant the bottom sprouts are the most mature. Between the sprouts (and at the top of the plant), large palmlike leaves grow sporadically to shelter the sprouts from excessive sun or heavy rains. The plants grow to a height of 2 to 3 feet, depending on the variety. Most Brussels sprouts are clipped off their stalks and packaged in containers for sale. But you can sometimes find sprouts attached to their stems at farmers' markets and roadside stands.

in the market

There are several varieties of Brussels sprouts, each planted to peak at various times in the fall-winter season; this provides a steady supply of the vegetable. The most common varieties—*Rampart, Content, Oliver, Rowena,* and *Valiant*—are virtually indistinguishable from one another.

choosing the best

Fresh Brussels sprouts should be displayed under refrigeration; if kept at room temperature, their leaves will turn yellow quickly. Although Brussels sprouts are commonly sold in pint or quart tubs, it's easier to choose sound sprouts if you can select them individually from a bulk display. Choose Brussels sprouts of comparable size so that they will cook evenly.

A bright green color is the best guide to freshness and good condition; yellowed or wilted leaves are a sure sign of age or mishandling. Old Brussels sprouts also have a strong, cabbagey odor. Avoid puffy or soft sprouts; choose small, firm, compact ones with unblemished leaves. Tiny holes or sootlike smudges on the leaves may indicate the presence of worms or plant lice. The stem ends should be clean and white.

▶ **When you get home** Don't wash or trim Brussels sprouts before storing them, except for removing any yellow or wilted outer leaves. Don't remove fresh outer leaves, since these contain the most nutrients. If you've purchased Brussels sprouts in a cellophane-covered container, take off the wrapping and examine the sprouts, then return them to the container, re-cover with the cellophane, and refrigerate. If you buy loose Brussels sprouts, store them in a perforated plastic bag.

preparing to use

Drop the Brussels sprouts into a basin of lukewarm water and leave them for 10 minutes; this easy step will eliminate any insects hidden in the leaves. Then rinse the sprouts in fresh water. Trim the stem ends, but not quite flush with the bottoms of the sprouts, or the outer leaves will fall off during cooking.

Pull off any wilted or blemished outer leaves. Many cooks cut an "X" in the base of each sprout; this helps the heat penetrate the solid core so that it cooks as quickly as the leaves.

serving suggestions

• Whole sprouts are perfect for shish kebabs: Steam them briefly, thread on skewers with meat or chicken and other vegetables, then grill.

• Halve or slice Brussels sprouts, steam, then toss with a vinaigrette or other salad dressing. Serve warm or at room temperature as a side dish or salad.

• Steam small Brussels sprouts and roast chestnuts separately. Then stir the two together in a skillet with some olive oil and balsamic vinegar to glaze them.

• Cut young, raw sprouts into lengthwise slices and add to salads.

▶ phytochemicals in brussels sprouts

• Brussels sprouts are among a handful of foods (including broccoli, cabbage, and cauliflower) with a rich reservoir of phytochemicals—such as indoles and isothiocyanates—that are thought to help thwart tumor development and to stimulate natural anticancer enzymes in the body.

• Brussels sprouts contain antioxidant flavonoids as well, which help to disarm damaging free radicals. Flavonoid phytochemicals contribute to this vegetable's high score on the ORAC (oxygen radical absorbance capacity) scale, which scientists use to measure a food's antioxidant power.

buckwheat

One of the earliest crops to be domesticated, buckwheat is thought to have originated in Central Asia. Some historians speculate that its earliest use as a food was most likely in China 5,000 to 6,000 years ago (it is still used there for making bread). It later became popular throughout Europe and eventually made its way to this country with the Dutch and German immigrants in the 17th century. These immigrants grew large quantities of buckwheat, which is a versatile, hardy, and easy-to-grow, short-season grain crop that can adapt well to poor soil. Although demand for buckwheat in this country as a food source is currently relatively small, its desirable nutritional value is slowly improving its popularity.

Interestingly, the "wheat" in the name buckwheat is misleading as it isn't related to wheat at all. In fact, buckwheat isn't a true grain, but rather the fruit of a leafy plant belonging to the same family as sorrel and rhubarb. It is often referred to as a pseudo-cereal, since the grain is used in ways similar to cereal grains. Its name comes from a Dutch word that translates as "beechwheat," most likely a reference to the plant's triangular fruits, which resemble beechnuts.

nutritional profile

Buckwheat contains plant protein and significant amounts of the amino acid lysine—which is lacking in most plant foods. Buckwheat is also an excellent source of iron and magnesium, and has a respectable amount of the B vitamin niacin.

in the market

Americans are probably most familiar with buckwheat as a flour used to make the pancakes called blini. But whole-grain buckwheat is widely available (in supermarkets as well as health-food stores), and can be cooked and offered as an alternative to rice. Buckwheat contains little gluten and may be a good grain choice for individuals who have a sensitivity to that protein substance. The forms of buckwheat on the market include:

Flour See Flour, Nonwheat (*page 324*).

Grits Sold as buckwheat cereal or cream of buckwheat, these finely ground, almost white, unroasted groats cook much more quickly than whole groats, developing a soft and creamy texture. They are best served as a breakfast cereal or as a rice-pudding-style dessert.

Groats Groats are the raw kernels of buckwheat. They come either hulled (with their inedible black shells removed) or unhulled. *Unhulled groats*—which are available in health-food stores—are used for sprouting (*see Sprouts, page 542*). *Hulled groats* come in two forms: *white (unroasted)* or *brown*

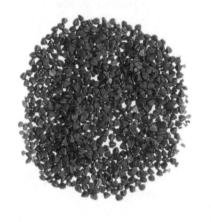

roasted buckwheat groats

BUCKWHEAT GROATS 1 cup cooked	
Calories	155
Protein (g)	6
Carbohydrate (g)	33
Dietary fiber (g)	4.5
Total fat (g)	1.0
Saturated fat (g)	0.2
Monounsaturated fat (g)	0.3
Polyunsaturated fat (g)	0.3
Cholesterol (mg)	0
Potassium (mg)	148
Sodium (mg)	7

KEY NUTRIENTS (%RDA/AI*)	
Niacin	1.6 mg (10%)
Iron	1.3 mg (17%)
Magnesium	86 mg (20%)

*For more detailed information on RDA and AI, see page 88.

(roasted). The white groats have a fairly mild flavor and can be substituted in dishes that call for white or brown rice. Brown, roasted buckwheat is known as kasha (*see below*).

Kasha Roasted, hulled buckwheat kernels that are either whole or cracked into coarse, medium, or fine granules are commonly known as kasha. Enjoy their toasty flavor as an accompaniment to meat or as the basis for a grain–and–vegetable main dish.

choosing the best

As with all grains, shop in markets that have a brisk turnover. If purchasing in bulk, from open bins, the grains should not have any stale or rancid odor, and they should look whole, rather than dusty or powdery. Buy only what you'll use within a short period of time.

If buying kasha in boxes, check the label to make sure you're getting the granulation you want. If possible, check for a "sell by" date as well.

► **When you get home** To prevent bug infestation, store buckwheat in tightly sealed containers. In the summer months, if you have room, place buckwheat in the refrigerator or freezer.

buckwheat & eggs

Many recipes for buckwheat dishes call for a beaten egg to be mixed into the groats before cooking. The addition of the egg keeps the grains separate as they cook, so that they have the consistency of rice rather than oatmeal. As grains cook and absorb water, their cell walls rupture and release the starches contained inside, thus causing the grains to stick together. Egg albumin—a protein—acts as a sealant, strengthening the outer cell walls of the groats and preventing them from rupturing.

The egg also supplies the buckwheat with essential amino acids, making a complete protein. It does, however, add fat and cholesterol—but only a little: ½ cup of cooked kasha prepared with 1 egg will have about 1 gram of fat and 43 milligrams of cholesterol. To avoid the added fat and cholesterol and still get the protein benefit, use just the egg white instead.

serving suggestions

- Add buckwheat to soups and stews as a thickener.

- Serve buckwheat instead of rice or in combination with brown, white, or wild rice.

- Combine cooked groats or kasha with tuna, chopped mushrooms, and a yogurt or vinaigrette dressing for a main-dish salad.

- Use cooled, cooked kasha as you would bulgur wheat, to make tabbouleh.

- Add cooked kasha to burger and meatloaf mixtures.

- Cook buckwheat grits in milk or a milk/water mixture for a hot cereal or serve them as a dessert with dried cherries stirred in.

cabbage

Cabbages have been cultivated for at least 2,500 years, most likely first in the eastern Mediterranean, though the cabbages eaten then had loose leaves and were probably a different variety from the types we consume today. During the Middle Ages, farmers in northern Europe developed compact-headed varieties with overlapping leaves (the cabbages familiar to us today) that were capable of thriving in cold climates and thus provided sustenance for people who had little else to eat during the winter. The cabbage continues to be a useful food that is easy to grow, is tolerant of cold, keeps well, and can be cooked in a wide variety of ways. A long-standing dietary staple, the cabbage is a sturdy, abundant, and inexpensive vegetable that is versatile and full of texture.

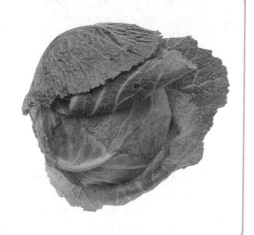

savoy cabbage

nutritional profile

Along with vitamin C, fiber, and the B vitamin folate, cabbages (like other cruciferous vegetables) are rich in potential cancer-fighting phytochemical compounds. Each type of cabbage has a different nutritional make-up—for example, red cabbage has more vitamin C than green cabbage, and compared with other types of cabbage, Savoy cabbage contains more beta carotene.

in the market

Hundreds of varieties of cabbage are grown throughout the world, but in American markets you will find three basic types: green, red, and Savoy.

Green This cabbage has smooth, dark to pale green outer leaves; the inner leaves are pale green or white. (Sometimes the outer leaves are tied around the head as the cabbage grows to keep the interior white; cabbage also turns white if it is kept in cold storage.) Three types of green cabbage—Danish, domestic, and pointed—account for most commercially marketed cabbage. *Danish* types—which are grown for late-fall sale, and for storage over the winter—are very compact and solid, with round or oval heads. *Domestic* types form slightly looser, round or flattened heads, with curled leaves that are more brittle than any of the Danish types. *Pointed* varieties, which are grown mainly for spring marketing, have small, rather conical heads and smooth leaves.

Red Similar in flavor to green cabbage, red cabbage has deep ruby-red to purple outer leaves, with white veins or streaks on the inside. Its texture may be somewhat tougher than green, but red cabbage has more vitamin C, providing 56 percent of the RDA in a 1-cup serving.

Savoy This cabbage has crinkled, ruffly, yellow-green leaves that form a less compact head than other types. Savoy cabbage has a more delicate texture and milder flavor than other varieties, making it a good choice for salads and coleslaw.

GREEN CABBAGE 1 cup raw chopped	
Calories	22
Protein (g)	1
Carbohydrate (g)	5
Dietary fiber (g)	2.1
Total fat (g)	0.2
Saturated fat (g)	0
Monounsaturated fat (g)	0
Polyunsaturated fat (g)	0.1
Cholesterol (mg)	0
Potassium (mg)	219
Sodium (mg)	16

KEY NUTRIENTS (%RDA/AI*)	
Vitamin C	29 mg (32%)
Folate	38 mcg (10%)

*For more detailed information on RDA and AI, see page 88.

chinese cabbages

This is a huge category that is connected more by the market term cabbage than it is by any botanical relationship. Every market and every region will have a slightly different name for the same vegetable, and the Chinese names for these vegetables are no help: They are all some form of *choy*, a word that simply means vegetable. Many of the so-called cabbages, though, do share some flavor characteristics. They all have pungent, sometimes mustardy or cabbagey flavors, and probably share some of the same health benefits as other cruciferous vegetables. The following is a list of some of the more common ones that you may even find outside a Chinese neighborhood.

Baby bok choy This miniature bok choy is shaped just like the big boy, but its stems and leaves are a more uniform green. Its taste is fresh, clean, sweet, and not very cabbagey.

Bok choy Bok choy (*photo, left*) is a loose, bulbous cluster of white to light green stems topped with darker green leaves. Look for firm, white stems and crisp, dark green, glossy leaves. Avoid any with brown spots on the leaves, as these have not been stored at a low enough temperature to prevent some loss in flavor. Separate the leaves from the stalks. Slice the stalks and steam or sauté. The leaves can be sautéed or steamed, either whole or sliced.

Choy sum This member of the Chinese cabbage family is also known as flowering cabbage, and in Japan it's called *saishin*. It has small yellow flowers and slim stalks with rounded leaves. Select firm stalks with crisp leaves.

Gai choy This broad-leafed cabbage has curved stems, a semi-enclosed head, and a strong, pungent, mustardy flavor. It is entirely edible, yet with some varieties of *gai choy* (such as *dai gai choy*), the leafy part is discarded while the stems are used for salting, pickling, or drying.

Napa Though the market name for this cabbage comes from a Japanese word (*nappa*), it has been so absorbed into American cuisine that most people probably think that the name comes from California's Napa Valley. There are several varieties of napa cabbage, but the two most common are michihili, a long cylindrical head with slightly open leaves at the top, and wong bok, the more familiar napa cabbage head, which is large and barrel-shaped, with tightly packed leaves. The leaves on both varieties are crinkly and white to light green. Napa cabbage should feel compact when you press on it. Like regular cabbage, it can be eaten raw or cooked and has a mild cabbagey flavor.

BOK CHOY
1 cup cooked

Calories	20
Protein (g)	3
Carbohydrate (g)	3
Dietary fiber (g)	2.7
Total fat (g)	0.3
Saturated fat (g)	0
Monounsaturated fat (g)	0
Polyunsaturated fat (g)	0.1
Cholesterol (mg)	0
Potassium (mg)	631
Sodium (mg)	58

KEY NUTRIENTS (%RDA/AI*)

Beta carotene	2.6 mg (24%)
Vitamin B$_6$	0.3 mg (17%)
Vitamin C	44 mg (49%)
Folate	69 mcg (17%)
Calcium	158 mg (13%)
Iron	1.8 mg (22%)

*For more detailed information on RDA and AI, see page 88.

Tuscan Relatively new to this country, Tuscan cabbage is available mostly at farmers' markets and specialty produce stores. It's a mild–flavored cabbage, with long, narrow, almost feathery leaves that are dark green with white ribs. It looks like a narrow version of kale, which is a close relative. There is also a *black Tuscan cabbage* (known as *cavalo nero* in Italy where it is much favored), whose leaves are such a dark purple that they appear black.

choosing the best

Look for solid, heavy heads of cabbage, with no more than three or four loose "wrapper" (outer) leaves. These wrapper leaves should be clean and flexible but not limp, and free of discolored veins or worm damage, which may penetrate the interior of the head. The stems should be closely trimmed and healthy looking, not dry or split. The inner and outer leaves should be tightly attached to the stems.

A head of cabbage should not look puffy, although Savoy types are normally looser and lighter than smooth-leaved types. Fall and winter cabbage from storage is usually firmer than the fresh–picked types sold in spring and summer. Don't buy halved or quartered heads of cabbage, even if well wrapped: As soon as the leaves are cut or torn, the vegetable begins to lose vitamin C.

preparing to use

Don't wash cabbage until you are ready to use it. The interior of a tight head of cabbage is nearly always clean, but if you want to rinse it, do so after cutting or chopping the vegetable.

➤ phytochemicals in cabbage

Mounting evidence suggests that consuming a diet rich in cabbage and its cruciferous relatives helps to ward off cancer. The protective effect of cabbage is likely due to its wealth of phytochemicals, such as glucosinolates, which are converted into disease-fighting indoles and isothiocyanates upon digestion.

• Indoles appear to protect against tumor growth, particularly in breast and prostate cancer.

• Isothiocyanates are believed to increase levels of protective enzymes that inhibit hormone-related breast and prostate cancer.

• An intensely studied isothiocyanate phytochemical called sulforaphane may elevate levels of cancer-fighting enzymes.

• Another type of isothiocyanate, called phenethyl isothiocyanate, is thought to counter destruction from carcinogenic agents.

When cutting cabbage into wedges, trim the stem but leave part of the core intact, as it will help hold the leaves together. However, when cabbage is to be cut up into smaller pieces, the first step is to quarter and core it. Using a large, heavy knife, cut the cabbage into quarters through the stem. Then cut out a wedge-shaped section from each quarter to remove the stem and core. If the core is tender, it can be cut up and cooked. Or, you can nibble on it raw while you're cooking.

To slice or shred cabbage, place a quarter-wedge on the cutting board so that it's resting on one of its cut-sides. Slice the wedge crosswise, gauging your cuts to produce wide ribbons or fine shreds, as desired. Or, grate cabbage by hand on the coarse side of a grater, or shred it in a food processor, using the grating disk.

Use a stainless steel (not carbon steel) knife when cutting cabbage; the vegetable's juices react with carbon steel and will turn the cut edges of green cabbage black, and red cabbage blue. To further preserve its bright color, red cabbage should also be cooked in a nonreactive (i.e., not steel, aluminum, or cast-iron) pot.

To remove single leaves for stuffing, cut the base of each leaf with a sharp knife, then carefully peel the leaf from the head to avoid tearing it. To prepare leaves for stuffing, remove them from the head and blanch them until they are limp (2 to 3 minutes). Allow the leaves to cool and then shave off the thick part of the central rib from the back of each leaf, or it may cause the leaf to break when you stuff it.

low-fat coleslaw

Coleslaw (from the Dutch *kool sla*, or cabbage salad) is a deli favorite, but unfortunately, it can be a nutritional disaster: 1 cup may contain up to 200 calories and 16 grams of fat. If you prepare coleslaw at home, you can ensure that it is tasty and nutritious, without a high fat content. To make a low-fat slaw: Shred both red and green cabbage (for color) and toss with ingredients such as shredded apple or pear, grated raw carrots, slivered bell peppers, chopped scallions, or chopped nuts. Toss in some caraway, celery seed, ginger, mint, thyme, parsley, or cilantro. For a mayonnaise style dressing, blend "light" mayonnaise with an equal amount of fat-free plain yogurt. Or make a vinaigrette with 1 part oil to 1 part vinegar. The coleslaw should be very lightly dressed, not swimming in dressing.

RED CABBAGE
1 cup raw chopped

Calories	24
Protein (g)	1
Carbohydrate (g)	5
Dietary fiber (g)	1.8
Total fat (g)	0.2
Saturated fat (g)	0
Monounsaturated fat (g)	0
Polyunsaturated fat (g)	0.1
Cholesterol (mg)	0
Potassium (mg)	183
Sodium (mg)	10

KEY NUTRIENTS (%RDA/AI*)

Vitamin B_6	0.2 mg (11%)
Vitamin C	51 mg (56%)

*For more detailed information on RDA and AI, see page 88.

SAVOY CABBAGE
1 cup raw chopped

Calories	19
Protein (g)	1
Carbohydrate (g)	4
Dietary fiber (g)	2.2
Total fat (g)	0.1
Saturated fat (g)	0
Monounsaturated fat (g)	0
Polyunsaturated fat (g)	0
Cholesterol (mg)	0
Potassium (mg)	161
Sodium (mg)	20

KEY NUTRIENTS (%RDA/AI*)

Folate	56 mcg (14%)
Vitamin C	22 mg (24%)

*For more detailed information on RDA and AI, see page 88.

cantaloupe

Fragrant, sweet, and luscious, the melon we refer to as "cantaloupe" (the most popular melon in the United States) is technically a muskmelon. True cantaloupe comes from Europe and has a hard surface quite unlike the soft, netted rind of our familiar fruit. The khaki-colored skin of what we know as cantaloupe has green undertones that ripen to yellow or cream.

Cantaloupes are thought to be Persian in origin, and evidence shows that they may have been cultivated by the ancient Greeks and Romans. During the Middle Ages, they spread through the Mediterranean region and were prevalent in Spain by the 15th century. Indeed it was Columbus who reputedly brought muskmelon seeds to the New World. It was not until some time after the Civil War, however, that cantaloupes became an important market crop in the United States.

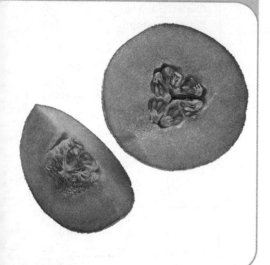

cantaloupe

nutritional profile

A perfect food for anyone trying to control their weight, cantaloupes have a high water content; offer a full, rich flavor and aroma; and contain very few calories. Cantaloupes supply a good amount of vitamin B_6 and potassium, and are an excellent source of vitamin C. Their major claim to fame, however, is revealed in the rich orange color of their flesh: They contain an exceptional amount of beta carotene. In fact, cantaloupes have more beta carotene than any other melon.

in the market

While there are many varieties of cantaloupe available for the home gardener, the cantaloupe found in the marketplace is generally the "Western shipping" type muskmelon, marketed as cantaloupe.

choosing the best

Since cantaloupes have no starch reserves to convert to sugar, they will not ripen further once they have left the vine. They're picked when they are ripe but still firm, to protect them during shipping. Invariably, some are picked too early, so it is important to know the characteristics of a ripe cantaloupe.

Unless the melon is cut, the only clue to ripeness is the condition of the rind. Cantaloupes should be slightly golden—not a dull green—under the rind's meshlike "netting," which should cover the whole rind; reject those with slick spots. The stem end should have a slight indentation (called a "full slip") if the melon was picked at the proper stage. The melon should be firm, but not rock hard. The blossom end will be slightly soft if the melon is ready to eat and, unless the fruit is chilled, a flowery, sweet fragrance will be apparent. Cantaloupes may be football-shaped or spherical, and while it's natural for the melon to be slightly bleached on one side from lying on the ground as it grew, it should not be flattened or lopsided.

CANTALOUPE / 1 cup	
Calories	62
Protein (g)	2
Carbohydrate (g)	15
Dietary fiber (g)	1.4
Total fat (g)	0.5
Saturated fat (g)	0.1
Monounsaturated fat (g)	0
Polyunsaturated fat (g)	0.2
Cholesterol (mg)	0
Potassium (mg)	547
Sodium (mg)	16

KEY NUTRIENTS (%RDA/AI*)	
Beta carotene	3.4 mg (31%)
Vitamin B_6	0.2 mg (12%)
Vitamin C	75 mg (83%)

*For more detailed information on RDA and AI, see page 88.

If your market sells cut cantaloupes, the fruit should be perfect for immediate consumption, as it will not improve once it is cut. With cut melons, you can check the color and texture of the flesh and usually smell the delectable fragrance of a ripe melon even through the tight plastic wrapping.

▶ **When you get home** You can improve the eating quality of a firm, uncut cantaloupe by leaving it at room temperature for 2 to 4 days; the fruit will not become sweeter, but it will turn softer and juicier. If during that time the cantaloupe has not reached its peak ripeness, it was picked immature and will not be worth eating. Once ripened (or cut), cantaloupe should be refrigerated and used within about 2 days. Enclose cut pieces in plastic bags to protect other produce in the refrigerator from the ethylene gas that the melons give off. Ripe cantaloupe is also very fragrant, and the aroma of a cut melon can penetrate other foods.

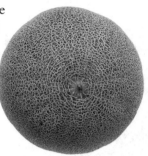

Persian melons very closely resemble cantaloupes, though they are larger and their rind is greener.

preparing to use

Simply cut the melon open and remove the seeds and strings. It can be served in many attractive ways: cut into halves, quarters, wedges, or cubes; or the flesh can be scooped out with a melon baller.

For melon rings, cut a cantaloupe into thick, crosswise slices, scrape out the seeds, and remove the rind, if desired.

serving suggestions

- Serve cantaloupe wedges with feta or goat cheese and cherry tomatoes.

- Add cantaloupe chunks to yogurt along with a couple of ice cubes and puree to make a smoothie.

- Combine cantaloupe and avocado for an interesting salsa.

- Freeze cantaloupe chunks, then pulse in a food processor to make an instant sorbet.

- Puree cantaloupe, peaches, orange juice, and lime juice, then chill for a cold soup.

- Add cantaloupe to skewers when grilling shrimp, scallops, or chicken.

- Halve and remove the seeds, then fill the centers of cantaloupe halves with part-skim ricotta and minced crystallized ginger.

- Wrap thin slivers of lean smoked turkey around cantaloupe wedges and serve with a drizzle of aged balsamic vinegar.

- Add cantaloupe chunks to chicken and pasta salad and toss lightly with lime or lemon vinaigrette.

carrots

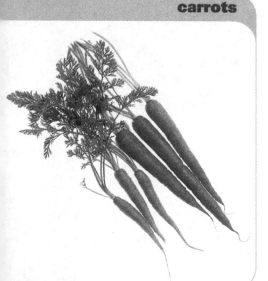

carrots

The carrot belongs to the *Umbelliferae* family, and is recognizable by its feathery leaves as a relative of parsley, dill, fennel, and celery—and the wildflower Queen Anne's lace, from which it first may have been domesticated. The carrot that we are familiar with today is quite different from its wild ancestor, which was a small, pale, acrid root. Early varieties of carrots were white, purple, red, yellow, and green, not orange.

Carrots were thought to be cultivated in the Mediterranean area before the Christian Era, probably for their purported medicinal value rather than as a food. By the 16th century, people in Europe were familiar with the carrot and writers of that time described many varieties. The elongated orange carrot, forerunner of today's familiar vegetable, was probably developed in the 17th century in the Netherlands and adjoining regions. When early European settlers came to Virginia, they brought carrot seeds with them for planting.

nutritional profile

Low in calories and virtually devoid of fat, carrots provide fiber, potassium, iron, and vitamin B_6, and spectacular amounts of beta carotene. Carrots are the leading source of this substance in the American diet. In fact, *carot*enoids, the group of plant pigments of which beta carotene is a member, are so named because they were first identified in carrots. Dietary beta carotene may reduce the risk of heart disease and certain types of cancer through its potent antioxidant activity.

In addition, dietary beta carotene is a safe source of vitamin A, because the conversion to vitamin A is regulated by the body's need for vitamin A. Essential for the functioning of the retina of the eye, vitamin A is synthesized in the body by the breakdown of carotenes, the orange pigments in carrots. Other carotenoids in carrots include alpha carotene and lutein. The deeper the orange color, the more carotenoids.

Carrots also contain a type of soluble fiber called calcium pectate, which studies suggest may help to lower LDL ("bad") cholesterol levels. Calcium pectate attaches to bile acids, which helps to remove harmful cholesterol from the body.

Eating excessive quantities of carrots can cause the skin to turn yellow because of the high intake of carotenoid pigments. This condition—called carotenemia—is perfectly harmless, and affected skin will return to normal within a few weeks if carrot consumption is reduced.

CARROTS / 1 cup cooked	
Calories	70
Protein (g)	2
Carbohydrate (g)	16
Dietary fiber (g)	5.2
Total fat (g)	0.3
Saturated fat (g)	0
Monounsaturated fat (g)	0
Polyunsaturated fat (g)	0.1
Cholesterol (mg)	0
Potassium (mg)	354
Sodium (mg)	103

KEY NUTRIENTS (%RDA/AI*)		
Beta carotene	17 mg	(169%)
Vitamin B_6	0.4 mg	(23%)
Iron	1 mg	(12%)

*For more detailed information on RDA and AI, see page 88.

in the market

There are many varieties of the good old-fashioned orange carrot, and they are interchangeable as far as the cook is concerned. There are a number of boutique carrots showing up now, including white, maroon, and baby carrots:

Baby carrots Available in farmers' markets and specialty food stores are bunches of carrots that are considerably smaller than others and that are loosely termed "baby" carrots. These "baby" carrots are actually fully mature specimens of a small carrot variety. A true immature, or baby, carrot would actually not have much flavor and not be worth eating. The bags of "baby" carrots available in supermarkets aren't baby carrots either. These are actually pieces of carrot that have been sculpted to resemble small carrots.

Beta III These super beta carotene-rich carrots (five times that of regular carrots) are the result of a four-year collaboration between a horticulturist and a geneticist.

Maroon carrots Also known as Beta-Sweet, these are sweeter than regular carrots. Although their exterior is maroon, the interior is bright orange. The texture of these carrots is more porous, like that of apples or celery.

Round carrots About the size and shape of large radishes, these orange carrots taste like regular carrots and are more of a curiosity than a culinary find.

White carrots These thin carrots are white in color and mild in flavor.

choosing the best

Carrots are usually sold one of three ways: in bunches with their tops still on, loose (with no greens), or in bags, also with no greens. Carrots in bunches with their tops are usually higher priced than bagged carrots. Some consumers see the tops as an indication of freshness, which indeed they are— if crisp and bright green. However, refrigeration and moisture-retaining packaging are the best preservers of freshness: If carrots are displayed unwrapped at room temperature, they will lose sweetness and crispness, with or without their leafy crown.

On the other hand, the bags that "clip-top" or "topped" carrots are packaged in often have thin red-orange lines printed on them. This decoration gives the illusion of brighter, fresher-looking carrots. Other bags have a dark band at their bottoms, thus obscuring the stem ends of the carrots, which provide an important visual clue to freshness. In certain states, however, carrots bags are required to have a "window" that affords the consumer a clear view of the contents. Look for well-shaped carrots; they should not be gnarled or covered with rootlets. Their color should be a healthy reddish-orange, not pale or yellow, from top to bottom (the darker the orange color, the more beta carotene is present). The top, or "shoulder," may be tinged with green, but should not be dark or black, both indications of age. However, the green part is likely to be bitter (it should be trimmed before eating); if carrots are very green on top, they should not be purchased. Also, avoid carrots that are cracked, shriveled, soft, or wilted.

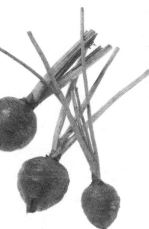

Round carrots look almost like big orange radishes.

Fairly young carrots are likely to be mild-flavored and tender, but, surprisingly, mature carrots are often sweeter, with a dense, close-grained texture. Regardless of a carrot's age, the smaller its core—the fibrous channel that runs the length of the vegetable—the sweeter the carrot, as the vegetable's natural sugars lie in the outer layers. Usually, you can't see the core until you cut the carrot, but any carrots that have large, thick "shoulders" (the top of the carrot) are likely to have large cores, too. Though the overall size of the carrot is not necessarily a clue to the size of the core, if the shoulders are disproportionately larger than the rest of the carrot, it may have a larger core and be less sweet.

▶ **When you get home** If you buy carrots with "tops," twist or cut off the stalks to about 1 inch above the root before storing. Otherwise, the greens will wilt and decay quickly; furthermore, moisture will be drawn from the roots, turning them limp and rubbery.

preparing to use

Although carrots may look clean, bacteria from the soil may be present on the surface. So, whether eating the carrots raw or cooked, be sure to scrub them with a vegetable brush under running water, or peel them with a swivel-bladed vegetable peeler or paring knife, then rinse thoroughly.

If you enjoy crunching on raw carrots, then do so. However, since carrots have tough cellular walls that the body cannot easily break down, cooking them just until crisp-tender actually makes their nutrients (including beta carotene) more accessible—although *over*cooking them may decrease the carotene level.

Proper cooking brings out the sweetness in carrots. They can be left whole, cut into short lengths, sliced, diced, or shredded. A food processor is handy for slicing or shredding.

carrot juice

One of the best-kept secrets of the cooking world is carrot juice. It's like a ready-made vegetable stock, with deep flavor, beautiful color, and virtually no fat. And if that isn't enough, it also carries with it a nice health bonus in the form of beta carotene (13 milligrams per cup, or 114 percent of the RDA), B vitamins (especially vitamin B_6, at 30 percent of the RDA), and potassium. Try carrot juice in place of some or all of the chicken stock in risottos or pilafs. Use it as the liquid in bread and pizza doughs, or homemade pasta. Add it to tomato-based pasta sauces, soups, and stews. Use it in smoothies and salad dressings.

Carrot juice is available in supermarkets in cans (it's usually in the canned fruit and vegetable juice area, though some stores seem to file it away as a health food). It is also available in the refrigerated compartments at health-food stores or at juice bars freshly "squeezed."

cauliflower

Cauliflower, as its name suggests, is indeed a flower, one growing from a plant that in its early stages resembles broccoli, its closest relative. However, while broccoli opens outward to sprout bunches of green florets, cauliflower forms a compact head of undeveloped white flower buds. As it grows on a single stalk, the head (known as the "curd") is surrounded by heavily ribbed green leaves that protect it from sunlight, so that the flower buds don't develop chlorophyll. With some types of cauliflower, however, the head pokes through the leaves and the grower periodically will tie the leaves over the head to shield it from the sun. Otherwise, exposure to sunlight would discolor the florets and also cause them to develop an undesirable flavor.

Cauliflower is believed to have originated sometime after the birth of Christ, in the Mediterranean and Asia Minor. It gradually made its way west, arriving in parts of Europe in the early 17th century. Its introduction to the United States is surprisingly recent: Cauliflower was not cultivated for commercial purposes in this country until the 1920s.

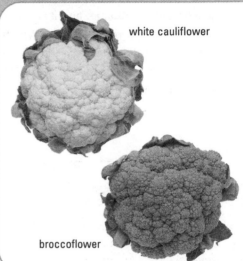

cauliflower

white cauliflower

broccoflower

nutritional profile

Cauliflower is an excellent source of vitamin C and a good source of the B vitamin folate and vitamin B_6. A substantial amount of both vitamin C and the B vitamins in cauliflower can be lost if the vegetable is cooked in too much water or for too long. The vitamin C is diminished by heat, and the B vitamins (because they are water-soluble) leach into the cooking water. For the highest vitamin C content, it's best to eat cauliflower uncooked, but for cooked cauliflower, steaming is best. (If you do cook cauliflower in water, try to save the water for soup or stock to conserve the B vitamins.)

in the market

While there are many different cultivars of *white cauliflower* grown, they are marketed simply under the name "cauliflower." There are also some variants available:

Broccoflower This genetic cross combines the physical features of cauliflower with the chlorophyll of broccoli, but tastes more like cauliflower than broccoli. With heads ranging from yellow-green to lime-green, broccoflower has a sweeter taste than conventional cauliflower.

Purple cauliflower This purple-headed type turns green when cooked.

choosing the best

For cauliflower, select clean, firm, compact heads that are white or creamy-white. A medium-sized head is 6 inches in diameter and weighs about 2 pounds—enough to serve 4 to 6 people after trimming off the leaves and

CAULIFLOWER 1 cup cooked	
Calories	29
Protein (g)	2
Carbohydrate (g)	5
Dietary fiber (g)	3.3
Total fat (g)	0.6
Saturated fat (g)	0.1
Monounsaturated fat (g)	0
Polyunsaturated fat (g)	0.3
Cholesterol (mg)	0
Potassium (mg)	176
Sodium (mg)	19

KEY NUTRIENTS (%RDA/AI*)	
Vitamin B_6	0.2 mg (13%)
Vitamin C	55 mg (61%)
Folate	55 mcg (14%)

*For more detailed information on RDA and AI, see page 88.

stem. Avoid heads that are soft, have brown coloring or small dark spots on the curds. (The size of the head doesn't affect its quality.) Any leaves that remain should be green and crisp. Small leaves growing between the florets are not a sign of poor quality; just pull them out before you cook the cauliflower. Some stores also sell packaged florets that have been trimmed off the head; these, too, should be free of bruises or spots.

For broccoflower, look for yellowish-green or pale-green heads that are firm with no space between the curds. The leaves should be fresh and green. As with regular cauliflower, there is no quality difference between large and small heads.

preparing to use

The head can be easily separated into florets for serving raw or cooked. (Raw cauliflower is milder tasting than raw broccoli.) For cooking, you can also leave the head whole, which some people prefer because of its appearance; however, it takes longer to cook than the florets and so more nutrients may be lost.

First, trim the cauliflower: Pull off any outer leaves and cut off the protruding stem end close to the head. If you find that the florets have started to turn brown at the edges, trim off these areas. To cook the head whole, remove the base of the core by cutting around the stem with a small knife; this step allows for faster, more even cooking.

To prepare florets, hollow out the inner core. Then you will be able to separate the head into florets, or slice off the florets around the inner core. Split any larger florets in two and slice up the inner core pieces. Rinse the cauliflower thoroughly before cooking.

Like broccoli, cauliflower contains plant acids that form odorous sulfur compounds as the vegetable is heated; these odors become more intense the longer the cauliflower cooks. Rapid cooking not only reduces the odors, but keeps the texture crisp, preserves the vegetable's white color, and reduces the loss of nutrients.

If possible, try to avoid cooking cauliflower in an aluminum or iron pot. When the chemical compounds in cauliflower come into contact with aluminum they turn the vegetable yellow, while an iron pot turns it brown or blue-green. To preserve its white color and to prevent cauliflower from turning a different color, add a tablespoon of an acid, such as lemon juice, lime juice, or vinegar to the cooking water.

➤ phytochemicals in cauliflower

Cauliflower (and its cruciferous cousins) is one of the few foods linked to a reduced risk of cancer by numerous population studies. Like broccoli, cabbage, and its other relatives, cauliflower is a reservoir of phytochemicals, such as isothiocyanates and indoles, which are thought to help detoxify cancer-causing agents and impede tumor development.

---

serving suggestions

• Toss cauliflower florets with a bit of olive oil and several cloves of unpeeled garlic. Roast, uncovered, in a 375° oven until golden brown and tender.

• Add chopped florets to pasta sauces.

• Combine mashed potatoes and cooked cauliflower or broccoflower. Add milk and heat for a quick soup.

• Add cooked cauliflower or broccoflower to macaroni and cheese.

• Season steamed cauliflower with dillweed or nutmeg, or toss with chopped fresh parsley, chives, or toasted almonds.

celery

Valued for its crisp texture and distinctive flavor, celery is as much a household staple as onions, carrots, or potatoes. Versatile and widely used as an appetizer, a salad ingredient, and a flavorful addition to many cooked dishes, celery is also a perfect snack food for people watching their weight. A bunch of celery is more accurately called a stalk, which is made up of individual ribs. These ribs are naturally crisp due to the rigidity of the plant's cell walls and the high water content within the cells.

Wild celery has been around for almost 3,000 years; it is believed to have originated in the Mediterranean, where it was used not as a food, but as medicine. It was also used by the ancient Greeks as an award in sports contests. Celery was first cultivated in the 16th century in northern Europe, though another 200 years passed before modern-looking varieties with large, fleshy ribs appeared. Celery has been commercially grown in the United States for more than 150 years.

nutritional profile

Because of its high water content, celery has hardly any calories: An 8-inch rib contains a mere 6 calories. Celery provides a good amount of potassium and vitamin C, and some insoluble fiber. Celery is an ideal food for people trying to control their weight because its fiber and high water content provide satiety (it can make you feel full), and its crunchy, chewy texture contributes to a feeling of satisfaction as well.

in the market

The celery that every American has seen in supermarkets, had in tunafish salad, or dipped into dips at a party is a type of celery called *Pascal*. This green celery, which dominates the market and is definitely not known by its name, is the result of years of effort to domesticate this ancient vegetable and turn it less stringy. There are several different varieties of Pascal and a number of Pascal clones, but they are all essentially the same. The only standouts, which are not that easy to find, are:

Chinese celery Also called Asian celery, this tall, skinny celery looks like a cross between parsley and celery. The stalks are fatter than parsley stalks and skinnier than celery stalks. It has a much more pronounced celery flavor than Pascal celery. Both the stems and leaves are used to add flavor to stir-fries and soups. Though it is difficult to find outside of Asian neighborhoods, this celery actually comes in a number of forms, mostly differing in stem and leaf color, from white to golden to deep green.

Golden celery Golden celery is light yellow, a color (or lack thereof) that occurs because the plant is grown under a layer of soil or paper to pre-

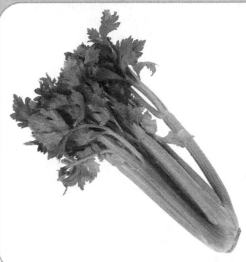

pascal celery

CELERY / 1 cup chopped	
Calories	20
Protein (g)	1
Carbohydrate (g)	4
Dietary fiber (g)	2.0
Total fat (g)	0.2
Saturated fat (g)	0
Monounsaturated fat (g)	0
Polyunsaturated fat (g)	0.1
Cholesterol (mg)	0
Potassium (mg)	344
Sodium (mg)	104

KEY NUTRIENTS (%RDA/AI*)

Vitamin C	8 mg (10%)

*For more detailed information on RDA and AI, see page 88.

vent chlorophyll from developing (much like white asparagus or Belgian endive). This pale celery is favored in Italian cooking and can often be found in Italian markets.

choosing the best

Light green celery ribs with a glossy surface tend to taste best. (Dark green ribs have slightly more nutrients, but are apt to be stringy.) If not wrapped, celery should be sprinkled with water to prevent wilting. Look first at the bunch—it should be compact and well shaped—and then examine the leaves, which should be green and fresh-looking. The leaves are a good guide to the celery's overall condition. The ribs and leaf stems should feel firm and crisp, as if they would snap when broken in half, and should be free of cracks or bruises.

Inspect both the outer and inner surfaces of ribs for discolored spots or bruises, or for patches that appear to be trimmed off—grocers sometimes slice off bruised or rotting areas, and such stalks won't keep as long as undamaged celery.

▶ When you get home Keep celery away from the coldest areas of the refrigerator—the back and the side walls—since it freezes easily, thus damaging the cell walls. Once thawed, the celery will be limp and watery. If the ribs have begun to wilt by the time you want to use them, refresh them by separating the ribs and submerging them in ice water for several minutes.

preparing to use

Should the outer ribs in a bunch be coarse and stringy, just peel them with a vegetable peeler. Trim off the leaves and knobby tops—and if you wish, save them to add flavor and texture to salads, broths, soups, and stews.

negative calories?

Does celery have "negative calories"? Celery is very low in calories, but not so low that chewing it burns more calories than the vegetable contains. It's true that a medium-sized rib has only 6 calories, but chewing celery burns about the same number of calories per minute as just sitting. Basically celery, like iceberg lettuce and cucumbers, is nearly calorie free—not because of the energy required to chew the vegetable, but because of its high water content. If you're on a diet, munching celery is better for you than eating a candy bar. But remember, no food has negative calories.

cheese

Rich, highly flavorful, and with an enormous range of textures and aromas, cheese is made in nearly every country where milk is produced and available—from the simple fresh cheeses that have graced the poor man's table since pre-biblical times, to today's sophisticated, gourmet cheeses.

Although its origins are obscure, it is believed that cheese was first made in the Middle East and dates back to the earliest domestication of animals, about 9000 B.C. By the time the Roman Empire rolled around, cheese had reached a place of luxury and status: Wealthy Romans even built special kitchens for cheesemaking and special areas where cheese could be matured (the poor folk had to bring their cheese to public smokehouses for curing). During the Middle Ages, innovative monks experimented with cheesemaking, and it is to them we owe many of the classic varieties of cheese sold today.

Cheese fell into some disfavor in Europe during the Renaissance, and was regarded with suspicion because people feared that it had occult powers that could make them ill—a not unreasonable fear, considering that pasteurization, which destroys disease-causing organisms in milk, didn't become widespread until the mid-19th century. Cheese's fall from grace eventually reversed, and by the 19th century it had moved from farm to full-scale commercial production.

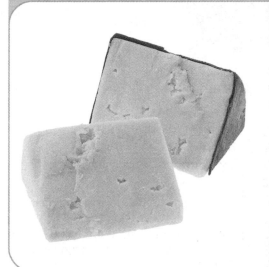

cheddar cheese

nutritional profile

Americans love their cheese. Per capita consumption in the United States is 30 pounds a year—that's more than a slice of cheese every single day. Unfortunately, this love affair may be more responsible for the high saturated-fat intake of the American diet than any other high-fat food.

Since about 8 pounds of milk are used to make 1 pound of most types of cheese, just an ounce (an average slice) of cheese contains more fat—most of it saturated—than a typical serving of ice cream. In fact, most cheeses derive 60 to 90 percent of their calories from fat. Therefore, vegetarians who replace meat with cheese are doing themselves no favor.

Despite this nutritional drawback, you needn't give up cheese: Just eat smaller portions. Because cheese is so savory and rich-tasting, a little can go a long way. (You might also consider trying some of the lower-fat cheeses; their flavor has improved considerably over the years.)

Like all dairy products, cheese is usually high in protein and an excellent source of the bone-building mineral calcium. To get calcium from cheese without a lot of fat, select higher-calcium cheeses that are also lower in fat (*see "Comparing Cheeses," page 224*), such as part-skim mozzarella cheese. Cheese also supplies other essential nutrients including vitamin A, vitamin B_{12}, riboflavin, phosphorus, and zinc.

in the market

Cheesemaking lends itself to experimentation, and the different kinds of cheese now available number in the thousands, with new types being created every year. The most familiar cheeses are made from cow's milk, with goat's milk and sheep's milk quickly gaining status. (There are, of course, in ethnic markets and elsewhere in the world, cheese made from other mammals' milk, such as camels, mares, and yaks.)

To turn milk into natural cheese, it is first cultured (like buttermilk or yogurt) with bacteria, then curdled—broken into curds (solids) and whey (liquid)—by the use of a culturing agent such as the enzyme rennin. The whey is drained off from the curds, which, depending on the type of cheese being made, may then be pressed to remove more moisture. This fresh cheese may then be aged, or ripened, to further dry it and develop its flavor; often, other ingredients are added to impart the unique characteristics associated with a particular type of cheese. Various natural cheeses are also injected or sprayed with mold or bacteria, washed with beer or brandy, smoked over fra-

COMPARING CHEESES

There are tremendous variations in the fat and sodium content of cheese even when the category or style is strictly defined (Roquefort is an example). So, take the following listing as a way of making some general comparisons, knowing there will be some examples with more or less fat than listed. The one exception to this is the fresh cheeses that are governed by labeling laws in this country, and for which there is an acceptable range of values. The quantities given for each type of cheese in the following chart are based on what a typical serving size should be, though most hover around 1 ounce in weight.

	Calories	Protein (g)	Total Fat (g)	Saturated Fat (mg)	Cholesterol (mg)	Sodium (mg)	Calcium (mg)
American cheese (2 slices)	138	8	10	6.5	27	499	241
Brie (1 ounce)	95	6	7.9	4.9	28	178	52
Camembert (1 ounce)	85	6	6.9	4.3	20	239	110
Cheddar cheese, shredded (¼ cup)	114	7	9.4	6.0	30	175	204
Cottage cheese, 1% (½ cup)	82	14	1.2	0.7	5	459	69
Fontina, diced (¼ cup)	116	8	8.8	5.6	23	289	250
Goat cheese, fresh (1 ounce)	82	6	6.5	4.5	14	113	43
Gouda (1 ounce)	101	7	7.8	5.0	32	232	199
Gruyère, shredded (¼ cup)	112	8	8.7	5.1	30	91	273
Monterey Jack, shredded (1 ounce)	123	8	10	6.3	29	177	246
Mozzarella, part-skim, shredded (¼ cup)	72	7	4.5	2.9	16	132	182
Neufchâtel cream cheese (1 ounce)	75	3	6.8	4.3	22	116	22
Parmesan, grated (¼ cup)	114	10	7.5	4.8	20	465	344
Provolone (1 ounce)	100	7	7.5	4.9	20	248	214
Ricotta, part-skim (¼ cup)	85	7	4.9	3.0	19	77	167
Roquefort (1 ounce)	105	6	8.7	5.5	26	513	188
Swiss cheese (1 ounce)	107	8	7.8	5.1	26	74	272

grant wood, or coated with herbs, spices, or ash. Cheese may be encased in a layer of wax to hold in moisture and prevent the cheese from drying out.

Some natural cheese varieties can be grouped according to their firmness or density; others are classified according to special techniques used in the process of making the cheese. The varieties included here represent those you might find in a specialty cheese shop or a gourmet shop; large supermarkets also carry many of these cheeses.

Cheeses can be divided into two broad categories: natural and processed. The latter, which are made from the former, are described in "Processed Cheeses" (*page 231*).

unripened ("fresh") cheeses

If you're looking for "real" cheese that's low in fat and sodium, this is a good place to start. Just a few steps from fresh milk, foods such as cottage cheese and farmer cheese do not have the concentration of fat and sodium that hard cheeses do. They can be made from fat-free milk and are easy to find in low-fat and even nonfat versions.

Cottage cheese The traditional "dieter's delight," and certainly a healthful food in its low-fat form, cottage cheese exhibits the first stage of all cheesemaking: the separation of milk or cream into curds and whey. To make cottage cheese, the curds are drained and sometimes pressed to form a soft, white, spoonable cheese. You'll find *creamed* cottage cheese (which has small curds and added cream), *reduced-fat (2%)* cottage cheese, *low-fat (1%)* cottage cheese, *fat-free* cottage cheese, and *dry-curd* cottage cheese. As with milk, however, the percentage of fat is a percentage by weight and does not give an accurate picture of the percentage of calories from fat. For example, creamed cottage cheese derives 39 percent of its calories from fat (as opposed to 4 to

---

facts & tips

Some cheeses contain a naturally occurring chemical called tyramine, which can cause vascular headaches—such as migraines—in people prone to them, because it causes blood vessels to dilate. Ripe cheeses, such as Camembert, Cheddar, and blue cheese, are high in tyramine. Cottage cheese and processed cheeses have very little or none.

---

low-calcium cheeses

Many people think cheese and calcium are synonymous. But the truth is that two cheeses—cottage cheese and cream cheese—are meager sources of calcium when compared to milk, yogurt, or other cheeses. To get the same amount of calcium in a cup of low-fat (1%) milk—25 percent of the RDA—you'd have to eat more than 2 cups of low-fat cottage cheese.

Though this isn't horrible (it's 368 calories and over 5 grams of fat), it's nothing compared to what's in cream cheese: To get 25 percent of the RDA, you'd have to eat over ¾ pound of cream cheese, with 1,336 calories and 134 grams of fat.

Instead, try 1 ounce of: part-skim mozzarella (182 milligrams of calcium), Swiss (272 milligrams), Parmesan (344 milligrams), or Provolone (214 milligrams). They all provide between 15 and 30 percent of the RDA for calcium for under 8 grams of fat.

5 percent fat by weight). On the other hand, low-fat (1%) cottage cheese derives 13 percent of its calories from fat. Cottage cheese usually is slightly salted, but is also available unsalted; there are even lactose-free versions.

Cream cheese This is the familiar creamy, white cheese liberally spread on toast and bagels. It comes in a range of fat contents: from 90 percent calories from fat for *full-fat* cream cheese to no fat in *fat-free* cream cheese. In between are *reduced-fat* cream cheese (also called Neufchâtel cheese or "⅓ Less Fat" cream cheese) and *low-fat (light)* cream cheese.

Farmer cheese (hoop, pot, or bakers' cheese) If cottage cheese is placed in a form and the liquid pressed out, it produces a firm, rather grainy white loaf, very low in fat with a mildly tart flavor. Farmer cheese can be sliced or crumbled, and is a good baking ingredient. Sometimes farmer cheese is combined with chopped chives or fruit to make a flavored cheese.

Goat cheese Fresh, unaged goat cheese is much milder than its aged counterpart. Made in many countries, it typically comes in small or large logs. *(See also "Goat & Sheep Cheeses," page 230.)*

Mascarpone This Italian curd cheese resembles the thickest whipped cream and is usually served as a dessert topping. It is made from cream and therefore is very high in fat.

Mozzarella The familiar pizza cheese is fresh in that it is not aged, but it undergoes a process that differentiates it from other fresh cheeses. The warmed curds are kneaded, and the resulting cheese can be separated into layers or strips. Freshly made mozzarella, sold in Italian grocery stores and now available in many supermarkets, is a soft, bland, delicate cheese. Factory-made mozzarella, which is drier and has more salt in it (for longer shelf-life), can be sliced or shredded and used as a topping for pizzas, pastas, and sandwiches. Because fresh mozzarella is so wet (it's still got quite a bit of liquid milk in it), it can be difficult to shred and may add too much moisture to dishes. Many cooks let mozzarella sit for a day or two to firm it up enough to shred.

Fresh mozzarella only comes in whole-milk form. Factory-made mozzarella comes in several versions: *Whole-milk, part-skim, low-moisture* (both whole-milk and part-skim), *reduced-fat, low-fat,* and *fat-free*. Part-skim mozzarella may sound like a low-fat product, but it gets about 55 percent of its calories from fat (compared with 71 percent for whole-milk mozzarella). Still, part-skim mozzarella is lower in fat than cheeses such as Cheddar and Swiss. The lowest-fat forms of mozzarella do not melt as smoothly as whole-milk or even part-skim mozzarella, but they can have 20 to 50 percent fewer calories than the full-fat version. Low-moisture mozzarella is slightly higher in calories and fat (and in protein and calcium) than regular mozzarella, simply because it contains less water.

Neufchâtel Although there are both a fresh and a soft-ripened French cheese by this name, American Neufchâtel is actually a cream cheese (but with a lower fat content than regular cream cheese). Some brands of cream

PART-SKIM MOZZARELLA ¼ cup shredded	
Calories	72
Protein (g)	7
Carbohydrate (g)	1
Dietary fiber (g)	0
Total fat (g)	4.5
Saturated fat (g)	2.9
Monounsaturated fat (g)	1.3
Polyunsaturated fat (g)	0.1
Cholesterol (mg)	16
Potassium (mg)	24
Sodium (mg)	132
KEY NUTRIENTS (%RDA/AI*)	
Vitamin B$_{12}$	0.2 mcg (10%)
Calcium	183 mg (15%)

For more detailed information on RDA and AI, see page 88.

cheese only say Neufchâtel on the label, whereas others may say "Neufchâtel cream cheese" and still others may simply be called "⅓ Less Fat" cream cheese.

Ricotta Whey remaining from making other types of cheese was originally the sole ingredient in ricotta, but American ricotta is now made from a combination of whey and whole or fat-free milk. Ricotta is like a fine-textured cottage cheese and can be eaten by itself, although it is more commonly used in Italian pasta dishes and desserts. It comes in *whole-milk, part-skim*, and *fat-free* forms. The part-skim version has about 40 percent less fat than the whole-milk cheese. Ricotta has, ounce for ounce, four times more calcium than cottage cheese, which it closely resembles.

String cheese Although snack-sized sticks of mozzarella are now sold under this name, true string cheese originated in Syria, and often comes in a braided rope. The flavor is similar to mozzarella, but saltier. Soaking string cheese in water before serving will remove some of the salt.

semisoft cheeses

This is the largest category of cheese, comprising many of the best-known cheeses from all over the world. They're especially beloved by cooks because they melt smoothly. Aged for just a few weeks, they remain relatively moist and delicate in taste—though if left to age further, they will become denser and stronger in flavor. Some of the better-known cheeses in this category are: American Munster, Bel Paese, Caciocavallo, Esrom, Havarti, Morbier, Oka, Port Salut, Provolone, Saint Paulin, Taleggio, and Tilsit

Unlike hard cheeses, which develop a tough rind, some semisoft cheeses have a wax or plastic coating applied to them. Typical of this style of semisoft cheese are: Edam, Gouda, Fontina, and Jarlsberg (which also comes in a harder version).

GOUDA / 1 ounce	
Calories	101
Protein (g)	7
Carbohydrate (g)	1
Dietary fiber (g)	0
Total fat (g)	7.8
Saturated fat (g)	5
Monounsaturated fat (g)	2.2
Polyunsaturated fat (g)	0.2
Cholesterol (mg)	32
Potassium (mg)	34
Sodium (mg)	232

KEY NUTRIENTS (%RDA/AI*)	
Vitamin B_{12}	0.4 mcg (18%)
Calcium	199 mg (17%)
Zinc	1.1 mg (10%)

For more detailed information on RDA and AI, see page 88.

low-fat cheese

Low-fat cottage cheese may be the all-time best-known diet food. However, there is virtually no aged cheese (with the possible exception of Sapsago) that can be classified as low in fat: Most cheeses get about 70 percent of their calories from fat. Cream cheese, although a fresh type, gets 90 percent of its calories from fat. And even whole-milk ricotta gets 60 percent of its calories from fat; creamed cottage cheese weighs in at 45 percent.

For many people, who can't bear to deprive themselves of this indulgence, cheese is a major source of fat and calories. So fat-free and "lite" versions can make a big difference. They may not compare to real Cheddar or Swiss, but many brands do taste better than they used to, and you may not be able to tell the difference when you tuck a slice in a sandwich. The typical fat-free and lite "singles" have 25 to 30 calories, compared to 100 in an ounce of most regular cheeses. And they still provide about 10 percent (that is, 100 to 150 milligrams) of your daily requirement of calcium—but also, unfortunately, about 10 percent of your recommended maximum daily sodium intake.

Some semisoft cheeses are protected not by a rind or a wax coating, but by being stored in brine. The prime examples of these so-called pickled cheeses are Feta and Brynza.

soft-ripened cheeses

These cheeses are sprayed on the surface with different strains of penicillin and then aged, during which time they develop soft, edible rinds. Despite their luxuriously creamy texture and delicious flavor, these cheeses are actually somewhat lower in calories than firm cheeses, such as Cheddar. The soft-ripened cheeses get 60 to 75 percent of their calories from fat. Some of the best-known soft-ripened cheeses are: Boursault, Brie, Brillat-Savarin, Camembert, Chaource, Coulommiers, Crema Danica, Explorateur, Reblochon, Robiola, and St-André. Cheeses known as double- and triple-crèmes have extra cream added and are higher in fat.

washed cheeses

"Washed" cheeses are aged in rooms where they pick up natural molds to form a soft rind, then are rinsed with salt water (or beer or brandy) to further sharpen their flavors, which are considerably more assertive than those of other semisoft and soft-ripened cheeses. Examples of washed cheeses include: Brick, Liederkranz, Limburger, Livarot, and Pont-l'Evêque.

firm cheeses

To many people, "cheese" means Cheddar, the predominant cheese in this category. Robust but not pungent in flavor, firm cheeses are popular for cooking—think of macaroni and cheese, fondue, and French onion soup. Because they dehydrate as they age, these cheeses are more concentrated sources of calcium than softer products.

Cheddar, originally an English cheese, is America's favorite cheese, accounting for about a third of the country's total cheese consumption. It

CHEDDAR / 1 ounce	
Calories	114
Protein (g)	7
Carbohydrate (g)	0
Dietary fiber (g)	0
Total fat (g)	9.4
Saturated fat (g)	6
Monounsaturated fat (g)	2.7
Polyunsaturated fat (g)	0.3
Cholesterol (mg)	30
Potassium (mg)	28
Sodium (mg)	175

KEY NUTRIENTS (%RDA/AI*)	
Vitamin B$_{12}$	0.2 mcg (10%)
Calcium	204 mg (17%)

*For more detailed information on RDA and AI, see page 88.

is moldy cheese spoiled?

Even if kept wrapped and refrigerated, cheese may develop fuzzy spots of multicolored mold on its surface. Does this mean you have to throw the cheese away? If it's a dry cheese—a firm or very hard variety such as Cheddar or Parmesan—and the mold is limited to a small spot, it is probably safe to cut off the moldy portion to a depth of about ½ inch and use the remaining cheese. However, with softer, moister cheeses, such as mozzarella, ricotta, or cottage cheese, threadlike branches of mold may have penetrated deep beneath the surface. Although many food molds are harmless, some are toxic or carcinogenic. In the case of softer cheese, it's better to throw it away.

ranges from white to deep orange in color; yellow and orange Cheddars are colored with annatto, a natural coloring that does not affect the taste of the cheese. Other members of the Cheddar family include: Caerphilly, Cheshire, Dunlop, Gloucester, Lancashire, Leicester, and Wensleydale.

Another large category of firm cheeses, those with holes in them, is known unofficially as Swiss-style cheese. This group includes: Appenzell, Emmentaler, Goutu, Gruyère, Jarlsberg, Maasdam, Piora, Raclette, and Sbrinz.

A great many of the firm cheeses are allowed to age, at which point they have lost enough moisture to become grating cheeses (*see below*). Examples of cheeses that come in both unaged (firm) and aged forms (grating) include: Asiago, Kashkaval, Manchego, Monterey Jack, and Parmesan.

very hard (grating) cheeses

As cheese ages, it loses moisture, becoming denser in texture and more concentrated in flavor (and calcium content). A boon to the fat-conscious cook, these cheeses, grated finely and used sparingly, can go a long way.

Most grating cheeses come in large, heavy wheels and are sold by the piece (an irregular chunk if the cheese is too hard for smooth slicing). To really enjoy the flavor of grated cheese, buy a chunk and grate it yourself. The flavor is markedly better than that of pre-grated cheese sold in a jar or a shaker bottle, which despite its preservative content can never have the robust flavor of just-grated cheese. These cheeses can be frozen if wrapped well and will grate easily without thawing, so you can always keep them on hand.

Grating cheeses include: Asiago, Dry Jack (Dry Monterey Jack), Grana Padano, Kashkaval, Kefalotyri, aged Manchego, Mimolette, Parmesan, Romano, and Sapsago.

blue-veined cheeses

Mold is usually considered an unwelcome intruder in our food, but blue cheese is a notable exception: Roquefort, Gorgonzola and Stilton—the great blues of France, Italy, and England respectively—are referred to as "the Kings of Cheeses." While there are good blue cheeses made in Denmark, Germany, and the United States, these three are the most popular worldwide.

The discovery of the delicious flavor of mold-ripened cheese, like the discovery of wild yeast as a dough leavener, was undoubtedly accidental; however, cheesemakers have learned how to carefully preserve the particular molds that give the best flavor. Blue cheeses are inoculated with these molds (which are related to penicillin) by different methods and then allowed to ripen in a controlled atmosphere until they are streaked with bluish-green veins and develop some of the finest flavors in the cheese world. The flavors are relatively mild in young blues, then intensify as the cheeses age.

Although blue cheeses get about 74 percent of their calories from fat, they are so strongly savory you need only use a small amount. They go particularly

PARMESAN / ¼ cup grated	
Calories	114
Protein (g)	10
Carbohydrate (g)	1
Dietary fiber (g)	0
Total fat (g)	7.5
Saturated fat (g)	4.8
Monounsaturated fat (g)	2.2
Polyunsaturated fat (g)	0.2
Cholesterol (mg)	20
Potassium (mg)	27
Sodium (mg)	465

KEY NUTRIENTS (%RDA/AI*)	
Vitamin B$_{12}$	0.4 mcg (15%)
Calcium	344 mg (29%)
Selenium	6.6 mcg (12%)

For more detailed information on RDA and AI, see page 88.

facts & tips

People who are allergic to penicillin should probably not eat blue cheeses and some other soft cheeses, since they may experience a reaction to the *penicillium* molds used to produce the cheese.

FRESH GOAT CHEESE 1 ounce	
Calories	82
Protein (g)	6
Carbohydrate (g)	0
Dietary fiber (g)	0
Total fat (g)	6.5
Saturated fat (g)	4.5
Monounsaturated fat (g)	1.5
Polyunsaturated fat (g)	0.2
Cholesterol (mg)	14
Potassium (mg)	8
Sodium (mg)	113

KEY NUTRIENTS (%RDA/AI*)

Vitamin A	87 mcg (10%)

For more detailed information on RDA and AI, see page 88.

well with low-fat foods such as fruits or salads. The sodium content of these cheeses ranges from about 400 to 500 milligrams per ounce, however.

In addition to the trio of best-known blues, other blue cheeses include: Bleu d'Auvergne, Blue Castello, Cabrales, Fourme d'Ambert, Maytag Blue, and Saga Blue.

goat & sheep cheeses

Goat's milk and sheep's milk cheeses have a pleasant tartness when young that can develop into a mild gaminess or a striking pungency as the cheese ages. You might like to try one of the milder cheeses, then progress to the stronger (longer-aged) varieties if the flavor appeals to you.

Chèvre This is simply the generic French name for goat's milk cheeses. They range from fresh, soft, cream-cheese types with just a faint tartness, to rock-hard, aged cheeses with an undeniable pungency. Some are treated with mold to form a soft rind, while others are formed into log shapes and coated with herbs or ashes. The mild Montrachet and the larger and slightly stronger Bûcheron are two of the most familiar French chèvres. Older, stronger French examples include Valençay (pyramid-shaped and sometimes coated with ash) and Crottin de Chavignol, one of the sharpest goat cheeses. Many American goat cheeses have come on the market in the last 30 years or so, often echoing their French forebears in shape and flavor. You may be able to find them in low-fat versions.

Sheep's milk cheeses Like goat's milk cheeses, these cheeses have distinctive, tangy flavors that those who are not fond of the taste describe as barnyardy. Many of them, by tradition, are also quite salty, since part of their production involves storage in brine. Sheep's milk is also higher in fat than whole cow's milk. The best-known cheeses made from sheeps' milk are: Brin d'Amour, Brynza, Feta, Kashkaval, Kasseri, Kefalotyri, Manchego, Pecorino Romano, Ricotta Salata, and Roquefort. Many of the sheep's milk cheeses that have gained global popularity are now made with cow's milk (feta is the best example), because sheep do not produce enough milk to meet the demand.

choosing the best

Use four of your five senses when choosing cheese: In addition to tasting the cheese, if possible, sniff it, feel it, and, above all, take a close look at it.

Soft-ripened cheeses such as Brie or Camembert should feel plump and full, and look fresh and white, not sunken, dry, or browned; there should be no sharp, ammonialike smell. A knowledgeable salesperson will help you choose a soft-ripened cheese you can serve immediately, or one that will ripen in a few days.

Semisoft and firm cheeses should look moist but not oily on the surface, and should feel resilient. Cheeses with holes should show a slight gleam (but not an oily slick) in their eyes.

When buying precut, packaged cheese, or fresh cheeses like cottage cheese, the "sell by" date and physical appearance of the cheese and the package are your best cues. Be sure the package is sealed.

▶ **When you get home** Cheese must be well wrapped to protect it from picking up other aromas in the refrigerator and also to prevent its flavor from migrating to other foods. Foil is the best wrapping; plastic wrap traps moisture that may cause cheese to mold more quickly. Placing the wrapped cheese in a covered container provides an extra measure of protection for strong-smelling cheese. Wax-coated cheeses need no further wrapping until they are cut (however, they will lose moisture, becoming more dense and flavorful over time). Check cheese for mold from time to time.

Generally, the softer the cheese, the more perishable it is. Ripe Brie will keep for just a few days, while Cheddar will keep for a month or more, and

processed cheeses

More than half the cheese produced in the United States goes into making processed cheese, which is most commonly sold as slices or spreads. Many consumers appreciate its uniformity of color, flavor, and texture (typified by its dependable melting quality). Processed cheese is marginally lower in protein, vitamin A, calcium, and iron than many natural cheeses, but is higher in sodium.

These products are made by melting one or more types of ground natural cheese with an emulsifier to form a smooth mass; pasteurization, an integral part of the process, improves the keeping quality of these foods. Pasteurized process cheese food may have added dairy ingredients other than cheese, such as cream or nonfat milk solids, and may be flavored with sweeteners, fruits, vegetables, or meat. Rather than being shaped into forms and sliced, processed cheeses are poured onto a chilled surface in their liquid state and cut into "slices" when the cheese re-congeals.

Pasteurized process cheese spreads have additional ingredients that make them soft and spreadable. It is sold in pots, tubes, and even aerosol cans. (When natural cheeses are blended without heating and flavored to make a spread, the product is called cold-pack or club cheese.)

American cheese is a term that can be applied to Cheddar, Colby, and other natural cheeses, but to most people it means the perfectly square slices that have been a lunchbox staple for decades. This American cheese is a pasteurized process cheese made from Cheddar or a combination of Cheddar and Colby cheeses.

Pasteurized process cheese spreads will keep indefinitely in their unopened jars at room temperature; once opened, they will keep for 3 to 4 weeks.

aged Parmesan can be stored for several months. Whole cheeses keep longer than cut ones: A whole Edam or Gouda can be stored in the refrigerator for a year or more.

If you buy a whole soft-ripened cheese (such as Brie or Camembert), let it ripen, if necessary, at room temperature for a few days. Once cut, such a cheese is unlikely to ripen properly. A properly ripe cheese will look plump and feel soft if you squeeze it gently. Once cut, it should appear to be melting slowly, but not be runny and liquid. An underripe cheese will have a chalky, hard center layer.

Keep cottage cheese and ricotta tightly covered in the original container; they should be good for about 1 week after the marked date. Storing the carton upside down—make sure it's tightly closed—will help seal out air and keep the contents fresh longer. Farmer cheese and cream cheese should keep for about 2 weeks.

preparing to use

All cheeses—except the unripened fresh cheeses—taste best at room temperature. As with wine, the subtleties of their flavor are "numbed" by cold. The textures of soft-ripened cheeses, especially, are at their best when at room rather than refrigerator temperature. When serving cheese, remove it from the refrigerator at least an hour before serving time (but keep it wrapped so the cut surfaces don't dry out). It's best to take out only the amount you think you'll need, so you don't end up repeatedly warming and chilling the cheese.

Cheese grates better when cold; if you're cooking with cheese, you might even put the cheese in the freezer for 15 to 30 minutes before grating or shredding it.

To make serving and cooking cheese easier, you might try a few inexpensive gadgets. A cheese plane, which looks like a pie server with a slit cut in it, shaves thin slices from Cheddar, Swiss, and the like. You can also buy a wire cheese cutter that adjusts for slices of different thicknesses. A rotary (drum) grater is very effective for finely grating hard cheeses; some have interchangeable drums for varying the coarseness of the shreds. Many types of cheese can be grated in a food processor fitted with the steel blade.

cheese & your teeth

It will never take the place of the toothbrush, but cheese may save you some cavities. Studies conducted in Britain and Canada have shown that eating Cheddar and other aged cheeses after eating sweets seems to somehow counteract the decay-causing action of the sugary food. The reason is not clear: The cheese may simply stimulate saliva production, helping to rinse the sugar away; some substance in the cheese may fight cavity-causing bacteria, or it may favorably change the acid-alkaline balance in your mouth. Still, considering the fat and calorie content of cheese, you're better off reaching for your toothbrush than for a piece of cheese after a meal or snack.

cherries

Tantalizingly sweet, tart, and juicy, cherries are a highly popular fruit. In fact, so popular are cherries that recent statistics reveal that the U. S. cherry industry produces more than 650 million pounds of tart and sweet cherries each year. Cherries are drupes, or stone fruits (they are related to plums and more distantly to peaches and nectarines), and as such, they contain pits. Still, the pits should not prevent you from enjoying their sweet flavor and satisfying texture. Their only other shortcoming is their brief season, which lasts less than three months. But during that time, they are in abundant supply.

nutritional profile

Low in calories, rich in flavor and nutrients, and requiring hardly any preparation, cherries are a perfect snack. They contain pectin, a type of soluble fiber, that is noted for its cholesterol-lowering properties. Cherries also provide vitamin C. Sour cherries (sometimes called "pie" cherries) are lower in calories and higher in vitamin C and beta carotene than sweet cherries. One cup of sweet cherries has only 104 calories, and both sweet and sour cherries supply a good amount of potassium.

in the market

There are two basic categories of cherry: sweet and sour. Sweet cherries are further differentiated by color: dark- and light-skinned cherries. Dark-skinned sweet cherries far and away dominate the market, with Bing being the most popular in this category.

Balaton This is a deep burgundy sweet-tart cherry that combines the tangy taste of sour cherries with the richness of sweet cherries.

Bing There are many commercial varieties of sweet cherries, but the leader is the Bing, developed first in Oregon by a pioneer grower, just over 100 years ago, who named it for one of his Chinese workmen. Bings are large, round, extra-sweet cherries with purple-red flesh and a deep red skin that verges on black when fully ripe. There are a number of other dark, sweet cherries that look just like Bings, but most people would not know the difference, because their taste and texture are quite similar.

Lambert The second most popular variety after the Bing is the Lambert, a small, heart-shaped red cherry similar in taste and texture to the Bing.

Morello This tart cherry is sometimes eaten fresh when fully ripe, but is ordinarily used in cooking. It has very dark red flesh and dark juice.

Rainier The Rainier, a sweet cherry with yellow or pinkish skin, is grown in limited quantities and is milder and sweeter than the Bing.

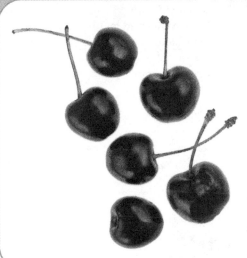

sweet cherries

SWEET CHERRIES 1 cup pitted	
Calories	104
Protein (g)	2
Carbohydrate (g)	24
Dietary fiber (g)	3.3
Total fat (g)	1.4
Saturated fat (g)	0.3
Monounsaturated fat (g)	0.4
Polyunsaturated fat (g)	0.4
Cholesterol (mg)	0
Potassium (mg)	325
Sodium (mg)	0

KEY NUTRIENTS (%RDA/AI*)

Vitamin C	10 mg (11%)

*For more detailed information on RDA and AI, see page 88.

SOUR CHERRIES 1 cup pitted	
Calories	78
Protein (g)	2
Carbohydrate (g)	19
Dietary fiber (g)	2.5
Total fat (g)	0.5
Saturated fat (g)	0.1
Monounsaturated fat (g)	0.1
Polyunsaturated fat (g)	0.1
Cholesterol (mg)	0
Potassium (mg)	268
Sodium (mg)	5

KEY NUTRIENTS (%RDA/AI*)	
Beta carotene	1.1 mg (10%)
Vitamin C	16 mg (17%)

For more detailed information on RDA and AI, see page 88.

Royal Ann Another light-skinned variety, the Royal Ann is often canned or made into maraschino cherries.

Sour cherries (pie cherries) Most commercially grown sour varieties—such as *Montmorency*, the best-known type—are canned or frozen for use as pie fillings or sauces, although you can occasionally find fresh sour cherries during the summer months at farmers' markets and roadside stands. Sour cherries are smaller than sweet cherries and are a bright scarlet.

▶ **Availability** Bing cherries are usually available from the end of May through early August, with their peak in June and July. Most Bing look-alikes appear in markets until mid-August. Keep in mind that the varieties appearing earliest and latest in the season are softer and less sweet than Bings. Any cherries sold after August probably come from cold storage.

choosing the best

Buy cherries that have been kept cool and moist, as flavor and texture both suffer at warm temperatures. Take a few cherries at a time in your hand and select only the best. If circumstances allow, taste one. Good cherries should be large (an inch or more in diameter), glossy, plump, hard, and dark-colored for their variety (good Bing cherries, for example, range from a purplish-mahogany color to nearly black). Reject undersized fruits or those that are soft or flabby. Sweet cherries should crackle when you bite into them.

Check carefully for bruises or cuts on the dark surface, and toss back cherries that are sticky through juice leakage. If you find many damaged fruits,

other cherry products

Dried cherries Dried cherries are made from both sweet and sour cherries. Like all dried fruit, they have a higher concentration of nutrients (and more calories) than their fresh counterparts. Use them as you would raisins.

Cherry juice Commercial cherry juice, available in supermarkets, is likely to be sweetened with either sugar or grape juice. While that's not necessarily bad, you can purchase unsweetened cherry juice concentrate (made from sour cherries) and sweeten it on your own. Stir 2 to 3 tablespoons of concentrate into 1 cup of cold water and sweeten to taste. Look for cherry juice concentrate in farmers' markets and health-food stores.

• Use cherry juice concentrate as a glaze for roasted or grilled meat.

• Use it as the acid component of a salad dressing.

• Add it to homemade or store-bought barbecue sauces.

• Substitute cherry juice concentrate for red wine in your favorite sangria recipe.

• Use cherry juice concentrate to season meat for hamburgers or meatloaf.

consider shopping elsewhere, as a number of spoiled cherries in a bin will start the others on the road to decay.

If they have stems they should be fresh and green; darkened stems are a sign of either old age or poor storage conditions.

Sour cherries sold fresh should be plump, firm, and a bright scarlet color.

▶ **When you get home** Loosely pack unwashed cherries in a refrigerator container, or pour them into a shallow pan in a single layer and cover with plastic wrap. Store them in the refrigerator. Fresh cherries in good condition should keep for up to a week, but check them occasionally and remove any that have begun to go bad.

You can extend the cherry season by freezing them. Rinse and drain the cherries thoroughly, either remove the pits or not, then spread them out in a single layer on a baking sheet and freeze. Once frozen, transfer the cherries to a heavy plastic bag. They'll keep for up to a year. Of course, cherries can be made into preserves, pickled, or stewed for longer storage.

> ➤ *phytochemicals in* **cherries**
>
> The intense color of cherries is attributed in part to the abundance of their anthocyanin phytochemicals, healthful plant pigments that are high in antioxidant capacity.

preparing to use

When serving fresh cherries, simply rinse them under cold water and drain; they're most attractive with the stems intact. To pit cherries for cooking, halve them with a paring knife and pry out the pit with the tip of the knife, or use an inexpensive cherry pitter (found in any kitchenware shop), which works like a hole punch. A partially unbent paper clip (or an old-fashioned V-shaped hairpin, if you can find one) will also do the job.

> ### serving suggestions
>
> • Halve and pit cherries (either sweet or sour), sauté briefly in a bit of oil, and serve over sliced cake or as a topping for pancakes or waffles.
>
> • Use sweet cherries to make fruit salsas for roasted meat or poultry.
>
> • Add chopped cherries (sweet or sour) to muffin batters.
>
> • Thread cherries and melon wedges on skewers and serve alongside grilled meat or fish.
>
> • Sprinkle chopped sweet cherries over frozen yogurt or sorbet.
>
> • Add fresh sweet cherries to a spinach salad along with toasted nuts and red onions.

chestnuts

Chestnuts are round, glossy, mahogany-colored nuts that are formed inside prickly burrs, which break open when the nuts are ripe. Rich and "meaty," they are a starchy food and can be served as a vegetable, mashed like potatoes. Not long after they are harvested, much of their starch turns to sugar, giving them a satisfying sweetness.

Grown in China and Japan for centuries, chestnuts have a long and esteemed history of cultivation. They made it to Europe by way of the Roman armies and soon became an important food source there. Chestnuts were also a dietary staple of Native Americans, who taught the early settlers to cook them in stews or grind them into flour for bread. In the early years of Colonial America, chestnuts supplied a year-round source of sustenance.

Although the entire eastern half of the United States was once covered with majestic wild chestnut trees, in the early 20th century virtually all of the American chestnut trees were destroyed by a blight. While efforts are underway to re-establish a disease-resistant variety of the native chestnut tree, most chestnuts we get today are from Europe.

nutritional profile

A low-fat, high-carbohydrate food, chestnuts supply protein, thiamin, vitamin B_6, vitamin C, and potassium. And interestingly, unlike other nuts, chestnuts supply a respectable amount of vitamin C.

in the market

Chestnuts are most commonly sold in their shells. They are also sold dried shelled (in Chinese and Italian markets), canned unsweetened, and as a flour (*see Flour, Nonwheat, page 324*).

▶ Availability Fresh chestnuts are most abundant in fall and winter.

choosing the best

Choose chestnuts that are heavy for their size, with smooth unbroken skin. If it rattles, the chestnut is old and has shriveled inside its skin.

preparing to use

Fresh chestnuts need to be roasted or boiled in order to peel them. Peeled chestnuts can be eaten as is, or used in a recipe that calls for cooked chestnuts. To facilitate the loosening (and later peeling) of the chestnut skin, use a small sharp knife to cut an "X" through the skin on the flat side of the nut. As the chestnut cooks, the skin will pull apart at the "X," making it easier to remove. If using dried chestnuts, soak in hot water for several hours to reconstitute.

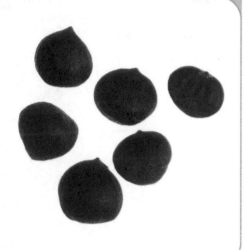

chestnuts

CHESTNUTS / 6 roasted	
Calories	124
Protein (g)	2
Carbohydrate (g)	27
Dietary fiber (g)	2.6
Total fat (g)	1.1
Saturated fat (g)	0.2
Monounsaturated fat (g)	0.4
Polyunsaturated fat (g)	0.4
Cholesterol (mg)	0
Potassium (mg)	299
Sodium (mg)	1

KEY NUTRIENTS (%RDA/AI*)	
Thiamin	0.1 mg (10%)
Vitamin B_6	0.3 mg (15%)
Vitamin C	13 mg (15%)

*For more detailed information on RDA and AI, see page 88.

chick-peas

Chick-peas are pale, round, cream-colored legumes that are used extensively in the Mediterranean, India, and the Middle East. They also have a strong foothold in American cuisine, by way of Latin American cuisine (where they are called *garbanzos*) and Italian dishes (where they are called *ceci*). It is thought that chick-peas originated in the Near East, and archeological records show that they were cultivated as far back as 7000 B.C.

nutritional profile

One of nature's perfect foods, these versatile legumes, with a firm yet creamy texture and a delicate nutlike flavor, are highly nourishing. They are rich in protein, fiber, complex carbohydrates, folate, iron, and zinc. One half-cup of cooked chick-peas provides 7 grams of protein, and only 2 grams of fat. It also provides 35 percent of the RDA for folate, a B vitamin that studies show helps to reduce certain birth defects. Chick-peas are no slouches when it comes to iron content, with ½ cup providing 30 percent of your daily iron requirement. The body's absorption of the form of iron (nonheme) found in chick-peas can be enhanced by consuming them with a dietary source of vitamin C.

Chick-peas are an excellent source of both soluble and insoluble fiber, which contribute to satiety (feeling full), a benefit for people who are trying to control their weight. Like other beans, chick-peas are digested slowly, which promotes a gradual release of blood glucose, which may be helpful in the control of diabetes. In addition, the soluble fiber in chick-peas may help to lower blood cholesterol levels.

Evidence indicates that a diet that contains generous amounts of legumes—which are nutrient-rich, low in fat, and high in complex carbohydrates—may help to reduce the risk of developing certain diseases.

in the market

There are two main varieties of chick-peas, *kabuli* and *desi*. Small, dark desi chick-peas have a yellow interior. Kabuli are large, and beige-colored throughout, with a thin skin. However, in the market, both are simply designated chick-peas. The kabuli chick-peas are the type most commonly found in American supermarkets.

Black chick-peas (Bengal gram) These chick-peas come from India where they are sun-dried until they turn a deep rust color. Like regular chick-peas, they have a deep, earthy aroma and a nutty flavor. Black chick-peas can be found in Indian markets and specialty food shops.

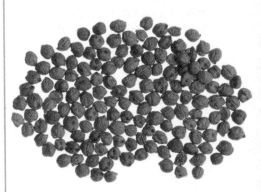

chick-peas

CHICK-PEAS / ½ cup cooked	
Calories	135
Protein (g)	7
Carbohydrate (g)	23
Dietary fiber (g)	6.2
Total fat (g)	2.1
Saturated fat (g)	0.2
Monounsaturated fat (g)	0.5
Polyunsaturated fat (g)	1.0
Cholesterol (mg)	0
Potassium (mg)	239
Sodium (mg)	6

KEY NUTRIENTS (%RDA/AI*)	
Folate	141 mcg (35%)
Iron	2.4 mg (30%)
Zinc	1.3 mg (11%)

*For more detailed information on RDA and AI, see page 88.

Chana dal These small split desi chick-peas are sold in Indian stores and look very much like yellow split peas. Chana dal have a sweet, nutty taste. In India, chana dal are used to make chick-pea flour (called *besan*), while in the United States, the larger kabuli chick-peas are used. Chana dal can be found in Indian stores and some specialty food shops.

Chick-pea shoots These feathery shoots of the chick-pea plant are excellent in salads. Like fresh green chick-peas, they can occasionally be found in local farmers' markets.

Flour See Flour, Nonwheat (*page 324*).

Green chick-peas Fresh and sweet, like green peas, these are young, tender, fresh chick-peas. They are only found in local farmers' markets.

choosing the best

Supermarket chick-peas are packed in 1-pound (or larger) bags. Look for bags with whole, unbroken chick-peas. Unfortunately, bags are not dated, so just buy what you think you'll need and restock when necessary. The older the chick-peas, the longer it takes to cook them.

preparing to use

For whole chick-peas, soak them overnight before cooking. Or quick-soak them by placing them in a saucepan with water to cover by at least 2 inches. Bring to a boil and boil for 2 minutes. Remove from the heat, cover, and let sit for 1 hour before cooking. Drain the chick-peas and cover with fresh water for the final cooking.

If you are using chana dal (split chick-peas), there's no need to presoak them before cooking.

serving suggestions

• For a soup, combine mashed cooked chick-peas and vegetable or chicken broth. Heat gently. Serve with a dollop of yogurt.

• For a lower-fat version of hummus, puree chick-peas with lemon juice, yogurt, and a touch of dark sesame oil.

• Add chick-peas to tuna salad.

• Stuff celery stalks with chick-pea puree seasoned with black pepper and lemon juice.

• Sprinkle chick-peas over the top of a pizza.

• Add chick-peas to chicken, beef, lamb, or pork stews.

• Add chick-peas to pasta sauces.

• For a cool summer soup, combine pureed chick-peas with buttermilk and ground coriander.

• Mash chick-peas with a little low-fat mayonnaise and use as a spread for sandwich wraps.

chicken

Chicken is the most versatile of meats. It can be prepared in many ways—roasted, broiled, grilled, or poached, in soups, stews, and pot pies—and with a variety of seasonings, toppings, and sauces. No wonder, then, that it is a staple in practically every culture's cuisine. In the United States, simple roast chicken is a favorite. In Italy, chicken is sautéed with tomatoes, mushrooms, and wine and served *alla cacciatore*. The Spanish combine chicken with shellfish and rice to produce paella, contributing to chicken's increased popularity. More and more people have made a conscious decision to eat less red meat and more poultry in an effort to lower the fat in their diets. When cooked, light-meat chicken without the skin is 33 to 80 percent leaner than trimmed cooked beef, depending on the beef's cut and grade. Chicken breast, the leanest part of the chicken, has less than half the fat of a trimmed Choice-grade T-bone steak. Moreover, the fat in chicken is less saturated than that in beef.

nutritional profile

Chicken is comparable to beef in quantity and quality of protein. Both foods supply approximately the same amounts of other vitamins and minerals, except that beef has slightly more iron and zinc. Although chicken is relatively low in fat, it depends on what cut you eat and whether or not you eat the skin (*see "Comparing Chicken," page 240*). Although dark-meat chicken (such as as thigh; *see nutrition box, at right*) is higher in fat, it also brings with it a higher concentration of minerals.

in the market

As with beef, chicken is graded for quality by the USDA only if the processors request and pay a fee for it. As a result, many processors have developed their own standards, and you often find ungraded chickens on the market. The chickens you do find on the market with a USDA grade are likely to be Grade A; lesser quality Grade B and C chickens are usually sold to food manufacturers for use in processed and packaged products. The fat content of the chicken is not a primary criterion for a top USDA rating (which is unlike the grading system for beef). Grade A birds are meaty, well-shaped, free of feathers, and have a layer of fat. The skin must be unbroken, free of cuts, tears, bruises, or blemishes. A chicken with a bruised wing could have the wing cut off and be rated Grade C, but if the rest of the bird were of better quality, it would be cut up and the parts sold as Grade A.

Chicken is divided into classes based on age and sex. The meat from small, young chickens is usually leaner than that from larger birds.

Broiler/fryers The most popular type of chicken, broiler/fryers are 6 to 8 weeks old and weigh 2½ to 5 pounds. They are meaty, tender, all-purpose birds, and despite their name, can be roasted, grilled, poached, steamed, or

CHICKEN BREAST	
3 ounces cooked, skinless	
Calories	140
Protein (g)	26
Carbohydrate (g)	0
Dietary fiber (g)	0
Total fat (g)	3
Saturated fat (g)	0.9
Monounsaturated fat (g)	1.0
Polyunsaturated fat (g)	0.7
Cholesterol (mg)	72
Potassium (mg)	218
Sodium (mg)	63

KEY NUTRIENTS (%RDA/AI*)	
Niacin	12 mg (73%)
Vitamin B_6	0.5 mg (30%)
Vitamin B_{12}	0.3 mcg (12%)
Iron	0.9 mg (11%)
Selenium	23 mcg (43%)

For more detailed information on RDA and AI, see page 88.

CHICKEN THIGH	
3 ounces cooked, skinless	
Calories	178
Protein (g)	22
Carbohydrate (g)	0
Dietary fiber (g)	0
Total fat (g)	9.3
Saturated fat (g)	2.6
Monounsaturated fat (g)	3.5
Polyunsaturated fat (g)	2.1
Cholesterol (mg)	81
Potassium (mg)	202
Sodium (mg)	75

KEY NUTRIENTS (%RDA/AI*)	
Riboflavin	0.2 mg (15%)
Niacin	6 mg (35%)
Vitamin B_6	0.3 mg (18%)
Vitamin B_{12}	0.3 mcg (12%)
Iron	1.1 mg (14%)
Selenium	24 mcg (45%)
Zinc	2.2 mg (20%)

For more detailed information on RDA and AI, see page 88.

sautéed as well as broiled and fried. They are not a good choice for stewing, however, as their meat will become dry and stringy.

Capons These are male chickens that have been surgically castrated. This practice results in large birds at a young age, so the meat remains tender. They are usually slaughtered when 15 to 16 weeks old, and they weigh 9½ to 10½ pounds. Capons have a large proportion of white meat but a thick layer of fat underneath the skin, which makes the white meat fattier than that of other chickens. They are best roasted.

Roasters These birds are a little older and larger than broiler/fryers. They are generally brought to market when they are 3 to 5 months old and weigh 3½ to 6 pounds. Roasters have tender, flavorful meat. They can be roasted, grilled, braised, or stewed.

Rock Cornish hens Developed in the 1800s in the United States by crossing a Cornish gamecock with the White Plymouth Rock chicken, Rock Cornish hens weigh ¾ to 2 pounds—the perfect size for serving one person, though a 2-pound bird could serve two people. These plump-breasted birds are very low in fat, and generally come onto the market at 5 or 6 weeks of age. You may occasionally find them fresh, but they are often sold frozen. The traditional way to serve Rock Cornish hens is stuffed and roasted, but they can also be broiled, braised, grilled, or sautéed.

Stewing chickens These mature hens are usually 12 months old and weigh 4 to 6 pounds. Their meat is flavorful but tough, making them excellent candidates for stewing, braising, and making stock.

Chicken parts According to the National Broiler Council, over 50 percent of chicken is purchased cut up as parts. You can purchase whole or half breasts with the bone in, or boneless, skinless chicken breast fillets. Drum-

COMPARING CHICKEN 3 ounces cooked

As a general rule of thumb, 4 ounces of raw boneless chicken will yield 3 ounces of cooked. For 3 ounces of cooked chicken from a bone-in piece, start with about 8 ounces raw. Before cooking, you should trim any visible fat. The chicken cuts are listed in by percentage of fat calories, with the highest at the top and the lowest at the bottom.

	Calories	Fat (g)	% Calories from Fat	Saturated Fat (g)	Cholesterol (mg)
Wing	247	17	62	4.6	71
Thigh, with skin	210	13	56	3.7	79
Drumstick, with skin	184	9.5	47	2.6	77
Thigh, skinless	178	9.3	47	2.6	81
Breast, with skin	168	6.6	35	1.9	71
Drumstick, skinless	146	4.8	30	1.3	79
Breast, skinless	140	3.0	19	0.9	72

sticks and wings are also sold separately. Chicken breasts can be baked, broiled, grilled, or sautéed. Drumsticks and wings can be baked, broiled, or grilled.

Free-range chickens These are chickens that have been allowed to run freely in the farmyard and scratch for their food, unlike most chickens, which are raised in coops. Some people think that free-range chickens have a better flavor because the exercise develops their muscles. Exercise also toughens muscles, but free-range chickens are usually slaughtered at a young age, so the meat remains tender. They are no more nutritious than other chickens, however, and may come at a premium price. In addition, they are processed in the same way as other chickens, and therefore are just as prone to salmonella contamination.

choosing the best

One way to get a really fresh chicken is to check the "sell by" date on the store's label. Chicken can reach the supermarket as early as the next morning after slaughter. The sell-by date is 7 to 10 days from slaughter and it's the last day recommended for sale. However, the bird will remain fresh for up to 3 days afterward if properly refrigerated.

When shopping for a whole chicken, look for a well-shaped bird with a plump, rounded breast, and more breast than leg. You can tell the approximate age of a bird by pressing against the breastbone; if it is pliable the chicken is young and will have tender meat. Chicken parts should be moist and plump. Both whole chickens and chicken parts should have a clean smell.

The color of the skin has no bearing on quality or nutritional value. The poultry industry turns out white and yellow chickens to suit consumer

chicken soup

Studies have shown that chicken soup—and other hot drinks—can help alleviate cold symptoms by increasing the flow of nasal secretions. The taste and aroma of chicken soup may also be part of the therapy. Nothing will cure a cold, but a bowl of hot soup offers as much relief as anything.

The start to any chicken soup is chicken broth, and because most canned chicken broths tend to be quite high in sodium (especially monosodium glutatmate), it's always best to make homemade broth, that way you can control the amount of salt you add and can remove fat from the broth after cooking.

To make homemade chicken broth: Use stewing chickens, chicken backs, or the leftover carcass from a roast chicken. Place the chicken in a large stockpot with yellow onions with the skins on (to add color), celery ribs, carrots, bay leaves, whole peppercorns, thyme, and salt. Cover with water and bring to a boil. Remove any scum that floats to the top, reduce to a simmer, and cover. Cook for 2 to 3 hours (keeping an eye on the water level). Strain the liquid to remove the vegetables, bones, and any meat pieces; discard. Let the broth cool completely and refrigerate. Remove any fat that congeals at the top.

preferences, which vary from region to region. The color of the skin depends on the breed and what the chicken was fed. If the chicken was fed substances containing yellow pigment, such as marigold petals, its skin will be yellow. No matter what the color of the skin is, make sure it does not appear transparent or mottled.

Frozen poultry should be rock-hard and show no signs of freezer burn or ice crystals inside the package. Choose packages from below the freezer line in the grocer's case. If there is frozen liquid inside the package, it is likely that the chicken has been defrosted and then refrozen. This does not mean that the chicken is spoiled, but the taste will suffer since the juices that make a bird flavorful have seeped out.

▶ **When you get home** Fresh chicken is highly perishable and should be stored immediately in the coldest part of your refrigerator. To minimize handling, keep the chicken in its original store wrapping. Be sure that the fluids from the package do not leak onto other foods in the refrigerator; if the package seems leaky, place it on a plate to prevent the contamination of other foods. Fresh raw chicken will keep in a home refrigerator for 2 to 3 days; once cooked, it will keep for 3 to 4 days.

If you buy whole birds with the giblets, store the meat and giblets separately since the giblets will spoil before the meat. Open the store wrapping and remove the giblets. Rinse the chicken, pat it dry with paper towels, and rewrap it loosely. The giblets should be discarded or stored in a container and used within a day. The giblets (but not the liver) can also be frozen and saved for making chicken broth.

To freeze chicken, remove it from the store wrapping, wash it, and pat it dry with paper towels. Wrap it in freezer paper or aluminum foil, taking care that odd-shaped parts are fully covered and the package is airtight. Do not try to freeze a whole bird in a home freezer; cut it into parts first.

preparing to use

Keep chicken refrigerated until you are ready to cook it. Wash the chicken in cold running water and pat it dry with paper towels. Pluck out any stray feathers remaining with your fingers or a pair of tweezers.

Never thaw frozen chicken at room temperature; the outside thaws first and becomes susceptible to bacterial growth during the time it takes for the inside to thaw. Leave it in the refrigerator to defrost on a plate to catch the drippings. Allow 3 to 4 hours of thawing time per pound of whole chicken; chicken parts may thaw more quickly. Use a microwave oven for thawing only if you plan to cook the chicken right away; if that is not possible, refrigerate it until cooking time.

serving suggestions

Because chicken is such a versatile meat, you can experiment with all manner of seasonings. Here are some ideas for flavoring a simple roast chicken. Although the chicken roasts with the skin on, you should remove the skin before eating the chicken, so seasonings such as these should be rubbed on the flesh of the chicken, under the skin.

• *Herbed chicken:* Mix a teaspoon or two of olive oil with ground dried rosemary, sage, or basil. Lift the skin and rub the mixture lightly over the flesh; replace the skin.

• *Asian chicken:* Combine soy sauce, honey, sherry, and a touch of sesame oil and rub it over the flesh under the skin. Place two or three whole scallions in the cavity, along with a few slices of fresh ginger and crushed garlic cloves.

• *Lemon chicken:* Place a halved lemon, small whole onion, garlic cloves, black pepper, and oregano in the cavity.

Cut away any visible fat on the chicken, but don't remove the skin before cooking. Researchers from the University of Minnesota found that it doesn't matter whether you remove the skin before or after cooking in terms of fat content. No significant amount of fat is transferred from the skin to the meat during cooking. Skinning poultry before cooking only leads to drier—not leaner—meat. Remove the skin before eating the chicken and be sure to remove any visible fat left on the meat.

Chicken breasts often have a tough white tendon under the fillet, a small tender piece that is tucked underneath the main part of the breast. If the breast is boneless, you can easily remove this tendon with a sharp paring knife. To tenderize boneless chicken breasts, pound them lightly between two sheets of aluminum foil or wax paper. This also flattens the breasts to a uniform thickness for even cooking.

Keep raw poultry away from other foods, especially salad greens or any food that will be served raw or cooked only briefly. Be sure to thoroughly wash your hands, the countertop, sink, cutting board, and utensils with hot, soapy water after handling raw chicken.

Marinate chicken pieces in the refrigerator, not at room temperature. Chicken can spoil if it sits out even for 3 hours on a warm day. Don't use the marinade as a sauce unless you bring it to a rolling boil for several minutes before serving. Better yet, make extra marinade and store it separately until you are ready to serve it.

serving suggestions

To marinate chicken parts, try one of these combinations:

• Red wine, Dijon mustard, crushed garlic, tarragon, pepper, and a dash of olive oil.

• White wine, lemon zest, chopped fresh dill, cayenne pepper, and a touch of olive oil.

• Lime juice and zest, minced garlic, minced chili peppers, chili powder, ground cumin, black pepper, and a small amount of olive oil.

• Orange juice, tarragon, cracked black pepper, and a small amount of olive oil.

• Yogurt, toasted cumin, chopped scallions, curry powder, and a dash of sesame oil.

kosher poultry

Kosher poultry is no more nutritious than regular poultry. Nor is it less likely to harbor salmonella or other bacteria. Kosher foods comply with a set of religious dietary laws, but they contain the same amount of fat and cholesterol as their nonkosher counterparts.

Kosher poultry is salted after slaughter to draw out the blood. This may kill some salmonella and other types of bacteria, but the birds are not salted long enough to kill all disease-causing bacteria. In addition, contamination can occur later on; like other poultry, kosher poultry is mechanically eviscerated and processed.

The salt used in koshering may increase the sodium content—500 milligrams of sodium in 8 ounces of kosher meat versus 150 milligrams in nonkosher, according to one study. This increase may be significant if you're on a low-sodium diet. Some kosher producers claim to wash the birds to remove excess sodium.

chili peppers

Noted for their fiery bite, chili peppers are members of the genus *Capsicum* and are thought to have originated in South America, after which they spread to Central America. While searching for the peppercorn plants that produce the spice known as black pepper, Columbus and his explorers discovered sweet and hot peppers in the West Indies and took samples back to Europe, where the peppers' popularity quickly grew. Currently, demand for chili peppers in the United State is considerable. In fact, there is a growing appreciation of chili peppers as evidenced by the aficionados and culinary daredevils who test their heat tolerance thresholds at chili pepper festivals.

The incendiary nature of chili peppers is due to a volatile substance called capsaicin, which varies in amount depending on the species of chili pepper. Producing an unmistakable sensation of heat (and often pain) in the mouth by targeting and stimulating pain receptors in the skin and mucous membranes, capsaicin can cause discomfort, sweating, watery eyes, and exhilaration. Some scientists theorize that in response to the discomfort produced by the chilies' "burn," the brain releases endorphins—substances that, at high levels, can create a sensation of pleasure. (Interestingly, the active ingredient in a range of new topical neuralgesic ointments happens to be capsaicin, which numbs pain receptors in the skin.)

nutritional profile

Pungent and fiery, chili peppers are distinguished from sweet peppers by their longer and thinner shape and their hot, burning flavor. They are a good source of vitamin C. Hot red chili peppers contain more beta carotene than their hot green counterparts.

in the market

Chili peppers are cultivated in a range of sizes, shapes, and degrees of hotness. While nearly all of them belong to one species—*Capsicum annuum*—the number of varieties is daunting, and the names are confusing, as they vary from region to region.

While the following listing can help you distinguish the most common chili pepper varieties, it can be tricky, if not impossible, to determine just how hot a pepper is. Even within an individual variety, the more mature the pepper, the hotter it will be—for example, a red Anaheim will pack more punch than a green one. Soil, climate, and other conditions also affect the amount of capsaicin in a pepper, so that peppers of the same variety—even those on the same plant—can differ in hotness. For a look at the relative heat of chili peppers, see the chart called "Scoville Units" (*page 246*).

jalapeños

GREEN CHILI PEPPERS
¼ cup chopped

Calories	15
Protein (g)	1
Carbohydrate (g)	4
Dietary fiber (g)	0.6
Total fat (g)	0.1
Saturated fat (g)	0
Monounsaturated fat (g)	0
Polyunsaturated fat (g)	0
Cholesterol (mg)	0
Potassium (mg)	128
Sodium (mg)	3

KEY NUTRIENTS (%RDA/AI*)

Vitamin C	91 mg (101%)

For more detailed information on RDA and AI, see page 88.

Ajis These searingly hot chili peppers range from green to yellow to orange to red. It is long (3 to 5 inches) and thin, and has a fruity flavor—which can be hard to appreciate in peppers as hot as this. Native to the Andes, the aji is an essential (and revered) ingredient in traditional Incan cuisine.

Anaheims Among the most commonly used chilies in the United States, with a bite ranging from mild to moderately hot, these long, slender, lobed peppers come in varieties also known as *New Mexico, long green, long red,* or *California.* Anaheims are eaten in both the green and red stages of development. When mature and red, they are often made into *ristras*—strands of peppers strung together on a cord—and left to dry. Green Anaheims are often used in American versions of the Mexican dish called *chiles rellenos* (the Mexican chili of choice is the poblano). The "heat" of Anaheims ranges widely, because Anaheim peppers grown in California tend to be milder than those grown in New Mexico.

Anchos Technically, ancho refers to a dried poblano pepper, but many distributors and markets also apply the term to the fresh version. Dried anchos are flat, wrinkled, and heart-shaped, ranging in color from oxblood to almost black. Considered one of the mild to moderately hot peppers (like poblanos), anchos are often soaked and ground for use in cooked sauces.

Bird peppers This is not a type of pepper, but a group of about a dozen wild chili peppers that have one thing in common: They are so small that birds can eat them whole (the birds do not taste the chilies' heat). The benefit of this is that when the seeds arrive at the other end of the birds' digestive system, they are out of their pods and are surrounded by natural fertilizer. Bird peppers favored by cooks include chiletepins (*page 246*), piquins (*page 247*), and Thai chilies (*page 247*).

Cascabels These moderately hot chilies are mostly available dried. In their fresh state, they are green or red and shaped like a small tomato. Dried, their skin turns a brownish-red and becomes translucent, and their seeds rattle around inside. The name cascabel means "jingle bell" in Spanish.

Cayennes Among the hottest chilies, cayenne peppers are long, thin, sharply pointed red pods that are either straight or curled at the tip; they grow to a length of 6 to 10 inches. (The chile de árbol is closely related and similar in shape, but grows only 2 to 3 inches in length and usually does not have a curled tip; it is also slightly less pungent.) Ground, dried cayenne is a popular spice.

Cherry peppers So-named for their resemblance to the familiar fruit, cherry peppers are round and red. They range in pungency from mild to moderately hot. They're sold fresh and pickled.

Chiles de árbol About 2 to 3 inches long and ½ inch wide, this hot pepper is a good substitute for cayenne.

> **▶ *phytochemicals in* chili peppers**
>
> Scientists are investigating the health benefits of capsaicin, the phytochemical that gives chili peppers their distinctive heat. Capsaicin appears to be an antioxidant and may exert additional cancer-fighting actions. Capsaicin is also under review for its potential to improve cardiovascular health by preventing blood clotting.

RED CHILI PEPPERS
¼ cup chopped

Calories	15
Protein (g)	1
Carbohydrate (g)	4
Dietary fiber (g)	0.6
Total fat (g)	0.1
Saturated fat (g)	0
Monounsaturated fat (g)	0
Polyunsaturated fat (g)	0
Cholesterol (mg)	0
Potassium (mg)	128
Sodium (mg)	3

KEY NUTRIENTS (%RDA/AI*)

Beta carotene	2.2 mg (20%)
Vitamin C	91 mg (101%)

For more detailed information on RDA and AI, see page 88.

Chiletepins These tiny, pea-sized peppers are a type of bird pepper. Their heat levels can range quite a bit, but they are moderately hot (quite similar to serranos).

Chipotles Also known as smoked jalapeños, chipotles are medium-hot with a deep, smoky flavor. They can also be found canned in adobo sauce.

Fresnos This variety—developed in Fresno, California, in the early 1950s—is similar to jalapeño peppers, but with thinner walls. Fresnos are available green in the summer, and then in their hotter red form in the fall.

Guajillos These long peppers measure about 6 by 1½ inches and have a sweet, medium-hot flavor. The guajillo is used in Mexican cooking.

Habaneros These lantern-shaped peppers, measuring about 2 by 2 inches, are *Capsicum chinense*, not *Capsicum annuum*. Their color is most often yellow-orange, but can be yellow, orange, or red. Habaneros hold the distinction of being the most fiery of all domesticated peppers; however, their heat can sneak up on you, so beware of taking a second bite if you think the first one wasn't hot (which is unlikely). Furthermore, rather than dissipating quickly, the heat of habaneros persists.

Hungarian wax peppers These are the hot version of sweet banana peppers (*see Peppers, Sweet, page 466*). They are never green—the peppers start out yellow and ripen to orange or red—and are mostly sold when yellow, either fresh or pickled in jars.

Jalapeños Probably the most familiar hot peppers—and almost as popular as the Anaheims—jalapeños are tapered, about 2 inches in length, and have slight cracks at their stem ends. They vary in degree of heat, sometimes tast-

---

SCOVILLE UNITS

In 1912, a pharmacist named Wilbur Scoville came up with a scoring system for the "heat" in peppers. This "heat" index measures the capsaicinoid content of peppers in parts per million. These parts per million are converted into Scoville Units: One part per million is equivalent to 15 Scoville Units. At the bottom of the scale are bell peppers, with a value of zero. At the top are habaneros, which register a blistering 200,000 to 300,000. (Pure capsaicin has a Scoville heat unit score of 16 million!)

Cherry	100-500	Yellow wax	5,000-15,000
New Mexico	500-1,000	Serrano	10,000-23,000
Ancho	1,000-1,500	Chile de árbol	25,000
Poblano	1,000-1,500	Aji	30,000-50,000
Pasilla	2,500	Cayenne	30,000-50,000
Cascabel	3,000	Piquin	30,000-50,000
Guajillo	3,000	Tabasco	75,000
Hungarian wax	2,500-5,000	Thai	50,000-100,000
Jalapeño	2,500-5,000	Habanero	200,000-300,000
Chipotle	10,000	Scotch bonnet	100,000-350,000

ing much like a green bell pepper and other times being very hot, with a bite that you notice immediately. Most often, these peppers are consumed at the mature green stage, but sometimes you will find fully ripe red jalapeños at the market. In addition, they are sold canned, sliced, and pickled, and are used in a wide array of products including sausage, cheese, and jelly. Canned types may be milder than fresh because they are usually peeled, seeded, and packed in liquid—but they will still pack a punch. Pickled jalapeños are always hot.

New Mexico green chilies These large chilies are similar in size to Anaheims, but they're hotter.

Pasillas In Spanish, *pasilla* means "little raisin," and this pepper is so named because of its deep black color and raisinlike aroma. It has a mild, smoky flavor.

Piquins These small orange-red chili peppers are a type of bird pepper and are respectably hot. They are most commonly sold dried. Because they are so small, you can use one whole pepper to add a small amount of heat to a dish, instead of having to cut into a larger pepper.

Poblanos These are ancho peppers in the green state; they look like small bell peppers at the stem end, tapering to a thin point at the blossom end. Ranging from fairly mild to hot, poblanos are usually roasted and peeled before using in casseroles, soups, and sauces, or stuffed with meat or cheese for *chiles rellenos*.

Scotch bonnets These chilies looks just like habaneros and are equally hot. There are botanical distinctions, but no culinary ones.

Serranos Very popular in Mexico and the southwestern United States, these 1- to 4-inch long torpedo-shaped chilies are primarily consumed fresh, usually in salsas. Serranos are very hot and are typically sold in their mature green state, though they are also sometimes available red.

Tabascos Made popular by the Louisiana hot sauce of the same name, these bright red-orange chili peppers are moderately hot and are named for the region they originally came from in Mexico. They are a different species—*Capsicum frutescens*—from most other peppers. Tabascos look like elongated Christmas tree lights.

Thai chilies These small bird peppers pack an incredible punch.

▶ Availability Fresh chili peppers are generally available year round. They are grown in California, New Mexico, and Texas; some are imported from Mexico. Dried chilies are also available at all times of the year. Most supermarkets sell canned or jarred chilies, and many now carry both fresh and dried chili peppers as well due to the rise in popularity of Mexican, Asian, and other "spicy" cuisines.

choosing the best

Fresh chili peppers should be well-shaped, firm, and glossy. Their skins should be taut and unwrinkled, and their stems fresh and green. Watch out for

facts & tips

People often reach for water or beer to cool a chili pepper's fire. However, milk may be a better choice. Because the pepper's fiery substance, capsaicin, is fat-soluble (which makes it stable and not easy to break down), casein, a protein in milk, bonds to the capsaicin and washes away the heat. This may be one of the reasons that in India spicy-hot curries are served with cooling yogurt-based side dishes called *raitas*.

soft or sunken areas, slashes, or black spots. Except for jalapeños, which often have shallow cracks at their stem ends, chili peppers should be free of cracks.

Dried chili peppers should be glossy and unbroken (wrinkled is fine), not dusty or fragmented.

▶ **When you get home** Store unwashed chili peppers, wrapped in paper towels, in the refrigerator for up to 3 weeks. Do not store them in a plastic bag, because trapped moisture will hasten spoilage. Check the chilies fre-

seasoning from peppers

Whole chili peppers are not the only means of enlivening dishes. You can also substitute a wide variety of seasonings and condiments made from hot peppers:

Cayenne This ground spice—very hot and orange-red or deep red in color—is based on very pungent peppers grown in Louisiana, Africa, India, and Mexico. Some spice companies also offer a ground spice labeled simply "red pepper." It may be made from other dried mild to medium-hot red peppers, but the term can also refer to the more pungent cayenne.

Chili oil This Asian condiment and cooking ingredient is vegetable oil that has been infused with heat from ground red chilies and then strained.

Chili paste There are red pepper-based Chinese chili pastes and there are several types of Thai chili pastes. They are all quite hot. The Thai pastes vary in color (including red, green, yellow, and brown) and each one has a particular flavor in addition to chili heat.

Chili powder Dried ground Anaheim peppers are the basis for the typical seasoning used to flavor chili con carne. Usually the peppers are mixed with other spices, such as garlic, cumin, and cayenne. There are also pure chili powders, which are made from a single type of chili pepper (and sometimes a combination of chilies), but they have no added seasonings.

Curry powder A number of variations of this Indian spice are available; all of them contain dried hot peppers as their base. The heat level varies, depending on how much chili pepper is used.

Hot pepper sauces There is no way to conveniently characterize the multitude of pepper sauce styles available. Broadly speaking, however, there are the vinegar-based Louisiana-style red sauces—of which Tabasco is the best-known example. There are the slightly fruity, sweet-sour Caribbean-style sauces. There are mustard- and Scotch Bonnet–based Jamaican hot sauces. There are garlicky Southeast Asian sauces. And then there is a world of proprietary commercial hot sauces competing with one another to be the hottest one in town.

Paprika Originating in Hungary, this spice is made by grinding dried mild to slightly hot red peppers into a powder. Sweet paprika contains just the pods; hotter versions may also include the ground seeds and ribs.

Tabasco sauce One company, based on Avery Island in Louisiana, is the only one that can call their hot spicy sauce Tabasco (the name is a registered trademark). The sauce is made by soaking Tabasco peppers with salt and letting the mixture age for at least three years. It is then mixed with vinegar and strained before it is bottled. (Similar hot sauces are made from other red chilies, such as cayenne.) The same Louisiana company also makes a green Tabasco sauce using green jalapeño peppers.

quently; immediately use any that have developed soft spots. If you've gotten more than you can use, you can hang them to dry and use them in their dried form. Store dried chili peppers in an airtight container at room temperature for several months or longer.

preparing to use

Wash the chilies just before using them. Then cut them open and remove the seeds and ribs, if desired, to temper the chilies' pungency. Since capsaicin, the chilies' heat-producing substance, is primarily concentrated in the pepper's interior walls or ribs and not in the seeds as is commonly believed, removing the ribs can help to reduce the chili pepper's bite. (Of course the seeds also impart considerable fire because they are in close contact with the ribs, so remove them, too.) Soaking the peppers in cold salted water for an hour will further diminish their hotness.

When cutting hot peppers, it is best to wear thin rubber gloves. If gloves aren't available, be sure to wash your hands very thoroughly with soap and water (a mild bleach solution is even better) after working with the peppers. And never touch your hands to your face—especially to your eyes—when they have come into contact with capsaicin. Don't forget to wash the utensils and cutting board after use, as you may taint other foods with undesired heat.

The same caveats apply for dried hot peppers, with one additional caution: When grinding them (by hand or in a food processor or blender), be careful not to inhale the fumes or let them waft into your eyes.

To add the mildest chili flavor to food, cut a few slits in a whole chili pepper, impale it on a toothpick or skewer, then add it to food that is already cooking. When the dish is done, remove and discard the toothpick and pepper.

With chili peppers, you will find that even those of the same type vary in hotness. Consequently, you may need to use a different amount each time you prepare a favorite recipe. Sample a bit of the pepper before deciding how much to use in a particular dish. It's a good idea to add chilies a small amount at a time, until the food reaches the degree of hotness you desire.

chocolate

The word "chocolate" is derived from the Aztec *cacahuatl*, meaning "bitter water," and refers to the extremely bitter unsweetened drink the Aztecs made from ground cocoa beans and spices. Chocolate made its way from its origins in Mexico to Europe, and by the mid-17th century, numerous chocolate shops existed where patrons could sip the exotic drink. The first chocolate processing factory was built in London in 1728. By the mid-1800s, chocolate's popularity had skyrocketed thanks to technological innovations that produced the first chocolate bars. Today chocolate is one of the world's most beloved foods, with more than one billion people worldwide consuming some form of it every day.

Chocolate is made from the beans of the cacao tree (whose botanical name is *theobroma*, which aptly means "food for the gods"). The beans (it takes approximately 400 cocoa beans to make 1 pound of chocolate) are processed to a sticky, bitter paste called chocolate liquor, which consists of 53 percent cocoa butter and 47 percent cocoa solids. The chocolate liquor is then used to create a variety of chocolate products, all varying in ratios of cocoa butter to solids, and with varying degrees of additives (such as milk and sugar).

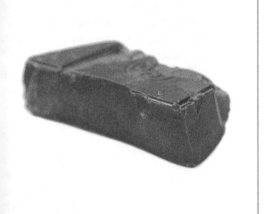

chocolate

nutritional profile

Chocolate contains copper, iron, zinc, and small amounts of protein. The fat in chocolate is from cocoa butter, and is comprised almost equally of oleic acid (a monounsaturated fat also found in olive oil) and stearic and palmitic acids (both saturated fats).

Though some people may assume that chocolate contains a lot of caffeine, this is simply a common misperception; in fact, chocolate contains only a small amount of caffeine. One ounce of milk chocolate contains about 5 milligrams of caffeine, 1 ounce of semisweet chocolate usually has 5 to 10 milligrams of caffeine, and a 6-ounce cup of cocoa usually has 10 milligrams. For comparison, a 6-ounce cup of coffee contains 100 to 150 milligrams.

in the market

Chocolate comes in all shapes and forms including unsweetened cocoa powder; bars of unsweetened, semisweet, and sweet chocolate for baking; chocolate chips or pieces; extra-creamy "designer" chocolates (they have a higher percentage of cocoa butter); and the everyday candy counter chocolate bar.

Unsweetened chocolate Primarily used in baking, unsweetened chocolate is just cocoa powder and cocoa butter with no sugar at all.

Dark chocolate There are several types of dark chocolate—bittersweet, semisweet, and sweet—whose names suggest a range of sweetnesses, but there are no established rules for labeling based on sugar content. *Bittersweet* and

SEMISWEET CHOCOLATE 1 ounce	
Calories	135
Protein (g)	2
Carbohydrate (g)	13
Dietary fiber (g)	0.9
Total fat (g)	11
Saturated fat (g)	6.3
Monounsaturated fat (g)	4.2
Polyunsaturated fat (g)	0.2
Cholesterol (mg)	0
Potassium (mg)	174
Sodium (mg)	1

KEY NUTRIENTS (%RDA/AI*)		
Copper	0.3 mg	(28%)
Iron	1.4 mg	(18%)
Zinc	1.1 mg	(10%)

*For more detailed information on RDA and AI, see page 88.

semisweet can be quite similar; though *sweet* chocolate is fairly reliably the sweetest of the three. Dark chocolates can be eaten on their own or used in cooking and baking. Depending upon the manufacturer, sweet chocolate is generally molded into bars. Semisweet and bittersweet chocolates are also available in bar form, but the bulk of commercially available semisweet chocolate is in the form of chips and pieces.

Milk chocolate This type of chocolate contains cocoa, varying amounts of sugar, milk powder, and flavorings such as vanilla, which are all blended with cocoa butter to give it its creamy texture and sweetness.

White chocolate This chocolate contains no cocoa solids and is made from cocoa butter, sugar, milk, and added flavorings. Because it contains no cocoa powder, the FDA states it is not real chocolate.

Coating chocolate (dipping chocolate, couverture) Sold in bars, this chocolate usually contains a minimum of 32 percent cocoa butter, which enables it to form a thin shell when used as a coating for candies. Unlike regular chocolate, which requires tempering (a melting and cooling process by which chocolate is stabilized), coating chocolate can just be melted and used as is for making and coating candies.

Organic chocolate Becoming increasingly more popular, organic chocolate is made from cocoa beans that have been grown without the use of pesticides.

Liquid chocolate These packages of pre-melted chocolate are a mixture of cocoa powder and vegetable oil. Because liquid chocolate is made with vegetable oil rather than cocoa butter, it doesn't taste strongly of chocolate and according to the FDA is not considered real chocolate.

Cocoa powder This is the general term for the portion of chocolate liquor that remains after most of the cocoa butter has been removed by a process that presses the chocolate liquor to extract the butter. The paste that results from this pressing is then cooled, ground, and sifted. Cocoa powder is sold unsweetened. (This is not to be confused with cocoa mixes, which contain sugar and sometimes other ingredients.) *Dutch process cocoa* is unsweetened cocoa powder that is treated with alkaline compounds to neutralize the natural acids. It is slightly darker in color and milder in flavor than natural cocoa.

➤ *phytochemicals in* chocolate

We've known that tea contains substances called catechins (types of antioxidant phytochemicals) that may protect against heart disease and even cancer. Now it turns out that dark chocolate, too, has large quantities of the same beneficial catechins: 1 ounce contains as much as ½ cup of brewed black tea.

---

carob

Carob (aka St. John's bread or locust bean) are the long (up to 12 inches), leathery pods that grow on a tropical tree. The tiny beans inside the pods are dried and ground into carob powder. Because it has a flavor reminiscent of chocolate, carob is sometimes used as a chocolate substitute. It is most often sold as a powder (toasted or untoasted) and in various chocolatelike products, such as chips for baking. Carob is mostly available in health-food stores. Though it is preferred by those with a sensitivity to chocolate, it offers no nutritional advantage. In fact, 1 tablespoon of carob chips is higher in calories and saturated fat than the same amount of chocolate chips.

choosing the best

Always look at the ingredient list of any bar chocolate or cocoa to make sure that you are buying real chocolate. Though there's no way to judge the quality of bar chocolate in its wrapper, you should still know what characteristics to look for in the chocolate you've bought. Bar chocolate that breaks cleanly and is shiny, dark, and fresh-smelling is of good or superior quality. The chocolate should smell rich and melt evenly on your tongue. Chocolate that appears grayish, dull, or crystallized may be old, contain a fat that is something other than cocoa butter, or have been improperly stored. Don't worry about slight traces of white on the surface of chocolate. These slight white areas on the surface (called "bloom") indicate that the chocolate has undergone temperature variation that will not influence taste or quality.

▶ When you get home Room temperature is preferable (about 65°), though you can store chocolate in the refrigerator. Chocolate will keep for several months at room temperature if it is well wrapped and kept away from heat or moisture. Do not freeze chocolate as this interferes with the characteristics of the cocoa butter and causes the chocolate to crumble.

preparing to use

When a recipe calls for sweet, semisweet, or bittersweet chocolate, you have a huge number of products to choose from. You'll probably find one that you prefer over another, but they are all pretty interchangeable in recipes. If a recipe calls for unsweetened chocolate, however, you should not substitute bittersweet, semisweet, or sweet.

If a recipe calls for pieces of chocolate (and you're using bar chocolate instead of chips), coarsely chop the bar with a sturdy chef's knife, or use the coarse holes of a box grater.

Most recipes, however, call for melting the chocolate. The safest way to melt chocolate is to finely chop it, place it in a bowl over a pan of hot water, and stir until melted. Be especially careful not to get any water in the bowl as this will cause the chocolate to seize and become granular.

You may melt chocolate in the microwave, but be aware that chocolate will hold its shape even though it is melted. Since you can't tell by looking at it, stir the chocolate several times when melting to prevent burning. Once melted, if you want to keep the chocolate fluid, place it in a bowl over a pan of warm water.

If cocoa powder is to be mixed in with the dry ingredients in a recipe, simply measure it the way you would flour or sugar and combine it with the dry ingredients. If it looks lumpy, sift it first before using it. If cocoa powder is to be combined with liquid ingredients, first stir a small amount of cold liquid into the cocoa powder to make a paste. Once it's pasty, you can stir the remaining liquid into it.

serving suggestions

• Finely chop chocolate or use mini chocolate chips and fold into sweetened ricotta cheese. Serve with pears.

• Dip bananas into melted chocolate, then into chopped sunflower or pumpkin seeds and freeze. Serve frozen.

• Fold chocolate chips into muffin batters.

• Stir a tablespoon or two of unsweetened cocoa powder into chili to give it richness and depth of flavor.

• Make your own cocoa mix: Combine 1 part unsweetened cocoa powder, 1 to 2 parts sugar (to taste), 6 parts nonfat dry milk. For one serving, combine 3 tablespoons cocoa mix with 1 cup of boiling water.

clams

For the most part, clams are caught in local waters. Easterners eat Atlantic clams, and Westerners enjoy Pacific varieties, but similar types of clams are harvested—dug from the sand at low tide or scooped from beds in deeper waters—on each coast.

Clams may be hard-shelled or soft-shelled. The edible portion may consist of the muscles that operate the shell; the siphon, or neck (through which the bivalve takes in water); and the foot, which it extends from the shell to propel itself through sand. In general, clams are sweet and a bit chewy; flavor and relative tenderness depend on the size and species.

In recent years, the danger of contamination has made it quite risky to eat raw clams. Raw shellfish may harbor various kinds of bacteria and other potentially harmful organisms. Although there are health risks associated with eating raw clams (*see the safety information on pages 119–122*), many people continue to eat this shellfish on the half-shell, as well as in chowders, pasta sauces, and baked.

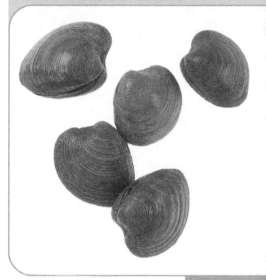

hard-shelled clams

nutritional profile

A remarkably rich source of iron, these bivalves also supply other minerals, including selenium and zinc. In addition, they are an excellent source of B vitamins in general, but an exceptional source of vitamin B_{12}—a half dozen cooked clams has only 166 calories but supplies 40 times the required daily amount of this vitamin.

in the market

Butter clams Small Pacific clams with a smooth shell, these are available primarily canned, especially as smoked clams.

Geoducks Pacific geoducks are large soft-shelled clams weighing 2 to 4 pounds each, with sweet, tasty flesh. They can be shucked, chopped, and sautéed, and also make a tasty chowder.

Manila clams These are very small West Coast clams sold as steamer clams.

Pismo clams Large Pismo clams, found off the California coast, are scarce and delicious.

Quahogs This hard-shelled clam is the largest eastern type, ranging from about 1½ to 6 inches across. The clams called *cherrystones* and *littlenecks* are not different species, but just smaller-sized quahogs: Cherrystones measure less than 3 inches across, littlenecks about 2 to 2½ inches (there is also a West Coast clam called a littleneck, though it's a different species). Full-sized quahogs are sometimes called *chowder clams*, as they can be tough and are best cut up and cooked.

Razor clams Long, skinny razor clams are named for their resemblance to an old-fashioned straight razor and the sharpness of their shells. They are commercially marketed on the West Coast, but not in the East. Razor clams are sometimes available in Asian and specialty seafood markets.

Steamers A third type of eastern clam is the soft-shelled steamer, which has a long siphon that projects from a thin, brittle shell. As the name suggests, this type of clam—about 2 inches long—is usually steamed, but it can also be shucked and then sautéed or deep-fried.

Surf clams Also called sea clams, skimmer clams, or chowder clams, surf clams are the most common eastern species. Large and comparatively tough, they are commonly cut up and used in recipes; most surf clams are canned.

▶ Availability Clams are available in one form or another (fresh, frozen, or canned) year round.

choosing the best

In many states, the harvesting of clams is monitored by the National Shellfish Sanitation Program. Packaged shellfish bear a sticker from the state agency; items sold in bulk have a tag that the fish dealer should show you on request (although there's no way of proving that the tag came with the shellfish you're buying). As with finfish, your nose and eyes can tell you a lot about the merchandise. Clams should smell briny-fresh.

Clams that are sold live offer specific signals of freshness: They should be tightly closed (so that you can't pull them apart) or should close tightly when the shell is tapped; don't buy clams with open or cracked shells. Clams that seem especially heavy for their size should be avoided as they may be full of sand. The protruding necks of soft-shelled clams should retract when you touch them.

Freshly shucked clams should smell perfectly fresh, with no trace of ammonia or "fishy" odor.

▶ When you get home Possibly the most perishable of all foodstuffs, clams are highly susceptible to bacterial contamination and growth once they die or get too warm. Therefore, when you buy live clams, it is imperative to keep them cold until you are ready to cook and serve them.

Store live clams in the refrigerator, covered with wet kitchen towels or paper towels. Don't put them in an airtight container or submerge them in fresh water, or they will die. The key is to keep them truly cold: if possible, at 32° to 35°. Within that range, clams should keep (in a live state) for about 4 to 7 days. Be sure to remove any that die (look for open shells) during that period so they do not contaminate the remaining clams. Shucked clams should be kept in tightly covered containers, immersed in their liquor; they, too, should keep for up to a week.

CLAMS / 6 cooked	
Calories	166
Protein (g)	29
Carbohydrate (g)	6
Dietary fiber (g)	0
Total fat (g)	2.2
Saturated fat (g)	0.2
Monounsaturated fat (g)	0.2
Polyunsaturated fat (g)	0.6
Cholesterol (mg)	75
Potassium (mg)	705
Sodium (mg)	126

KEY NUTRIENTS (%RDA/AI*)	
Vitamin A	192 mcg (21%)
Thiamin	0.2 mg (14%)
Riboflavin	0.5 mg (37%)
Niacin	3.8 mg (23%)
Vitamin B$_{12}$	111 mcg (4,624%)
Vitamin C	25 mg (28%)
Vitamin E	2.2 mg (15%)
Iron	31 mg (393%)
Selenium	72 mcg (131%)
Zinc	3.1 mg (28%)

*For more detailed information on RDA and AI, see page 88.

You can freeze shucked raw clams in their liquor in airtight containers. Most types of frozen raw or cooked clams will keep for 2 months if the freezer is set at 0° or colder. Be sure to thaw frozen clams in the refrigerator, not at room temperature.

preparing to use

Unless you have experience shucking live clams, it's safer and faster to have this service performed by the fish seller. If that isn't possible, or you want to store the clams unshucked, then do it yourself—just be sure you have the right tools: A clam knife is about the size of a paring knife, but has a stronger, wider blade and a rounded tip. It's not uncommon for the knife to slip while you're applying pressure to open a shell, so wear a pair of rubber or work gloves to protect your hands.

To shuck clams First, discard any clams with broken or gaping shells—they have died and are not fit to eat. To prepare the remainder, scrub the shells (with a stiff brush, if necessary) and rinse under cold running water.

All clams should be rinsed—and preferably also swirled about—in several changes of cold water to loosen the grit they accumulate. Some people like to take this a step further and purge the grit by soaking clams in salt water— usually a gallon of cold water to which 2 teaspoons of salt have been added. You can also try using a cup of cornmeal instead of, or in addition to, the salt. Let the clams sit in this solution in the refrigerator for 2 to 3 hours.

Hard-shelled clams are easier to open if you place them in the freezer for 10 minutes beforehand. Hold a clam in your gloved palm, rounded-side up, with the shell's hinge toward your wrist. Working over a bowl to catch the juices, push the knife blade between the shell halves from the front. Twist the knife when it is well inside to separate the shell halves. Cut the muscles on each side of the hinge, then cut the interior muscles to free the clam. When opening soft-shelled clams, you'll also need to pull off the dark membrane that covers the edible "neck" of the clam.

serving suggestions

• Instead of serving melted butter with steamers, make a Thai-style dipping sauce with lime juice, soy sauce, fresh ginger, and a bit of sugar.

• Make Manhattan-style clam chowder, but stir in chopped mild green chilies and some ground cumin.

• Make a clam sauce for pasta with chopped clams, clam broth, and garlic. Thicken the sauce with cornstarch instead of butter.

• Cook rice with two-thirds water and one-third white wine. When the rice is cooked, stir in chopped cooked clams, a little bit of Parmesan, and lots of chopped parsley.

coffee

Botanical evidence places the first wild coffee plants in Abyssinia, on the central plateaus of what is today Ethiopia. The fruit of these wild plants was eaten by nomadic herdsmen, who crushed it together with animal fat, then formed it into balls that they carried with them. The resulting food was high in protein—and one suspects the herdsmen found that, as a bonus, they were able to stay awake longer and were in a generally more cheerful mood.

The coffee plant made its way to what is now Yemen where, as early as the 6th century A.D., it became a cultivated crop. From there the culture of coffee moved to Constantinople and eventually to Europe—in part through the offices of the extremely social Suleiman Aga (ambassador from the Ottoman Empire to the court of Louis XIV), who threw flamboyant coffee parties for the French nobility.

In the early 18th century, through a series of political and romantic intrigues, a stolen coffee plant made its way to the West Indies and from there to Central and South America. About 150 years later, coffee seed from Brazil was introduced in Kenya and Tanganyika, several hundred miles south of coffee's original home in Ethiopia.

The source of all this intrigue and gustatory devotion is the coffee plant, a small tree (or large shrub) with shiny, dark green leaves and jasmine-like white flowers. The coffee plant bears a deep-purple fruit called a cherry, which contains two seeds, or beans.

Coffee is grown around the world in the Coffee Belt—in the frost-free band between the Tropics of Cancer and Capricorn—and the best coffees are grown at the higher altitudes. The relatively cooler temperatures at the high altitudes slow the growth of the coffee cherry and as a result produces a denser, harder bean, with more flavor.

nutritional profile

While coffee offers minimal nutritional value, its main claim to fame is the reason why so many of us have to have our early morning cup of java: caffeine. Known chemically as 1,3,7-trimethylxanthine, caffeine gives coffee its jolt; it's a natural substance that functions as a mild stimulant. The effects of caffeine vary from person to person, with large amounts (1,000 milligrams or more) causing adverse effects such as insomnia, restlessness, nervousness, and trembling. Too much caffeine can also temporarily boost heart rate and cause palpitations. While the U.S. Food and Drug Administration considers caffeine to be "Generally Recognized as Safe," studies on the effects of caffeine have been knocked back and forth over the years like a tennis ball, yielding some conflicting information.

Neither coffee nor other products that contain caffeine are classified by drug dependence experts as addictive. Some people, however, do experience

coffee beans

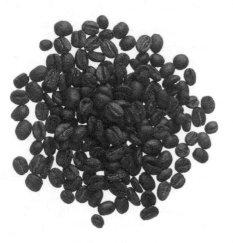

facts & tips

The amount of caffeine in any single serving of coffee depends on a number of factors, including the variety of coffee bean, where the bean was grown, the year the bean was grown, the type of roast, the fineness of the grind, the brewing method, the length of brewing, and the proportion of coffee to water.

some temporary caffeine withdrawal, which can cause fatigue, mild headache, irritability, and drowsiness, feelings that last no more than a day or two when coffee consumption is abruptly ceased. Tapering consumption gradually over several days can help to prevent the symptoms of caffeine withdrawal.

in the market

There are two principal botanical varieties of coffee grown: *Coffea arabica* and *Coffea robusta*. Robusta is a hardier, more economically attractive plant that can be grown at lower altitudes. Unfortunately, it also produces a lower quality bean. All top-quality coffees come from arabica plants, while robusta beans are used in so-called "commercial" coffees, which are sold as instant or preground in cans. The only coffees worth looking into are the arabica coffees sold by the bean. "Commercial" coffees have no differences worth mentioning and are uniformly inferior to arabica coffees.

the bean

Arabica, or "specialty," coffee beans are labeled according to one or more of several criteria. First, some beans are known only by the country of origin, but most are further pinpointed by a regional name; for example, Ethiopian Harrar is grown near the city of Harrar in Ethiopia. Sometimes the origin name will be the port through which the beans are exported, for example, Mocha, which is exported through the Yemenese port of Mocha.

Other coffees are known not by regional names, but only by their countries and grades. Unfortunately, grading systems are complicated, not at all standardized, and usually designed to confuse. Here are some basic guidelines: Grade names that imply high altitude, hardness or density of beans, and "washing" are all desirable.

Another clue to getting around in a coffee store is knowing the difference between "straight" coffees and "blends." A straight Mexican Altura Coatepec, for example, should be nothing but beans of *that* grade (altura) from *that*

the caffeine controversy

Over the years, coffee has been suspected of great mischief but acquitted on nearly all counts regarding the possible adverse effects that it has on heart disease, blood cholesterol, cancer, bone disease, and other illnesses. In fact, some studies have revealed a protective effect linked to coffee consumption.

Research suggests that drinking 2 to 3 cups of caffeinated coffee a day may reduce the risk of developing gallstones (lumps composed mainly of cholesterol, possibly caused by fatty diets). These results may be due to the beneficial effects of caffeine on the gallbladder and/or to the antioxidant effects of a phytochemical in coffee called caffeic acid. Or perhaps it may not be the caffeine at all, since there are a number of other possibly beneficial phytochemicals in coffee as well.

However, it would be unwise to start drinking more coffee on the basis of this research. For now, enjoy the satisfying flavor, aroma, and appeal of drinking coffee, with or without caffeine.

region (Coatepec) in *that* country (Mexico). Blended coffees, on the other hand, can be a number of different bean types mixed together and are usually labeled as "blends" or "styles." Often a blend will be the proprietary blend of the specialty store or the roaster. Beans are usually blended to create a better, more balanced, coffee (like the classic blend of Mocha-Java, for instance). Sometimes, unfortunately, the coffees are blended to save the merchant money: Thus, a Hawaiian Kona Blend coffee may have a very small percentage of Kona beans and a high percentage of another, cheaper bean.

the roast

An extremely important factor to consider in buying coffee is its roast. The coffee bean has no coffee taste at all until it has been roasted; the roasting process brings out the coffee essence—more or less, depending on the length of roasting time. Most straight coffees sold in this country are roasted to a medium-brown roast. Darker roasts—like French and Espresso—are also available, but the coffee beans thus roasted are almost always blends, since most coffee dealers believe that the dark roast obscures the individual flavor characteristics of straight coffees, and feel that a blend is just as good.

Full city This is not a roast name that you will see in stores, but it is a term that roasters use and it is the roast most common in urban America. The bean is medium-dark brown with a dry surface.

Viennese This roast is somewhere between full city and French. It is often a blend of two roasts, usually dark and medium in a ratio of 1 to 2.

French The bean is the color of semisweet chocolate with an oily surface. French roast coffee with chicory added becomes New Orleans-style coffee.

Italian or **Espresso** The bean is almost black and is very oily. This is the heaviest, most bittersweet of all roasts.

choosing the best

It is important to buy coffee from a store that has a brisk turnover, because beans should be as fresh as possible. When roasted coffee beans are exposed to air, their volatile aromatics start to dissipate, or oxidize, and the coffee begins to go stale. Whole-bean coffee will maintain its freshness and peak of flavor for 7 to 10 days after roasting, with dark (oilier) roasts deteriorating somewhat more quickly than lighter roasts. Ground coffee, exposing its vastly increased surface area to the air, begins to go stale almost immediately.

Coffee beans sold in vacuum-sealed bags or cans will stay fresh indefinitely as long as the container is closed. Once opened, the same rules apply.

▶ **When you get home** For the best shelf-life of the coffee you buy, it's best to buy unground beans. And, especially for dark roasts, you should store them in the refrigerator or freezer. If you have the specialty store grind the beans for you, then the ground coffee should definitely be stored in the freezer, in an airtight container.

corn

An important nutritional resource for thousands of years, corn was probably first cultivated in areas of southern Mexico or Central America, perhaps as early as 3400 B.C., and it became a dietary staple of indigenous peoples throughout the Americas.

In America's northeast, the local Native Americans called corn, squash, and beans "the three sisters," which they planted together to form the foundation of their diet. When European colonists arrived in the New World in the 17th century, the grains they brought with them didn't grow well, and initially they depended upon corn for their survival. The early settlers learned from the natives how to prepare corn dishes such as corn fritters, corn pone, succotash, corn bread, corn chowder, and even popcorn (the settlers ate popcorn as a breakfast cereal with milk and maple syrup).

The corn of that day was a starchier, less-tender version of the sweet corn that now ranks as one of America's favorite fresh vegetables—though technically it's not a vegetable but a grain, the seed of a type of grass. Today, in spite of being America's favorite, much of the world's corn crop (and at least 80 percent of this country's crop) is devoted to a category of corn called field corn. Field corn, which is not intended for human consumption, is picked at a mature, predominantly starchy stage and then dried to a more hardened state. From there its uses are varied: as animal feed, in an array of processed foods (from cornstarch to whiskey), or in nonfood products, such as fuel or plastics.

nutritional profile

One of America's favorite foods, corn provides rich texture and flavor. Most varieties are good sources of carbohydrates, fiber, B vitamins (thiamin and folate), and a handful of minerals (potassium, iron, and magnesium). They also have some vitamin C. Only yellow corn, however, contains beta carotene as well as the carotenoids lutein and zeaxanthin. These two carotenoids are associated with healthy eyes and may be helpful in preventing cataracts and age-related macular degeneration.

Although corn contains protein, it's low in the essential amino acids lysine and tryptophan (though combining corn with legumes, such as its succotash partner lima beans, can complete the protein picture). And though corn contains a reasonable amount of the B vitamin niacin, most of it is in a form that is unavailable to the body. However, when corn is combined with an alkaline substance, such as lime (which is used to process corn for corn tortillas), much of the niacin is released.

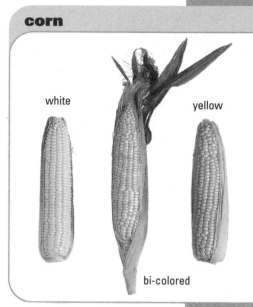

corn

white

yellow

bi-colored

YELLOW CORN 1 cup kernels, cooked	
Calories	177
Protein (g)	5
Carbohydrate (g)	41
Dietary fiber (g)	4.6
Total fat (g)	2.1
Saturated fat (g)	0.3
Monounsaturated fat (g)	0.6
Polyunsaturated fat (g)	1
Cholesterol (mg)	0
Potassium (mg)	408
Sodium (mg)	28

KEY NUTRIENTS (%RDA/AI*)	
Thiamin	0.4 mg (29%)
Niacin	2.6 mg (17%)
Vitamin C	10 mg (11%)
Folate	76 mcg (19%)
Iron	1 mg (13%)
Magnesium	53 mg (12%)

*For more detailed information on RDA and AI, see page 88.

serving suggestions

• Skip the butter on corn-on-the-cob and use wedges of lemon or lime instead.

• Add corn kernels (raw or cooked) to turkey burger mixtures.

• Add corn kernels to pancakes as they cook.

• Remove the silk on corn-cobs but leave the husks on. Brush the kernels with a combination of olive oil and spices (try cumin and black pepper), put the husks back in place, and grill or roast the corn.

in the market

Most varieties of sweet corn—there are more than 200—have yellow kernels; smaller local crops often include white or bicolor corn (which has a mixture of white and yellow kernels). Other interesting types of corn available include:

Baby corn These novelty vegetables are merely undeveloped ears of sweet corn; they can be eaten cob and all. However, because they are so young, they do not have much corn flavor and their sugars haven't developed yet. Although you can occasionally find them fresh, people are probably most familiar with the canned version used in Chinese cuisine.

Corn shoots As the name suggests, these are just the beginnings of the corn plant. They are very sweet and tender and taste very distantly like the grains that would eventually grow on them. They are available almost exclusively in upscale farmers' markets.

Indian Summer This is like the decorative dried "Indian corn" that is a familiar sight on front doors in the Thanksgiving season, but the difference is that this is sold fresh and is an edible sweet corn. Like its dried counterpart, this corn has a mixture of yellow, white, red, and purple kernels.

Supersweets Corn genetics has produced varieties called "supersweets," bred to have more than twice the sugar content of regular corn. Much of the corn now grown in Florida is a supersweet variety known as *Florida Sweet*. Some supersweet varieties also convert their sugar into starch more slowly after the corn is picked—a highly desirable trait in corn that must be shipped to distant markets. Supersweets, like standard sweet corn, may be yellow, white, or bicolor.

▶ Availability Fresh corn is available year round. However, to appreciate corn at its best, you should get it when it's not long off the corn plant. This means buying it when local crops are available; usually this means mid to late summer, and sometimes early fall, for most of the country.

choosing the best

For corn, freshness means staying cool, since warmth converts the sugar in the kernels into starch. In the supermarket, therefore, corn should be displayed in a refrigerated bin; at a farmstand or a farmers' market, it should be kept in the shade or on ice. Shop early in the day for the best selection of locally grown corn; ideally, it should have been picked the morning you buy it. The corn should not be piled high in the bin, or it will generate its own heat, hastening the conversion of sugar to starch. If you're making a trip to the country to get fresh-picked corn, take along an ice chest or cooler in which to pack it.

Check that the husks are fresh-looking, tight, and green (not yellowed or dry); strip back part of the husk to see whether tightly packed rows of plump kernels fill the ear. The kernels at

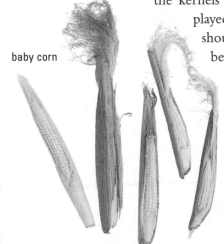

baby corn

dried corn & corn products

Chicos Chicos are dried sweet yellow corn kernels. They can be reconstituted in the same manner as you would cook dried beans.

Corn flour and **cornmeal** See Flour, Nonwheat (*pages 325, 327*).

Grits Grits is the word used to describe any cracked grain, but most people associate it with the Southern staple, hominy grits, which is cooked into a mush and served hot for breakfast or as a side dish; mush can also be chilled, cut into squares, and fried (much like its Italian relative, polenta). The most common type of corn turned into grits is white hominy, though there are also yellow-corn grits. Grits come in a range of granulations, from fine to coarse.

Hominy (posole) These are large, dried white or yellow corn kernels whose hull and germ have been removed. Traditionally this is done by soaking the corn in a solution of lime (or lye) and water to loosen the skin. Although removing the hull is also accomplished mechanically, it's the lime or lye solution that gives the southwestern and Mexican versions of hominy, called posole, their distinctive flavor. The whole kernels can be cooked as a side dish, or added to soups and stews. Dried hominy is also typically ground into grits.

Nixtamal This Mexican cousin to posole is dried corn that is soaked in a lime (or lye) and water bath to loosen its skin, but the bran and germ are not stripped from it. This is the type of corn that is turned into the flour (masa harina) used to make tortillas.

Popcorn Popcorn is a type of "field corn" with thick-walled kernels; when heated, steam is trapped inside the dried kernels, causing them to "explode." Although popcorn is itself low in calories and virtually fat-free, its nutritive value is undermined if it is popped in oil or if salt and butter are added. Microwave popcorns are usually no healthier; many are packed in highly saturated coconut or palm kernel oil; some also come with additional butter. Even the "light" microwave versions get 45 percent of their calories from fat.

Samp This is hominy that has been broken up into coarse pieces, not ground into smaller, more uniform pieces, as for grits.

serving suggestions

• Add chicos or posole to any bean dish where the beans are being cooked from scratch (the dried corn will then cook in the same amount of time).

• Use fine white-corn grits in place of yellow cornmeal in an Italian polenta recipe.

• Cook whole hominy (or use canned, rinsed) and toss with sliced scallions, diced red bell pepper, and a lime vinaigrette for a side salad.

WHITE HOMINY GRITS
1 cup cooked

Calories	145
Protein (g)	3
Carbohydrate (g)	32
Dietary fiber (g)	0.5
Total fat (g)	0.5
Saturated fat (g)	0.1
Monounsaturated fat (g)	0.1
Polyunsaturated fat (g)	0.2
Cholesterol (mg)	0
Potassium (mg)	53
Sodium (mg)	0

KEY NUTRIENTS (%RDA/AI*)

Selenium	7.5 mcg (14%)

For more detailed information on RDA and AI, see page 88.

the tip should be smaller (large kernels at the tip are a sign of overmaturity), but still plump rather than shrunken. Pop a kernel with your fingernail: Milky juice should spurt out. If the liquid is watery, the corn is immature; if the skin of the kernel is tough and its contents doughy, the corn is overripe. The stalk of a freshly picked ear of corn will be green and moist; if it is opaque and white, or dry and brown, the corn is several days old and will not be very sweet. The silk should be moist, soft, and light golden, not brown and brittle.

▶ **When you get home** To best enjoy fresh corn's flavor, "the sooner the better" is a rule of thumb. Try not to store corn for more than a few hours; cook it as soon as possible after it is picked, and be sure to refrigerate it the moment you get home if you are not cooking it immediately. (At room temperature, sweet corn loses its sugar six times faster than at 32°—up to half its total sugar in one day.) Refrigeration also helps the corn retain its vitamin C content.

If the corn is unhusked, leave it that way to keep it moist until you are ready to cook it. If the ears are already fully or partially husked, place them in a perforated plastic bag. If you have more corn on hand than you can use within a day or two, parboil it for just a minute or two (this step stops the conversion of sugar to starch); then you can refrigerate it for up to 3 days. Finish the cooking process by dropping the corn into a pot of boiling water and boiling it for a minute. Or, cut the kernels from the cob and reheat them in a small saucepan.

preparing to use

Unless you are grilling or roasting corn in its husk, strip off the husk and snap off the stalk ends (or leave them on to use it as "handles," if you like). Pull off the silk, using a dry vegetable brush to remove strands of silk caught between the kernels.

If you prefer to eat the kernels off the cob, there are two basic ways to remove them:

To cut whole kernels from the cob, hold an ear of corn vertically, resting the tip on the bottom of a large, wide bowl (to catch the kernels as you work). Slide a sharp knife down the length of the cob to slice off the kernels. Don't press hard, or you will also cut off part of the cob.

For cream-style corn, slit each row of kernels with a sharp knife, then run the back of the knife down the length of the cob, to squeeze out the pulp and juice, leaving the skins of the kernels on the cob.

crab

Crabs belong to a broad spectrum of crustaceans (animals with a shell). They have many legs (10), the front two of which have scissorlike pincers. Although crabs have historically been associated with nasty dispositions—perhaps because they fearlessly brandish their pincers at humans and are all too happy to take a nip out of an innocent swimmer's toe—they are a much prized seafood. There are freshwater crabs and saltwater crabs, the latter being the more plentiful and commercially available.

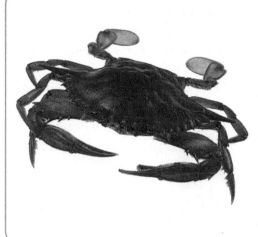

crab

nutritional profile

Crabmeat is a good source of low-fat protein, niacin, and zinc, and it also supplies folate, iron, and a large amount of the antioxidant mineral selenium. But its biggest claim to nutrient fame is its vitamin B_{12} content, with 3 ounces of cooked crabmeat providing over 250 percent of the required amount.

In addition, crabmeat provides heart-healthy omega-3 fatty acids, which reduce blood clotting, thereby lessening the chance of a fatal heart attack. They may also make the heart less susceptible to dangerous, sometimes fatal, rhythm abnormalities. Moreover, although crabmeat is high in dietary cholesterol, it is low in saturated fat, which many major health organizations hold to be more of a risk factor for heart disease than dietary cholesterol.

in the market

Found in the Atlantic and the Pacific, these crustaceans can be divided into two categories: swimming crabs (such as the blue crab) and walking crabs (such as the rock crab). Although there are dozens of different crabs in both categories, only a handful dominate the market. By far the commonest fresh crab is the blue crab.

Alaska king crab The Alaska king crab, the largest of all crabs, is mostly sold as cooked and frozen meat from the legs and claws.

Blue crabs In the East, the hard-shell Atlantic blue crab (sold as soft-shell crab in the seasons when it is molting) is the premier variety. Like all other members of the swimming crab family, blue crabs (whose scientific name translates as "beautiful swimmers") are characterized by having their last pair of legs flattened into swimming paddles. Live hard-shell blue crabs are marketed when they are about 5 to 7 inches across.

Dungeness crab The Pacific coast from California to Alaska is the source for the Dungeness crab, one of the larger species. Most weigh between 1½ and 3 pounds, but the largest can weigh as much as 4 pounds. Winter and early spring are the prime seasons for live Dungeness crab.

Jonah crabs A delicious East Coast crab, it's mostly available locally, from New York north to Nova Scotia.

CRABMEAT 3 ounces cooked	
Calories	87
Protein (g)	17
Carbohydrate (g)	0
Dietary fiber (g)	0
Total fat (g)	1.5
Saturated fat (g)	0.2
Monounsaturated fat (g)	0.2
Polyunsaturated fat (g)	0.6
Cholesterol (mg)	85
Potassium (mg)	276
Sodium (mg)	237

KEY NUTRIENTS (%RDA/AI*)	
Niacin	2.8 mg (18%)
Vitamin B_{12}	6.2 mcg (259%)
Folate	43 mcg (11%)
Iron	0.8 mg (10%)
Selenium	34 mcg (62%)
Zinc	3.6 mg (33%)

*For more detailed information on RDA and AI, see page 88.

Rock crabs This is an umbrella term for several members of the walking crab family, including Jonahs and Dungeness crabs.

Snow crabs Snow crabs are harvested in both the North Atlantic and the North Pacific; like Alaska king crabs, their meat is mostly sold cooked and frozen, so it is available year round.

Soft-shell crabs These are crabs in the process of molting: As crabs grow, they shed their hard shells several times and grow new, larger shells to accommodate their bigger bodies. When the new shell is just forming, it is quite soft and the crab can be eaten shell and all. Many crabs go through this process, but only the blue crab is sufficiently meaty to be of commercial (or culinary) interest.

Stone crabs Another East Coast species, the Florida stone crab is unusual in that only its meaty, thick-shelled claws are eaten: When the crab is caught, just one leg is removed and the crab is thrown back—it has the ability to regenerate the missing leg.

▶ **Availability** Fresh hard-shell crabs are available locally year round. Soft-shell crabs are available from late spring through early fall, but their peak season is mid-summer. Stone crabs are caught from October through March.

questionable delicacy

Open up a crab and you will find the so-called mustard, or crab butter (hepatopancreas), which some consider a delicacy. This organ in the crab performs the usual functions of the liver in any animal—filtering toxins from the system—and may contain high concentrations of PCBs and other contaminants if the crab was harvested from contaminated waters. Therefore, it's safest to discard it.

choosing the best

Crabs are sold live, and their meat—delicately sweet, firm yet flaky—is also available fresh cooked, frozen, and canned. Fresh crabmeat is sold as lump, backfin, or flake. Lump crabmeat, which consists of large, choice chunks of body meat, is the finest and most expensive. Backfin is smaller pieces of body meat. Flake is white meat from the body and other parts and is in flakes and shreds. Some fresh-cooked crab is pasteurized after cooking, which helps it keep longer. Canned crab is often imported from Asia and may come from a variety of species.

As with finfish, your nose and eyes can tell you a lot about the merchandise. Crabs should smell briny-fresh, and look bright and clean. Shells should be hard (except for soft-shell crabs) and moist. Live crabs should be active, moving their legs when touched. Choose crabs that feel heavy for their size.

Cooked crab should smell perfectly fresh, with no trace of ammonia or "fishy" odor, and should have bright orange-red shells. Crabmeat should be snowy-white (meat from some parts of the crab may be tinged with brown or red). Cooked crabs should be purchased the same day they were cooked. Fresh-cooked crab should not be displayed alongside raw fish or shellfish, as bacteria can migrate from the raw to the cooked.

▶ **When you get home** It's best to cook and eat live crabs the same day they are purchased. Fresh-cooked crabmeat will keep for 2 days, refrigerated.

preparing to use

If you plan to boil live hard-shell crabs, you can simply drop them headfirst into boiling water. If you plan to cook them by another method, such as broiling, they need to be killed first. If you want the fish seller to perform this task for you, be sure to make your purchase shortly before you plan to cook the crabs; or you can do it at home using a heavy chef's knife.

To kill a crab Place it belly-side up on a cutting board, lay the knife lengthwise on the belly of the crab, and strike it firmly with a mallet to cut the crab in half. Break off the shells, first the bottom belly flap and then the top shell; remove and discard the spongelike gills. Then twist off and crack the legs and claws to extract the meat. Remove the body meat as well, pick over all the meat for shell bits, and it is ready to cook. Soft-shell crabs can be killed by cutting off their eyes and about ⅛ inch of their head with a sharp knife or large shears. Lift up the side flaps and remove and discard the soft, spongy gills. With your fingers, remove the tail flap. If you prefer, your fish seller can do this for you, but have it done only a few hours before you plan to cook the crab.

Before using cooked crabmeat, check for any stray pieces of cartilage or shell. Pick over the crabmeat and discard any shell or cartilage you may find. Chances are, even if you've purchased crabmeat that is clean, it will still have a little shell or cartilage in it.

serving suggestions

· Sprinkle a small amount of shredded crabmeat and corn over pancakes as they cook for a savory brunch or lunch.

· Substitute crab for some of the clams in Manhattan clam chowder.

· Toss shredded crabmeat with diced mild green chilies, cooked black beans, and chopped tomatoes, and wrap in flour tortillas.

· Steam crabs and serve with Thai dipping sauce made with lime juice, soy sauce, and a touch of brown sugar.

adding flavor to crabs

Crabs are often cooked in what is called "crab boil," which is simply water seasoned with a traditional combination of spices. The spice mixture can be purchased in any area where live crabs are sold (or by mail order). Or, you can make your own by adding to the salted cooking water a few whole mustard seeds, dill seeds, coriander seeds, allspice berries, a whole clove, bay leaves, and a pinch of cayenne or crushed red pepper.

The spices can be added directly to the water, or, for easy removal, placed in a square of cheesecloth and tied with a piece of string. Add a squeeze of lemon juice to the water as well.

If you do not salt the water too heavily, use the cooking water as a base for a seafood soup after cooking the crabs and removing the spices.

This same mixture can be used to add flavor to lobster or shrimp.

cranberries

The cranberry, which is one of only a handful of commercially valuable fruits native to North America, was used long before the early settlers arrived in America. The Native Americans used cranberries for medicinal purposes and as a natural dye for rugs, blankets, and clothing. They also distributed cranberries as a symbol of peace at tribal feasts. In addition, they mashed cranberries with deer meat to make pemmican, which kept for long periods of time and served as a convenient form of sustenance and nourishment during the winter months.

The early settlers called the tart fruit "crane berries" because of the resemblance of the blooming cranberry flower to the head of a sand crane. Cranberries were plentiful in Massachusetts in 1620 and there is speculation that they may have been served at the first Thanksgiving dinner, although we have no way of knowing that to be true.

While most people tend to regard cranberries as merely a garnish for Thanksgiving turkey, they are actually a more versatile food and can be used in grain dishes, casseroles, and stews—not to mention all manner of desserts.

nutritional profile

Cranberries are low in calories and a good source of vitamin C. Because they are so tart, cranberries are often processed into sweetened sauces or juices. If the berries are heated during processing, their vitamin C content is diminished. Also, the amount of sugar in store-bought cranberry sauce increases the calories to 209 per ½ cup. Sweetened cranberry juice cocktail sold in supermarkets is also heavily sweetened, and often contains very little actual cranberry juice.

in the market

The wild cranberries favored by early settlers have been largely replaced by cultivated varieties that are larger, glossier, and more flavorful. The United

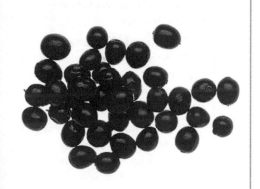

cranberries

CRANBERRIES / 1 cup raw	
Calories	47
Protein (g)	>1
Carbohydrate (g)	12
Dietary fiber (g)	4.0
Total fat (g)	0.2
Saturated fat (g)	0
Monounsaturated fat (g)	0
Polyunsaturated fat (g)	0.1
Cholesterol (mg)	0
Potassium (mg)	67
Sodium (mg)	1

KEY NUTRIENTS (%RDA/AI*)	
Vitamin C	13 mg (14%)

For more detailed information on RDA and AI, see page 88.

serving suggestions

• Stir cranberries into meat and poultry stews to provide tartness and some thickening.

• Make your own cranberry sauce and use it in place of store-bought jams or jellies.

• Poach apples or pears in cranberry juice.

• Add cranberry juice to a meat braise in place of some of the broth or other liquid.

• Stir chopped cranberries into rice or other grain pilafs.

• Combine chopped cranberries with a little sugar and horseradish and use as a condiment.

States harvests approximately 36,000 acres of cranberries a year. Most cranberries are from Wisconsin and Massachusetts.

There are over 100 varieties of cranberries in the United States with the majority being *Early Blacks, Howes, Searles,* and *McFarlins*. They range in size from large to small, but there is no appreciable difference in their flavor. The indicator of ripeness—a deep red, or rosy hue—is the same for all types.

▶ Availability Only about 10 percent of the commercial crop is sold fresh; the rest is used either in juice or canned cranberry sauce. Fresh cranberries are available year round, but are more plentiful beginning in September and through December, for the holiday season. Frozen cranberries have become increasingly more available.

choosing the best

Cranberries are usually sold in bags, and since they're firmer than most other berries, they're likely to be in good condition. Check them for firmness and good red color; the bag should contain a minimum of pale berries and debris.

▶ When you get home Cranberries store well and can be easily frozen: You can put bags of cranberries in the freezer with no further preparation. You can cook with the frozen berries without thawing them.

preparing to use

It's easy to clean and pick over cranberries by placing them in a basin of cold water; twigs, leaves, and unripe berries are easy to spot because they float to the surface. The process should be done quickly, though—you don't want to soak the berries.

Cranberries are too tart to eat raw or in any unsweetened form, but they can be combined with sweeter fruits, such as apples or pears, so that very little additional sugar is needed.

➤ *phytochemicals in* cranberries

Cranberries are a rich source of procyanidins, phytochemicals that appear to prevent bacteria from sticking to the urinary tract and causing an infection. Researchers speculate that regularly drinking a 10-ounce glass of cranberry juice may deliver enough procyanidins to help ward off a urinary tract infection. (This advice is based on a Harvard study in which the subjects drank a 10-ounce glass of cranberry juice cocktail daily. To increase the amount of actual cranberry juice consumed, try unsweetened cranberry juice or cranberry juice concentrate; see "Other Cranberry Products," below.) Procyanidin phytochemicals may offer protection against cancer and cardiovascular disease as well.

---

other cranberry products

Dried cranberries Dried cranberries (sometimes called craisins) are available in bulk and packaged. They are usually sweetened and can be substituted for raisins or other dried fruits in compotes, cookies, and muffins.

Cranberry juice Cranberry juice sold in supermarkets is full of sugar, since cranberries are naturally too tart to make a drinkable juice. These juices are labeled "drink" or "cocktail" rather than juice, since the proportion of juice to sugar is too low to allow them to be called juice. However, in health-food stores, you can find unsweetened cranberry juice concentrate. Stir 2 to 3 tablespoons of concentrate into 1 cup of cold water and sweeten to taste. Use the concentrate to add tartness to barbecue sauces, meat glazes, salad dressings, and smoothies and other drinks.

cucumbers

The cucumber belongs to the same vegetable family as pumpkin, zucchini (a close look-alike), watermelon, and other squash. First cultivated in Thailand centuries ago, the plant spread easily throughout India and Asia. It is said to have been prized by the ancient Romans, who are believed to have introduced the plant to Europe. Some historians speculate that it was Columbus who brought the cucumber to America, where it was eventually grown by both Native Americans and colonists from Florida to Canada. Today "cukes," as they are popularly called, grow in a wide variety of shapes and sizes, from the inch-long ones called gherkins to mammoth greenhouse varieties that reach 20 inches or longer.

nutritional profile

Cucumbers are generally low in nutrients (though they do have some potassium), but their skins are a surprisingly good source of lutein, a carotenoid that has been linked with eye health.

in the market

There are two basic types of cucumbers, those eaten fresh (called slicing varieties) and those cultivated for pickling. The *slicing cucumbers* most commonly seen in supermarkets are field-grown varieties that are usually 6 to 9 inches long and have glossy, dark-green skin and tapering ends. After harvesting, the skin is often waxed for longer shelf-life.

Pickling cucumbers, on the other hand, rarely make it to the market fresh. There are numerous varieties, and they all tend to be smaller and squatter than the typical slicing cucumber. One of the best known pickling cucumbers is the diminutive, bumpy-skinned *gherkin*.

On the fresh (slicing) cucumber scene, in addition to the typical supermarket cucumber, there are a number of unusual types available:

Armenian (snake melon, snake cucumber) These extra-long, twisted cucumbers have thin, dark green skin that's marked with paler green longitudinal furrows. As it ripens, the fruit turns yellow and releases an aroma not unlike its relative the muskmelon. This slicing cucumber is mild in flavor.

Hothouse Most of these varieties originated in Europe (they are sometimes called European or English cucumbers), and they tend to be thin, smooth-skinned, and 1 to 2 feet in length. The majority are also seedless, or nearly so. For that reason, many people find hothouse cucumbers easier to digest (they're sometimes called burpless) and milder (or blander, depending on your tastebuds) in flavor than field-grown varieties. Hothouse cukes are usually more expensive than supermarket cucumbers.

Japanese cucumbers (kyuri) Dark green and slender, with tiny bumps and thin skin, Japanese cucumbers have small seeds; both the skin and seeds are generally consumed. They have a crisp texture and sweet flesh.

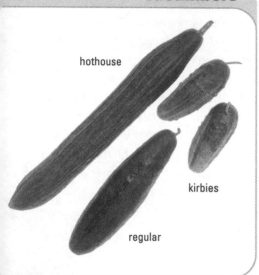

cucumbers

hothouse

kirbies

regular

CUCUMBERS / 1 cup sliced	
Calories	14
Protein (g)	>1
Carbohydrate (g)	3
Dietary fiber (g)	0.8
Total fat (g)	0.2
Saturated fat (g)	0.1
Monounsaturated fat (g)	0
Polyunsaturated fat (g)	0.1
Cholesterol (mg)	0
Potassium (mg)	176
Sodium (mg)	2

Kirby The vast majority of kirbies grown are turned into commercial dill pickles, but they are also sold fresh. Many cooks prefer kirbies because they are usually unwaxed and have thin skin, crisp flesh, and tiny seeds.

Lemon About the size of a lemon, with pale lemony skin that turns golden-yellow as the cucumber matures, this cucumber has a very delicate, sweet flavor and crisp texture.

Persian (Sfran) Similar to the slicing cucumber, but shorter, squatter, and more compact, Persian cucumbers are crunchy and watery.

▶ Availability The familiar dark green slicing varieties and hothouse cucumbers are available year round, as are Armenian and Japanese cucumbers. Other specialty cucumbers tend to be more seasonal.

choosing the best

Cucumbers and coolness are natural partners—at least in the sense that the vegetable must be kept cool, or it will quickly wilt to soggy limpness. (Overchilling or freezing, however, will reduce the inside of a cucumber to slush.) At the supermarket, cucumbers should be kept under refrigeration; at a farmers' market or roadside stand, they should always be displayed in the shade. Hothouse cucumbers are usually sealed in a tight plastic wrapping.

No matter what kind you buy, look for cucumbers that are very firm and rounded right to the ends; avoid any that have withered, shriveled tips. Although the overall size varies with the type, slender cukes typically have fewer seeds than thick or puffy ones. Beware of cucumbers that bulge in the middle, since they are likely to be filled with large seeds and have watery, tasteless flesh. Waxed or not, cucumber

serving suggestions

· Combine diced cucumbers with scallions, yogurt, and chopped cilantro, basil, or dill for a cooling accompaniment to serve with spicy food.

· Sauté cucumber slices in olive oil with garlic for a quick side vegetable.

· Combine diced cucumber, watermelon, and crumbled feta cheese for an interesting salad.

· Halve and seed cucumbers and stuff with a mixture of chopped smoked salmon, capers, lemon juice, and a little olive oil.

· Make an Armenian-style salad: Combine diced cucumbers, minced garlic, and yogurt.

· Make a slaw with thin wedges of apple, diced cucumbers, and toasted walnuts. Dress the slaw with a lemon vinaigrette.

· Make traditional Spanish gazpacho with cucumber, tomatoes, red onion, and roasted green peppers, and a splash of wine vinegar. Toss in a blender and pulse until chunky. Serve chilled.

the quest for straight cucumbers

Unlike the long cylindrical cucumbers of today, cucumbers of the 18th and early 19th centuries grew bent and twisted. Unhappy with crooked cucumbers, George Stephenson—the inventor of the locomotive and an avid cucumber gardener—developed a device to force them to grow straight. He placed young cucumbers inside a hollow, long glass cylinder—which he aptly called a cucumber glass—and as they grew, the cucumbers took on the shape of the tube. Fortunately for modern gardeners, today's varieties grow practically straight on their own.

skin should be a rich green—not extremely pale and definitely not yellow (except, of course, for "lemon cucumbers"). Watch out for bruises or dark spots.

▶ **When you get home** Store cucumbers in the refrigerator crisper. Uncut, waxed cucumbers will keep for about 1 week. Check unwaxed cukes every day or so and discard any that show signs of decay. Wrap cut cucumbers tightly in plastic wrap and use within a day or two of purchase.

preparing to use

If a cucumber is unwaxed, you can leave the skin on; it's best to wash the cucumber before eating it, though. But most people prefer to peel waxed cukes; slice off the ends first, to make the job easier.

Even if the seeds are small, some people prefer to remove them before serving cucumbers. Simply halve the cucumbers lengthwise and scoop out the seeds with the tip of a teaspoon. Then slice, dice, julienne, or grate the flesh.

There are several ways to remove the bitterness cucumbers sometimes have. Try cutting off the ends and peeling the skin. If that doesn't work, sprinkle the peeled cucumbers with a pinch of salt, a pinch of sugar, and a few drops of vinegar, and let stand for 20 to 30 minutes.

dates

Native to the Middle East, dates are as old as civilization and have been culti-vated for more than 4,000 years. Crowning the tops of towering palm trees that can grow 100 feet high and yield 1,000 dates each year, they grow in heavy clusters of oblong brown fruits—as many as 200 in a cluster that weighs up to 25 pounds. The date palm tree, along with offering dates, is used to make thread, baskets, lumber, mattresses, rope, and other household items. The word "date" alludes to its shape and comes from the Greek *daktulos*, meaning finger. While much of the world's date crop is grown in the Middle East, the United States also supplies a large amount from California and Arizona, where date orchards—called gar-dens in the industry—were introduced in the early 1900s.

nutritional profile

With up to 70 percent of their weight coming from sugar, dates are among the sweetest of fruits. Dates are unusual because, unlike most other fruit, they contain hardly any vitamin C. Still, they are low in fat and rich in potassium and fiber. Dates also supply some iron.

in the market

Dates are classified into three categories—soft, semisoft, and dry—according to the softness of the fruit. Dry dates (also called bread dates) are not dates that have been deliberately dehydrated, as is the case with other kinds of dried fruits; they simply contain relatively little moisture when ripe. You're more likely to find dry varieties in health-food stores.

Barhi Barhi dates, named for the hot Arabic winds called "Barh," are medium-sized, thin-skinned fruit with soft, tender flesh and a syrupy flavor.

Deglet Noor A semisoft date, deglet noor is the variety most often available—it accounts for 95 percent of U.S. production. It has firm flesh and a color range from light red to amber.

Halawy These soft dates are thick-fleshed, caramel-y, and sweet. Their appearance is wrinkled and the skin ranges from yellow to amber.

Khadrawy Similar to the Halawys, these soft dates have a caramel-like texture and sweet flavor.

Medjool These semisoft dates, sometimes called the Cadillac of dates, are sweet, moist, meaty, and firm-textured.

Thoory This is a dry date with firm skin and chewy flesh.

Zahidi The Zahidi, a semisoft date, is called "Nobility." It has a large seed and crunchy fibrous flesh, and is often processed for sliced dates and date sugar products.

▶ Availability Dates are harvested in late fall and early winter, but because they store well, they are available throughout the year.

dates

barhi

deglet noor

medjool

DATES / 2 ounces pitted	
Calories	156
Protein (g)	1
Carbohydrate (g)	42
Dietary fiber (g)	4.3
Total fat (g)	0.3
Saturated fat (g)	0.1
Monounsaturated fat (g)	0.1
Polyunsaturated fat (g)	0
Cholesterol (mg)	0
Potassium (mg)	370
Sodium (mg)	2

choosing the best

Dates are sold in both fresh and dried form. It isn't always easy to tell the difference between the two, since fresh dates may appear somewhat wrinkled, and both types are usually packaged in cellophane or plastic containers. The dates that are commonly available in stores are fresh or partially dried, and do not contain any preservatives.

Both fresh and dried dates should be smooth-skinned, glossy, and plump; they should not be broken, cracked, dry, or shriveled (although they may be slightly wrinkled). Avoid those that smell sour or have crystallized sugar on their surface. Dried dates should not be rock hard.

▶ **When you get home** Dried dates keep extremely well, since they are often pasteurized to inhibit mold growth.

preparing to use

Dates sold as pitted may occasionally contain a pit; the labels on their packages often carry warnings as to this possibility. Check each date before you eat it.

To prepare unpitted dates for eating or cooking, slit each date open and push out the pit. To chop dates, either snip them with scissors or cut them with a knife. In either case, dip the blades into water frequently to keep the dates from sticking. For easier slicing, separate dates and place them in the freezer for an hour to firm them.

If dried dates seem excessively dry, you can plump them by soaking them in hot water or juice for about 15 minutes.

---

chinese dates

The Chinese date, or jujube (not to be confused with the chewy jelly candy of that name), is neither a variety of date, nor a member of the same botanical family. It does, however, strongly resemble a true date in color and texture, and is used in much the same way. Unlike true dates, fresh Chinese dates are an excellent source of vitamin C: 2 ounces provide 43 percent of the RDA. In their dried form, the vitamin C is diminished, but, as with other dried fruit, there is a higher concentration of nutrients, including riboflavin, thiamin, iron, and potassium.

---

serving suggestions

- Stir-fry noodles with shredded pork or duck, sweet bell peppers, and diced dates.

- Stuff ravioli with a mixture of part-skim ricotta cheese and chopped dates.

- Add diced dates to homemade apple or pear pies.

- Stir chopped dates into peanut butter and use as a sandwich spread.

- Make a low-fat shake with dates, yogurt, and a splash of lemon.

- Stuff cored apples with dates and bake.

- Combine chopped dates with cooked lentils and chicken for a main-dish salad.

- Use chopped dates in place of raisins in baked goods.

- Add chopped dates to a cheese sandwich.

duck

In Colonial times, wild duck was an important part of the dinnertime menu. But it's fair to say that duck hasn't come close in popularity to chicken or turkey in many years. Americans now eat an average of only about ¾ pound of duck annually per capita (compared to 55 pounds per person for chicken, for example). Perhaps this is because duck is considered sophisticated fare—more difficult to prepare than chicken or turkey and with a more complicated flavor. Ducks also have a large chest cavity (so they contain a smaller proportion of meat to bone), and all of their meat is dark. And most people wouldn't consider turning to duck if they're watching their fat intake.

Much of this reputation, however, turns out to be unjustified, though there are certainly some legitimate reasons that it has been slow to gain popularity. Duck is hard to find (in supermarkets, anyway), and it is a high-maintenance bird to roast, because the skin must be constantly pricked to release the fat. But there is one strike against it that is undeserved: Though most people think of duck as too fatty to eat, duck meat (the breast in particular) is actually leaner than chicken. A 3-ounce serving of skinless cooked duck breast has 30 percent less than the same amount of skinless chicken breast.

nutritional profile

After the skin has been removed, ducks, like other types of poultry, are a good source of protein, iron, selenium, and B vitamins.

in the market

The most widely sold domestic duck is the white Pekin, which was brought to the United States from China in the 19th century. Young white Pekin ducks are often sold as Long Island ducklings, although only about a third of domestic ducks are raised on Long Island, New York. The majority come from duck farms in the Midwest.

Mallard Rarely available unless you or someone you know hunts or has access to a specialty store, these small birds (close in size to a Cornish hen) are best eaten medium-rare.

Moulard Prized for their large, dark, sweet breast meat, these birds are often twice as large as Pekin ducks and quite difficult to find. The breasts, or magrets, can be cooked like steak, though they're much leaner. The breast meat is now more readily available in specialty and high-end butcher shops.

Muscovy This variety is often used in restaurants. It is small and gamy with more pronounced flavor than the Pekin. Generally weighing between 3 and 4 pounds, a 3¼-pound bird will feed two to three. These are best cooked to medium-rare or pink.

Pekin The Pekin is the most widely available duck. Fed on a diet of corn and soy, the Pekin is milder in flavor than other varieties. It is heavy-boned and yields proportionally less meat per pound than some other varieties. The

DUCK BREAST (PEKIN) 3 ounces cooked, skinless	
Calories	119
Protein (g)	24
Carbohydrate (g)	0
Dietary fiber (g)	0
Total fat (g)	2.1
Saturated fat (g)	0.5
Monounsaturated fat (g)	0.7
Polyunsaturated fat (g)	0.3
Cholesterol (mg)	123
Potassium (mg)	n/a
Sodium (mg)	89

KEY NUTRIENTS (%RDA/AI*)	
Niacin	8.8 mg (55%)
Iron	3.8 mg (48%)
Selenium	25 mcg (45%)

*For more detailed information on RDA and AI, see page 88.

facts & tips

Current official analysis for duck breast does not include a number of nutrients that are known to be significant in duck as a whole. It's quite likely that duck breast, too, has good amounts of the following nutrients: thiamin, riboflavin, vitamin B$_6$, vitamin B$_{12}$, and zinc.

ducklings are 8 weeks old or younger, and weigh from 3 to 6 pounds, a large percentage of that weight being fat. A 4½-pound bird will feed two to three.

▶ **Availability** Ducks are available fresh on a limited basis from late spring through late winter, but 90 percent of the duck supply is sold frozen. Duck breasts (magrets) are sometimes available in specialty food markets. If available, they are generally fresh.

choosing the best

If you purchase a fresh duck, check that the skin is clean, odor-free, feather-free, and off-white (not yellow). Frozen ducks should be plump-breasted and wrapped in airtight packages. If you buy the duck in a supermarket, check the "sell by" date.

▶ **When you get home** As with other poultry, keep duck in its original wrapping but overwrap it with aluminum foil to catch any leakage. Store fresh duck in the coldest part of the refrigerator. (Wrap and store any giblets separately.)

Because duck is widely available frozen, there is no sense in freezing fresh duck. Store-bought frozen duck should be placed in the freezer in its original wrapping. Date the package and use it within 3 months. (Some frozen birds carry an expiration date.)

preparing to use

To defrost a frozen whole duck, place it on a dish in the refrigerator; a 5-pound bird will thaw in 24 to 36 hours. Alternatively, you can submerge the duck in a pot or sink full of cold water. (Warm water thaws the bird too quickly and can cause bacteria to flourish.) Change the water every 30 minutes. Thawing takes about 3 hours.

Before cooking a fresh or thawed whole duck, check for any feathers and remove them, and also remove any visible fat (especially from the cavity). Then rinse the bird and pat it dry. Prick the skin all over without piercing the flesh. For roasting, leave the bird whole. Remove the skin before eating. For broiling or grilling, choose skinless duck breasts.

COMPARING POULTRY 3 ounces cooked

Skinless duck breast is a surprisingly low-fat source of protein, despite its reputation. Here's how it stacks up against chicken breast and turkey breast. All examples are skinless.

	Calories	Fat (g)	% Calories from Fat	Saturated Fat (g)	Cholesterol (mg)
Turkey breast	115	0.6	5	0.2	71
Duck breast	119	2.1	16	0.5	123
Chicken breast	140	3.0	19	0.9	72

eggplant

Thought to have originated in China or India, eggplant is a member of the nightshade family and therefore related to potatoes, tomatoes, and peppers. Apparently, it was introduced to Europe in the 12th century, when Arab traders brought it into Spain. The early plants that English-speaking people came into contact with bore egg-shaped fruits, most likely white ones, hence the vegetable's name.

By the 18th century, the eggplant was established as a food in Italy and France (where it is known as aubergine). Sometime in the 17th century, eggplant was brought to America, and by the early 1800s it was grown for use as an ornament. Today, eggplant is cultivated in most warm regions of the world, and is widely used in Asian and Middle Eastern cookery, as well as in many Mediterranean dishes. Americans have learned to appreciate its exceptional adaptability and it appears as a main dish, an appetizer, or a side dish. Its robust flavor and "meaty" texture also make it a perfect vegetarian main-dish choice.

nutritional profile

A high-fiber, virtually fat-free vegetable with only a small amount of vitamins and minerals, eggplant's primary virtues lie in its culinary applications.

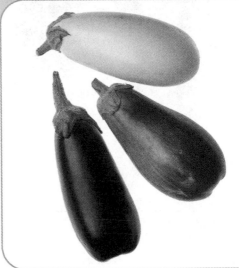

american eggplants

in the market

In the United States, the familiar dark purple eggplants (called *American eggplants* or *globe eggplants*) come in a variety of sizes—from 1 to 5 pounds—and are the most common type sold commercially. They also come in two basic shapes, squat and tear-shaped (in both cases with the bottom wider than the top). A multitude of other shapes, sizes, and colors is also available, including some highly unusual "heirloom" varieties that are bright orange.

Baby eggplants These are small, young eggplants in the shape of a tennis ball. They can be from a number of different varieties and come in a number of colors, including purple, violet, white, and canary yellow.

Chinese Long and slim, these eggplants are distinguished by their pale purple skin. The flesh is soft and white. Some examples of Chinese eggplant can be quite long and crooked.

Cluster eggplants These pea-sized green eggplants are sold in a cluster still attached to its stem. They are not really suitable for cooking, but make wonderful pickles.

Graffiti These eggplants come in both purple and white varieties and have a shape similar to the standard American eggplant. The purple graffiti is covered with white striations (and looks like a huge cranberry bean). The white version has very pale purple striations.

EGGPLANT / 1 cup cooked	
Calories	26
Protein (g)	1
Carbohydrate (g)	6
Dietary fiber (g)	2.4
Total fat (g)	0.2
Saturated fat (g)	0
Monounsaturated fat (g)	0
Polyunsaturated fat (g)	0
Cholesterol (mg)	0
Potassium (mg)	208
Sodium (mg)	3

Green Goddess This hybrid is elongated in shape with unusually pale green skin. It has a very mild flavor.

Italian These resemble a scaled-down version of the large purple American eggplant. A true Italian eggplant has a finer flesh and a thinner skin than conventional purple eggplants, though in some markets, it is simply the size of the eggplant that prompts the use of the market term "Italian eggplant."

Japanese These eggplants are long and narrow, with a much darker purple skin (though there is also a white variety of Japanese eggplant). Its flesh is sweeter and less astringent than American eggplant.

Rosa Bianco This Italian heirloom variety is a squat, violet eggplant tinged with white. Like other Italian eggplants, its flesh is creamier than that of American eggplants.

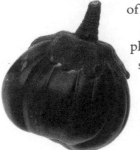

rosa bianco eggplant

Thai These small, round, firm eggplants are green-and-white striped and are usually a little bit bigger than a golf ball. The skin is thin and covers creamy-white flesh that has a subtle flavor and soft texture. The seeds tend to be bitter and should be removed.

Tiger These small spherical eggplants have orange and green skin, with occasional dark vertical stripes (hence the name tiger). The flesh is ivory-white and the flavor delicate.

White Increasingly, you will find these smooth-skinned, ivory-white eggplants sold in supermarkets. Their shapes and sizes are similar to American eggplants, but they have firmer, moister flesh. Some varieties include: Cloud Nine, Casper, and Ghostbuster.

▶ **Availability** American, Chinese, and Japanese eggplants are available year round, but some of the more exotic "heirloom" eggplants are only available in the fall and early winter.

choosing the best

Look for a symmetrical eggplant with satin-smooth skin and no blemishes; tan patches, scars, or bruises on the skin indicate decay, which will appear as discoloration in the flesh beneath. An eggplant with wrinkled or flabby-looking skin will probably be bitter. If you press the vegetable gently with your thumb, the indentation should refill rapidly if the eggplant is fresh.

A good eggplant will feel fairly heavy; a light one may be seedy. The stem and calyx (cap) should be bright green. A medium-sized American purple eggplant, 3 to 6 inches in diameter, is likely to be young, sweet, and tender; oversized specimens may be tough, seedy, and bitter.

---

serving suggestions

• Steam halved Italian or small American eggplants. Drizzle with a dressing of sesame oil, soy sauce, and vinegar. Let sit at room temperature and serve as an appetizer.

• Cut eggplants into thick lengthwise slices, brush lightly with olive oil, and grill.

• Bake whole eggplants (poked with a couple of holes to let steam escape), then mash with lemon juice, parsley, garlic, and a touch of peanut butter or tahini (sesame butter).

• Bake halved eggplants until soft but still firm enough to hold their shape. Scoop out the flesh and mash with crumbled feta cheese, fresh herbs, and fresh tomatoes. Return the mixture to the eggplant shells, top with a light sprinkling of Parmesan, and broil.

▶ **When you get home** Ideally, an eggplant should be stored at about 50°. Cold temperatures will eventually damage it, as will warm conditions. You can store an uncut, unwashed eggplant in a plastic bag in the refrigerator crisper for 3 to 4 days. If the eggplant won't fit easily in the crisper, don't try to squeeze it in; the vegetable is so delicate that any undue pressure will bruise it. The skin is also easily punctured, leading to decay.

preparing to use

Wash the eggplant just before using, and cut off the cap and stem. (Use a stainless steel knife for cutting eggplant; a carbon steel blade will blacken it.)

Eggplant may be cooked with or without its skin. If the eggplant is large, the skin may be tough, so you may want to peel it with a vegetable peeler. White varieties tend to have thick, tough skins, and should always be peeled. (If you're baking the eggplant, the flesh can be scooped from the skin after cooking.)

Many recipes call for salting eggplant before cooking it. This step draws out some of the moisture and produces a denser-textured flesh, which means the eggplant will exude less water and absorb less fat in cooking. Salting also seems to help reduce the vegetable's natural astringent taste. Rinsing the eggplant thoroughly after salting will remove most of the salt; however, if you are following a sodium-restricted diet, you should not use this method.

To salt eggplant Cut it in half lengthwise (or slice or dice it, depending on the recipe) and sprinkle the cut surfaces with salt; ½ teaspoon is sufficient for a pound of eggplant. Place the salted eggplant in a colander and let stand for about 30 minutes. You can then rinse the eggplant, squeeze out the excess moisture, and pat dry with paper towels.

sexing an eggplant

A good eggplant should not be seedy. Some people believe that they can predict the seed content of an eggplant by determining its sex (supposedly indicated by the size and shape of the scar at the blossom end). According to the theory, male eggplants have fewer seeds than female ones. But this method is a myth. An eggplant is self-pollinating; that is, it has both male and female characteristics and can reproduce on its own. A better way to judge seediness is by size. Small- and medium-sized eggplants have fewer seeds than large, overmature eggplants, which are practically guaranteed to be seedy.

eggs

When Americans began to be cholesterol-conscious, the egg was one of the first foods they stopped eating: Following a gradual decline since World War II in per capita consumption of fresh eggs came a markedly steeper drop of some 22 percent between 1980 and 1990. However, with a revised cholesterol count (*see "The Cholesterol Issue," opposite page*) and an increased awareness that dietary cholesterol is not the criminal it was once thought to be, the per capita consumption of eggs has been steadily increasing—though it is still well shy of the 400 eggs a year of 1945!

nutritional profile

The egg is an inexpensive source of high-quality protein (about 6 grams in a large egg) and an important source of vitamin B_{12}, riboflavin, and selenium. These attributes should make it one of nature's near-perfect foods, but the egg has one drawback: Its yolk contains about two-thirds of the total suggested daily maximum intake of cholesterol.

Egg whites, though, can be used freely: It is the yolk that contains all of the fat and cholesterol (as well as the major concentration of calories, B vitamins, and minerals). The white is almost pure protein—protein that is considered nearly perfect because of its exemplary balance of amino acids. Even if you are very concerned about your consumption of cholesterol, you can still take partial advantage of the egg's culinary usefulness and nutritional value by cooking with egg whites alone.

Along with certain kinds of fish (salmon, mackerel, sardines), egg yolks are one of the few foods that naturally contain Vitamin D. About 7 percent of the RDA for vitamin D can be found in one large yolk. Egg yolks also contain vitamin A and the carotenoids lutein and zeaxanthin, which may function as antioxidants against free-radical damage. Studies suggest that lutein and zeaxanthin may help protect your eyes from the development of cataracts.

in the market

Most supermarkets carry just one or two types of eggs: white and/or brown hen's eggs. Most white eggs come from the Single Comb White Leghorn breed of hen. Brown eggs, which are preferred over white eggs by consumers in New England and some other parts of the country, are produced by Rhode Island Red, New Hampshire, and Plymouth Rock hens. The color of the shell—and, for that matter, the color of the yolk—has no bearing on the egg's quality or nutritional value. Duck, goose, or quail eggs are available at some gourmet shops or, locally, direct from the farm.

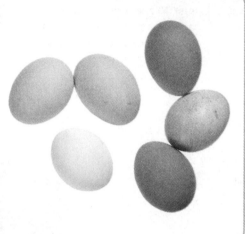

eggs

EGGS / 1 large	
Calories	75
Protein (g)	6
Carbohydrate (g)	1
Dietary fiber (g)	0
Total fat (g)	5
Saturated fat (g)	1.6
Monounsaturated fat (g)	1.9
Polyunsaturated fat (g)	0.7
Cholesterol (mg)	213
Potassium (mg)	61
Sodium (mg)	63

KEY NUTRIENTS (%RDA/AI*)	
Vitamin A	96 mcg (11%)
Riboflavin	0.3 mg (20%)
Vitamin B_{12}	0.5 mcg (21%)
Selenium	15 mcg (28%)

*For more detailed information on RDA and AI, see page 88.

choosing the best

USDA egg grades—AA, A, and B—indicate freshness as well as other aspects of quality. Federal grading is not mandatory, but most eggs sold in the United States are inspected by the USDA, marked with that agency's seal, and assigned a grade. Some packers comply with state standards comparable to the federal grading rules; some states also have their own grading seals. Eggs that do not bear the USDA grade seal must be Grade B or better. Most eggs that are assigned Grade B end up in egg products rather than being sold fresh.

Grading is based on the condition of the inside and outside of the egg, including the cleanliness, soundness, shape, and texture of the shell, the thickness and clarity of the albumen (white), the size and shape of the yolk, the presence of blood spots, and the size of the air cell or pocket (eggs dry as they age, so the fresher the egg, the smaller the air pocket). The interior of the egg is evaluated by one of two methods: candling and breakout. Candling, or rotating the eggs over a high-intensity light, shows the size of the air cell and the condition of the yolk (this process was originally performed with candles, hence its name).

The breakout method is just what it sounds like—breaking a random sample of eggs and evaluating them visually and with special measuring devices. USDA-graded eggs are also required to be washed with a disinfectant and then sprayed with oil to replace the natural protective coating that is washed away.

Almost all the eggs you'll find in the supermarket will be graded AA or A, and the two are very nearly comparable. Eggs are also sorted by size (actually by weight) when they are graded, and packed as Peewee, Small, Medium, Large, Extra Large, or Jumbo. There is a difference in weight of 3 ounces per dozen between each size and the next. Medium eggs are appropriate for

facts & tips

A healthier variety of eggs is available in the market: Eggs enriched with omega-3 fatty acids. The eggs are the same as traditional eggs, except for their enhanced levels of omega-3s, which are polyunsaturated fats that may lower the risk of cardiovascular disease, according to research. To produce omega-3-rich eggs, hens are fed a diet with higher levels of omega-3 fatty acids than traditional feed. (Though these eggs are indeed healthier, they are not intended as an important dietary source of omega-3s; for this, you are better off with a serving of salmon.)

the cholesterol issue

In the years since cholesterol became a widespread concern, research has shown that saturated fat has a greater effect on blood cholesterol levels than dietary cholesterol does—and eggs are not a major source of saturated fat. A whole large egg contains about 5 grams of total fat (31 percent of that is saturated fat). By comparison, 3 tablespoons of grated Cheddar cheese has 7 grams of fat, with close to 64 percent of that saturated.

Another point in favor of the egg: Differences in the way cholesterol is measured have resulted in an updated and lower cholesterol content for eggs. A study performed by the Egg Nutrition Board (whose values were accepted by the USDA) found that a large egg contains between 213 and 220 milligrams of cholesterol—nearly 25 percent less than the formerly accepted figure of 275 milligrams.

In response to these findings, the American Heart Association has raised acceptable egg intake for healthy people from three whole eggs (or egg yolks) a week to one egg per day—provided that the total amount of dietary cholesterol for that day still stays under the recommended 300 milligram maximum. People who have elevated cholesterol still need to limit themselves to one whole egg (or egg yolk) per week.

many cooking uses, but baking recipes, which tend to be more specific in their requirements, often call for large eggs.

Grading tells you a lot about the eggs you buy. Still, the way the eggs are handled after they leave the packing plant can determine their condition when you take them home. Refrigeration is vitally important to freshness: Eggs age as much in one day at room temperature as they do in one week of refrigerated storage. Therefore, buy eggs only at stores that keep them in chilled cases. Look for a date or freshness code on the carton. All USDA-inspected eggs are required to carry a three-digit number that indicates what day of the year they were packed (i.e., January 1 is 001; December 31 is 365). Look for the highest-numbered carton you can find. If kept refrigerated, the eggs should be good for 4 to 5 weeks from the packing date. In some states and localities, egg cartons must be marked with expiration dates after which they should not be sold.

When eggs are sold at a farm or at a nearby outlet, they may be displayed in "flats," or cardboard trays. It's best to be sure of their source when buying eggs locally; they may not be graded or dated, so the seller's reputation is your only assurance of quality. And the eggs should always be kept under refrigeration if that farm-fresh quality is to be preserved.

Check eggs carefully before purchasing, looking for cracks, breaks, or excessive dirt. Gently jiggle each egg to make sure the egg is not cracked at the bottom and stuck to the carton. Get them home and into the refrigerator quickly.

▶ When you get home Store eggs in their original carton in the coldest part of the refrigerator. (The molded rack in the refrigerator door is *not* a good place to store eggs; they're exposed to warm air every time the refriger-ator is opened.) The carton also protects the eggs from aromas of strong-fla-vored foods in the refrigerator; eggs can absorb odors right through their porous shells. Large-end-up—the way the eggs come in the carton—is the best way to keep them: The yolk remains centered in the white, away from the air pocket at the large end of the egg.

Although fresh eggs will keep for 4 to 5 weeks, their quality declines with time; the whites become thinner and the yolks flatter. For best flavor and appearance, use eggs that are less than one week old for frying or poaching; reserve older eggs for hard-cooking, scrambling, and baking.

Hard-cooked eggs can be refrigerated for up to 1 week. Since the cooking washes the protective coating from the shells, it's best to store the cooked eggs in a carton or covered container. Mark unshelled hard-cooked eggs with a penciled "X" to distinguish them from fresh eggs. (If you forget which is which, place the eggs on their sides and spin them. A hard-cooked egg, with its yolk immobilized in the center, will spin smoothly and easily, while a raw egg will wobble.) You can also peel hard-cooked eggs and place them in a bowl with cold water to cover them.

preparing to use

In cooking, the two parts of the egg perform different functions. The yolk acts as a fat and, to some degree, as a protein, enriching, thickening, and emulsifying mixtures; it also adds color and flavor. Egg whites take in air when beaten, trapping air bubbles. The protein coagulates when heated, creating the structure that causes a cake to rise while baking. Egg white serves as a binder and as a thickener as well.

Separating eggs Practiced cooks break eggs by rapping them sharply downward on the edge of a bowl and then using the pieces of shell to hold the yolk as the whites are allowed to flow into a bowl beneath. However, current safety issues suggest that you can reduce the risk of salmonella contamination—from any bacteria that might be on the shell—by using an egg separator instead. Using an egg separator is also easier for the novice cook.

Beating egg whites Whites will beat to a fuller volume if eggs are brought to room temperature first. To do this quickly, place them in a bowl of warm water for a few minutes. Beat the eggs just before you need them, not in advance. The other ingredients, the baking pans, and the oven should be ready. Use a large, deep bowl, and be sure it's free of grease. Begin beating with a whisk, an egg beater, or an electric mixer at slow speed; once the eggs are foamy, gradually increase the speed and beat until the whites are firm but not dry. When you lift the mixer out of the eggs, it should pull the whites into glossy peaks that neither fold over nor break; when you tilt the bowl, the whites should not slide. (If the recipe directs you to beat the eggs to soft, not stiff, peaks, the tips of the peaks should curl over as you lift the beater from the bowl.) Where a recipe calls for adding sugar to the egg whites, add it very gradually, just about a tablespoonful at a time, or it may decrease the volume of the beaten whites.

Either lemon juice or cream of tartar—both acidic ingredients—may be added when beating egg whites. They help to stabilize the beaten whites so they do not deflate so readily. Either ingredient will slow the aeration of the egg whites, so do not add lemon juice or cream of tartar until the whites have been beaten to the foamy stage.

serving suggestions

Frittatas and omelets make it possible to use a minimum number of eggs—especially if you omit some of the egg yolks and increase the number of whites used. You can also add healthful, nutrient-rich ingredients. Try some of these suggested fillings:

· Diced cooked sweet potatoes, minced scallions, diced plum tomatoes.

· Shiitake mushrooms sautéed with rosemary, black pepper, and a bit of olive oil.

· Black beans, crumbled turkey bacon, toasted cumin, diced carrots.

· Chopped fresh fennel, cubed boiled potato, sun-dried tomatoes, diced green beans.

· Chick-peas, diced preserved lemon, sautéed red onion, shredded chicken.

· Part-skim mozzarella, steamed broccoli, raisins, hot pepper flakes.

endive & chicory

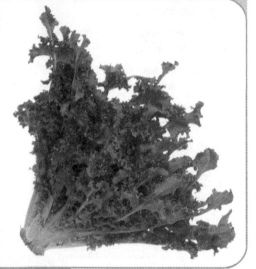

Both endive and chicory belong to a large group of plants of the genus *Chicorium*. There are two main branches to the genus—*C. endivia* and *C. intybus*. On the endivia side—the true endives—are escarole, curly endive, and frisée. On the other side are Belgian endive and radicchio. However, in the marketplace, the term chicory gets applied to endives and vice versa. In spite of this confusion, these plants are all chicories.

nutritional profile

An abundance of vitamins and minerals are found in the green chicories (but not in the pale, blanched Belgian endive). They are an admirable source of beta carotene, riboflavin, vitamin C, vitamin E, folate, and potassium. And they also provide calcium, iron, and magnesium. In addition, chicory contains nondigestible complex carbohydrates called fructo-oligosaccharides (FOS), which may promote the growth of healthy bacteria, also known as "friendly flora," in the colon.

in the market

Belgian endive (witloof endive, French endive) Belgian endive are the shoots of the witloof chicory plant. There is a curious process involved in growing these pale, bittersweet vegetables. It begins in the field, where the seeds are sown and the plants are allowed to put down roots and actually grow a chicory plant. The tops of the plants are mowed off to a point that does not kill the plant but allows the roots to continue growing. The roots are then dug up and moved to cold frames where the plants are forced to grow tight, compact heads called *chicons*. When ready to harvest, the *chicon*, which is the Belgian endive that will arrive in the marketplace, is cut from the top of the chicory root by hand. There are both *white Belgian endive* and *red Belgian endive*. Both are bullet-shaped, but the white has white flesh and very pale yellow tips; the red has the same white flesh with bright red-purple tips (the color of radicchio). Because the cultivation of Belgian endive is labor-intensive, it is usually quite expensive.

Chicory Though this is the overall name for the group of plants that includes endives, the green sold as chicory comes from the *C. intybus* side of the family. It comes in a loose head of curly-edged, bitter-tasting greens. It looks a lot like curly endive, but its leaves are more uniformly green and broader. It also tends to be more bitter.

CHICORY / 1 cup chopped	
Calories	41
Protein (g)	3
Carbohydrate (g)	8
Dietary fiber (g)	7.2
Total fat (g)	0.5
Saturated fat (g)	0.1
Monounsaturated fat (g)	0
Polyunsaturated fat (g)	0.2
Cholesterol (mg)	0
Potassium (mg)	756
Sodium (mg)	81

KEY NUTRIENTS (%RDA/AI*)	
Beta carotene	4.3 mg (39%)
Riboflavin	0.2 mg (14%)
Vitamin C	43 mg (48%)
Vitamin E	4.1 mg (27%)
Folate	198 mcg (50%)
Calcium	180 mg (15%)
Iron	1.6 mg (13%)
Magnesium	54 mg (13%)

For more detailed information on RDA and AI, see page 88.

Curly endive Curly endive, a true endive, comes in a loose-headed bunch with ragged edges. The heart of the curly endive is yellow while the outer leaves are green. When added to a salad, its bitter flavor works well as a counterpoint to other, sweeter salad greens.

Escarole (Batavian endive) This member of the chicory family comes from the endive side. It grows in loose, elongated heads and has broad, wavy leaves with smooth edges. The flavor is slightly bitter, but milder than chicory—though the inner leaves, as with chicory, do not have as sharp a bite as the outer leaves. Escarole can be torn and added to a salad or cooked like a cooking green.

Frisée This is another name for curly endive (the word *frisée* means curly in French), but by tradition it is usually sold (and used) in its young, tender form. The leaves are small, very delicately frilly, and light green to yellow-white.

Radicchio See Radicchio (*page 499*).

choosing the best

For the leafy heads (such as chicory, curly endive, and escarole), look for crisp green leaves without any bruises. Belgian endive, delicate and light-sensitive, is usually displayed in boxes, wrapped in dark-colored paper. If the heads at the top of the box have emerged from the wrappings, don't purchase them. Exposure to light causes the vegetable to discolor and turn bitter. Reach deep into the box and choose small, pale heads for the sweetest flavor. The layers of paper also encourage shoppers to handle the endive with care—as it bruises easily. Avoid any heads with brown spots, this indicates bruising.

preparing to use

Belgian endive requires no advance preparation; simply separate the leaves or slice the whole head. Chicory, curly endive, escarole, and frisée should be well-washed before using.

BELGIAN ENDIVE 1 cup sliced	
Calories	15
Protein (g)	1
Carbohydrate (g)	4
Dietary fiber (g)	2.8
Total fat (g)	0.1
Saturated fat (g)	0
Monounsaturated fat (g)	0
Polyunsaturated fat (g)	0
Cholesterol (mg)	0
Potassium (mg)	190
Sodium (mg)	2

serving suggestions

- Spoon a low-fat cheese spread into whole Belgian endive leaves and serve for an appetizer.

- Add torn pieces of escarole, curly endive, chicory, or frisée to vegetable soups.

- Steam escarole and chicory and dress with a warm vinaigrette.

- Make a frisée salad with cooked turkey bacon, crisp croutons, and a warm vinaigrette.

- Stir steamed chopped greens into rice or mashed potatoes.

- Stuff chicken breasts with cooked escarole.

- Combine sliced Belgian endive with sliced apples and dress as you would a coleslaw.

- Stir chopped greens into a low-fat ricotta filling for manicotti or ravioli.

exotic fruits

Interest in unusual fruits—especially from tropical countries—has been steadily rising for the past decade or so. Though not necessarily more nutritious than standbys like apples or peaches, these uncommon fruits can add variety and interest to your diet. The following guide sorts out some of the myriad possibilities available. Some of them are new to the marketplace and some have been around for a while, but most of them tend to be difficult to find. Browsing fruit stands in ethnic neighborhoods may help turn up some of these unusual offerings. Be sure to check out other entries in this book for fruits that have become more commonplace in American markets, such as Mangoes (*page 388*) and Papaya (*page 438*). See also Melons (*page 390*).

Because the following exotic fruits are uncommon, information about their nutritional make-up is in many instances either incomplete or lacking. Therefore, no nutritional profiles or charts accompany these entries; rather, information on any key nutrients is summarized in the text. (Unless noted otherwise, nutritional information is for the food in its raw state.)

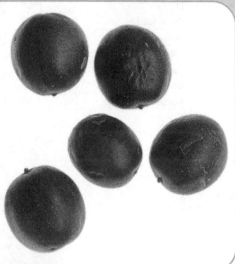

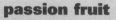
passion fruit

in the market

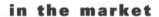

This country's strict laws governing the import of fresh fruits and vegetables has meant that some of the fruits grown in tropical countries (where the pest-control standards don't measure up) may never make it to our shores. However, many of these tropical fruits are available in dried and canned form and are worth seeking out. In addition, some tropical fruits are now being cultivated in Hawaii and may soon make it onto the mainland.

Ackee A bright red fruit, ackee bursts open at the bottom when it's ripe, exposing its pale yellow pulp and several large glossy black seeds. One of two fruits—the other being breadfruit—made famous by the infamous Captain Bligh, ackee was imported to Jamaica from West Africa in the 18th century. It has since been adopted by the Jamaicans as their national fruit. The edible portion of ackee looks and tastes like scrambled eggs, and in Jamaica it is traditionally cooked with salt cod. It is difficult to find fresh ackee—it was illegal in this country until only a few years ago—but the canned form is available in Caribbean markets. One of the main reasons that most ackee is canned is that underripe or improperly processed ackee can cause vomiting (and in extreme cases, death).

Canned ackee has a respectable amount of vitamin C (about 38 percent of the RDA), plus dietary fiber and some folate.

Atemoya This delicious dessert fruit is the result of a cross between a cherimoya and a sweetsop, or sugar apple. From the outside, an atemoya looks something like an artichoke carved from clay; inside, it has cream-colored flesh with the flavor and texture of a vanilla or fruit custard. Grown in this country, atemoyas are also imported from South America and the West Indies. Look for a pale-green fruit that is slightly tender to finger pressure but that has not cracked open (which the fruit often does as it ripens). Keep the atemoya at room temperature for a day or two if it is not already softened and ready to eat when you bring it home. Once it is ripe, you can refrigerate the fruit for a day or two; it tastes best chilled. To serve, cut the atemoya in half through the stem end and scoop out the flesh with a spoon. Or, use cubed atemoya in a fruit salad.

Atemoyas have decent amounts of fiber, riboflavin, and vitamin C.

Breadfruit The size of a large melon, weighing 2 to 5 pounds, breadfruit (as its name implies) is a starchy, somewhat bland food that is notable for its high carbohydrate content, which is comparable to many vegetables: A 4-ounce portion (about one-fourth of the edible part of a small fruit) contains 31 grams of carbohydrate, which account for close to 100 percent of the calories. The fruit is also a good source of vitamin C, thiamin, and potassium.

Breadfruit has been an important staple for many years in the Pacific islands and the Caribbean. (The infamous Captain Bligh of the *H.M.S. Bounty* was en route to Tahiti to get breadfruit trees for the English colonies of St. Vincent and Jamaica when his crew mutinied.) Though it is a tree fruit covered with a scaly green rind, the starchy consistency of its pale-yellow flesh has made it better-suited for eating as a vegetable. The flesh resembles that of a potato when unripe, and can be used like a potato at this stage. As breadfruit ripens slightly, it softens, and is creamier and stickier (but still starchy) when cooked. After further ripening, breadfruit turns very soft, but its sweetness never matches that of the mango and papaya.

Imported from the Caribbean, breadfruit can be found in grocery stores in West Indian and Caribbean neighborhoods. Choose a hard, firm, evenly colored specimen. If you want the fruit to reach the soft, creamy stage, ripen it at room temperature until it gives to the touch. You can then refrigerate it for a day (but no longer) if not using it immediately. Breadfruit, like potatoes, can be baked in its skin, or it can be peeled, cut up, and boiled. Ripe breadfruit can be made into a sweetened, baked pudding.

Buddha's hand Also known as fingered citron, this citrus fruit grows in a cluster of fingerlike sections and looks vaguely like a human hand. Like other citrons, this fruit is not used for its pulp or juice (which it has none of), but for its fragrant yellow rind. The rind is used to flavor liquors and liqueurs, and is also candied.

Cactus pear (Indian pear, prickly pear, sabra) The prickly pear cactus grows in many parts of the world, and its large egg-shaped berry—a pinkish- or yellowish-brown fruit covered with spines—is popular in Mexico and the American Southwest, all over the Mediterranean, in South Africa, and in Israel (whose natives are nicknamed "sabras" for their supposed resemblance to cactus fruit: prickly on the outside and sweet on the inside).

cactus pear

You can eat the melony-flavored fruit by itself, or use it in fruit salads or drinks. Choose cactus pears that are soft but not mushy; let them ripen at room temperature for a few days if they are firm when you buy them, then refrigerate. To eat the juicy flesh, which is full of seeds (edible in some types, too hard to chew in others), you have to get past the prickly skin. Wear thick rubber gloves, use tongs, or hold the fruit impaled on a fork to protect yourself, then cut off the ends of the fruit, slit it lengthwise in several places, and peel the skin off.

The cactus pear has dietary fiber, vitamin C, and a respectable amount of magnesium.

Canistel (egg fruit, yellow sapote) One of several fruits called sapote, the canistel is a yellow, smooth-skinned fruit whose shape varies from egg-shaped to peach-shaped to persimmon-shaped. The flesh is yellow-orange and has been described by some as having the consistency of a hard-boiled egg yolk. The flavor, similar to other sapotes, has a richness that suggests custard: In this case it tastes like a sweet potato custard. Grown primarily in the tropics, there are local crops of canistel available in Florida, the only state to successfully grow the fruit.

cherimoya

Cherimoya Sometimes called a custard apple or sherbet fruit, the cherimoya looks like an oversized green pinecone. It is grown in South and Central America and the Caribbean, and recently has been cultivated in California and Florida. The cherimoya is a wonderful dessert fruit, with sweet, juicy, custardlike flesh whose flavor echoes that of other fruits: Depending on the variety, it may have hints of pineapple, papaya, banana, mango, or strawberry. Select fruits of any size with uniform yellow-green color, and let them ripen at room temperature until just softened (like a ripe peach) but not mushy, then chill and serve cold. The easiest way to eat this seed-filled fruit is to spoon it from the shell.

The fruit is a good source of fiber, riboflavin, and vitamin C.

Durian This fruit has to be the single most challenging tropical fruit: It has such a pungent odor that it has been likened to extremely dirty feet. In Southeast Asia, where the fruit grows, signs in hotel rooms strictly forbid guests from opening a durian in their room. The durian is quite large—it can reach the size of a basketball—and is covered with sharp spikes. The interior contains soft and sweet yellow flesh. If you can get past its overwhelming odor, the taste of the fruit is extremely complex, ranging from grapefruit to Parmesan to banana—the flavors are not blended, but present themselves in a succession of tastes. Some have even suggested that there's an onion flavor, as well. While fresh durian is sometimes available in local Chinatowns, it's more likely to be canned or frozen.

In spite of its stinky reputation, durian is an exceptional source of B vitamins, most notably thiamin. It also has good amounts of vitamin C, fiber, and potassium.

Feijoa This egg-shaped, egg-sized green fruit (it resembles a fuzzless kiwifruit), native to South America, is grown today in New Zealand and California. Its dense, pale yellow flesh has a slightly gritty texture like that of a Bosc pear, with a tart flavor and a strong fragrance. A ripe feijoa should feel like a ripe pear. Also known as pineapple guava, feijoa is frequently mislabeled in produce markets as common guava. Feijoa can be halved and eaten with a spoon, used in fresh fruit salads, or cooked in compotes. The edible skin may be bitter; if so, peel the fruit before serving. And, like pear, the fruit will discolor when cut and exposed to the air. So rub with lemon juice or submerge in a bowl of water with lemon juice mixed in.

Guava A tropical fruit believed to have originated in Central America, the guava plant was domesticated more than 2,000 years ago. It thrives in a variety of soils, propagates easily, and bears fruit relatively quickly. Considered the "apple of the tropics," guava is common throughout most tropical regions, where it enriches the diet of millions of people.

The average guava is 2 to 4 inches in diameter with knobby skin that can vary from yellow to yellowish-red to deep purple. The flesh may be pale yellow (almost white in appearance) or soft salmon to bright red, and the flavor ranges from sweet to sour. While guava is grown throughout the world, it is often plagued by fruit-fly infestations, which cuts down on the amount of guava imported to this country. Domestic crops are grown in Hawaii, California, and Florida. Though there are numerous varieties of guava grown in tropical regions worldwide, the following are available in the United States: *Blitch* (tart-flavored with light pink flesh and numerous seeds), *Red Indian* (red-fleshed with numerous seeds), *Ruby* (sweet, red-fleshed, with few seeds), *Strawberry* (small purple fruit whose flavor is reminiscent of the strawberry), and *Supreme* (white-fleshed, with few seeds). Though fresh guavas can be hard to find, many supermarkets and any Hispanic market sells cans of guava paste, which is a cooked down puree of guava.

Guava is an excellent source of vitamin C: Just a single guava (about 4 ounces) provides more than twice the RDA. Guava also contains a variety of carotenoids, most notably lycopene.

Jackfruit This huge fruit is a relative of the breadfruit and is considered the largest fruit in the world (it can weigh up to 80 pounds). Shaped like a rugby football, and covered with small bumps and spines, it has blandly sweet, banana-flavored, yellow flesh. The unripe flesh, which is starchier, is treated more like a vegetable than a fruit. A ripe jackfruit will have a yellow-brown skin and the fruit will have a slight give; unfortunately, the ripe fruit also smells like decayed onions. However, cooks in this country are unlikely to encounter a fresh jackfruit; it is more commonly sold dried or in cans in markets that specialize in Indian or Southeast Asian products.

Kumquats Diminutive citrus fruits that can be eaten skin and all, kumquats are as decorative as they are tasty. The egg-shaped orange fruits are about 1½ inches long and often come with their shiny dark-green leaves

serving suggestions

Cut ripe jackfruit (or canned jackfruit) into cubes and toss with an equal amount of cubed banana. Sprinkle with ground cardamom and some brown sugar, and toss with plain yogurt and chopped cilantro. Serve as a refreshing side dish alongside curried dishes.

attached. Kumquats are in best supply in the winter and may be found in supermarkets as well as Asian grocery stores and gourmet markets.

Choose plump, shiny, fully orange fruits; be sure to wash them before serving, since the skin as well as the pulp is eaten. To mingle the flavors of the sweet rind and tart flesh, squeeze the kumquats between your fingers before biting into the fruit. Add kumquat slices to fruit salad and use the whole or sliced fruit as an edible garnish. You can also use kumquats in cooked dishes that call for oranges.

Kumquats are an excellent source of vitamin C: Just a 4-ounce serving (about 5 kumquats) supplies 47 percent of the RDA in only 71 calories.

Longan These grape- to plum-sized Asian fruits, which are related to lychees, are sometimes called "dragons' eyes," because peeling their thin brown shells reveals a transparent, jellylike fruit with a large, dark seed in its center. Look for fresh longans in Asian markets in late summer; choose heavy fruits with uncracked shells. Longans are most commonly eaten raw (serve them on their stems, like grapes), but they can also be poached. You can also buy dragons' eyes in their dried form in Chinese markets.

Fresh longans are among the richer sources of vitamin C, with 4 ounces supplying over 100 percent of the RDA.

Loquat This golden-skinned tropical fruit resembles an apricot, but its firm, sweet-tart flesh—which can be orange, yellow, or white—tastes something like plums or cherries (in fact when loquats were first introduced to this country from Asia, they were marketed as Japanese plums). Choose large loquats that are tender and fragrant. Stem, peel, and seed them before eating out of hand or cooking.

Like other yellow-orange fruits, loquats are a good source of beta carotene.

Lychee Related to longans, lychees sometimes appear on the dessert menu at Chinese restaurants. Once stripped of their nubbly, reddish-brown shells, these fruits look like large white grapes, each with a single large, glossy seed within its pale flesh. They have a sweet, flowery fragrance and flavor. Fresh lychees can be found in Asian markets in the summer months. Select heavy, uncracked fruits with the stems still attached; the redder the shells, the fresher the lychees. Unpeeled, the fruit can be stored for up to 3 weeks in the refrigerator. Serve whole lychees one at a time (they need to be peeled), or peel several and sprinkle with a little lime or lemon juice to heighten the flavor. They can also be cut up and combined with berries or other soft fruit, or poached. Canned and dried lychees (the latter has a raisinlike texture) are also sold in Asian grocery stores.

Lychees are rich in vitamin C: Just 4 ounces (about 10 fruits) supply almost 100 percent of the RDA.

Mangosteen This clementine-sized, red-skinned fruit has seeded segments much like a tangerine, but the flesh is bright white to light pink. The flavor is deep and fruity, and is said to resemble a combination of grapes and strawberries. Though it is grown in Hawaii, the fresh fruits are consumed locally, and imports from other parts of the world are severely restricted.

Monstera The familiar houseplant called split-leaf philodendron is the source of this unusual fruit. It grows like an elongated pinecone; when ripe, the hexagonal plates on its surface split apart, exposing a creamy, tart-sweet fruit that looks something like a banana, with a pineapple-banana flavor. Monstera, called *ceriman* in Spanish-speaking countries, grows in Florida and California and is sometimes sold in gourmet produce markets in northern U.S. cities. If you buy it, let it ripen at room temperature; do not eat it until it is fully ripe (when the surface scales fall off), or it will irritate the mouth and throat.

Passion fruit An egg-shaped tropical fruit that is also called a purple granadilla, the passion fruit has a brittle, wrinkled, purple-brown rind enclosing flesh-covered seeds, something like those of a pomegranate (*granadilla* means "little pomegranate" in Spanish). The seeds are edible, so you can eat the orange pulp straight from the shell, but passion fruit is more commonly sieved and its highly aromatic pulp or juice used as a flavoring for beverages and sauces. Native to Brazil, passion fruits are now grown in Hawaii, Florida, and California; these crops, along with imports from New Zealand, keep passion fruit on the market all year. Choose large, heavy specimens. If the skin is not deeply wrinkled, keep the fruit at room temperature until it does wrinkle; the leathery rind, however, will not soften much. Ripe passion fruit can be refrigerated for a few days.

Passion fruit has about 110 calories per 4-ounce serving, but supplies 38 percent of the RDA for vitamin C. It is also a good source of riboflavin, niacin, iron, and potassium. And if eaten with the seeds, it is an excellent source of dietary fiber.

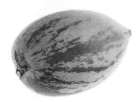

pepino

Pepino Its melonlike flavor could fool you about the pepino's place in the plant kingdom: It is a member of the nightshade family, like peppers and tomatoes. The heart-shaped golden fruit is marked with purple stripes or patches. Pepinos, which range from plum-sized to cantaloupe-sized, have fragrant yellow flesh surrounding a central pocket of seeds, like a melon. Choose aromatic fruits (the size does not affect the flavor) that give to gentle finger pressure. Avoid those with greenish undertones; ripen the fruit at room temperature for a few days, if necessary, until it is fully golden-yellow. Serve pepino like melon, with a squeeze of lemon or lime, or use it in fruit salads. There are also *purple pepinos,* which are shaped like regular pepinos, but are more slender. The golden flesh tastes similar to regular pepinos, with the sweet taste underscored by a hint of cucumber.

Pitaya (apple cactus) This South American cactus fruit has a grainy, white flesh. Not currently available fresh in this country, it is available canned or jarred in specialty food markets.

Pomelo (pummelo) An ancestor of today's grapefruit, the pomelo is a citrus fruit that looks like a super-sized grapefruit with a narrower end. It

serving suggestions

Use mashed white sapote in a banana bread recipe. Scoop the ripe flesh out of the sapote skin and measure out the same amount of sapote as the mashed bananas called for in the recipe.

originated in Southeast Asia and today is grown in California. Pomelos have yellow or greenish-yellow skin, with fibrous flesh separated into segments by membranes. Their flavor may range from very tart to very sweet. Look for pomelos in gourmet produce shops and Asian markets from late fall through mid-winter; select heavy, fragrant fruits and store them in the refrigerator. The segments inside a pomelo can be a bit difficult to get to. The rind surrounding the flesh is extremely thick; you have to cut off some of it and then remove the rest of it before you even get to the fruit inside. Then, you have to pull off the membranes that surround the segments, because unlike grapefruit, the membranes are tough and inedible. The pulp is also quite thick-skinned compared to a grapefruit. But don't be misled by this: The "flavor cells" are very juicy. Although you can use the pomelo segments the way you would grapefruit, the fruit is most often eaten out of hand. Maybe this is because it is quite a labor-intensive fruit to prepare for cooking.

Like all citrus fruits, pomelos are an excellent vitamin C source, providing more than 75 percent of the RDA in 4 ounces (about ½ cup of sections).

Rambutan The rambutan, another tropical fruit that is rarely found fresh in this country (though it's grown in Hawaii), looks more like a sea anemone than a fruit. Similar to a lychee or a longan, this grape-sized fruit is covered with hairlike tentacles. Inside it has a sweet, milky-white, grapelike flesh that surrounds a single, large black seed.

Sapodilla Native to the lower Americas, this small fruit (2 to 4 inches in diameter) has a rough brown skin and yellow to brownish flesh. Its texture is like a very ripe pear and its flavor has been described as being a mixture of brown sugar and root beer. The sapodilla tree can grow to over 100 feet, and its principal commercial use is as a source of chicle: This gummy latex substance, found in the tree's bark, is used as a component of chewing gum.

Sapote Several quite different fruits have come to be called sapote or sapota. The *white sapote*, common in tropical markets, is a nearly seedless, orange-sized fruit with a green to yellow skin and mild, creamy-textured white flesh. It has been grown in California since the 19th century and also grows in Florida, but it is still relatively scarce in northern U.S. markets. *Mamey sapote* are about the size of a large sweet potato (which they vaguely resemble), with pink-orange flesh and hints of berry flavor. The *black sapote*, grown in Florida, looks like a green persimmon (not surprising because it is a relative of this fruit). It is also called chocolate pudding fruit, because its flesh is chocolatey-brown and it tastes a bit like chocolate, but only when perfectly ripe (unripe black sapotes can be bitter). Choose firm sapotes to ripen at room temperature for a few days; refrigerate them once they are soft. Some sapotes can be eaten out of hand, but others are best peeled and seeded.

Soursop (guanabana) A relative of the atemoya (*see page 284*), these tart, juicy fruits are heart-shaped with a rough green skin that has soft fleshy spines. Though it's rare to find fresh soursop, you can reliably find cans of guanabana juice in Hispanic markets.

Starfruit (carambola) A ready-made garnish, the golden-yellow starfruit, when sliced crosswise, yields perfect five-pointed, star-shaped sections—hence its name. Its sweet-tart flavor is like a blend of several fruits—plums, pineapple, grapes, and lemons. This elliptical, deeply ribbed fruit, 2 to 5 inches long, originated in Southeast Asia but is now grown in Florida. Look for shiny, well-shaped fruit. The skin on unripe fruit is green, but ripening at room temperature will turn it a deep, glowing gold and the fruit will develop a fragrant aroma. Slice the unpeeled fruit and remove the seeds; use the slices as a garnish for salads, poultry, desserts, or beverages. Starfruit slices can also be sautéed and served as a condiment or dessert topping.

Starfruit is an excellent source of vitamin C, supplying 27 percent of the RDA in 1 cup sliced.

Tamarillo This subtropical "tree tomato" is, in fact, related to the tomato (as well as to the potato and eggplant). It looks like an elongated plum, with skin colors ranging from purplish-red or crimson to orange; its dark orange flesh has a plumlike texture but an acidic, somewhat astringent flavor. It tastes vaguely like a tomato. There is also a *golden tamarillo,* with yellow skin, which tends to be a bit sweeter. Tamarillos grown in California are available in late fall and winter; in other months, you can find imports from New Zealand. Look for well-colored fruit that gives just slightly to finger pressure; ripen at room temperature, if necessary. Tamarillos are best cooked before using. They can be sweetened and used as a dessert, or used unsweetened and cooked (like tomatoes) with savory foods and seasonings. Either way, they must be peeled. Immerse them in boiling water for 3 to 5 minutes, as you would peaches, to loosen the skins.

Tamarind Also known as tamarindos or Indian dates, the tamarind fruit is actually a thick, sticky pulp (with a consistency similar to dried fruit) that surrounds seeds inside a hard, brittle seed pod. The pulp is both tart and sweet, like a sour apricot. You can eat the pulp straight out of the pod, which you can occasionally find whole in Hispanic markets (and some Indian markets). However, the process of getting the pulp out of tamarind pods is a bit labor-intensive, so most people who cook with it (it makes wonderful sweet-tart drinks and sauces) buy bricks of tamarind pulp. There are also numerous tamarind purees and concentrates available in jars.

ugli fruit

Ugli fruit This poor citrus fruit—bred by crossing a grapefruit with an orange or tangerine—is indeed ugly. The grapefruit-sized fruit has a puffy, saggy skin that looks like it's several sizes too big, but the pinkish-orange flesh is sweeter than grapefruit and nearly seedless. Ugli fruit originated in Jamaica (where it's called HOO-gli), and is now grown in Florida. There has been a marketing push to rename it Uniq fruit, but it hasn't stuck. Choose heavy fruit that gives slightly to finger pressure. Use ugli fruit as you would grapefruit or oranges.

exotic vegetables

Restaurant chefs and farmers' markets have had a profound impact on the American cook's interest in trying something new. In addition to the multitude of domestic heirloom vegetables, our marketplaces have also begun swelling with exotic imports from around the world.

Some of these exotic vegetables are available only in ethnic neighborhoods, but many of them have migrated to supermarkets across the nation. The following list is only a small sampling of the vegetables that are out there. There is also a good collection of exotics in Cabbage (*page 210*) and Roots & Tubers (*page 512*). See also "Chinese Squash" (*page 547*).

Because these vegetables are uncommon, information about their nutritional make-up is in many instances either incomplete or lacking. Therefore, no nutritional profiles or charts accompany these entries; rather, information on any key nutrients is summarized in the text.

in the market

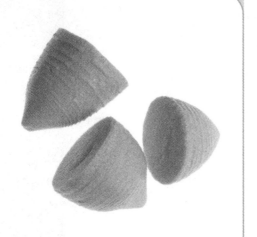

bamboo shoots

Bamboo shoots You've probably eaten crisp strips of bamboo shoots in Chinese dishes. They are literally the shoots—the young, sprouting stems—of a bamboo plant, which is a type of grass, not a tree. Sometimes the shoots are cut when they first appear, but they may also be "hilled"—piled with soil as they grow, which prevents the development of the green pigment chlorophyll so the shoots remain pale. In supermarkets, you can usually find only canned bamboo shoots, which have been peeled and cut into strips. However, Chinese grocery stores often carry the fresh, whole shoots, which are cone-shaped and about 4 inches long. Canned bamboo shoots, after rinsing, can be added directly to stir-fries; they are precooked and need only to be heated through. Fresh bamboo shoots should be boiled until tender, then husked and cut up; they can be stir-fried or served as you would asparagus.

Cardoon Plants of the thistle family produce the familiar globe artichoke and also the celerylike cardoon. When the thick, silvery stalks are cooked, their flavor is reminiscent of artichokes, but they can also be eaten raw, like fennel or celery. Cardoons have long been popular in Italy, and can often be found in Italian markets in the United States in the winter and early spring. Look for slender, supple but firm stalks that are velvety-gray, not

cardoon

moist-looking and green like celery. Trim the bases and tops of the stalks, then cut them into strips to serve raw or into short pieces or squares for cooking. Cut the base into large chunks. Serve raw cardoon with other crudités for dipping; dress the cooked vegetable with lemon juice or a vinaigrette, and serve it hot or cold.

Like celery, cardoon is very low in calories—only 32 in 1 cup. For a vegetable, it is rather high in sodium—1 cup contains over 250 milligrams. It also supplies fair amounts of folate and magnesium.

Chinese broccoli See Broccoli (*page 203*).

Chinese celery See Celery (*page 221*).

Chrysanthemum leaves Called *tung ho* in Chinese and *shungiku* in Japanese, these Asian greens are used fresh in salads (when the leaves are young) and in stir-fries and soups. They have a spinachlike texture and earthy-floral flavor. The leaves are usually blanched to make them more tender and they are generally added to dishes at the last minute, as overcooking will make them bitter.

Fiddleheads A spring delicacy, fiddleheads are the young fronds of certain types of ferns. Although the word "fiddlehead" could refer to any fern shoots, only one variety, the ostrich fern, is considered edible. These tightly curled green shoots are picked before their leaves unfurl; gathered from the wild, they are rare and expensive. Once available only in the areas where they grew (Maine is noted for its fiddleheads), the highly perishable greens are now flown in to city markets during their short season. Choose small, bright green, tightly coiled fiddleheads; they should still have their brown scales. Use them within a day or two of purchase. Rub off the brown scales, then wash the greens and blanch or steam them as you would asparagus.

Fiddleheads are a quite decent source of beta carotene: 4 ounces (about 1 cup) have 2.5 milligrams (23 percent of the recommended daily intake).

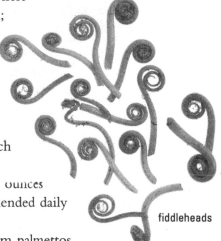

fiddleheads

Hearts of palm This delicate white vegetable comes from palmettos, small palm trees that grow in Florida (there are also some South American palm species). Harvesting the heart, or terminal bud, often kills the plant, so it is an expensive food; for the same reason, some conservationists object to its use. The entire palm heart, weighing 2 to 3 pounds, is sometimes sold fresh in the United States. If you can find fresh palm heart, it will be husked and cut into cylinders; the layered, ivory-white flesh is firm-crisp and has the consistency of slightly soft coconut. However, you are much more likely to find canned hearts of palm, which are available in supermarkets. You can use either fresh or canned hearts of palm as is, without cooking. They are delicious cut into thin slices and tossed into a salad.

Lotus root Once you've seen slices of lotus root in a dish, there's no mistaking it for anything else. The large, sausage-shaped rhizome of an aquatic

serving suggestions

Make an Asian chopped salad: Toss together slivered hearts of palm, diced water chestnuts, and shredded napa cabbage. Make a salad dressing with olive oil, Chinese black vinegar (or balsamic vinegar), and grated fresh ginger.

plant (a relative of the common water lily), lotus root is pierced with 10 air tunnels so that when cut crosswise, the white slices look something like snowflakes—or strangely symmetrical rounds of Swiss cheese. The starchy yet crisp flesh is slightly sweet; it may be sliced or grated to use in salads, stir-fried, or cooked in soups or stews. Thin, lacy slices make a nice garnish. Fresh lotus root needs to be peeled before cooking.

Nopales (cactus pads) The "leaves" of the Mexican prickly pear cactus, nopales are eaten as vegetables. Succulent yet crisp, they exude a sticky substance (as okra does) when cooked. Their delicate flavor resembles that of bell peppers or asparagus. Look for nopales in Mexican grocery stores and specialty produce markets; choose small, bright-green pads that are resilient, not limp or dry. They will likely be de-spined (or of a spineless variety), but you will still need to trim the "eyes" just in case there are any tiny prickers remaining. A vegetable peeler works well for this. Trim the outside edges of the pads as well. Steaming is one of the best ways to cook cactus pads; they can then be served with lemon juice as a vegetable side dish, or cooled and used in salads. You can also find canned nopales.

Nopales are a good source of vitamin C (1 cup cooked provides 16 percent of the RDA), potassium, and magnesium.

Seabeans (sea asparagus, pousse-pierre, glasswort) Seabeans look like delicate green coral, with thin, jointed sprigs that are crisp and quite salty. This sea vegetable has been around for millennia: Ancient Greeks and Romans ate it in salads or steamed as a vegetable. And in Colonial America, it was called chicken's claws. Originally gathered in the wild, seabeans are now being commercially cultivated. The green itself can be eaten as a vegetable (though a salty one) and it has historically been put up as a pickle. Wild seabeans are available in the summer months, but cultivated seabeans are available year round.

Seaweed Consisting of long stems and frondlike leaves, the various types of seaweed, or sea vegetables, are large forms of algae. Fresh seaweed tastes rather like greens with an overlay of seawater flavor. Dried seaweed is commonly sold at Japanese grocery stores and health-food stores. Seaweeds have a naturally salty flavor from their high mineral content and are sometimes crumbled or shredded and used as a seasoning rather than served as a vegetable. (However, a high percentage of the seaweed harvested in this country goes toward creating thickening and stabilizing agents for processed foods.)

Of the dried seaweed, perhaps the type many Americans are most familiar with is *nori,* a dark green seaweed dried in square sheets and used to wrap sushi rolls. Nori is traditionally toasted over a flame or in an ungreased skillet before use. You can also buy nori that is already toasted. Both nori and *laver,* which the Irish (and Welsh) cook into flat cakes called laverbread, are actually the same plant. *Kombu* and *wakame,* popular foods in Japan, are types of kelp,

nopales
(cactus pads)

**serving
suggestions**

Cut steamed nopales into thin slices. Toss with lemon juice and some hot sauce. Place nopales, some crumbled goat cheese or feta, cooked black beans, and shredded lettuce in flour or corn tortillas and roll up.

a brown algae. The Japanese use kombu to make a flavorful broth, while wakame is cooked in soups or stir-fried and served over rice. *Irish moss* is red algae and the source of carrageenan, which is a common commercial thickening agent. The Scots collect a type of seaweed called *dulse* and make soup from it.

Seaweed is high in fiber, and some varieties are rich in vitamin C and beta carotene. But its greatest claim to fame is as a concentrated source of minerals, including potassium, calcium, magnesium, iron, and iodine. However, you have to eat a good-sized serving—not just the tiny amount that's wrapped around sushi—to get any significant benefit. (Some types, such as kombu and wakame, are also high in sodium.)

Tomatillo (husk tomato) Its name means "little tomato" in Spanish, and this small, round vegetable-fruit does look like a large green cherry tomato—but a tomato that's enclosed in a papery light brown husk. Their tart, lemony flavor contributes to Mexican *salsa cruda* and *salsa verde* (a cooked green sauce). Fresh tomatillos can be found in some supermarkets and most Hispanic grocery stores: Select hard specimens (like unripe tomatoes) with clean, dry husks. Husk and wash off the stickiness that is usually found between the husk and the vegetable. Canned tomatillos are common in Hispanic stores, and can be used in many of the same ways as the fresh. In addition to the common green tomatillo, there are now a number of varieties available in farmers' markets, including *pineapple tomatillo* (sweeter than other tomatillos with overtones of pineapple) and *purple tomatillo* (purple-skinned fruit, but with a flavor and flesh color similar to a regular tomatillo).

tomatillos

fats & oils

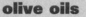

olive oils

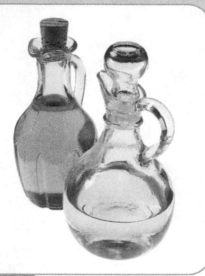

Dietary fats and oils are found in virtually all foods. Butter, suet, and lard are fats from animals, while oils (such as cooking oils and salad oils) are from seeds, nuts, fruits (olives are fruit), and vegetables. Fats and oils belong to a group of substances called lipids, which are biological chemicals that do not dissolve in water. The difference between fats and oils is that, at room temperature, fats are solid while oils are liquid.

The addition of fats and oils to foods enhances their flavor and texture and makes cooking easier. Most people enjoy what's known as the satisfying rich, smooth, creamy "mouth feel" of fats, which is why certain foods like ice cream and chocolate are so appealing.

nutritional profile

Fats and oils are made up of basic units called fatty acids, with each particular type of fat or oil a mixture of saturated and unsaturated fatty acids—terms referring to the degree of saturation by hydrogen atoms (*see "Fats," pages 24–26*). Unsaturated fats are further classified as either monounsaturated or polyunsaturated.

Some fatty acids promote good health while others may actually contribute to diseases. But in a healthful diet, all fats and oils should be used sparingly. In addition to recommending an overall reduction in consumption of fat, health authorities recommend that Americans consume less saturated fat—which is found in the greatest quantity in animal fats as well as tropical oils (coconut, palm kernel, and palm oils).

Foods derived from animals also contain dietary cholesterol, a fatlike substance that is considered harmful to health. Dietary cholesterol is not found in any oils derived from plants, including margarine prepared from plant oils.

The fat composition of fats and oils varies (*see "Comparing Fats & Oils," opposite page*). Animal fats are high in saturated fats, but they have unsaturated fats as well. And all oils contain some saturated fats—ranging from tropical oils at the high end, to olive oil, nut oils, safflower oil, and canola oil at the low end. The oils at this far end of the spectrum are high in unsaturated fats.

Any unsaturated vegetable oil will lower total and LDL ("bad") cholesterol while maintaining—or even slightly raising—levels of HDL ("good") cholesterol. But of the two main types of unsaturated fats—monounsaturates and polyunsaturates—the polyunsaturated fats may be more susceptible to harmful oxidation, which can contribute to heart disease. Health experts agree that substituting foods rich in monounsaturated and polyunsaturated fats for saturated fats helps to decrease harmful LDL cholesterol levels and thus reduce the risk of heart disease.

in the market

grain & seed oils

Many seed oils come in two forms: roasted and cold-pressed. A good example of this is sesame oil, which comes in both a toasty-tasting, dark brown form, as well as a light-colored, almost bland, cold-pressed form. Grain oils, on the other hand, are almost never roasted.

Canola oil (rapeseed oil) This bland-tasting oil has the distinction of being rich in alpha-linolenic acid (ALA), a polyunsaturated fatty acid related to the heart-protective omega-3 fatty acids found in fish. Canola oil is suitable for sautéing, baking, and salad dressings.

Corn oil Made from the endosperm of corn kernels, corn oil is relatively tasteless and odorless and is used in the production of many margarines. It can be used in baking and with its high smoke point (the temperature at which oil begins to smoke and burn), it is also good for sautéing and stir-frying.

COMPARING FATS & OILS

The fat in each type of fat or oil is made up (primarily) of three types of fatty acids: saturated, monounsaturated, and polyunsaturated. Each fat or oil has its own specific ratio of these fatty acids. The list below is not alphabetical. Instead, it is organized by percentage of saturated fat, from the least at the top to the most at the bottom. (Note that the percentages do not add up to 100% because other fatlike substances make up the total composition.)

	Saturated Fat %	Monounsaturated Fat %	Polyunsaturated Fat %
Canola oil	7	59	30
Hazelnut oil	7	78	10
Almond oil	8	70	17
Safflower oil	9	12	75
Walnut oil	9	23	63
Flaxseed oil	10	17	69
Sunflower oil	10	84	4
Avocado oil	12	71	13
Corn oil	13	24	59
Olive oil	14	74	8
Pistachio oil	14	49	33
Sesame oil	15	40	41
Soybean oil	15	11	45
Peanut oil	17	46	32
Lard	40	42	14
Butter	62	29	4
Coconut oil	87	6	2

Cottonseed oil Cottonseed oil is used commercially in some margarines and salad dressings, and in many fried products.

Flaxseed oil Cold-pressed flaxseed oil can be found in the refrigerated section of health-food stores. For more information, see Flaxseed (*page 322*).

Grapeseed oil Extracted from the seeds of grapes, this oil is used to make margarine or salad dressings. It is also used by chefs because it has an extremely high smoke point.

Pumpkin seed oil Made from roasted pumpkin seeds, this is an extremely full-flavored oil with a deep green-black color. Because of its robust flavor, it is best used in combination with lighter oils.

Rapeseed oil This oil comes from the seeds of the same plant that gives us the vegetable called broccoli rabe. The oil is sold commercially as canola oil (*see page 297*).

Rice bran oil Used commercially for frying foods such as potato chips, this oil has long been a staple in Japan. Rice bran oil has a light, nutty flavor and can be used both for sautéing and in salad dressings.

Safflower oil Flavorless, colorless, and relatively odorless, safflower oil is extracted from the seeds of the safflower. It has a high smoke point (making it excellent for frying) and contains more polyunsaturates than any other oil.

Sesame oil Sesame oil comes in cold-pressed and roasted forms. The dark-brown roasted oil is usually sold in the Asian foods section in supermarkets. Cold-pressed sesame oil, which is light in color and delicate in flavor, is available in health-food stores. The roasted oil is generally used as a flavor accent, added during the final minutes of cooking. In combination with a lighter flavored oil, it works well in salad dressings and sauces. The cold-pressed oil is good for both salad dressings and sautéing.

Soybean oil Extracted from soybeans, this oil is used extensively in the manufacturing of margarines. Because of its high smoke point and relatively inexpensive cost, it is often used for sautéing.

Sunflower oil Pale yellow in color and light in flavor, sunflower oil has a relatively low smoke point. It is used in salad dressings and baking.

Wheat germ oil Cold-pressed from whole grains of wheat, this oil has a nutty flavor and can be used along with a lighter oil for salad dressings.

fruit oils

Avocado oil This oil is made by dehydrating avocado flesh, then pressing or extracting the oil with solvents. Along with olive oil and canola oil, it

---

trans fats

To make vegetable oils solid at room temperature (for margarines and vegetable shortening) and to prolong the shelf-life of crackers, cookies, chips, and other foods that contain vegetable oils, manufacturers hydrogenate—that is, add hydrogen to—vegetable oils. This process both solidifies the oils and makes them more stable. Unfortunately, hydrogenation alters many of the oils' unsaturated fatty acids, making them more saturated and changing their structure in other ways that makes them into trans fatty acids, often called "trans fats." Studies have shown that trans fats act like saturated fats, raising total blood cholesterol levels.

Though food labels specify how much saturated fat is in foods, trans fats have not been counted or identified on labels. The Food and Drug Administration (FDA) is planning to include such information in the near future. In the meantime, if you use lots of margarine, consider a few of the useful tips found in "Margarine Pointers" (*page 300*).

is an exceptional source of monounsaturated fats. Avocado oil is used in salad dressings.

Olive oil See Olives & Olive Oil (*page 421*).

nut oils

As with seed oils, nut oils can come both roasted and unroasted (cold-pressed). The cold-pressed forms are more commonly found in health-food stores, while the roasted forms tend to be sold in specialty food and gourmet stores. In general, the toasted varieties are full-flavored and best used sparingly, without heating. Most nut oils are subject to rancidity and should be stored in the refrigerator.

Almond oil Made from roasted almonds, almond oil has the flavor of almonds. Use it in baked goods, pastas, drizzled over vegetables, or on grilled bread. The unroasted form is usually labeled "Sweet Almond Oil." Very light in flavor, without any real nut taste, sweet almond oil is often used by chefs to oil molds of unbaked desserts. It has a high smoke point, making it good for stir-frying.

Hazelnut oil The most common form found in the market is derived mainly from unroasted Italian hazelnuts (aka filberts). However, a roasted version from American hazelnuts is also available. Full of flavor, hazelnut oil is excellent for seasoning desserts as well as salads.

Macadamia nut oil With its light, delicate macadamia flavor, this oil is especially good with fish, chicken, vegetables, or baked goods. It has a high smoke point and can be used for sautéing or stir-frying. Roasted macadamia oil has a fuller, somewhat nuttier flavor than unroasted and should not be heated; use it as a finishing oil to drizzle over cooked foods.

Peanut oil While most American peanut oils are mild flavored, Chinese and health-food store varieties tend to have a full peanut flavor and aroma. Available both roasted and unroasted, peanut oil is delicious in salad dressings and sauces. Use the unroasted variety for frying because of its higher smoke point.

Pecan oil Roasted pecan oil has a deep, nutty flavor. It makes a nice salad dressing when used in combination with a lighter, less flavorful oil. It can also be drizzled on vegetables or pasta.

Pine nut oil Made from ground and roasted pine nuts, a little goes a long way. Use it to drizzle over pasta, vegetables, or bread.

Pistachio oil This cold-pressed oil, derived from pistachios, has a deep green color and a rich, full-bodied flavor. Use it along with a lighter oil to flavor salads or drizzle over fish or vegetables. A roasted pistachio oil is also available and has a slightly more pronounced toasted flavor.

Sweet almond oil See almond oil (*above*).

---

serving suggestions

- Replace some or all of the melted butter in a baking recipe with avocado oil.

- Instead of sautéing vegetables in butter, steam them and then drizzle some flavorful nut oil over the cooked vegetables.

- For a butter that's lower in saturated fat, soften butter and beat it together with olive oil or any of the other flavorful oils. Store in the refrigerator and use as you would butter.

- Replace the butter in your mashed potatoes with olive oil.

- Use avocado oil, walnut oil, hazelnut oil, or pistachio oil in a pasta salad.

- Substitute a small amount of roasted sesame oil for tahini (sesame seed paste) in hummus recipes.

- Drizzle pumpkin seed oil over baked, broiled, or steamed fish.

- For added flavor use a fragrant nut oil in a carrot cake recipe.

- Steep herbs or spices in a mild oil and use it for sautéing.

Walnut oil This highly fragrant oil is frequently used in salad dressings in combination with a less flavorful oil. Walnut oil can also be used for sautéing, in baked goods, and drizzled over vegetables or fish. However, roasted varieties have a fuller, deeper flavor and should be used with finished dishes, not heated.

margarine & vegetable shortening

Margarine As in butter, 100 percent of margarine's calories come from fat, but the fat is largely polyunsaturated. It's good for spreading and cooking. None of the major brands have any cholesterol, since almost all are made from vegetable oils (though the Food and Drug Administration does allow lard—which is animal fat—to be used).

Vegetable-oil spreads These contain less than the 80 percent fat by weight required in a margarine, but this does not necessarily add up to them being more healthful than regular margarine.

Diet or **reduced-calorie margarines** One way to cut fat is to use a "diet" margarine. Though all of its calories still come from fat (about 45 per-

facts & tips

Diet margarines have less fat by weight because they make up the difference with water—up to 55 percent. Thus, when you heat the margarine, you end up with 45 percent of the fat you thought you were cooking with. So instead of cooking with diet margarine, start with a smaller amount of regular margarine—or better still, olive oil.

margarine pointers

How much saturated fat a margarine or spread contains depends on which vegetable oil it contains and how it was processed. When shopping for a margarine or spread, let the ingredients list be your guide:

• Most margarine products tell how much saturated and polyunsaturated fats they contain. Look for a product with at least twice as much polyunsaturated as saturated fat. If a brand doesn't give you a breakdown of fats, be suspicious.

• Although all the oils commonly used in margarines are high in polyunsaturated fat and low in saturated fat, they vary substantially. Those lowest in saturated fat are safflower, sunflower, corn oil, and soybean oil, in that order.

• The softer or more fluid a margarine is, the less saturated it is

likely to be. For this reason, liquid "squeeze" margarines or tub margarines are almost always better than stick margarines.

• Margarine with water listed as the first ingredient has one-third to one-half less fat than the average margarine.

• Watch the sodium content, which tends to be relatively high. Salted margarine is just as undesirable as salted butter. Unsalted varieties are available.

• If a hydrogenated or partially hydrogenated oil is listed first, the product is likely to be more saturated because of hydrogenation—a process that transforms the unsaturated fatty acids in vegetable oils into a more saturated (and therefore less healthy) kind of fat called "trans fats" (*see "Trans Fats," page 298*).

cent fat by weight), it is diluted with water, so it has half the fat and calories of regular margarine per tablespoon. It is not, however, suitable for cooking.

Butter-margarine blends These are anywhere from 15 to 40 percent butter. Thus they contain some of butter's cholesterol and saturated fat, as well as its taste.

Sprinkle-on powders Made from carbohydrates, these powders are virtually fat- and cholesterol-free. They melt well on hot, moist foods like baked potatoes. But they can't be used in recipes or for sautéing.

Vegetable shortening This solid fat is made from vegetable oils such as cottonseed and soybean. It is made solid by the process of hydrogenation. Solid vegetable shortening is used primarily for baking and can be stored at room temperature.

tropical oils

Coconut oil This tropical oil is semisolid at room temperature and highly saturated. It is often used in commercial baked goods.

Dende This deep-orange oil comes from the fruit of the red palm (but not the same palm as the source for palm oil). It is a common ingredient in Brazilian dishes.

Palm oil This tropical oil is semisolid at room temperature and highly saturated (though less so than the other tropical oils). Palm oil is made from the fruit of the oil palm, and the nut inside the palm fruit is also used to make an oil called *palm kernel oil*. Palm kernel oil is extremely high in saturated fat and is used chiefly in soapmaking.

animal fats

Butter Made by churning cream until it reaches a solid state, butter comes in *sweet (unsalted)* and *lightly salted* varieties as well as *whipped* and *reduced-calorie*. Whipped butter, which is packed in tubs and comes sweet and lightly salted, has had air beaten into it, making it soft and easy to spread. Reduced-calorie butter, with about half the calories of regular butter, has (in addition to cream) water, fat-free milk, and gelatin. If you're trying to follow a "heart-healthy" diet, you should limit your use of butter, since most of its calories come from saturated fat, and it contains a fair amount of cholesterol. Of course, if your diet is sensibly low in fat and cholesterol, a daily pat of butter won't hurt you.

Ghee This is butter that has been slowly cooked so that the milk solids settle to the bottom of the pan and after about 45 minutes of cooking turn golden-brown. The transparent butter on top is then strained through several layers of cheesecloth until not a speck of solids remains. The resulting ghee has a rich, nutty flavor. Ghee is generally used in Indian cooking for sautéing and also flavoring desserts.

Lard Made from rendered and clarified pork fat, processed lard is about the consistency of vegetable shortening and is often used in South American cooking. In the South, lard is sometimes used in biscuits and pie dough, as it is very rich and makes an extremely tender, flaky crust.

Suet This solid white fat found around the kidneys and loins of beef, sheep, and other animals is often used in British recipes for pastries, puddings, and mincemeat. (In this country we often feed it to birds.)

choosing the best

While many oils are available in local supermarkets, chances are you'll have to go to a specialty food or health-food store to find some of the less common oils. Wherever you shop for them, remember that oils tend to go rancid if not stored properly, so purchase them in a store that keeps them away from direct sunlight and heat.

▶ **When you get home** Check the labels to see what is advised, but most fats should be stored in the refrigerator if you are not going to use them in a short amount of time.

cholesterol-lowering spreads

The FDA has approved new brands of margarine that can actually lower total blood cholesterol by an average of 10 percent, when eaten in sufficient quantities daily. The good news is that they lower LDL ("bad") cholesterol levels without adversely affecting HDL ("good") cholesterol levels.

The spreads can lower cholesterol because they contain plant chemicals called sterols, whose cholesterol-lowering abilities have been the subject of study for the past 50 years. Through improved techniques, plant sterols (as well as stanol ester, a fat-soluble derivative of plant sterols) have been incorporated into various margarinelike spreads. Sterols and stanols work because they resemble cholesterol and are able to "fool" your intestines. Your body mistakes them for dietary cholesterol and tries to absorb them, but these substances actually block sites where cholesterol is absorbed.

These cholesterol-lowering spreads are intended to be taken in daily doses (each of them is slightly different) in order to have a salutary effect. However, since these products derive their calories from fat, these doses should not be in *addition* to the daily amount of fat consumed. Instead, they should be a *substitute* for the fats that would otherwise have been consumed, such as butter, other margarines, cream cheese, or cheese.

The one drawback is the price. A week's supply (about 6 ounces, the equivalent of 1½ sticks of margarine) can cost up to four times the amount for butter or margarine. These spreads are of course cheaper than cholesterol-lowering drugs, but don't lower blood cholesterol levels as much.

Caveat: Everybody needs professional medical advice about risk factors for heart disease. If you are overweight or sedentary; are a smoker; have hypertension or diabetes; have "high" total cholesterol; have low HDL ("good") cholesterol; or have other coronary risk factors, don't assume that eating a cholesterol-lowering spread will cancel them out. And, of course, you need to know what your blood cholesterol levels are in the first place.

fennel

With its rounded pale green bulb, short stalks, and dark green feathery fronds, fennel could be mistaken for a plump bunch of celery. The texture, too, is similar, but fennel's flavor emphatically sets it apart from celery and other stalk vegetables. The overlapping layers of bulb, the stalks, and the fronds all impart a mild, sweet flavor akin to licorice or anise. Because of its flavor, fennel is called "anise" in many markets; however, the vegetable is an entirely different plant from the herb anise.

A member of the parsley family, fennel is also known, in Italian neighborhoods, as *finocchio*. Europeans, particularly the Italians and the French, have been enthusiastic about fennel for many years—they cultivate more of it than anyone else—but the vegetable is becoming more widely appreciated in the United States.

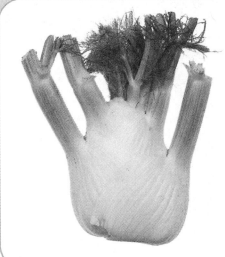

florence fennel

nutritional profile

Like celery, fennel is filling and yet very low in calories. One cup of fennel is only 27 calories. Vitamin C and potassium (and small amounts of folate) can be found in fennel.

in the market

Baby fennel This is a smaller, younger, slightly more tender version of Florence fennel. Young fennel is sometimes available in farmers' markets.

Florence fennel This is the type of fennel most available in supermarkets. It has a squat, creamy-colored round bulb, with short green (celerylike) stalks and dark green feathery fronds.

Wild fennel Small, with almost flat bulbs and lots of feathery fronds, this is occasionally available in farmers' markets and specialty grocery stores.

choosing the best

No matter what size fennel you're shopping for, the bulbs should be firm and clean, the stalks straight, and the feathery fronds fresh and green; if flowers are

FENNEL / 1 cup raw	
Calories	27
Protein (g)	1
Carbohydrate (g)	6
Dietary fiber (g)	2.7
Total fat (g)	0.2
Saturated fat (g)	--
Monounsaturated fat (g)	--
Polyunsaturated fat (g)	--
Cholesterol (mg)	0
Potassium (mg)	360
Sodium (mg)	45

KEY NUTRIENTS (%RDA/AI*)

Vitamin C	10 mg (12%)

For more detailed information on RDA and AI, see page 88.

fennel seeds

The fennel seeds used as a kitchen herb come from a variety of fennel called common fennel, which does not develop a bulb as do other fennels. The plant is actually grown not as a vegetable, but for its seeds. Fennel seeds are small, oval, and dull brown with a strong licorice flavor. This flavor is often associated with Italian-style sausages, because the seeds are added to the sausage meat.

present on the stalks, the bulb is overmature. The top of the bulb should be compact, with the stalks closely spaced rather than spread out. If the stalks are cut off (which may indicate that the fennel is not perfectly fresh), the cut ends should be fresh-looking, not dry and white. Avoid bulbs that show any brown spots or signs of splitting.

preparing to use

If you've bought a fennel bulb with the stalks attached, trim them off at the point where they meet the bulb. Set aside the stalks to use in soups and stews (they are too tough to eat as a vegetable, but they still have flavor), and save the feathery fronds to use as an herb (as you would use dillweed).

Halve the fennel bulb and trim the base (but not too closely, or the layers will fall apart). Then cut the bulb either into slices (lengthwise), dice, or chunks (for braising or for use in soups), or into slivers or sticks (for stir-frying, sautéing, or eating raw). You can also carefully remove individual layers of the fennel bulb and cut each into strips or squares. If cutting the bulb into lengthwise slices, leave the central core intact so that it holds the layers together; if halving, quartering, or slivering the bulb, cut out the dense core, or cut around it and discard.

If you've bought wild or baby fennel, there's no need to separate the stalks from the bulb, as they are both tender. Simply slice the two together and either stir-fry, sauté, or steam.

serving suggestions

- Thinly slice fennel bulbs and toss with lemon juice and a good olive oil; top with shaved Parmesan for a salad.

- Serve sliced fresh fennel with goat cheese and fresh figs as an antipasto (or even a dessert).

- Wrap chunks of fennel in foil along with a few garlic cloves and a drizzle of olive oil and bake at 400° until tender.

- Add fresh fennel and fennel seeds to lean ground pork, shape into patties, and broil or grill.

- Cook fennel and potatoes together until tender and mash with a little olive oil.

- Use fennel in place of celery in stuffings, soups, and salads.

- Sauté fennel with apples and onions for an interesting side dish.

- Add diced fresh fennel to your favorite salsa.

- Add fennel and fennel seeds to broth when poaching fish or shellfish. Or add chunks of fennel to fish or seafood chowders.

figs

One of the earliest foods to be cultivated, figs were prized as early as 2900 B.C. for their medicinal value. They were also reputed to have been Cleopatra's favorite fruit and a training food for Olympic athletes. (And where would prudish artists have been without the fig leaf?) Fig trees were introduced to California in the 18th century by Spanish missionaries.

Characterized by their sweet flavor and soft texture, figs consist of a pliable skin enclosing a sweet, even softer, fleshy interior filled with edible seeds. Interestingly, though most people think of the fig as a fruit, in reality it is actually a flower inverted into itself, with the blossom being the inside of the fruit, and the seeds being drupes, the "real" fruit.

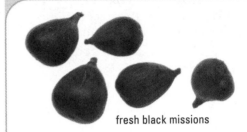

figs

fresh black missions

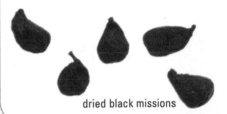

dried black missions

nutritional profile

Both fresh and dried figs contain important nutrients, with dried figs being more nutrient-dense (as well as higher in calories) than the fresh form. Figs are an exceptional source of fiber (due to the tiny seeds that fill the fruit) as well as the source of some potassium. Their high fiber content helps to aid digestion and promote heart health, with their soluble pectin fiber helping to lower cholesterol levels.

in the market

There are hundreds of fig varieties, but only about half a dozen are grown commercially in the United States, with California being the only important fig-growing state.

Adriatic This Mediterranean transplant has a high sugar content, making it a favorite for drying and using in fig bars and fig pastes. The fresh fig has light green skin and pale pink flesh.

Black Mission Named for the mission fathers who introduced the fruit to California, the Black Mission has dark purple skin (which deepens to black when dried) and pink flesh.

Brown Turkey This fig, with purplish skin and red flesh, is sold fresh and dried.

Calimyrna A large greenish-yellow fig when fresh, the Calimyrna is the California version of the Smyrna (Cali + Myrna = Calimyrna). In their dried form, Calimyrnas have a delicious nutlike flavor and tender, golden skin, making them the most popular dried form to eat out of hand.

Kadota The Kadota has greenish-yellow skin and purple flesh and is practically seedless (making it a favorite with those who make fig preserves). It dries to a light golden color.

Smyrna This is the same fig as the Calimyrna. The only difference is that the Calimyrna is grown in California and other Smyrnas are not.

FRESH FIGS / 2 medium	
Calories	74
Protein (g)	1
Carbohydrate (g)	19
Dietary fiber (g)	3.3
Total fat (g)	0.3
Saturated fat (g)	0.1
Monounsaturated fat (g)	0.1
Polyunsaturated fat (g)	0.1
Cholesterol (mg)	0
Potassium (mg)	232
Sodium (mg)	1

▶ **Availability** Fresh figs do not keep well, making their season very short. However, the figs grown in this country have staggered harvests, which makes them available from June through September.

choosing the best

A "fancy" produce item, fresh figs are packed carefully and thus should be in good condition when displayed in the market. Color differs with variety, but healthy figs will always have a rich color; ripe Mission figs, for example, will be nearly black. Look for shapely, plump figs with unbruised, unbroken skins and a mild fragrance; a sour smell indicates spoilage. They should be just soft to the touch, but not mushy. If the figs seem somewhat shriveled, as if they are beginning to dry, they will be particularly sweet. Size is not an indicator of quality, but you'll probably want to choose uniformly sized fruits if you are planning to serve them as individual portions for dessert.

▶ **When you get home** To ripen slightly underripe figs, place them on a plate at room temperature, away from sunlight, and turn them frequently. Keep ripe fresh figs in the refrigerator.

preparing to use

Wash fresh figs and remove the hard portion of the stem end. Halve or quarter the fruit. Thick-skinned Calimyrna figs are usually peeled; Mission figs do not need to be, as they have thin, edible skins.

a unique pollination

Unlike Mission and other types of figs, the Calimyrna fig—the most popular dried fig—is not self-pollinating and relies on an unusual method of pollination to produce mature edible fruit. Early growers of the Calimyrna were puzzled because the fruit would drop off the tree before maturing. Eventually, a researcher discovered that Calimyrna figs would remain on the trees if they received the pollen from an inedible fig called the caprifig. Each caprifig has a colony of small fig wasps, called Blastophaga, living inside it. When the wasp larvae mature and break out of each caprifig, they search for another fig to serve as a nest in order to reproduce. Calimyrna growers intervene just prior to this point and place baskets of caprifigs in their orchards. Female wasps then work their way into the Calimyrna figs, carrying a few grains of caprifig pollen on their wings and bodies. Once inside, the wasps discover that the structure of the Calimyrna figs is not suitable for laying eggs and they depart, leaving the pollen behind.

dried figs

Once they are harvested, fresh figs last only about a week. As a consequence, about 90 percent of the world's fig harvest is dried. Even though dried figs do not have the texture of fresh, they offer a dense nutritional package. Most notably, they boast an impressive amount of dietary fiber—over 9 grams in a serving of four figs. Dried figs are also a good source of vitamin B_6, vitamin E, potassium, and antioxidant phytochemicals.

Of course, ounce for ounce, dried figs are higher in calories than fresh, and the bulk of their calories—almost 90 percent of them—is derived from natural sugar. But they are undoubtedly one of the best snacking and dessert foods available.

All of the main fig varieties are available dried, though the more common types are Black Mission, Calimyrna, and Kadota. In specialty markets, you can occasionally find what are called string figs, which are Greek figs that have been dried and flattened into disks, then strung on a long reed. In biblical times, these strings were carried by travelers as a portable source of energy.

Dried figs can be stored at cool room temperature or in the refrigerator; just be sure that they are well-wrapped after opening so that they do not become too dry and hard.

Before preparing dried figs for cooking, place them in the freezer for an hour to make them easier to slice. When chopping dried figs, dip the knife into hot water from time to time, to prevent the fruit from sticking to it. Before using chopped figs in batters, toss the pieces with a little flour to keep them from sinking to the bottom.

Reconstituting dried figs: If you like dried figs plumped, simmer them in boiling water, wine, or fruit juice for 2 minutes; add a drop of almond extract if desired.

DRIED FIGS / 4 large

Calories	194
Protein (g)	2
Carbohydrate (g)	50
Dietary fiber (g)	9.3
Total fat (g)	0.9
Saturated fat (g)	0.2
Monounsaturated fat (g)	0.2
Polyunsaturated fat (g)	0.4
Cholesterol (mg)	0
Potassium (mg)	541
Sodium (mg)	8

KEY NUTRIENTS (%RDA/AI*)

Vitamin B_6	0.17 mg (10%)
Vitamin E	1.8 mg (12%)

*For more detailed information on RDA and AI, see page 88.

serving suggestions

- Serve quartered fresh figs with a dollop of lightly sweetened ricotta.

- Stir chopped dried figs into peanut butter or reduced-fat cream cheese for a sandwich spread.

- Add chopped dried figs to grain dishes.

- Make a salad of thinly sliced fresh figs, crumbled feta cheese, and lettuce, and dress with olive oil and lemon juice.

- Roast sliced fresh figs with sliced sweet potatoes and red onions tossed in a little olive oil.

- Use chopped dried figs in place of raisins.

- Skewer chunks of fresh figs and grill. Serve with sweetened yogurt.

- Poach whole dried figs in red wine and serve as a condiment with roast poultry or pork.

fish

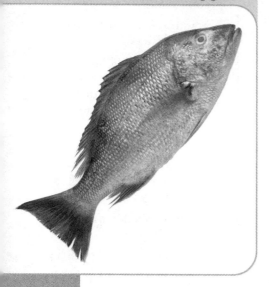

red snapper

The great resources of our oceans, lakes, and rivers have yielded important sustenance in the form of fish for thousands of years. Unfortunately, within the past few years or so, researchers are becoming concerned that our supply of fish is dwindling. With the advent of high-tech fishing methods, the number of fish in the ocean has begun to go down, with commercial fishermen catching them at faster rates than the fish can reproduce. In order to address the problem of the depletion of popular eating fish, farm-raised fish are becoming more prevalent, with trout and salmon being among the most popular. Aquaculture, the science of breeding and raising fish on fish "farms," is making a rapidly growing contribution to the market supply of both fresh and saltwater species.

Fish fall into two main categories: freshwater and saltwater. *Freshwater fish* are from rivers, lakes, and streams. Some of the more popular types of freshwater fish include lake and rainbow trout, bass, carp, lake perch, catfish, and pike. Freshwater fish tend to have smaller bones and require a bit more care when picking away the minuscule bones, which is often a source of frustration for diners. *Saltwater fish,* on the other hand, have larger bones (easier to de-bone) and are found in the ocean, gulfs, and seas. The more commonly consumed saltwater fish include salmon, mackerel, haddock, sea bass, cod, flounder, red snapper, swordfish, and tuna.

Fish are also divided according to their bone and body structure and are either "flat" or "round" fish. Shaped like an oval platter, *flatfish,* such as flounder, swim horizontally on their sides, along the bottom of the ocean, while *"round" fish,* such as striped bass, red snapper, and salmon, have thicker, more bullet-shaped bodies, and are more typically "fish" shaped. A round fish is more complicated to fillet than a flatfish, but it yields thicker fillets and meaty steaks, if the fish is reasonably large.

Another distinction among the various kinds of fish is their fat content, with fish being either lean or fatty. *Lean fish* (such as sea bass, brook trout, cod, flounder, and red snapper) typically have a mild flavor, making them adaptable to every sort of cuisine, and most of them are similar enough in taste and texture that you can substitute one variety for another. *Fatty fish* include some of the more popular fish, such as salmon and tuna. They tend to have a wider distribution of fat, and their flesh is darker, firmer in texture, and has a more distinctive flavor than lean fish.

More than 200 species of fish are caught in American waters alone, and hundreds more are available worldwide. The varieties that appear in markets have shifted over the years. Some traditionally popular species, such as striped bass and swordfish, are relatively scarce (and therefore expensive) due to overfishing and pollution.

FLOUNDER/SOLE 3 ounces cooked	
Calories	100
Protein (g)	21
Carbohydrate (g)	0
Dietary fiber (g)	0
Total fat (g)	1.3
Saturated fat (g)	0.3
Monounsaturated fat (g)	0.2
Polyunsaturated fat (g)	0.6
Cholesterol (mg)	58
Potassium (mg)	293
Sodium (mg)	89

KEY NUTRIENTS (%RDA/AI*)	
Niacin	1.9 mg (12%)
Vitamin B_6	0.2 mg (12%)
Vitamin B_{12}	2.1 mcg (89%)
Vitamin E	2.0 mg (13%)
Magnesium	49 mg (12%)
Selenium	50 mcg (90%)

*For more detailed information on RDA and AI, see page 88.

nutritional profile

It's simplest to think of fish, both from a health standpoint and a cooking standpoint, as lean or fatty. Lower-fat (or lean) fish have less than 5 percent fat by weight; fatty fish are more than 5 percent fat by weight.

Only a few so-called fatty fish are truly high in fat, with more than 10 grams of fat per 3 ounces cooked. These fish—which include Boston mackerel, salmon, sardines, and shad—are very rich in the polyunsaturated fatty acids called omega-3s. *(See "Comparing Fish," page 311, for how fish stack up for omega-3 content.)* Omega-3s make platelets in the blood less likely to stick together and may reduce inflammatory processes in blood vessels (and elsewhere). By reducing blood clotting, omega-3s thereby lower the chance of a fatal heart attack. Omega-3s can help decrease levels of triglycerides, the major type of fat that circulates in the blood. They may also make the heart less susceptible to dangerous, sometimes fatal, rhythm abnormalities. Since this is one instance where fat may help protect the heart, the American Heart Association advises eating at least two servings of fish a week, particularly fatty fish such as salmon and herring. In addition, there's promising research showing that fish oil may help relieve inflammatory symptoms of autoimmune diseases such as rheumatoid arthritis or psoriasis.

Along with heart-healthy fat, fish are very good sources of high-quality protein minus the artery-clogging saturated fat present in other high-protein foods. So called "heme" iron, the form of iron that is most readily and easily absorbed by our bodies, is present in fish. Depending on the type, fish also contain significant amounts of B vitamins, especially thiamin, niacin, vitamin B_6, and vitamin B_{12}. Salmon, sardines, and mackerel are important sources of bone-strengthening vitamin D, and a 3-ounce serving of canned sardines with bones contains over 25 percent of a day's requirement of calcium.

in the market

The following listing covers species of fresh fish that are available nationwide or in many areas of the country. Names of fish often vary with the region: For instance, various types of North American flounder are locally called "sole"—French sole, Pacific sole, sand sole, lemon sole, even Dover and English sole—even though no North American fish is truly a sole. Some flounders are given market names like sanddab, fluke, plaice, or turbot. The following listing is broken into "fatty fish" (over 5 percent fat by weight) and lean fish (under 5 percent). These designations are for fish caught in the wild. Generally speaking, their farm-raised counterparts are

fish oil capsules

Fish oil capsules have become increasingly popular, but they may not have the same benefits as fish, since fish is rich in other nutrients. And the capsules come with potential adverse effects, including an excessive reduction in the ability of your blood to clot, which increases the risk of hemorrhagic stroke. People with bleeding disorders, those taking anticoagulant medications, or those with uncontrolled hypertension (who are already at high risk for a stroke) should definitely not take fish oil capsules. In addition, the capsules can cause nausea, diarrhea, belching, and a bad taste in the mouth. They are also a concentrated source of calories.

If you have rheumatoid arthritis or psoriasis, fish oil capsules might be worth a try, despite any adverse effects. But be sure to consult your doctor first. Anyone else who wants the benefits of omega-3s should ignore the capsules and eat fish—ideally, at least two servings a week.

Also, be aware that, as with other dietary supplements sold in the United States, the quality and purity of fish oil capsules is left up to manufacturers—so there is no guarantee that the capsules you buy actually contain omega-3s or even fish oil, or that they are free of contaminants.

higher in fat. For an explanation on the forms fish take in the market, see "Market Forms of Fish," (*page 313*).

fatty fish

Anchovies Anchovies are small saltwater fish of the herring family. Rarely eaten fresh, they are usually sold in cans or jars and are used as a seasoning. Anchovies are a classic ingredient in salade Niçoise and Caesar salad, and are also a popular pizza topping. The tiny fillets are heavily salted and packed in oil; whole anchovies are also sold in bulk, packed in salt. Pureed anchovies go into tubes of anchovy paste, a convenient flavoring.

Butterfish Called butterfish in the eastern United States, and Pacific or California pompano in the West, this small silvery saltwater fish is usually sold whole, drawn, or dressed. Suitable for broiling, baking, or panfrying, it has a delicate flavor and soft, rather dark flesh that firms and lightens when cooked.

Carp This freshwater fish is a favorite with two diverse ethnic groups: Chinese cooks like to poach or steam it whole, while Eastern European Jews use it in making gefilte fish and also serve it poached, with a sweet-and-sour sauce. The flesh of carp is somewhat coarse, and parts of the fish can be tough. It is also a difficult fish to skin and bone, so you may prefer to buy fillets, although it is commonly sold dressed or split lengthwise. Try this fish baked, broiled, steamed, or poached.

Chilean sea bass (Patagonian toothfish) Chilean sea bass is not actually a member of the sea bass family. With its snow-white flesh, firm, rich texture, and melt-in-your-mouth flavor, Chilean sea bass has become extremely popular. Originally found off the southern coast of Chile to the Antarctic, it's now caught throughout most of the southern hemisphere.

Eel While they resemble snakes, eel are actually true fish, with tiny scales and gills. They are freshwater fish and have rich, firm, sweet-tasting flesh. Fresh eel are occasionally available, though they are more reliably found smoked. Have your fish dealer skin them for you as their skin is very tough and difficult to remove.

Herring This huge family of fish has over 100 varieties. Small young herring are commonly sold as sardines. Fresh herring is occasionally available but you're more likely to find it smoked and salted, or pickled.

Mackerel See Mackerel (*page 386*).

Pompano Sometimes called Florida pompano, this silvery fish is caught in the Atlantic off the southern U.S. coast, but overfishing has limited the supply so that pompano these days is fairly expensive. You can buy whole fresh or frozen pompano. Its rather oily, firm, white meat has a delicate flavor and is best cooked by broiling, grilling, or baking in parchment.

Sablefish Though it is commonly called "black cod," this northern Pacific fish is not a cod, nor is it a butterfish, another name often applied to sablefish fillets. A high fat content gives it a soft texture and a rich taste that is surprisingly mild. Fillets, fresh or frozen, are the most common market form,

POMPANO 3 ounces cooked	
Calories	180
Protein (g)	20
Carbohydrate (g)	0
Dietary fiber (g)	0
Total fat (g)	10
Saturated fat (g)	3.8
Monounsaturated fat (g)	2.8
Polyunsaturated fat (g)	1.2
Cholesterol (mg)	54
Potassium (mg)	541
Sodium (mg)	65

KEY NUTRIENTS (%RDA/AI*)	
Thiamin	0.6 mg (48%)
Riboflavin	0.1 mg (10%)
Niacin	3.2 mg (20%)
Vitamin B_6	0.2 mg (12%)
Vitamin B_{12}	1.0 mcg (43%)
Selenium	40 mcg (72%)

*For more detailed information on RDA and AI, see page 88.

but sablefish is also sold whole (weighing about 3 to 15 pounds) or cut into steaks. The fish is excellent broiled, though baking, poaching, and steaming are also suitable methods. It is also available smoked.

Salmon See Salmon (*page 518*).

Sardines The word "sardine" actually refers to more than 20 varied species of small, slender, soft-boned saltwater fish found worldwide and ranging in size from 3 to 6 inches. Sardines as we know them in the United States, however, are actually members of the herring family. Fresh sardines are occasionally available, but sardines are more commonly found salted, smoked, or canned in oil, tomato sauce, or mustard sauce. Some are packed whole, while others are skinned, boned, and sold as fillets.

Shad This member of the herring family is famous for its tasty roe as well as its rich flesh: Shad is one of the fattiest of all fish. Like salmon, shad is a fish that lives most of its life in salt water, but spawns in fresh water. Shad is at its best in the spring, when it enters inland waters on both the Atlantic and

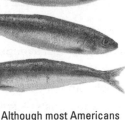

Although most Americans only know canned sardines (which in this country are a species of herring), you can find them fresh in the market.

COMPARING FISH 3 ounces cooked

Like meat and poultry, most fish loses about 25 percent of its weight when cooked. Therefore, 3 ounces of cooked fish starts out as 4 ounces raw. These fish are not organized alphabetically, but by omega-3 fatty acid content, highest at the top and lowest at the bottom.

	Calories	Fat (g)	Saturated Fat (g)	Cholesterol (mg)	Omega-3s (g)
Mackerel, Boston	223	15	3.6	64	2.2
Salmon, Atlantic	175	11	2.1	54	1.6
Herring	173	9.9	2.2	66	1.4
Tuna, white, canned*	109	1.0	0.3	36	1.3
Salmon, canned	76	6.2	1.4	37	1.1
Bluefish	135	4.6	1.0	65	1.0
Halibut	119	2.5	0.4	35	0.8
Striped bass	106	2.5	0.6	88	0.7
Pompano	180	10	3.8	54	0.5
Trout, rainbow	144	6.1	1.8	58	0.5
Tuna, yellowfin	118	2.5	0.7	49	0.3
Catfish	129	6.8	1.5	54	0.2
Flounder	100	1.3	0.3	58	0.2
Grouper	100	1.1	0.3	40	0.2
Haddock	95	0.8	0.1	63	0.2
Snapper	109	1.5	0.3	40	0.2
Swordfish	132	4.4	1.2	43	0.2
Tuna, light, canned*	99	0.7	0.2	26	0.2
Cod	89	0.7	0.1	47	0.1
Roughy	77	0.8	0	22	0

*water-packed

Pacific Northwest coasts to spawn. Females bear large sacs of roe weighing up to ¾ pound each, which are considered a great delicacy (some people prefer the roe to the fish itself). Female shad average about 8 pounds, males about 4 pounds. This fish has rich, sweet flesh but is unfortunately very bony—it has 360 bones, to be exact. It's best to buy fillets if you are not familiar with this fish, as it is difficult to bone. Sometimes the roe is sold with the fish, and sometimes it is marketed separately. Because of its high fat content, shad remains moist and delicious when baked or broiled.

Whitefish The term "whitefish" is sometimes loosely used to describe various white-fleshed fish, but true whitefish is a freshwater species related to trout and abundant in the Great Lakes. It has particularly sweet, moist, delicate flesh and is a favorite for smoking. Whitefish for market average around 4 pounds and are sold dressed and in fillets. This fish can be baked, broiled, or poached (leave the skin on fillets to hold them together while cooking).

scavenger fish

Should you be wary of scavenger fish? No. It's not really true that scavenger fish or bottom feeders—catfish and flounder as well as shrimp, crab, and lobster—feed mainly off waste. They eat whatever swims or floats by them. And even when dead organic matter is consumed by these bottom-feeding fish, they digest it and use it to form proteins, fats, and carbohydrates. They are not necessarily more likely to be contaminated than other fish.

lean fish

Bass A number of different freshwater and saltwater species are called "bass." The freshwater basses (which are really members of the sunfish family), such as largemouth and smallmouth bass, are not commercially fished. The saltwater basses include sea bass (*page 316*) and striped bass (*page 318*).

Bluefish This plentiful Atlantic fish is a great fighter, making it popular with sport fishermen. However, it ranges over a wide area during its lifespan and may be exposed to many contaminants, including PCBs and mercury. Some large bluefish have been found to contain PCB residues that exceeded the "level of tolerance" considered safe by the FDA, and even small bluefish may not be safe to consume too often. Although its exceptionally rich flavor has given bluefish a "high-fat" reputation, it actually has only 4.6 grams of fat per 3-ounce cooked serving. The bluefish you'll find in the market average 3 to 6 pounds; they are sold whole, dressed, and as fillets. The rather dark flesh is best baked or grilled (the flesh lightens when cooked).

Catfish Best known in the South, this tasty freshwater fish has become increasingly popular in recent years and is now one of America's favorite fish. Though once caught in rivers and streams, it is now farmed in ponds and sold fresh and frozen all over the country. The fish has a smooth but tough skin that can be difficult to remove, so it's preferable to buy fillets or nuggets. Although traditionally fried, catfish are also delicious baked, grilled, poached, sautéed, or in stews.

Cod Among the five most popular fish eaten in the United States, Atlantic cod is one of the mainstays of New England fisheries. A similar fish, called Pacific cod, is caught on the West Coast. (Haddock and pollack, described on the following pages, are also members of the cod family.) Cod is sold whole—at a weight of up to 10 pounds—dressed, and in fillets and steaks. The flesh is firm, white, and mild in flavor, and this very lean fish can be cooked by almost any method: Try it broiled, baked with tomato sauce, or in chowder. Small cod (under 3 pounds) are sometimes marketed as *scrod;* they are sweeter and more tender than full-grown cod. In Europe, especially Spain and Portugal, very little fresh cod makes it to the marketplace, since the majority of the catch is destined to become *bacalao,* or salt cod. Though the fish itself is quite salty, the method of preparing it removes most of the salt.

Flounder This widely available flatfish, which can be found on nearly every American coastline, has a mild flavor and light texture that have made it a longstanding favorite. The flounder family includes the true sole (caught only in European waters), European *turbot,* and *fluke.* Winter flounder from New England is sometimes called *lemon sole,* and other flounders are offered as *gray sole, petrale sole* (a Pacific flounder), or *rex sole.* If you see Dover sole on a restaurant menu, it may be imported from England (and will be priced accordingly) or it may be a type of Pacific flounder that is sometimes called by this name in the United States. Flounder is sold whole, dressed or filleted, fresh and frozen. This very low-fat fish can be broiled, sautéed, stuffed and baked; the whole fish can also be steamed.

market forms of fish

Unlike beef, with its myriad cuts and grades and elaborate nomenclature, the forms in which you'll find fish in the market are simple and few.

Whole fish comes to you just as it was caught. You'll likely have the fish seller prepare it for you, drawing or dressing it or cutting It into steaks or fillets. If the fish is filleted, about half the total weight of a whole fish will be discarded as fins, scales, skin, head, and bones.

A whole **drawn** fish has been eviscerated through a small opening so that it is not split. The gills and usually the scales are removed, but the head and tail are left intact.

A whole **dressed** fish has been split and then eviscerated; it is also scaled, and the fins, head, and tail are cut off. The backbone (which runs through the center of the fish) can be removed if you want to stuff the fish.

Fillets are the meaty sides of the fish, cut away from the backbone. Most of the other bones are also taken out when the fish is filleted, but fine bones called "pins" may remain; these can be removed before or after you cook the fish. Lean fish fillets are usually sold without their skin. If both sides of the fillet are left connected at the top, it is called a butterfly fillet; if joined at the bottom, it's a kited fillet. Fillets are the most popular form of fish in the United States. They can be cooked in many different ways—sautéed, steamed, broiled, poached—and are easy to eat because they are basically boneless.

Steaks are thick, cross-cut slices from dressed large round fish such as salmon, or from large, thick flatfish like halibut. Steaks are usually surrounded by a band of skin and have a section of the backbone in the center. The exception to this is steaks from very large fish, such as tuna or halibut, where the steak is actually a fraction of the full cross-cut. Dense fish steaks can be grilled or broiled, braised, or cut up for use in chowder; steaks of fish with more delicate flesh are good for poaching and baking.

Fish fingers are strips of fillets or steaks that are ideal for a quick sauté.

Grouper See Sea Bass (*page 316*).

Haddock A smaller member of the cod family, this lean North Atlantic fish can be substituted for cod in most recipes, although its flesh may be slightly softer.

Halibut A flatfish, like flounder, halibut is found in both the North Atlantic and northern Pacific waters. This very large fish is usually marketed in fillets or steaks, more commonly frozen (or thawed) than fresh. Poach, bake, broil, or sauté halibut steaks as you would salmon; you can also substitute firm, white-fleshed halibut fillets in flounder or sole recipes.

Lingcod A popular Pacific coast fish, lingcod is not a true cod, but has tender, delicate white flesh like its namesake. Whole lingcod, which weigh 3 to 10 pounds and up, are usually sold dressed, and markets also carry fillets and steaks. Try this fish baked, poached, or grilled.

Mahi-mahi This is the Hawaiian name for a fish that is also called "dolphin" or "dolphin fish" because of its resemblance to the porpoise (which is a mammal). Caught primarily in Pacific waters, it is most often sold in fillets or steaks, fresh or frozen, with the skin attached to hold the fish together during cooking. Mahi-mahi has dense, sweet, moist flesh something like swordfish, and it can be cooked in the same ways: baked, broiled, and poached. Despite its rich flavor, mahi-mahi is a lean fish.

Monkfish You won't find whole monkfish for sale at your market; this saltwater fish is so ugly that the head is cut off, and its thick, tapering tail section is sold whole or in fillets. Also called goosefish or anglerfish (*lotte* in French), monkfish has appeared on many American restaurant menus in

canned fish

Not only are canned versions of fish a convenient way to add fish to your diet, but if you choose carefully, they provide the same health benefits as fresh fish, being low in calories, fat, and sodium, and high in protein, B vitamins, and omega-3 fatty acids.

If possible, choose canned fish packed in water, not oil. This applies primarily to tuna, because salmon is so fatty it doesn't need a fatty packing liquid. Sardines do not come in a water-packed version.

The vegetable oil that is commonly used in canned tuna doubles the calories in the fish and adds up to 10 times more fat. Only 15 percent of the calories in water-packed tuna come from fat, compared to over 60 percent in the oil-packed version. Draining the oil removes about a third of the calories and half the fat, but can also remove the valuable omega-3 fatty acids.

One study found that while draining water-packed tuna removed only about 3 percent of the omega-3s, draining oil-packed tuna removed 15 to 25 percent of these valuable nutrients.

Added salt is another nutritional concern with canned fish. Processors usually add four to 10 times the amount of sodium naturally found in fresh fish. Fortunately, "low-salt" and "no-salt-added" varieties are available. "Low-salt" tuna usually has about 50 percent less sodium, and tuna marked "no-salt-added" contains 90 percent less.

Some canned fish have an added health benefit that might not be obvious. The canning process softens the bones of salmon and sardines. If the bones are eaten, these fish can supply significant amounts of calcium—200 to 325 milligrams per 3 ounces.

recent years (it has long been popular in France). Its texture and flavor are often compared to lobster, and you can substitute this lean fish for lobster meat or scallops in many recipes. (Monkfish is sometimes referred to as "poor man's lobster.") It can be poached, sautéed, stir-fried, cut into medallions, or used in chowders and soups.

Mullet Most of our saltwater mullet comes from Florida, with silver and striped mullet the most common species. This fish has distinctive areas of dark and light meat: The dark meat is strong-flavored and oily, while the light flesh is mild and sweet. Buy mullet dressed for baking, broiling, grilling, or sautéing; it is also sometimes sold in fillets.

Orange roughy This small saltwater fish is mostly imported from New Zealand and sold in the form of frozen fillets. It has become quite popular, probably because its firm, slightly sweet white flesh possesses an adaptable "neutral" flavor like that of flounder. Orange roughy can be cooked by almost any method and substituted for other mild-flavored, white-fleshed fish such as cod, haddock, and halibut.

Perch Although some species of saltwater fish are called perch (*see rockfish, below*), the true perch is a freshwater fish; yellow perch and walleye from the Great Lakes are the most familiar American types. Most perch are caught by sport fishermen. Weighing 3 pounds or less, this fish has firm, flaky white flesh and is sold whole, dressed, and as fillets. Small perch is most commonly sautéed, but can also be baked, broiled, or poached.

Pike This slender freshwater fish, also called pickerel, comes from the Great Lakes and other northern U.S. and Canadian lakes. Its intricate bone structure can make filleting this fish difficult. The flesh is flaky and somewhat dry, so it's best to bake pike with a moist stuffing or a sauce, or poach it; small whole fish are often sautéed. Pike is one of the leanest of all fish, with less than 1 gram of fat per serving.

Pollack (Alaska and Atlantic) Tons of mild white *Alaska pollack* from the Pacific go into fish sticks and surimi (ground up pollack that is flavored and shaped to imitate such shellfish meat as crab, lobster, and scallops), making it one of the top ten fish in the American diet. *Atlantic pollack,* a different species, is richer and more flavorful. Though sometimes called Boston bluefish, it is not related to true bluefish. It has a dark layer of flesh just under the skin on one side, which can be removed for a milder flavor. Cook this lean fish as you would cod—bake, broil, poach, sauté, or use it in chowders and soups.

Porgy (scup) This mild, delicate-tasting fish has a big following on the East Coast. It can be found dressed, whole, and occasionally filleted, and is often served panfried.

Rockfish (ocean perch) Fish of this large family go by many names. The Atlantic species is called *Atlantic ocean perch, rosefish,* or *redfish;* some of the many Pacific varieties may be called *rockfish, rock cod, Pacific ocean perch,* or even Pacific red snapper (although they are quite different from cod, fresh-

HALIBUT / 3 ounces cooked	
Calories	119
Protein (g)	23
Carbohydrate (g)	0
Dietary fiber (g)	0
Total fat (g)	2.5
Saturated fat (g)	0.4
Monounsaturated fat (g)	0.8
Polyunsaturated fat (g)	0.8
Cholesterol (mg)	35
Potassium (mg)	490
Sodium (mg)	59

KEY NUTRIENTS (%RDA/AI*)		
Niacin	6.1 mg	(38%)
Vitamin B_6	0.3 mg	(20%)
Vitamin B_{12}	1.2 mcg	(49%)
Iron	0.9 mg	(11%)
Magnesium	91 mg	(22%)
Selenium	40 mcg	(72%)

*For more detailed information on RDA and AI, see page 88.

water perch, and true red snapper). All types of rockfish/ocean perch have mild, firm, white flesh and have become very popular throughout the United States. Market size is 2 to 5 pounds and the fish are sold mostly in the form of thick fillets, which can be cooked by just about any method.

Scrod This is young cod (*see Cod, page 312*).

Sea bass Various species, including the large, diverse family of fish known as groupers, are marketed under this name (sometimes spelled "seabass"). Most have firm, lean, white flesh. One of the most popular species is *black sea bass,* a small fish (usually under 5 pounds) found in the Atlantic; it is marketed mostly in the Northeast and is popular as a steamed or fried dish in Chinese restaurants. Usually sold fresh and whole, and sometimes filleted, it can also be baked, broiled, or poached. *Red* and *black groupers* are taken from southern Atlantic waters and the Gulf of Mexico. Weighing from 3 to 20 pounds, they are sold fresh as steaks or fillets, which are best broiled, poached, sautéed, or stuffed and baked. Grouper is also good in soups and stews. The same cooking methods are also suitable for *white sea bass,* a West Coast fish from a different family that typically weighs 10 to 15 pounds and is sold whole, pan-dressed, or in thick fillets or steaks.

Sea trout See Weakfish (*page 318*).

Shark (mako, dogfish) If you aren't a fish lover, you may nevertheless find this notorious predator appealing as food. Shark has a lean, meaty, "unfishy" texture, a mild flavor, and is free of bones, due to its cartilaginous skeleton. *Mako shark,* which can weigh up to 1,000 pounds, are similar to swordfish in texture and flavor. *Dogfish* is a small shark (averaging about 2 feet long) with firm, rich flesh. Other types of shark, such as thresher, blue, and blacktip, also appear on the market. Shark is usually sold in thick steaks; sometimes in fillets. The meaty flesh holds up well in grilling and can also be baked or poached. (Fresh shark may have a slight odor of ammonia, which can be lessened by soaking the fish in salted water, milk, or water and lemon juice for a few hours, then rinsing it before cooking. If shark has a strong ammonia odor, it has not been properly treated after it was caught; pass it up.)

Skate (ray) This flat, kite-shaped ocean creature is a relative of the shark. Like the shark, it has tough skin instead of scales, and a cartilaginous skeleton rather than bones. Usually just the triangular "wings" (not the body itself) are eaten; it's easiest to buy skate skinned and filleted. Skate flesh has striations of muscle that make it resemble crabmeat in texture; its flavor is similar to that of scallops or other shellfish. Try skate baked, broiled, sautéed, or poached. Like shark, skate may have a slight odor of ammonia when you buy it. If it does, follow the suggestions given for preparing shark, above. Unlike most seafood, skate improves with a little aging: Storing it in the refrigerator for a day or two will tenderize it.

Smelt This small, delicately flavored fish is related to salmon. Some species live in fresh water, while others are found in the Pacific and the Atlantic. *Rainbow smelt* and *eulachon* are the major commercial species.

SNAPPER 3 ounces cooked	
Calories	109
Protein (g)	22
Carbohydrate (g)	0
Dietary fiber (g)	0
Total fat (g)	1.5
Saturated fat (g)	0.3
Monounsaturated fat (g)	0.3
Polyunsaturated fat (g)	0.5
Cholesterol (mg)	40
Potassium (mg)	444
Sodium (mg)	49

KEY NUTRIENTS (%RDA/AI*)	
Vitamin B$_6$	0.4 mg (23%)
Vitamin B$_{12}$	3.0 mcg (124%)
Selenium	42 mcg (76%)

*For more detailed information on RDA and AI, see page 88.

Because smelt are small and are usually eaten whole, they are most commonly sold dressed or drawn. The soft bones are edible, but the fish is also easy to bone once it's cooked. Smelt are very often deep-fried or sautéed, but they can also be broiled, grilled, or baked.

Snapper There are a number of snapper species in U.S. waters, and *red snapper,* caught off the southeastern coast, is by far the best known. Because this fish is in great demand, other species (such as mutton snapper and silk snapper) may be falsely advertised as red snapper in markets and restaurants. You can recognize the real thing by its bright red skin (usually left on the fillets to identify it) and its light-colored flesh. Because red snapper tends to be expensive, you're more likely to find it in a restaurant than in your fish market. If you can buy a dressed 4- to 6-pound fish, show it to best advantage by baking, grilling, poaching, or steaming it whole; bake or broil fillets.

Sole See Flounder (*page 313*).

pickled & smoked fish

Since fish is one of the most perishable of all foods, it's not surprising that techniques for preserving it were developed before the advent of refrigeration. Pickling and smoking are two time-honored methods. Not only do they help preserve the fish, they also alter and enhance its texture and flavor: Pickled herring and smoked salmon are delicacies quite different from either fish in its fresh state.

Oily fish such as salmon, sturgeon, sablefish, and butterfish are favorites for smoking; trout and whitefish are American smoked favorites. Finnan haddie is a famous Scottish smoked haddock specialty. Herring is sometimes smoked but more commonly pickled. You can choose from Dutch maatjes herring (lightly sugar-cured), German Bismarck herring (pickled in vinegar with onions), English kippers and bloaters (salted, cold-smoked herring), and Jewish-style schmaltz (fat) herring in sour cream sauce.

In addition to cold- and hot-smoked salmon, Scandinavians prepare gravlax, salmon cured with salt, sugar, and herbs. Lox is salmon cured in brine, while the salmon that is sold as "Nova Scotia" or "Nova" is cold-smoked. British kippered salmon is brined and then hot- or cold-smoked.

Various types of smoked and pickled fish are sold by the pound at the deli counters of many grocery stores, in fish markets, and in gourmet shops; less-expensive packaged versions are found in the dairy case of many supermarkets. When sold in bulk, these products will not have nutritional labels, so be aware that they can be very high in sodium (667 milligrams of sodium in 3 ounces of smoked chinook salmon, 740 milligrams in the same size serving of pickled herring, for example). Since smoked and pickled fish are made from fatty fish, they are relatively high in fat (only 4 grams for the salmon, but 15 grams for the herring). Delectable smoked sablefish is especially high in fat, with nearly 17 grams of fat in a 3-ounce, 219-calorie serving.

Although pickling and smoking do preserve fish to some extent, they do not eliminate the need for proper storage. Unless canned or vacuum-packed, these products should be stored in the refrigerator, where they will keep for about a week. Smoked salmon can be frozen if carefully wrapped, but its texture may change slightly. Also, unless the fish is hot-smoked for a long period of time, or actually cooked, the process of curing, salting, or pickling will not necessarily kill dangerous organisms that may be present in the fish. Freezing at -4° for at least 3 days will destroy parasites, but this is not appropriate for all types of preserved fish.

Striped bass The striped bass, also called striper or rockfish, is a large fish with firm, well-flavored flesh. Once abundant on both coasts, striped bass has become much rarer because of overfishing and contamination with PCBs, and commercial fishing is now banned in most Eastern states and in California. Fish farms, where bass are harvested year-round, are becoming the principal source of this fish.

Swordfish Highly prized by sport fishermen, swordfish can be found on both U.S. coasts. This large saltwater fish has meaty, rich-tasting flesh. Unfortunately, like many fish, swordfish has been severely overfished. Another drawback to swordfish is that many fish have been found to contain large concentrations of mercury. Other big fish, such as shark, are also susceptible to mercury contamination, but swordfish have been found to contain the highest levels. Since this problem was discovered, the FDA has monitored both domestic and imported swordfish very closely. Swordfish is usually sold in boneless loins (a lengthwise quarter-section of the whole fish), steaks, or chunks, fresh or frozen. Its exceptionally firm flesh makes it a good choice for kebabs; or, broil, poach, or bake swordfish steaks.

Tilapia Tilapia is sometimes called sunshine snapper, cherry snapper, Nile perch, mouthbrooder, or St. Peter's fish. Tilapia is an important farm-raised fish, which was once largely imported, but is now being farmed in this country. This firm-fleshed, mild tasting fish can be prepared like flounder or snapper.

Tilefish Caught in deep Atlantic waters, tilefish average about 10 pounds. This fish was not very popular until a few years ago, but now is increasingly available and worth seeking out for its firm, pinkish-white flesh that has some of the sweetness of lobster or scallops. You'll find whole tilefish and fillets in the market. Tilefish can be substituted for other white-fleshed fish such as cod, where its sweet flavor will be a bonus. Use tilefish in chowders, or bake, broil, poach, or steam it.

Trout (freshwater) Related to salmon, trout are freshwater fish that, in markets, range from 1½ to 10 pounds whole. *Rainbow trout,* the most frequently available, is sold fresh or frozen throughout the country all year. It is an immensely popular game fish, but only farm-raised rainbows are sold commercially. *Steelhead trout* is an ocean-going rainbow trout that breeds (and tastes) like salmon; it is now also farmed. Trout generally have mild, sweet flesh, though texture, flavor, and fat content vary. Usually, the larger the fish, the higher the fat content. Smaller trout are sold whole or dressed. They are often panfried, but can also be broiled, grilled, or baked; try poaching or baking whole larger fish (or steaks or fillets).

Tuna See Tuna (*page 578*).

Weakfish (sea trout) This fish's name comes from its fragile mouth, which tends to break when the fish is hooked. The sweet, pale flesh is also

mercury in fish

The FDA warns pregnant women—and those who might become pregnant or who are nursing—not to eat shark, swordfish, king mackerel, or tilefish because these may contain mercury, which can damage the brain and nervous system of the fetus. The FDA also advises pregnant women to eat no more than 12 ounces of fish a week and to vary the types of fish they eat.

rather tender, and should be handled carefully in cooking. Weakfish average 1 to 3 pounds and are abundant on the Atlantic and Gulf coasts. Weakfish are sold whole, dressed, and in fillets, and can be substituted for striped bass, or for less flavorful fish such as cod and pollack. Bake whole large weakfish, and grill, broil, or steam smaller fish and fillets.

▶ Availability Because of more sophisticated fishing methods and improved refrigeration and shipping, fishermen are able to bring fish to market that were previously either uncatchable or too perishable. We also rely increasingly on farm-raised fish as well as imports from Canada, Latin America, and even New Zealand.

Most fish markets, therefore, now offer many kinds of fresh fish. It's true that a handful of species—including tuna, pollack, cod, salmon, and flounder—account for at least three-quarters of all the fish we eat. But other varieties are growing in popularity, and many are available nationwide or over a fairly large area of the country.

choosing the best

Since government inspection is not mandated for seafood, it is up to the consumer to find a reliable source for fresh, wholesome fish. You have to trust your senses when shopping for fish: Overall quality can be judged by sight, smell, and touch. Start by locating a good fish dealer, either a fish market or a supermarket fish department with a good reputation, a clean appearance, and a knowledgeable staff. Ask questions about unfamiliar fish (and expect informed answers), and let the dealer know if seafood you've bought is ever unsatisfactory: You are entitled to return it if it is less than perfectly fresh.

Schedule your shopping so you can get seafood home and into the refrigerator as quickly as possible. Make the fish store (or fish counter) the last stop of your shopping trip. In warm weather, or when you may be delayed on the trip home, have the fish packed in ice.

Your nose will tell you instantly whether the fish in the shop are fresh; on walking in the door, you should smell only a saltwater scent, not a "fishy," sour, or ammonialike odor. When buying prepackaged fish, take a closer sniff: Off-odors will penetrate the plastic. The date on the label will help you choose the freshest fish in the display, but don't place total faith in it: Ask the fish dealer when it was packaged.

Fish decays much faster than beef or chicken, so it must be kept very cold to forestall bacterial growth. It should be displayed on top of clean ice, with metal trays or sheets of paper or plastic to shield the delicate flesh of fish steaks or fillets from direct contact with the ice. (Whole or dressed fish, protected by their scales, can safely be placed directly on ice, and should be covered with some ice as well.) Fish should not be stacked too deeply or displayed under hot lights.

Whole fresh fish should have tight, shiny scales, and should not feel slippery or slimy. The eyes should be bright and clear, not clouded or sunken in their

RAINBOW TROUT 3 ounces cooked	
Calories	144
Protein (g)	21
Carbohydrate (g)	0
Dietary fiber (g)	0
Total fat (g)	6.1
Saturated fat (g)	1.8
Monounsaturated fat (g)	1.8
Polyunsaturated fat (g)	2.0
Cholesterol (mg)	58
Potassium (mg)	375
Sodium (mg)	36

KEY NUTRIENTS (%RDA/AI*)	
Thiamin	0.2 mg (17%)
Niacin	7.5 mg (47%)
Vitamin B_6	0.3 mg (20%)
Vitamin B_{12}	4.2 mcg (176%)
Selenium	13 mcg (23%)

*For more detailed information on RDA and AI, see page 88.

sockets. Gills should be clean and tinged with pink or red, never brownish or sticky. The surface of a steak or fillet should look freshly cut, and the fish should not be sitting in a pool of liquid. (Prepackaged fish should not contain excess liquid, either.) The flesh should look moist, slightly translucent, and dense, not flaky. Pass up steaks or fillets that are dried out at the edges.

Whether whole or cut, fresh fish is firm and resilient: If you poke it with your finger, the flesh should spring back, not remain indented.

Frozen fish can be of very high quality, but only if it has been handled properly. Sometimes fish are flash-frozen on the boat just after they are caught; later the fish are thawed and sold as fresh. The quality may be comparable or even superior to fresh fish, and such fish needs no special treatment (except that it should not be refrozen when you get it home). When buying prepackaged frozen fish, be sure that the fish is still solidly frozen when you buy it. Watch out for excessive quantities of ice crystals or water stains on the package, or for cloudy liquid in the package if the wrapping is clear. Avoid fish with freezer burn, which will appear as whitened, cottony-looking patches.

▶ When you get home It's best to use fish within a day of buying it, although it can be kept an extra day or two if it is of very high quality and was very fresh when purchased. Whole or drawn fish will keep longer than steaks or fillets.

Place it, still in the wrapper from the market, in a glass or enamel pan in the coldest part of the refrigerator. Fill a plastic bag with crushed ice and place it on top of the fish. Check the fish daily and pour off any liquid that may have accumulated in the bottom of the pan. Replace the ice.

If you want to freeze fish yourself, you'll need a freezer that stays at 0°. Fish for freezing should be perfectly fresh and of high quality. Thawed fish is sometimes sold as fresh, so be sure to ask the dealer if you suspect this, because fish that has been frozen should not be refrozen. The faster the fish freezes, the better, so freeze whole fish only if they weigh less than 2 pounds; cut larger fish into fillets or steaks. Freeze whole fish and fillets individually.

Rinse and dry the fish and wrap it tightly in heavy-duty freezer paper or plastic wrap. Overwrap the package with foil or a freezer bag, then label and date the package and freeze it quickly. (Packaged fresh fish should be rinsed and rewrapped.) Freeze fish that you've purchased frozen (and that has not been thawed) in its original wrapping. Frozen lean fish keeps longer than frozen fatty fish. Use frozen fatty fish within 6 weeks, frozen lean fish will keep for up to 3 months.

preparing to use

Fish can be just as easy to prepare as chicken breasts. If you buy dressed fish, fillets, or steaks, there is virtually no additional preparation necessary. Just rinse the fish quickly (or dip it briefly in cold water), then pat it dry before cooking. Always check for bones remaining in a fillet (this is likely with round fish) by running your finger across the fillet; if you feel the tips of any bones, pull them out with tweezers.

If you want to thaw frozen fish, place it in the refrigerator overnight; do not thaw it at room temperature; the fish may be subject to bacterial contamination. As with raw meat or poultry, you must thoroughly wash all surfaces and utensils (and your hands) used to prepare raw fish; be particularly careful not to bring cooked food into contact with raw fish or with utensils that were used to prepare it.

Don't marinate fish at room temperature; place the fish and marinade in the refrigerator.

the scoop on caviar

Most people eat caviar, if at all, in small amounts and rarely. As an occasional treat, caviar is not bad; it has fewer calories and more nutrients than the same amount of potato chips.

Whether it's the expensive "real" kind, made from sturgeon roe, or the cheaper roes of salmon, lumpfish, and whitefish, caviar is high in protein: 4 grams per tablespoon. A tablespoon also contains 133 percent of the RDA for vitamin B_{12}, 24 percent for iron, along with vitamin A, vitamin E, and some magnesium. As for calories, there are 40 per tablespoon, or fewer than 80 per ounce. There are no nutritional differences between one type of caviar and another, but there are differences in taste, texture, color, and price.

A tablespoon of any fish roe contains 94 milligrams of cholesterol, almost a third of the recommended maximum daily allowance. However, caviar has a moderate fat content—about 2 grams per tablespoon—and, like other fish, it supplies some omega-3s (about 1.1 grams, which is comparable to some of the better sources, such as mackerel).

Fresh sturgeon caviar labeled malossol (Russian for "lightly salted") contains approximately 4 percent salt as a preservative, which works out to about 240 to 300 milligrams of sodium per tablespoon. The sodium content of economy-class caviars (which may be made from "injured" eggs) can go as high as 700 milligrams per tablespoon.

flaxseed

One of the oldest known cultivated plants, flaxseed is thought to have originated in Mesopotamia, where it was cultivated as long ago as 5000 B.C. The flax plant has provided not only sustenance for humans, but has also been prized for fiber used for clothing: It's the source of linen. Ancient Egyptian burial chambers contained flaxseeds as well as wall paintings depicting the cultivation of flax and the manufacture of cloth made from flax fiber. Flaxseed gradually spread across Africa, Europe, and finally to North America. It is currently enjoying a resurgence of popularity, probably due to its interesting health benefits.

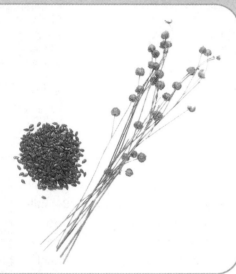

flaxseed

nutritional profile

Flaxseed supplies an essential fatty acid, alpha-linolenic acid (ALA), which may contribute to a wide range of health benefits including cell membrane health, the production of prostaglandins (hormonelike substances that indirectly exert anti-inflammatory actions), and, most notably, cardioprotective abilities. A long-term study of 76,000 nurses (as well as other research) shows that ALA may prevent heart attacks. Not many foods are rich in it—only canola, flaxseed, and soybean oils, as well as walnuts and purslane (*see page 355*). In this study, nurses who over the years had consumed the equivalent of a daily tablespoon of canola oil, half an ounce of walnuts, or a little ground flaxseed had a one-third to one-half less risk of a fatal heart attack than those consuming little ALA.

In addition, ALA is converted by the body into the type of omega-3 fatty acids found mainly in fish. These "long chain" omega-3s, as they are sometimes referred to, make platelets in the blood less likely to stick together and may reduce inflammatory processes in blood vessels. Thus they reduce blood clotting, thereby lessening the chance of a heart attack. Unfortunately, the conversion of ALA to long chain omega-3s is a far less efficient process than getting the omega-3s directly from fish; still, every little bit helps.

Flaxseed is also high in fiber, including a type of soluble fiber that helps to lower cholesterol levels. The insoluble fiber in flaxseed keeps your digestive system running smoothly and helps to prevent constipation. Because flaxseed is rich in fiber, you should increase water intake along with it.

A caution: In rare instances people may have an allergic reaction to flaxseed and go into anaphylactic shock, as someone might from bee stings or nuts.

in the market

Flaxseed is available in *whole-seed* form, as flaxseed *meal*, and as flaxseed *oil*. All forms are available in health-food stores, and flaxseed oil can also be found in stores selling supplements.

FLAXSEED / 1 tablespoon	
Calories	47
Protein (g)	2
Carbohydrate (g)	4
Dietary fiber (g)	3.3
Total fat (g)	4.1
Saturated fat (g)	0.4
Monounsaturated fat (g)	0.8
Polyunsaturated fat (g)	2.7
Cholesterol (mg)	0
Potassium (mg)	82
Sodium (mg)	4

choosing the best

If you buy the whole seeds in bulk from a health-food store, sniff them to make sure they have not turned rancid. Over-the-hill flaxseeds will smell like oil paint. Ground flaxseed, with its increased surface area, is much more prone to rancidity than the whole seeds. It's best to buy whole seeds and grind them at home.

Flaxseed oil easily turns rancid. Therefore, you should buy oil that comes in an opaque bottle and from a store that keeps their flaxseed oil refrigerated.

▶ When you get home Transfer whole seeds to an airtight container and store in the refrigerator. The whole seeds should keep well for up to 1 year. Grind only as much as you need at one time; if you have leftover ground flaxseed, freeze in a sealed container for up to 6 months.

If you do buy the pre-ground meal, store it in the freezer. Sniff the meal before using it.

Store flaxseed oil in the refrigerator. If the oil goes rancid, discard it.

preparing to use

Your body can't derive any nutritional benefit from flaxseed if you consume the seeds whole (they pass right through your body), so ground (milled) flaxseed is best. You can buy prepared flaxseed meal, but because of its high fat content, the ground seeds can go rancid quickly. You're better off grinding your own, using a coffee grinder or mini food processor.

serving suggestions

• Stir coarsely ground flaxseeds into cooked cereals or sprinkle it into yogurt.

• Make a pesto with fresh basil, garlic, ground flaxseed, flaxseed oil, and grated Parmesan cheese. Toss with hot pasta.

• Use ground flaxseed in baked goods, but don't replace more than about one-fifth of the flour in a recipe or the texture will suffer.

• Substitute flaxseed oil for other oils in salad dressings.

• Use ground flaxseed to replace one-fourth of the flour in pancake or waffle mixes.

• Stir a tablespoon of flaxseed oil into your morning orange juice.

➤ phytochemicals in flaxseed

Flaxseed is the richest source of lignans, which provide fiber. Some lignans are also a type of phytoestrogen (isoflavonoids are another type). In the process of digestion, bacteria convert lignans into estrogenlike substances called enterodiol and enterolactone. These may have antitumor effects. Phytoestrogens are also found in other plants, including soy, certain herbs, whole grains, and other seeds.

Lignans and other flaxseed components may also have antioxidant properties—that is, they may reduce the activity of free radicals, which cause damage at the cellular level. Studies have shown that flaxseed can reduce tumors in lab animals. So far there's no convincing evidence of a similar action in humans, though some ongoing studies may provide answers.

In addition, lignans may play some role in lowering cholesterol and possibly in maintaining bone density. (Flaxseed oil usually does not contain lignans, though some processors do add some lignans back into the oil.)

flour, nonwheat

There are many reasons to cook with flours made from plants other than wheat—such as other grains, beans, seeds, tubers, and roots. For people who are allergic to gluten (the protein formed when wheat flour is made into batter or dough) or to wheat itself, these flours offer excellent alternatives. Some types of flour also add unusual flavors, or are especially good at thickening liquid mixtures, such as sauces and soups (arrowroot and tapioca are in this category).

There are some obstacles to deal with when nonwheat flours are used for baking. Because they produce little or no gluten when mixed with liquid, these flours need special treatment in order to form a workable dough or batter that will rise, hold its shape, and have a pleasing texture. If a wheat or gluten allergy is not the problem and the other flour is being used to boost flavor or nutrition, a suitable formula might be: As a starting point, use 1 part nonwheat flour for 4 parts of wheat flour.

nutritional profile

Nonwheat flours also have their own merits aside from their lack of gluten: Some are particularly high in protein, or in amino acids that wheat lacks. Some contain more dietary fiber than wheat, or offer phytochemicals that wheat does not. Nonwheat flours provide an array of essential vitamins and minerals and generally confer the same benefits as the grain or bean from which they are derived. Similar to wheat flour, unrefined nonwheat flour tends to have the highest vitamin, mineral, fiber, and phytochemical content since all of the healthful parts of the grain or bean are used.

in the market

bean & legume flours

Any dried bean or legume can be finely ground into flour. There are some pre-ground bean flours available, or you could make your own using a wheat mill or grinder. Some of the more common bean flours include:

Chick-pea flour This flour has a rich culinary tradition in both Indian cuisine—where it is known as *besan* or *chana* and is used in pancakes, stews, and curries—and in Italian cuisine where *farina di ceci* (chick-pea flour) is used to make pasta and a polentalike dish. Chick-peas are also used in some blended flours, such as *garfava flour* (a combination of chick-peas and fava beans) and *dhokra flour* (a combination of rice, lentils, and chick-peas).

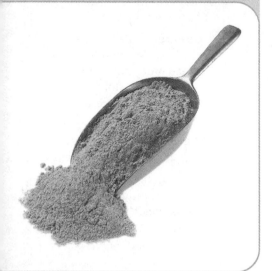

buckwheat flour

BUCKWHEAT FLOUR ⅓ cup	
Calories	133
Protein (g)	5
Carbohydrate (g)	28
Dietary fiber (g)	4.0
Total fat (g)	1.2
Saturated fat (g)	0.3
Monounsaturated fat (g)	0.4
Polyunsaturated fat (g)	0.4
Cholesterol (mg)	0
Potassium (mg)	229
Sodium (mg)	4

KEY NUTRIENTS (%RDA/AI*)	
Thiamin	0.2 mg (14%)
Niacin	2.4 mg (15%)
Vitamin E	3.1 mg (21%)
Iron	1.6 mg (20%)
Magnesium	99 mg (24%)
Zinc	1.2 mg (11%)

*For more detailed information on RDA and AI, see page 88.

Lentil flour Indians use a flour made from a certain type of lentil (called *urad dal*) to make the dough for a crispy, fried wafer called pappadum.

Soy flour Made from roasted soybeans that have been ground into a fine powder, soy flour is a rich source of protein, isoflavones, folate, iron, and magnesium. Soy flour contains almost three times the amount of protein as wheat flour. Soy flour may be used in a number of ways, including adding it to sauces and gravies as a thickener, or to pancake batter for a nutty flavor and protein boost. Though it can be used to enrich breads and other baked goods, it cannot completely replace wheat flour because it has no gluten. Soy flour is available in *defatted, low-fat,* and *full-fat* forms, with the full-fat flour containing natural soybean oils.

grain flours

Amaranth flour The seeds of the amaranth plant (*see Amaranth, page 158*) boast a higher percentage of protein than most other grains, and have more fiber than wheat and rice. They are also higher in the amino acid lysine, which gives this flour a more complete protein than those made from other grains. Amaranth flour has a slightly peppery taste and can be used in savory quick breads and other baked goods. However, it can be expensive and is not widely available.

Barley flour This mild-flavored flour made from barley grain contains some gluten (though not enough to use it on its own in baking).

Buckwheat flour A common ingredient in pancake mixes, buckwheat flour is also used to make Japanese soba noodles. It is available in *light, medium,* and *dark* varieties, depending on the kind of buckwheat it is milled from. The dark flour boasts the strongest flavor. You can make your own buckwheat flour by processing whole buckwheat groats in a blender or food processor.

Corn flour This is made from whole cornmeal—either *blue, white,* or *yellow*—ground to a floury consistency. Blue corn flour made from roasted blue corn is called *atole.* You can make corn flour yourself by processing cornmeal in a blender or food processor.

Masa harina Made from hominy (lime- or lye-treated corn), this flour is used to make corn tortillas. It is made with either *yellow* or *white* corn.

Millet flour This yellow flour is high in protein and easy to digest. It is traditionally used to make the Indian flatbread called *roti.*

Oat flour Milled from either the entire oat kernel or the endosperm only, oat flour is frequently used in ready-to-eat breakfast cereals. You can make your own to use in baking by grinding rolled oats in a food processor or blender (1¼ cups of rolled oats will yield 1 cup of oat flour).

Pumpernickel flour (dark rye meal flour) Made from the whole rye grain, including the bran, this is used for making pumpernickel bread.

Quinoa flour Higher in fat than wheat flour, quinoa flour makes baked goods moister. You can make your own quinoa flour by processing whole

FULL-FAT SOY FLOUR ⅓ cup	
Calories	122
Protein (g)	11
Carbohydrate (g)	9
Dietary fiber (g)	2.7
Total fat (g)	5.8
Saturated fat (g)	0.8
Monounsaturated fat (g)	1.3
Polyunsaturated fat (g)	3.3
Cholesterol (mg)	0
Potassium (mg)	706
Sodium (mg)	4

KEY NUTRIENTS (%RDA/AI*)	
Thiamin	0.2 mg (14%)
Riboflavin	0.3 mg (25%)
Vitamin E	2.4 mg (16%)
Folate	98 mcg (24%)
Iron	1.8 mg (22%)
Magnesium	120 mg (29%)
Zinc	1.1 mg (10%)

*For more detailed information on RDA and AI, see page 88.

quinoa in a blender; stop before the flour is too fine—it should be slightly coarse, like cornmeal.

Rice flour Both white and brown rice are used to make rice flour. *White rice flour* is very fine-textured as it is made from polished white rice, while *brown rice flour* contains the bran, giving it a coarser texture. Brown rice flour also provides more fiber than white.

Rye flour In combination with wheat flour, rye flour (which contains some gluten) is most commonly used in breads. *Light, medium,* and *dark* varieties (with dark having the strongest flavor) are available. Light rye flour may be labeled *"bolted,"* which means the flour has been sifted to remove the bran and germ. Dark rye flours are often *"unbolted,"* and so contain a good deal more fiber. When adding rye flour to bread recipes, use less of the dark flour than you would of the light flour, or the flavor will be too dominant.

Sorghum flour Sorghum is a cereal grain that isn't consumed much in this country, though it's a staple grain elsewhere in the world. Sorghum flour works well in breads when combined with wheat flours.

Teff flour Made from the ancient grain teff, this flour has a nutty flavor and can be used to make pancakes, waffles, and quick breads. Ethiopians use a

starches

There are several high-starch plants and tubers that are used to make flour-like substances that are more often than not called "flour" instead of starch. These starches are generally not used in baking (though they can be) but are used to coat foods for frying or for thickening liquids. In some cases, the vegetable itself is dried and ground to a powder. In other cases, starch is extracted from the plant.

Arrowroot flour The rootstalks of a tropical plant are the source of this flour, often used as a thickener for sauces and desserts; the finely powdered arrowroot turns completely clear when dissolved (giving gloss to sauces), while adding no starchy flavor. Because arrowroot flour is easy to digest, it is also used as an ingredient in cookies intended for infants and young children.

Cornstarch This silky ingredient is made from only the endosperm (starchy part) of the corn kernel. It is used to thicken sauces and to create baked goods with a particularly fine texture. In England, cornstarch is called corn flour.

Potato flour (potato starch) Steamed potatoes are dried and then ground to a powder to make this gluten-free flour, which is commonly used in baked goods for Passover (when wheat flour may not be used). There are also pastas made from potato flour.

Tapioca flour (cassava, manioc) Milled from the dried starch of the cassava root, this flour thickens when heated with water and is often used to give body to puddings, fruit pie fillings, and soups. It can also be used in baking. Gari flour, made from fermented, roasted, and ground cassavas, is used in Nigerian cooking. It has a slightly sour flavor.

Water-chestnut flour (water-chestnut powder) This Asian ingredient is a fine, powdery starch that is used to thicken sauces (it can be substituted for cornstarch) and to coat foods before frying to give them a delicate, crisp coating.

White sweet potato flour Made from steamed and dried (not roasted) white sweet potatoes, this can be used as a thickener, added to pancake and quick-bread batters, or for pasta.

fermented batter made with teff flour to make their staple pancakelike flat-bread called *injera*.

Triticale flour A hybrid of wheat and rye, triticale is higher in gluten than other nonwheat flours but still needs to be combined with a wheat flour to produce a satisfying texture in baked goods. A close relative of wheat, it should not be eaten by those with gluten allergies.

nut & seed flours

Nut flours are ground from the solids that remain after nuts have been pressed for oil. Seed flours are generally made by grinding the endosperm only, making a defatted or partially defatted flour. The flours can be used in baking as well as for breading fish or chicken for sautéing. Nut and seed flours include: *almond flour, hazelnut (filbert) flour, peanut flour, pistachio flour, pumpkin seed flour, sesame seed flour, sunflower seed flour,* and *walnut flour.* There is also a flour made from chestnuts, but because it is naturally low in fat, *chestnut flour* is ground from the whole nut.

nut & grain meals

Meals are really just flours with an exceptionally coarse grind. Many grains come in this coarse form.

Cornmeal Ground from either *yellow, blue,* or *white* corn, cornmeal is often sold de-germed in order to extend its shelf life, but you can find *"unbolted" cornmeal,* which contains both the bran and germ. Cornmeal is widely used in breads, pancakes, and muffins. More finely ground cornmeal becomes corn flour.

Millet meal This is coarsely ground whole-grain millet and is used in breads and for cereal. You can purchase already ground millet meal or grind your own in a spice or coffee grinder.

Nut meals These meals are ground from whole nuts (unlike nut flours, which are ground from defatted nut solids). As a result, nut meals are pastier (and oilier) than nut flours.

▶ Availability If you can't find these products in your supermarket, try a specialty food shop, a health-food store, gourmet shop, or Asian grocery store; they are also available by mail-order.

choosing the best

Because flour can become rancid or buggy as it sits around, shop for it in markets that do a brisk turnover.

▶ When you get home Low-fat flours, like potato, arrowroot, tapioca, water-chestnut, white rice, and cornstarch, can be stored at room temperature for 6 to 12 months in a tightly covered container, because there's no fat to go rancid. Whole-grain and nut flours, on the other hand, should be refrigerated in a tightly covered container (or in the freezer for longer storage).

POTATO FLOUR / ⅓ cup	
Calories	211
Protein (g)	4
Carbohydrate (g)	49
Dietary fiber (g)	3.5
Total fat (g)	0.2
Saturated fat (g)	0.1
Monounsaturated fat (g)	0
Polyunsaturated fat (g)	0.1
Cholesterol (mg)	0
Potassium (mg)	591
Sodium (mg)	33

KEY NUTRIENTS (%RDA/AI*)	
Thiamin	0.1 mg (11%)
Niacin	2.1 mg (13%)
Vitamin B$_6$	0.5 mg (27%)
Iron	0.8 mg (10%)

*For more detailed information on RDA and AI, see page 88.

flour, wheat

The primary use of flour is in baked goods, such as bread, cakes, and muffins, and as the main ingredient in pasta and noodles. But flour plays other roles in cooking—it's used to thicken soups, stews, and gravies; meats are often coated with flour before panfrying to help them brown better; and cake and muffin pans are floured before adding batter to prevent sticking.

For thousands of years, flour was milled by grinding kernels of grain between stones. Although you can still find stone-ground flour, today most flour is milled by the roller process, in which seeds are alternately put through a series of high-speed steel rollers and mesh sifters. The rollers crack the grain, allowing the endosperm to be separated from the bran and germ. The endosperm is then ground to the desired consistency. For whole-grain flours, the bran and germ are returned to the flour at the end of the process.

nutritional profile

The vast majority of the wheat flour we eat is white, or refined, flour. White flour has been stripped of the bran and germ of the wheat kernel, and thus also most of its fiber and many of its nutrients. White flour is usually enriched with a few vitamins and minerals, sometimes even with fiber, but not all of the nutrients are replaced. Typically, white flour is enriched with iron and the B vitamins niacin, riboflavin, and thiamin, providing generous quantities of these nutrients. In addition, large amounts of folate are often added.

Unlike refined flour, whole-wheat flour is made from the entire wheat kernel—bran, germ, and endosperm. Because all of the healthful parts of the grain are used, vitamins, minerals, fiber, and phytochemicals are plentiful in whole-wheat flour. Just ⅓ cup is an excellent source of the B vitamins thiamin and niacin, plus tremendous quantities of the minerals copper, iron, and selenium. Whole-wheat flour also contains decent amounts of fat-soluble vitamin E (about 6 percent of the RDA in ⅓ cup) embedded in very small amounts of healthful unsaturated fat from the wheat kernel's germ layer; this means whole-wheat flour must be refrigerated (or frozen) in order to prevent the oils from going rancid.

in the market

Among grains, wheat flour is unique because it has the potential to produce gluten, a protein that imparts strength and elasticity to dough and influences the texture of baked goods. The gluten content of a flour depends on whether the flour is made from a hard or soft wheat; hard wheats are higher in protein than soft wheats, and thus produce more gluten. Most flour is a mixture of hard and soft wheat.

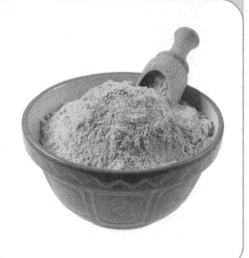

whole-wheat flour

ENRICHED WHITE FLOUR ⅓ cup	
Calories	150
Protein (g)	4
Carbohydrate (g)	32
Dietary fiber (g)	1.1
Total fat (g)	0.4
Saturated fat (g)	0.1
Monounsaturated fat (g)	0
Polyunsaturated fat (g)	0.2
Cholesterol (mg)	0
Potassium (mg)	44
Sodium (mg)	1

KEY NUTRIENTS (%RDA/AI*)	
Thiamin	0.3 mg (27%)
Riboflavin	0.2 mg (16%)
Niacin	2.4 mg (15%)
Folate	64 mcg (16%)
Iron	1.9 mg (24%)
Selenium	14 mcg (25%)

*For more detailed information on RDA and AI, see page 88.

Because the production of flour isn't standardized, flours from two manufacturers may use different milling procedures and consist of different blends, which will produce varying results in the kitchen. For example, all-purpose flours sold in the southern region of the United States contain a higher proportion of soft wheat, good for making the light, airy biscuits that are popular there. In northern states, by contrast, the preference is for breads rather than biscuits, and the all-purpose flour used in bread-making contains a higher proportion of hard wheats.

white flour

Refined white flour consists of the ground endosperm of the wheat kernel. White flour is popular because it produces lighter baked goods than whole-wheat flour and has an unequaled ability to produce gluten.

When the bran and germ are removed from the wheat kernel, vitamins and minerals are decreased, along with dietary fiber. Therefore, most white flour is enriched to replace some of the missing nutrients; if a flour has been enriched, the label will say so. There are many types of white flours:

All-purpose flour (plain, white) Made from a blend of hard and soft wheats, this type of flour has a "middle of the road" protein and starch content that makes it suitable for either breads or cakes and pastries. All-purpose flour is available presifted. This aerates the flour to make it lighter than standard all-purpose flour. However, all flour, whether labeled presifted or not, has a tendency to settle and become more compact in storage, so the benefit of presifting isn't always apparent.

Bleached flour When freshly milled, flour is slightly yellow. To whiten it, manufacturers could let the flour age naturally, but most choose to speed up the process by adding chemicals (such as benzoyl peroxide or acetone peroxide) to bleach it. This process gives the flour more gluten-producing potential, but naturally aged flours develop more gluten as well.

Bread flour This is made entirely from hard wheat; a high gluten content helps bread rise higher because the gluten traps and holds air bubbles as the dough is mixed and kneaded. (It's also available in whole-wheat form.)

Bromated flour Some manufacturers add a maturing agent such as bromate to flour in order to further develop the gluten and to make the kneading of doughs easier. Other maturing agents include phosphate, ascorbic acid, and malted barley.

Cake flour Finer than all-purpose flour, cake flour is made entirely from soft wheat. Because of its low gluten content, it is especially well suited for soft-textured cakes, quick breads, muffins, and cookies.

Durum flour Since it has the highest protein content of any flour, durum flour can produce the most gluten. It is frequently used for pasta.

Farina Farina is milled from the endosperm of any type of wheat, except for durum wheat (which is milled to make semolina, see below). Farina is primarily used in breakfast cereals and pasta.

WHOLE-WHEAT FLOUR ⅓ cup	
Calories	134
Protein (g)	5
Carbohydrate (g)	29
Dietary fiber (g)	4.8
Total fat (g)	0.7
Saturated fat (g)	0.1
Monounsaturated fat (g)	0.1
Polyunsaturated fat (g)	0.3
Cholesterol (mg)	0
Potassium (mg)	160
Sodium (mg)	2

KEY NUTRIENTS (%RDA/AI*)	
Thiamin	0.2 mg (15%)
Niacin	2.5 mg (16%)
Iron	1.5 mg (19%)
Selenium	28 mcg (51%)

*For more detailed information on RDA and AI, see page 88.

Gluten flour Made so that it has about twice the gluten strength of regular bread flour, this flour is used as a strengthening agent with other flours that are low in gluten-producing potential.

Instant flour (instant-blending, quick-mixing, granulated flour) Instant flour pours easily and mixes with liquids more readily than other flours. It is used to thicken sauces and gravies, but is not appropriate for most baking because of its very fine, powdery texture and high starch content.

Pastry flour (cookie flour, cracker flour) This flour has a gluten content slightly higher than cake flour but lower than all-purpose flour—making it well-suited for fine, light-textured pastries.

Self-rising flour Soft wheat is used to make this flour, which contains salt, a leavening agent such as baking soda or baking powder, and an acid-releasing substance. However, the strength of the leavener in some flours deteriorates within 2 months, so purchase only as much as you need during that period. Self-rising flour should never be used in yeast-leavened baked goods.

Semolina This is the coarsely ground endosperm (no bran, no germ) of durum wheat. Its high protein content makes it ideal for making commercial pasta, and it can also be used to make bread.

bugs in flour

Grain products in all stages of growth, processing, and packing are prey to beetles, moths, weevils, and their eggs. These insects are perfectly harmless—in fact, the FDA allows wheat flour to contain an average of 50 insect fragments per 50 grams (about ½ cup).

Infestation often occurs in the fields or in warehouses. Insects and their residues—including eggs—probably inhabit flour by the time it reaches your shelves. If you find evidence of insects in a new purchase, you can always take the flour back to the store for a refund. It might be easier, however, to simply sift or pick out any fragments.

whole-wheat flour

Since roller-milling separates the bran and the germ from the endosperm, the three components actually have to be reconstituted to produce whole-wheat flour. (The germ and bran are visible in the flour as minute brown flecks.) You may also find it called *graham flour* in the supermarket.

Because of the presence of bran, which reduces gluten development, baked goods made from whole-wheat flour are naturally heavier and denser than those made with white flour. Many bakers combine whole-wheat and white flour in order to gain the attributes of both. *Whole-wheat pastry flour* is also available.

For *stone-ground whole-wheat flour,* the kernels of wheat are crushed between two heavy, rotating stones, so that the bran and germ remain. Because oil in the germ is released during this process, stone-ground flour is more susceptible to rancidity. Nutritionally, there is no difference between stone-ground flour and roller-milled flour.

In addition to regular whole-wheat flours, there are a number of whole-grain flours made from close relatives of wheat.

Kamut flour Because of its very low gluten content, this flour is tolerated by many people with wheat allergies. Use it for bread baking.

Spelt flour Made from the ancient grain spelt, this low–gluten flour is well tolerated by many with wheat allergies. Use it for bread baking.

choosing the best

If buying in bulk, shop at a market that does a brisk turnover. Look for flour that is clean. Buy what you'll need for a couple of months and store it in the freezer.

Choose the flour you buy based on how you plan to use it. When buying packaged flour, buy a brand you like, since there is little difference between the brands.

▶ When you get home Flour doesn't keep forever and is more susceptible to spoilage than you might think. If flour is stored improperly or for too long, it can develop an off flavor or give unpredictable results in baking. Give flour the sniff test if it's been kept for any length of time. If it smells off, discard it. Flour can absorb moisture from the air. The fat from the germ in whole-grain flours can go rancid with time.

White flour can be stored at room temperature for 6 to 12 months in a tightly covered container. Whole-wheat flour keeps for less than a month at room temperature, so store it in a tightly covered container in the freezer; it will stay fresh for up to a year. You can use the flour directly from the freezer, although it is best to bring it to room temperature before using as the cold temperature of the flour may increase the rising times in bread.

preparing to use

When measuring flour, use a dry measure. These are the metal or plastic cups rather than the glass or plastic see-through liquid cups. To get an accurate measure, scoop the flour into the cup, then level the top with the back of a knife. Don't pack the flour down or you'll wind up using more than what's called for in the recipe.

If sifted flour is called for, use either a sifter specifically made for this purpose or a fine-meshed sieve. Sifting flour is not done to remove debris, but rather to lighten the flour so it isn't packed down. If a recipe calls for 1 cup of sifted flour, sift the flour into a bowl or onto a piece of waxed paper, then scoop it into the cup, leveling the top. If a recipe calls for 1 cup of flour, sifted, measure the flour first and then sift; this is often done when flour is combined with other ingredients.

beating the bugs

Once in a while, bug problems can get out of hand, especially if grain products aren't stored properly. Follow these tips:

• Store whole-grain flours in your freezer to prevent insect eggs from hatching.

• If you find evidence of bugs, remove the infested items from your home as soon as possible. If left in the kitchen garbage, the insects could contaminate other foods.

• Empty the cabinet and wash all surfaces with soap and water; pay special attention to cracks and crevices. Vacuum-clean the cabinet, if possible.

• Transfer other grains from the same cabinet to glass containers with tight-fitting lids. Watch these problem areas carefully.

• Continue to check for infestation. The bugs may reappear if you don't clean well enough. If you haven't seen anything for 2 months, your cabinet is probably insect-free.

game

From venison, quail, and pheasant to boar, elk, and ostrich, game is turning up on more and more restaurant menus and in specialty food stores and mail-order catalogues. Up until about 100 years ago, game was popular and widely available, even in city markets. Most of today's game is not hunted in the wild but is farm-raised, making the meat less tough and "gamy" (strong-flavored) than it would be in animals that consume a traditional "wild" diet of tree bark, leaves, and grasses.

nutritional profile

Game animals (both wild and farm-raised) are high in protein and minerals, like their domesticated counterparts. But game is lower—sometimes significantly lower—in fat and cholesterol, even if it's farm-raised. One of the reasons for the lower fat content is that in game animals (especially wild game) the fat is concentrated on the back or under the spine, rather than being dispersed as marbling throughout the meat.

in the market

There are many different game animals, but they can be divided into two basic categories: feathered and furred.

feathered game

After duck and goose, the most popular domestic game bird in the United States is pheasant. It is followed in popularity by two of its relatives, quail and partridge.

Duck Most duck sold in this country is domesticated, but there are some wild birds available on the market (*see Duck, page 273*).

Emu A cousin of the ostrich, emu is lower in fat than the already lean ostrich. It is best grilled, broiled, or panfried, and its flavor is comparable to very lean beef or duck breast, although not as rich.

Guinea fowl (guinea hen) This small bird, ranging in size from 12 ounces to 4 pounds, is a relative of the chicken and partridge. Although its meat is dark, guinea fowl dries out quickly if overcooked. It can be braised or roasted. If roasting, cover with a layer of fat to prevent drying out. Guinea fowl has a delicate, gamy flavor.

Ostrich Originally from Africa and southwest Asia, ostrich is now being farmed in the United States. Weighing up to 250 pounds, this huge, flightless bird has meat that is dark and very lean. Its flavor and texture can be compared to very lean beef or duck breast. Ostrich can be grilled, broiled, or panfried.

Partridge This small bird (about 1 pound) resembles a baby pheasant, but has darker meat and a stronger flavor. Young partridge is best roasted; older birds should be braised.

PHEASANT 3 ounces cooked	
Calories	151
Protein (g)	27
Carbohydrate (g)	0
Dietary fiber (g)	0
Total fat (g)	4.1
Saturated fat (g)	1.4
Monounsaturated fat (g)	1.3
Polyunsaturated fat (g)	0.7
Cholesterol (mg)	75
Potassium (mg)	297
Sodium (mg)	42

KEY NUTRIENTS (%RDA/AI*)	
Riboflavin	0.2 mg (13%)
Niacin	7.7 mg (48%)
Vitamin B_6	0.8 mg (49%)
Vitamin B_{12}	1 mcg (40%)
Iron	1.3 mg (16%)
Selenium	16 mcg (29%)
Zinc	1.1 mg (10%)

*For more detailed information on RDA and AI, see page 88.

Pheasant The domestic bird weighs 2 to 3 pounds, and a hen is considered more tender and flavorful than a cock. Baby pheasant, usually sold frozen, is considered a delicacy.

Quail More mildly flavored than its cousins, the quail is a tiny bird—weighing about 5 ounces—that has almost no fat. The bobwhite, or American quail, is hunted in the wild (and is popular in the South), and there are several other varieties raised on quail farms. Sautéing is usually the preferred cooking method, but you can also roast quail.

Squab (pigeon) These young, domesticated pigeons are generally less than 4 weeks old and have never flown. They have dark, tender juicy meat and usually weigh less than 1 pound. Squab can be roasted, grilled, or braised.

furred game

These animals range from large (deer, buffalo, boar) to small (rabbit, hare, opossum, squirrel). Buffalo, rabbit, and deer are the most common animals raised on game farms.

Beefalo A cross between domestic cattle and bison, beefalo, while lean, is not quite as lean as bison. Beefalo is best broiled or roasted.

alligator

While alligator tends to be a regional specialty, found in Louisiana and the Gulf states, it is making an appearance on restaurant menus and in some specialty shops. The tender white tail meat compares in flavor and texture to veal, while the pink body meat is stronger in flavor and tougher. The dark tail meat is too tough for anything other than braising. Alligator meat is relatively low in fat, with about 16 percent of its calories from fat and a total of 3.5 grams for a 3-ounce serving.

COMPARING GAME 3 ounces cooked

As with most meats and poultry, a general rule of thumb is that 4 ounces of raw, boneless will yield 3 ounces of cooked. For 3 ounces of cooked from a bone-in piece, start with about 8 ounces of raw. Before cooking, trim any visible fat. All numbers listed below are for skinless, boneless meat. The beef and chicken values are here for comparison.

	Calories	Fat (g)	% Calories from Fat	Saturated Fat (g)	Cholesterol (mg)
Feathered game					
Chicken (dark meat)	178	9.3	47	2.6	81
Emu	124	1.9	14	0.7	65
Ostrich	120	1.7	12	0.5	62
Pheasant	151	4.1	25	1.4	75
Quail	152	5.1	30	1.5	79
Squab	152	5.1	30	1.3	102
Furred game					
Beef (sirloin)	183	8.5	42	3.3	76
Boar	136	3.7	25	1.1	66
Elk	124	1.6	12	0.6	62
Goat	123	2.6	19	0.8	64
Rabbit	175	7.2	37	2.1	73
Venison	134	2.7	18	1.1	95

Bison (buffalo) Except for color, individual cuts of buffalo meat resemble those of beef. But buffalo is one of the leanest meats, with about two-thirds the calories of similar beef cuts. Steaks are good broiled; larger cuts can be roasted; and you can also try buffalo burgers.

Boar Boar tastes like pork, though richer and sweeter, but with significantly less fat and fewer calories.

Deer (venison) Originally "venison" meant the meat of any hunted animal, but it now refers to deer and other antlered animals, such as moose and elk. The best meat comes from young males; as with beef and lamb, the loin and ribs provide the tenderest cuts. Roasting or broiling is preferred for tender cuts. If the meat is from an older animal, braising is best.

Goat The best goat meat comes from kids, baby goats that are usually not more than 6 months old. Mature goat meat is tougher and more gamy in flavor than kid (think mutton versus lamb). Goat can be prepared in any manner suitable for lamb.

Rabbit A young rabbit weighs about 3 pounds, has tender meat that tastes somewhat like poultry, and is excellent roasted or stewed. The meat of hare, a larger rabbit relative, is tougher and gamier; it should be marinated, then braised or stewed.

▶ **Availability** Farm-raised game is usually available at any time of year in frozen form. Fresh meat, particularly from large animals, is more seasonal.

choosing the best

Whether you buy game meat from a specialty food shop or at a supermarket, try to check on how old the animal was when it was slaughtered: Age is the critical factor that determines taste and tenderness as well as the best cooking method. Most often, the game you buy will come frozen. Be sure the package is intact and that it doesn't contain any frozen liquid; this might indicate that the meat has been thawed and refrozen. With fresh game, the meat should be moist and springy to the touch; it should never feel soft.

▶ **When you get home** The rules for other meats apply here. Keep frozen game in a 0° freezer. Store fresh game in the coldest part of the refrigerator and use it within 1 or 2 days.

preparing to use

Game is traditionally aged by hanging it for anywhere from a few days to a few weeks, which tenderizes the meat and improves its flavor. Meat you buy from a reputable retailer will have been properly aged. Before cooking, trim away visible fat, which can impart a disagreeable flavor to some game meats.

VENISON
3 ounces cooked

Calories	134
Protein (g)	26
Carbohydrate (g)	0
Dietary fiber (g)	0
Total fat (g)	2.7
Saturated fat (g)	1.1
Monounsaturated fat (g)	0.8
Polyunsaturated fat (g)	0.5
Cholesterol (mg)	95
Potassium (mg)	285
Sodium (mg)	46

KEY NUTRIENTS (%RDA/AI*)

Thiamin	0.2 mg (13%)
Riboflavin	0.5 mg (39%)
Niacin	5.7 mg (36%)
Vitamin B$_6$	0.3 mg (19%)
Vitamin B$_{12}$	2.7 mcg (113%)
Iron	3.8 mg (48%)
Zinc	2.3 mg (21%)

*For more detailed information on RDA and AI, see page 88.

garlic

One of the world's oldest and most venerable medicinal foods, garlic has been praised over the centuries for its legendary healing powers as well as its notable culinary flexibility. Garlic indisputably holds center stage in the world of folklore, where it is reputed to bring good luck, protect against evil, ward off vampires, sorcerers, werewolves, and the like. The ancient Egyptians depicted garlic in papyrus documents that indicate it was used for 22 different ailments; they also fed garlic to the workers who built the pyramids, to increase their stamina. And in ancient Greece and Rome, garlic was valued for its anti-venom attributes; in China, it was used as a general cure-all; and during the Middle Ages, it was believed to ward off the plague.

Like the onion, garlic is a member of the *Allium* genus—it is classified as *Allium sativa*—and it consists of a bulb wrapped in a loose, crackly outer skin. Each garlic bulb has several small sections called cloves, which are individually enclosed by tight-fitting papery sheaths. Garlic's beguiling and characteristic pungent flavor is used to enhance a wide range of dishes. In the United States, statistics show that annual garlic consumption is over 3 pounds per person.

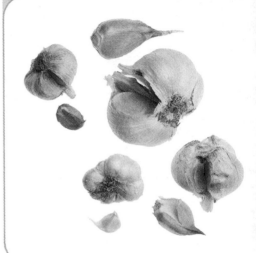

garlic

nutritional profile

Garlic contains a smattering of vitamins and minerals, but because we use it primarily to season dishes, and therefore consume it in small amounts, it doesn't contribute much to our nutritional requirements.

Garlic contains other substances, however, that have attracted the attention of both researchers and consumers because of their possible health benefits (*see "The Power of Garlic?" page 336*). Some scientists argue that garlic's benefits come from allicin—a chemical that breaks down into sulfur compounds when garlic is chewed or crushed and gives garlic its strong smell. However, one study from the University of California at Irvine showed that allicin is unlikely to survive in the digestive tract and would be destroyed in the bloodstream, so it's highly improbable that it could reach your cells and accomplish anything. Of course, some compound other than allicin might have beneficial effects, but no one knows what it is.

GARLIC / 3 cloves	
Calories	13
Protein (g)	1
Carbohydrate (g)	3
Dietary fiber (g)	0.2
Total fat (g)	0
Saturated fat (g)	0
Monounsaturated fat (g)	0
Polyunsaturated fat (g)	0
Cholesterol (mg)	0
Potassium (mg)	36
Sodium (mg)	2

in the market

Some 300 varieties of garlic are grown around the world, but most garlic is simply labeled "garlic." There are, however, a growing number of specialty garlics, especially in farmers' markets. There are two large categories of garlic grown: hard-neck and soft-neck. *Hard-neck garlics* have a thick, unbendable stem in the center of the scallionlike greens that grow out of the garlic bulb. You can identify hard-neck garlics in the market, because they will still have a portion of the hard stem sticking out of the head of garlic. *Soft-neck garlics* do not have this central stem, merely the greens. When the greens dry, they are strong but pliable, making this the type of garlic that is traditionally woven into garlic braids. Soft-neck garlics are also the most common type found in the supermarket.

Artichoke garlics Though they have an intriguing name, artichoke garlics are actually the main type of garlic sold in supermarkets. Some farmers' markets may carry a few of the more unusual cultivars, such as Red Toch and Chinese Cauldron. Artichoke garlics are soft-neck garlics.

Chileno This is a reddish-skinned, sharp-tasting garlic imported from Mexico.

Garlic chives This is actually a separate, but related plant. See Green Herbs (*page 349*).

Porcelain garlics These are large, beautiful heads of garlic with a small number (4 to 8) of large cloves. If you didn't know better, you might think you were getting elephant garlic. But unlike elephant garlic (which is not a true garlic), porcelain garlic is quite pungent. Porcelain is a hard-neck garlic.

Purple stripe This hard-neck garlic, as the name suggests, has rosy purple and white stripes on the skin.

Rocambole This popular garlic is sought after by cooks for its rich, well-balanced garlic flavor. It's a hard-neck variety of garlic and has large, even-sized cloves that are easy to peel.

Silverskin garlics These soft-neck garlics are the types most often sold in braids.

choosing the best

Look for garlic sold loose, so you can choose a healthy, solid bulb. Garlic bulbs should be plump and compact with taut, unbroken skin. Avoid those with damp or soft spots. A heavy, firm bulb indicates that the garlic will be fresh and flavorful. If the bulb feels light, or gives under your fingers, the contents may have dried to dust. Check out the clove formation. A bulb of garlic may contain a "standard" eight cloves, or as many as 40: Choose a bulb with large cloves if you're a garlic lover—peeling a large number of small ones to flavor your favorite dishes can be tedious.

▶ **When you get home** Garlic has the potential to sprout. If it does, the compounds responsible for its pungency will partly seep into the new sprouts, leaving the bulb itself diminished in flavor. Cloves that have sprouted can still be used, although you may need to include more of them in your recipe to compensate for the milder taste. To prevent sprouting, garlic should be kept in a dark but airy spot. A loosely covered container, out of the sun and away from the stove or other heat source, will make a good storage place.

preparing to use

To peel garlic cloves, place them on a cutting board and lay the flat side of a broad knife on top. Hit the knife with your closed fist: A fairly gentle impact is all that's required to split the peel without smashing the cloves. Some specialty garlic varieties have very thick skin that easily pulls off without smashing the clove.

To chop garlic, cut the cloves in half lengthwise. Make several cuts the length of the clove with the tip of the knife, then cut crosswise. The more finely the garlic is chopped, the more flavorful it will be.

garlic & oil: a warning

If not handled properly, garlic-in-oil preparations carry the risk of botulism. Garlic can pick up the bacterium that causes botulism from the soil in which it grows; then once the garlic is covered in oil, spores will have an ideal oxygen-free environment in which to germinate. The resulting toxin cannot be detected by taste or smell.

Commercial garlic-in-oil products are safe when they contain an antibacterial or acidifying agent, such as phosphoric or citric acid. Those products that do not contain such ingredients, and thus require refrigeration, have been banned by the FDA. Although these products should no longer be available, if you do find one that says "keep refrigerated," or that doesn't list a bacterial inhibitor on the label, do not buy it. And be sure to discard similar preparations you may have at home.

There is still a risk from home-made preparations. If you're making a garlic-in-oil or garlic-in-butter blend, be sure to keep it refrigerated and do not store it longer than 10 to 14 days. Or, prepare a fresh batch each time you need it.

serving suggestions

• Roast small, red-skinned potatoes in olive oil with rosemary sprigs and whole, unpeeled cloves of garlic.

• Wrap whole bulbs of unpeeled garlic in foil and bake at 350° for 45 minutes, or until tender. Squeeze the garlic from the bulbs, mash, and spread on bread.

• Chop a whole bulb of garlic, place in a saucepan, and cover with water by about 1 inch. Sprinkle with a little salt. Cover and cook until the broth is fragrant. Use as a nonfat vegetarian broth for savory soups.

• Cut French bread into 1-inch slices and broil until toasted on both sides. Rub a cut clove of garlic over one side of the toasts and brush with some olive oil.

ginger

The ginger plant (*Zingiber officinale*) is believed to have originated in southern Asia, where it has long been valued for its purported medicinal properties and varied culinary applications. The ginger plant is currently grown in Asia, the East Indies, Mexico, Jamaica, and Africa and is most prized for its rhizome (an underground stem), which is often incorrectly referred to as a root.

Ginger (along with other pungent spices) was used in medieval European cookery as a preservative, and it also doubled as a method of camouflaging meat that was old or bad. Easy to ship and transport, the Spanish explorers brought ginger from the East Indies into Spain in the 16th century, where it was considered a delicacy and sold in various parts of Europe. Second to pepper, ginger was the most traded commodity in Europe. Considered to be one of the world's favorite spices, it continues to enjoy worldwide popularity.

Ginger imparts a piquant, stimulating flavor to an endless variety of dishes, from gingerbread (rumor has it that Queen Elizabeth I invented the first gingerbread man), ginger tea, gingerale, gingersnap cookies, candied ginger, and ginger beer.

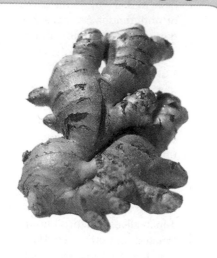

mature ginger

nutritional profile

The nutrients in ginger are insignificant (there is some potassium) given the small quantities of ginger usually consumed.

in the market

Fresh ginger can be found in a variety of forms, but the most common form of fresh ginger in the market is what is technically called mature ginger.

Mature ginger This is what most people know as ginger. The skin is thin, light brown, and papery. Mature ginger is more fibrous and stronger in flavor than young ginger.

Young ginger Sometimes called *spring ginger,* this looks like the ginger everyone is used to seeing, but the skin is very thin and pale, and needs no peeling. Very tender (not fibrous) and milder in flavor than mature ginger, it is generally available in Asian markets in the springtime.

choosing the best

When shopping for fresh (mature) ginger, look for knobs with plump, smooth, somewhat shiny skin. If it's wrinkled or cracked, the ginger is past its prime, and while still usable, is not as flavorful or as pungent. Shop for ground ginger and other forms of processed ginger in a store that has a rapid turnover and stores the products out of the heat or sunlight.

▶ **When you get home** Fresh ginger should be stored in the refrigerator. If you've bought more than you'll need in a couple of weeks, slice and place

FRESH GINGER 2 tablespoons sliced	
Calories	8
Protein (g)	>1
Carbohydrate (g)	2
Dietary fiber (g)	0.2
Total fat (g)	0.1
Saturated fat (g)	0
Monounsaturated fat (g)	0
Polyunsaturated fat (g)	0
Cholesterol (mg)	0
Potassium (mg)	50
Sodium (mg)	2

it in a jar of vinegar. Though the ginger will have lost some of its flavor (it leaches into the vinegar), it can still be used in stir-fries; it will have a bit of a pickled taste. The vinegar, on the other hand, will have a pronounced ginger flavor and can be used in salad dressings, sauces, and marinades.

preparing to use

If the skin is thin, it is not necessary to peel fresh ginger before grating, slicing, mincing, or shredding. If the skin is thick, however, it is preferable, although not absolutely necessary, to peel it first. A sharp paring knife is the best tool to use for navigating around all the knobs and bumps.

To juice fresh ginger, grate it (peeled or unpeeled) on the fine holes of a box grater or on a special grater made just for ginger. Grate the ginger into a bowl, then squeeze the pulp to extract as much of the spicy juice as possible. Discard the pulp.

other ginger products

Crystallized ginger (candied ginger) Slices of peeled young ginger are cooked in a sugar syrup until they've crystallized and are then coated in coarse sugar. This sweet-spicy form of ginger is sold as thick slices or already chopped. Both make a great addition to baked goods and desserts.

Ginger juice Fresh ginger is grated and squeezed to extract its juice. The juice is then packed in bottles along with citric acid and xanthan gum to preserve its flavor. Use ginger juice in baked goods, stir-fries, salad dressings, sauces, marinades, and drinks.

Ground ginger Fresh ginger is dried, then ground to a powder. This is commonly used in baking, but it can be used to add a very distinctive heat to savory dishes as well. It cannot, however, be substituted for fresh.

Preserved ginger Thick slices of peeled ginger are packed in a sugar-salt mixture, where they eventually turn translucent. They are traditionally stored (and sold) in "ginger jars."

Red candied ginger Slices of ginger are packed in a sweet sugar syrup that's been tinted red with food coloring.

Sushi ginger Thin slices of young ginger are pickled in a mixture of vinegar, sugar, and water. Called *gari* in Japanese, this is the traditional accompaniment (along with wasabi) to sushi and sashimi. Although you can get white sushi ginger, it is more commonly tinted a light pink.

serving suggestions

- Add slices of peeled fresh ginger to stews.
- Add minced preserved ginger to homemade or store-bought barbecue sauces.
- Garnish soups with thin strips of fresh mature or young ginger.
- Whisk ginger juice together with soy sauce and dark sesame oil to make an Asian salad dressing.
- Add ginger juice to lemonade or limeade.
- Add grated fresh ginger to a gingerbread recipe.
- Sprinkle minced crystallized ginger over fresh fruit.
- Stir grated ginger or ginger juice into your favorite jam or jelly to spice it up.

goose

Before turkey was introduced to Europe in the 16th century, goose was the bird of choice on European tables. Though not popular in the United States, this rich-tasting bird with its moist, dark meat is still the favorite for festive occasions in Britain, Scandinavia, and central European countries.

nutritional profile

Like duck, goose has a reputation for being extremely fatty. This is certainly true of goose with the skin on, but 3 ounces of roasted goose without skin is not as bad as its reputation would suggest: It has about 11 grams of fat, which is 48 percent of its calories. And to put this into perspective, 3 ounces of cooked, skinless dark-meat chicken has over 9 grams of fat, which is 46 percent of its calories.

Although goose is not a particularly healthful choice as far as fat is concerned, it does have a wealth of B vitamins and handsome amounts of vitamin E, iron, selenium, and zinc.

in the market

Domestic geese usually weigh between 6 and 14 pounds; those under 9 pounds are younger birds—less than 6 months old—and are usually more tender than older birds.

▶ Availability Like ducks, geese are generally sold frozen, though you can sometimes find fresh birds for Thanksgiving and Christmas. Because frozen birds are shipped to market from July through December, they can be hard to find in the spring and the early part of summer. Geese usually have to be ordered from a butcher—they are not readily available in supermarkets.

choosing the best

Check to see that the goose you are buying is free of feathers and that it has a clean smell. Frozen birds should be solidly frozen and there should be no tears in the wrapping.

preparing to use

As with all poultry, rinse the goose inside and out. If roasting, pat it dry with paper towels and then carefully prick the skin all over without piercing the flesh. This allows the fat to be released during cooking. Exercise care when roasting: A goose releases even more fat than a duck does and the fat can begin to smoke. Add a small amount of water to the pan to reduce the chance of the fat catching fire. (For this reason, broiling goose isn't recommended.)

GOOSE / 3 ounces cooked	
Calories	202
Protein (g)	25
Carbohydrate (g)	0
Dietary fiber (g)	0
Total fat (g)	11
Saturated fat (g)	3.9
Monounsaturated fat (g)	3.7
Polyunsaturated fat (g)	1.3
Cholesterol (mg)	82
Potassium (mg)	330
Sodium (mg)	65

KEY NUTRIENTS (%RDA/AI*)	
Riboflavin	0.3 mg (26%)
Niacin	3.5 mg (22%)
Vitamin B$_6$	0.4 mg (24%)
Vitamin B$_{12}$	0.4 mcg (17%)
Vitamin E	2.4 mg (16%)
Iron	2.4 mg (31%)
Selenium	17 mcg (31%)
Zinc	2.7 mg (25%)

*For more detailed information on RDA and AI, see page 88.

serving suggestions

• The rich, dark meat of goose is nicely complemented by fresh, tart flavors. Good side dishes for goose are applesauce and braised onions, or a colorful cabbage slaw made from red and green cabbage, carrots, and a sweet-and-sour dressing.

• Use leftover goose in a salad: Shred the goose and toss it with chicory, roasted peppers, and artichoke hearts dressed with orange juice and balsamic vinegar.

grapefruit

Grapefruit's ancestry is a bit unclear. Some research places the discovery of grapefruit in Barbados in the 18th century, suggesting that it was a natural mutation of a tropical fruit called the pomelo (*see page 289*). But other theories hold that grapefruit was developed from a cross between an orange and a shaddock, a citrus fruit with thick skin, many seeds, almost no juice, and a very sour taste. One way or the other, seeds of the grapefruit made their way to Florida in the 19th century. The original Florida grapefruit was probably much less palatable than the grapefruit of today; but over the years, growers have continued to hybridize the grapefruit to bring out the qualities that the public is looking for. A century ago, the seedless grapefruit was developed and since then sweeter, less-bitter varieties have been developed.

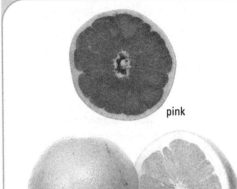

grapefruit

pink

white

nutritional profile

White, red, and pink grapefruit are rich in vitamin C and fiber. As with many fruits and vegetables, the darker or more intensely colored the fruit or vegetable, the higher the nutrient content, and this is true for grapefruit, with pink and red grapefruit containing beta carotene and lycopene, two carotenoids with antioxidant properties.

Like the fresh fruit, grapefruit juice is an excellent source of vitamin C: Just 1 cup has 94 milligrams, over 100 percent of the RDA. However, when you choose the juice over the fruit, you miss out on the benefits of fiber. In fact, the fiber in grapefruit juice is pectin, a type of soluble fiber that may help to lower LDL ("bad") cholesterol levels.

A prevailing myth circulating over the years is that grapefruit contains an enzyme that digests fats and burns them away, leaving you svelte and trim. While grapefruit contains no fat-burning enzymes and is hardly a miracle weight-loss food, it is a tangy low-calorie food that is perfect for people trying to control their weight.

in the market

Grapefruit comes in white (actually yellow), pink, and red varieties—colors that refer to the flesh. All three types are similar in taste and texture. Most grapefruits sold as table fruits are seedless; varieties that have seeds are often used for making grapefruit juice. The commonest white grapefruit on the market is the white Marsh seedless.

Duncan This large, yellow-skinned Florida grapefruit is very juicy and flavorful. Because it is very seedy it is generally used for juicing.

Lavender Gem A grapefruit-tangelo hybrid, the Lavender Gem resembles a mini grapefruit with either a lemon-yellow rind or a pink blush. The flesh is pinkish-blue with some small seeds. These grapefruits are delicate in flavor.

WHITE GRAPEFRUIT ½ medium	
Calories	39
Protein (g)	1
Carbohydrate (g)	10
Dietary fiber (g)	1.3
Total fat (g)	0.1
Saturated fat (g)	0
Monounsaturated fat (g)	0
Polyunsaturated fat (g)	0
Cholesterol (mg)	0
Potassium (mg)	175
Sodium (mg)	0

KEY NUTRIENTS (%RDA/AI*)	
Vitamin C	39 mg (44%)

For more detailed information on RDA and AI, see page 88.

Marsh seedless The *white Marsh* is the most popular variety of grapefruit. With yellow-white flesh and yellow skin, this grapefruit is both sweet and acidic. Other Marsh grapefruits include the *pink Marsh,* which generally has yellow skin with a pink blush. The pink flesh is slightly less acidic and sweeter than that of the white Marsh. The *ruby red Marsh* has yellow to pale red skin and red flesh. It is less acidic than the white Marsh and is considerably sweeter.

Melogold This cross between a pomelo and a grapefruit was the result of research conducted by two scientists from University of California at Riverside in the late 1950s. Their size varies, but they can be very large. Melogolds are juicy and taste likes oranges, with grapefruit overtones. They have a smooth, easy-to-peel rind and contain practically no seeds.

Oroblanco Another cross between a pomelo and a grapefruit, oroblanco (which means white gold in Spanish) is sweet and juicy without any bitterness or acidity. Oroblancos have yellow skin, a thick rind, and are nearly seedless.

Star Ruby Both tart and sweet, the Star Ruby has smooth yellow skin with a pink blush and deep red flesh. The general rule of thumb is the redder the flesh, the sweeter the fruit.

Sweeties Yet another cross between the grapefruit and a pomelo, these look like green grapefruits and, as their name suggests, they are sweet.

serving suggestions

• Combine grapefruit and orange segments with arugula or watercress and sliced red onion for a tasty salad.

• Sprinkle brown sugar over the top of halved grapefruits and broil. Serve warm.

• Make a grapefruit salsa with diced red grapefruit, scallions, chopped mint, and a touch of honey and serve with grilled poultry or fish.

• Blend cranberry juice with fresh-squeezed grapefruit juice. Add seltzer for a refreshing and not-too-sweet fruit soda.

• Add a slice of grapefruit, instead of tomato, to a turkey sandwich.

• Add diced grapefruit to your favorite tuna or chicken salad.

• Dice grapefruit and combine with spicy mustard. Use to top a turkey burger.

choosing the best

Since grapefruit is not picked until fully ripe, you never have to worry about getting a "green" one. Under certain growing conditions, the lemon-yellow skin may revert to green after it is ripe, but the fruit will lose none of its tangy sweetness.

Look for round, smooth fruits that are heavy for their size (they will be juicy). Coarse-skinned grapefruits or those that are puffy, soft, or pointed at one end are inferior; glossy fruits with slightly flattened ends are preferable. Gray-brown "russeting" or other skin defects are superficial and do not affect quality. At room temperature, you may be able to detect a mildly sweet fragrance, but it will not be apparent if the fruit is chilled.

▶ **When you get home** Grapefruits can be left at room temperature for a week, and are juiciest when slightly warm rather than chilled. For longer storage, they should be held in the refrigerator crisper, where they will keep for 6 to 8 weeks. Leave them at room temperature for a while before you juice them or eat them.

preparing to use

For serving from the "shell," halve grapefruit crosswise. Use a grapefruit spoon with a serrated tip to scoop out the sections, or prepare the fruit using a sharp paring knife or a curved-blade grapefruit knife, running it between each segment of flesh and the membrane "dividers." (Grapefruits, like other citrus fruits, may be called "seedless" if they contain no more than six seeds, so don't be surprised if you have to remove a few seeds.)

You can also peel a grapefruit as you would an orange; use your hands or pare the skin with a sharp knife. Then pull apart the segments with your hands and, if desired, remove the membranes from each segment.

Often, recipes call for peeling a grapefruit and separating the segments from the membranes. To do so, cut a thin slice from one end of the grapefruit so that it will stand on a work surface. With a chef's knife or paring knife, cut downward around the grapefruit removing both the peel and the bitter white pith underneath. Working over a bowl to catch the juice, use a paring knife to cut between the flesh and the membranes to release each segment.

RED GRAPEFRUIT ½ medium	
Calories	37
Protein (g)	1
Carbohydrate (g)	9
Dietary fiber (g)	1.4
Total fat (g)	0.1
Saturated fat (g)	0
Monounsaturated fat (g)	0
Polyunsaturated fat (g)	0
Cholesterol (mg)	0
Potassium (mg)	156
Sodium (mg)	0

KEY NUTRIENTS (%RDA/AI*)

Vitamin C	46 mg (51%)

For more detailed information on RDA and AI, see page 88.

the grapefruit effect

The potent compounds in fruits and vegetables can also have adverse effects. Grapefruit juice, for example, appears to inhibit an enzyme in the small intestine that helps to metabolize a number of medications. When one of these drugs is taken, the result is to boost its concentration in the bloodstream. This increases the risk of side effects and, in a few cases, can cause serious reactions.

Individual responses can vary widely, however: The problem doesn't occur in all people, doesn't happen with all grapefruit juice (oddly enough), and is most likely to occur when the drugs are taken with the juice. Whole grapefruit may or may not have the same effect as the juice.

The drugs known to be affected include some of the cholesterol-lowering drugs referred to as "statins"; certain calcium channel blockers taken for high blood pressure and angina; certain tranquilizers; cyclosporin, an immunosuppresant medication; and some antiviral drugs used to treat HIV infection. Other medications may also have interactions with grapefruit juice. If you are taking a prescription drug and you also eat grapefruit or drink its juice, check with your physician or pharmacist about the latest information on drug-nutrient interactions.

grapes

Grapes were first cultivated over 8,000 years ago; however, fossils indicate that the cultivation, or at least the consumption, of grapes goes back perhaps to the Neolithic Era. Native American wild grapes grew along stream banks, but compared with the table grapes we are familiar with today, they were sour. In the 18th century, as more Spanish settlers came to California, sweeter European grape varieties were introduced and used for eating fresh, as well as for making raisins and wine.

Grapes can grow in almost every type of climate, and while they do particularly well in regions like the Mediterranean (where they have long been established), they are now cultivated on six continents. A large percentage of the grapes grown in the United States are processed—more than half for wine, more than a fourth for raisins, and the remainder for juice and canning.

Grapes develop sugar as they ripen, but will become no sweeter once picked, so timing the harvest is of the utmost importance. And to ensure that they reach the consumer in full, handsome clusters, table grapes are harvested by hand (although grapes intended for processing can be shaken from the vines with mechanical pickers). Today, even though modern equipment is employed in certain aspects of grape growing, much of viticulture (as grape-growing is called) is still done by hand. Grapes grow on woody vines that are not raised from seeds, but are propagated from cuttings or grafted onto existing rootstocks. The vining plants must be staked or trellised as they grow, to support the heavy bunches of fruit. Leaves and shoots are pruned from the vines and, depending on the variety, the flower clusters or the berries themselves must be thinned by hand to improve the quality of the fruit.

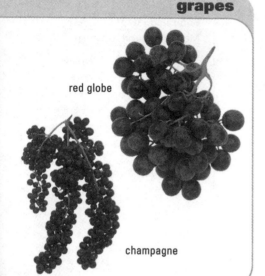

grapes

red globe

champagne

THOMPSON SEEDLESS 1 cup	
Calories	114
Protein (g)	1
Carbohydrate (g)	29
Dietary fiber (g)	1.6
Total fat (g)	0.9
Saturated fat (g)	0.3
Monounsaturated fat (g)	0
Polyunsaturated fat (g)	0.3
Cholesterol (mg)	0
Potassium (mg)	296
Sodium (mg)	3

KEY NUTRIENTS (%RDA/AI*)	
Thiamin	0.2 mg (12%)
Vitamin B$_6$	0.2 mg (10%)
Vitamin C	17 mg (19%)

*For more detailed information on RDA and AI, see page 88.

nutritional profile

While table grapes have only low to moderate amounts of vitamins and minerals, some varieties are good sources of vitamin C, and their juiciness and natural sweetness, combined with a low calorie count, make them an excellent snack and dessert food.

in the market

There are two basic types of grapes, American and European. Today, both are grown in the United States, but the European grapes are certainly more popular and versatile. Seeded varieties are thought to have better flavor than seedless, but Americans—who tend to eat grapes as a snack rather than as a dessert—seem to prefer the convenience of seedless grapes. The list that follows covers the major (and a few minor) varieties of grapes, both seeded and seedless, grown in this country.

european varieties

Our familiar table grapes are derived from a single European species, *Vitis vinifera*. Varieties of vinifera grapes were grown by the ancients, and now are made into the world's great wines and dried to produce raisins. They have relatively thin skins that adhere closely to their flesh; when seeds are present, they can be slipped out of the pulp quite easily (some varieties are seedless).

It is believed that Spanish missionaries moving north from Mexico established vineyards in California in the late 18th century, and by 1860 commercial cultivation of several varieties had been established there.

Today, California produces the majority of European varieties of grapes in the United States. Although a large proportion of the California crop is used for winemaking and raisins, the remainder is sufficient to provide a bountiful supply of fresh fruit for American tables during the greater part of the year. The major varieties are harvested in different seasons, and the period of market availability for some types is extended by imported grapes.

Black Beauty (Beauty Seedless) These are the only seedless black grapes. They are spicy and sweet, resembling Concords in flavor.

Calmeria These pale green oval grapes are so elongated that they are sometimes called Lady Finger grapes. They have a mildly sweet flavor, comparatively thick skin, and a few small seeds.

Cardinal A cross between the Flame Tokay and the Ribier, these large, dark red grapes have a pearly gray finish, a full, fruity flavor, and few seeds.

Champagne (Black Corinth) These grapes are tiny, purple seedless fruits with a deliciously winy sweetness. They are called champagne grapes because someone thought the cluster of small grapes resembled champagne bubbles. In their dried form, these grapes are called currants (which are not the dried fruit of the currant plant, but a mispronunciation of the grape's name, Corinth).

Emperor Second only to Thompson Seedless in quantity grown, these small-seeded red grapes may vary in color from red-violet to deep purple. Their flavor is mild and somewhat cherrylike (they have a lower sugar content than many other table grapes). Thick-skinned Emperors are good shippers and stand up well to consumer handling. They also store well, lengthening their period of availability.

Exotic These blue-black grapes are seeded and firm-fleshed, and resemble Ribiers.

Flame Seedless Round, deep red, and seedless, these grapes, a relatively new variety, are sweet-tart and crunchy.

> ### ➤ phytochemicals in grapes
>
> Red wine, as well as red and purple grape juice, is a concentrated source of flavonoid phytochemicals that are being studied for their potential to interfere with the harmful process that attaches LDL ("bad") cholesterol to artery walls.
>
> Note that grapes, grape juice, and red wine have different types and concentrations of phytochemicals, so what is true for one wine is not necessarily true for grape juice or another wine.
>
> And, with increasing scientific evidence for the heart-protective effects of moderate amounts of alcoholic drinks, there is much controversy over whether the protection that wine (especially red wine) provides is derived from something other than its alcohol content. The jury is still out on this, though it seems wine's alcohol content may turn out to be its most important health feature.

Italia (Italia Muscat) This variety has taken the place of the older Muscat varieties, which today are mainly used for making wine. Muscats are large, greenish-gold, seeded grapes with a winy sweetness and fragrance; the Italias have a milder flavor than the older varieties.

Perlette Seedless These round, crisp, green grapes have a frosty-white "bloom" on their surface.

Queen These large, firm grapes are rusty-red in color and have a mildly sweet flavor.

Red Globe These very large red grapes have a crisp texture and large seeds. The flavor is quite delicate.

Red Malaga Ranging in color from pinkish-red to purple, these grapes are crisp and mildly sweet. Their rather thick skins make them good shippers.

Ribier These large, blue-black grapes, which grow in generous bunches, have tender skins. They are sweeter than the look-alike Exotic and arrive at market later in the summer.

Ruby Seedless These deep-red, oval grapes are sweet and juicy.

Thompson Seedless These oval, amber-green grapes are the most popular fresh variety grown in the United States (and also the foremost variety used for processing into raisins).

Tokay (Flame Tokay) A sweeter version of the Flame Seedless, these are large, elongated, crunchy, orange-red grapes.

american varieties

Two species native to the United States are *Vitis labrusca* and *Vitis rotundita*. Labrusca grapes are the ones that Viking explorer Leif Ericson found growing so abundantly on the East Coast of North America, which resulted in his naming the newfound territory "Vinland." Later settlers tried and failed to establish European grapes (for winemaking) in the eastern United States; in the late 18th century, Easterners started to domesticate native varieties, which were obviously well suited to the local climate. Today, labrusca is the primary type of American grape grown.

American varieties are sometimes called slipskin grapes, as their skins separate readily from the flesh; their seeds are tightly embedded in the pulp. The most familiar American variety is the Concord, followed by the Catawba.

Although they can be grown in many parts of the country, commercial production of American varieties is still concentrated in the East: New York State is the major grower. Pennsylvania, Michigan, Arkansas, and the state of Washington also produce some American grapes. Nearly all of the crop is processed into jam, jelly, juice, wine, and other food products; cream of tartar, an ingredient in some types of baking powder, is made from Concord grapes. A small quantity of these grapes reach the market as table grapes, but since they do not ship well, they are generally sold locally.

All American grape varieties ripen in the fall and are available only in September and October.

Catawba Second to the Concord in popularity, the purplish-red Catawba is named for a river in Maryland, where it was discovered in the 1820s. It is a medium-sized, oval, seeded grape with an intense, sweet flavor. The Catawba is mainly used to make juices and is rarely found in the market as a table grape.

Concord This variety originated in the 1840s near the Massachusetts town whose name it bears. A typical labrusca grape, Concords are round, blue-black grapes with a powdery bloom. Their thick skin and heady, sweet aroma surpass their bland-to-sour flavor. They are most commonly used in grape preserves and juice. Grapes sold as white Concords are actually Niagaras.

Delaware These small, pinkish-red grapes have a more tender skin than other American varieties. They are sweet and juicy.

Niagara These large, amber-colored grapes have a grayish bloom. Niagaras may be either round or egg-shaped. They are somewhat coarse-fleshed, and are less sweet than most other American varieties. They are often sold as white Concord grapes and are used to make white grape juice.

Scuppernong The first cultivated wine grape in this country was discovered in North Carolina on the banks of the Scuppernong river in the early 16th century. Today the Scuppernong is mostly turned into jams, jellies, juices, and local wines.

Steuben These blue-black grapes are similar to the Concord, but have a less winy flavor.

CONCORD GRAPES 1 cup	
Calories	62
Protein (g)	1
Carbohydrate (g)	16
Dietary fiber (g)	0.9
Total fat (g)	0.3
Saturated fat (g)	0.1
Monounsaturated fat (g)	0
Polyunsaturated fat (g)	0.1
Cholesterol (mg)	0
Potassium (mg)	176
Sodium (mg)	2

grape juice

Grape juice is made by crushing grapes. If the juice is purple, its color comes from the skin, which is included in the processing. Virtually any type of grape can be used to make juice, but Concord grapes are the main variety used.

Because of its high sugar content, grape juice has more calories than other fruit juices. An 8-ounce glass has 128 to 155 calories (depending on whether or not it is made from concentrate), compared with 100 calories in grapefruit juice or 110 calories in orange juice.

When buying grape juice—or any fruit juice—check the wording on the label. If it is simply called "grape juice," it must be 100 percent juice. Grape "drinks," "beverages," "punches," or "blends" usually contain very little fruit juice; they are mainly a mixture of water and sugar, such as corn syrup. These products are not necessarily bad for you, but they may be a waste of money. Sometimes, they cost more than real grape juice.

If you find grape juice too sweet, thin it with a little apple juice.

choosing the best

Because they are thin-skinned and easily damaged, grapes should be displayed no more than two bunches deep and under refrigeration. The bunches may be wrapped in tissue paper or enclosed in perforated plastic bags. Loose bunches are easiest to evaluate, but the wrapped grapes are better protected from damage caused by customer handling.

Grapes are not picked and shipped until ripe, so unripe grapes are not usually a problem for the consumer. You can, however, use color as a guide to the sweetest fruit. Green grapes should tend toward a translucent yellow-green rather than an opaque grass-green; all fruit on a bunch of red grapes should be predominantly crimson; and blue grapes should be darkly hued, almost black. Once they have been picked, grapes will not ripen further: If you spot a bunch with many underdeveloped, very green fruits, leave it in the store.

A bunch of grapes in the market should look as inviting as those in a still-life painting: plump fruit with a silvery white "bloom," tightly attached to moist, flexible stems (except Emperor grapes, which should have brown, woody stems). The powdery bloom, more visible on dark-colored grapes than on pale ones, is an important sign of freshness; it fades with time and handling. Avoid wrinkled, sticky, or discolored grapes on withered, brown, limp, or brittle stems.

▶ When you get home Before storing grapes at home, remove any spoiled fruit. Place unwashed grapes in a perforated plastic bag and store them in the refrigerator. They should keep for about a week.

preparing to use

Wash grapes under cold water just before serving and remove any damaged fruit. Leave the bunch whole, or divide it into smaller branches for serving. This is easily done with a pair of scissors. If seeding is required, halve each grape and pick out the seeds with the tip of the knife.

grape leaves

Young, tender grape leaves are used as wrappers for rice and other fillings in Greek and Middle-Eastern cooking. The leaves are also used to wrap some French cheeses and to protect small game birds from the intense heat of broiling or grilling. Bottled or canned grape leaves are sold in Greek and Middle-Eastern groceries. If you have grapes growing on your property, you can use your own leaves as long as they are unsprayed. Fresh leaves should be blanched or steamed to soften them; canned leaves, usually packed in brine, should be rinsed to reduce their sodium content. One way to enjoy grape leaves is to fill each one with a spoonful of stuffing made from cooked rice, currants or pine nuts, lemon zest, and dill, then fold the leaves around the filling and place them snugly in a pan so they do not unfold. Poach the wrapped rolls in broth. Serve the rolls at room temperature or chilled.

green herbs

There are a handful of herbs that have soft, green leaves or stalks and are eaten in their fresh form in greater quantity than other herbs (for example, ¼ cup of parsley is a reasonable amount to consume, whereas ¼ cup of oregano is not). These herbs are treated differently by the cook and as a bonus, because they are eaten fresh, they bring with them more health benefits than dried herbs or spices.

nutritional profile

Green herbs contain varying amounts of carotenoids, insoluble fiber, and an array of vitamins and minerals. Notably, fresh mint, chives, and parsley offer some folate and ¼ cup of chopped parsley furnishes more than 20 percent of the day's requirement of vitamin C. Sorrel supplies a good amount of vitamin C as well, which along with the herb's oxalate content, contributes to its slightly sharp taste. Oxalate compounds are believed to hamper the absorption of certain minerals (such as iron, calcium, and zinc), and when consumed in large quantities may fuel the formation of particular types of kidney stones in susceptible people.

in the market

Many of the following herbs are available in supermarkets, though the unusual varieties are more often found in farmers' markets and specialty produce stores. Most of them are also available in dried form, though generally speaking, their flavors range from mild to nonexistent, depending on the herb.

Basil Pasta with pesto—the entrancingly fragrant Genovese sauce made from fresh basil, olive oil, pine nuts, and Parmesan—is one of the glories of Italian cuisine and a healthful dish, too. The most common form of sweet basil has large, pointed green or reddish-green leaves. There are numerous other varieties, some of which are: *anise basil, cinnamon basil, dark opal basil* (dark purple leaves, but with a taste like sweet basil), and *lemon basil*. As you might guess, in many cases, their names are indicative of their taste. So-called *holy basil* has smaller leaves with purple markings; it's often called for in Thai recipes. However, holy basil is quite pungent and is rarely eaten raw. Dried basil has lost quite a bit of the fragrance and pungency of the fresh herb, but it retains a certain delicate flavor that does well in sauces and soups.

Chives Chives are the leaves of a bulb plant in the onion family. In fact, the word chive comes from the Latin word for onion (*cepa*). The slender, hollow, grass-green leaves have a very delicate but pronounced onion flavor. They are best used fresh, but frozen and freeze-dried chives are not unreasonable substitutes.

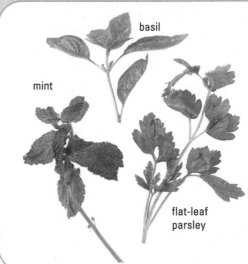

green herbs

basil

mint

flat-leaf parsley

SORREL / ½ cup	
Calories	15
Protein (g)	1
Carbohydrate (g)	2
Dietary fiber (g)	1.9
Total fat (g)	0.5
Saturated fat (g)	--
Monounsaturated fat (g)	--
Polyunsaturated fat (g)	--
Cholesterol (mg)	0
Potassium (mg)	259
Sodium (mg)	3

KEY NUTRIENTS (%RDA/AI*)		
Beta carotene	1.6 mg	(15%)
Vitamin C	32 mg	(35%)
Iron	1.6 mg	(20%)
Magnesium	69 mg	(16%)

For more detailed information on RDA and AI, see page 88.

Cilantro Mexican and Indian food—to name just two of many cuisines in which this herb is used—would not be the same without cilantro, also called coriander leaf or Chinese parsley. The leaves, which resemble those of flat-leaf parsley (and are in the same botanical family) are strongly aromatic; the root is also used in cooking, especially in Thailand, where it is an essential ingredient in many curry pastes. Cilantro's distinctive flavor is not to everyone's taste—in fact, it seems to be a "love it or hate it" seasoning. Some researchers believe that there is a genetic component to an individual's reaction to cilantro. The herb was used in ancient times as an appetite stimulant, and for cilantro aficionados, it still serves that purpose admirably. Dried cilantro is available but it has very little flavor.

Culantro (saw-leaf herb) An herb popular in Latin America and the Caribbean, this herb is often mislabeled cilantro, though it looks quite different. The flavors of the two herbs, however, are similar; though culantro is more pungent than cilantro. The leaves of culantro are long, narrow, and serrated (they look like skinny dandelion leaves). You can use culantro the way you would cilantro.

Dill Though native to the Mediterranean, dill as a seasoning is probably most connected with the cuisines of Scandinavia and Central Europe. Fresh dill leaves are used to flavor the salmon dish called gravlax; and dill seeds are what give dill pickles their distinctive flavor. Dill leaves are feathery fronds, which resemble the fronds of the fennel plant, a relative of dill. Dried dill (called dillweed) has very little flavor.

Garlic chives (Chinese chives) Like regular chives, garlic chives belong to the onion family, though they are different in appearance. Whereas regular chives are hollow, garlic chives are flat and look like large blades of grass. They are more pungent than regular chives and have a hint of garlic in their flavor. Garlic chives can be *green, yellow* (these are not a separate type, but are green chives that have been deprived of light to turn them yellow; they have a milder flavor), or *flowering* (these are chives that are allowed to form a bud, but are picked before they flower).

COMPARING GREEN HERBS **¼ cup chopped raw**

With the exception of sorrel (*see nutrition box, page 349*), most of these herbs are eaten in fairly small quantities.

	Beta carotene (mg)	Vitamin C (mg)	Folate (mcg)	Iron (mg)	Potassium (mg)
Basil	0.3	2	7	0.3	49
Chives	0.3	7	13	0.2	36
Cilantro	0.4	4	7	0.2	59
Dill	0.1	2	3	0.2	16
Mint	0.6	3	24	2.7	104
Parsley	0.5	20	23	0.9	83

Lovage This herb looks just like celery leaves and also tastes like a more pungent celery.

Mint There are 20 or so "pure" mint species (there are thousands more hybrids, since mint is a prolific and aggressive plant). But the three most common species are *Mentha piperita* (peppermint), *Mentha spicata* (spearmint), and *Mentha suaveolens* (apple and pineapple mint). The type of mint most commonly found in supermarkets is *spearmint* (also called garden mint). *Peppermint* is the strongest-tasting of all the mint species and the one used to make peppermint oils and candies. Most of the other mint varieties are the province of farmers' markets, specialty produce markets, and the home gardener. Some of the more unusual varieties of mint include ginger mint, grapefruit mint, and eau de cologne mint. Mint leaves tend to be oval and either slightly pointed or rounded at the tip. They can be wrinkled or smooth, but they are all slightly serrated. Mint flavor is fairly well preserved in the dried form.

Parsley This is the most common fresh herb in American supermarkets. There are two main types: *curly parsley* and *flat-leaf (or Italian) parsley*. Curly parsley is favored by restaurants for decorating plates, but flat-leaf parsley is the choice of most cooks, because it has a much more pronounced parsley flavor. There is also a type of parsley grown for its roots; *parsley roots* are cooked like carrot or parsnip. Although dried parsley is available, it has no flavor.

Sorrel (spinach dock) Sorrel, whose leaves look like arrow-shaped spinach, has a memorable tart flavor, which some have likened to rhubarb. Though sorrel can be treated as a salad green, its classic European use is as a puree that is turned into either a soup, or a sauce to serve over fish (traditionally salmon, whose rich flavor pairs beautifully with the tartness of the sorrel).

▶ Availability Most of these green herbs are available all year. The availability of unusual varieties sold in farmers' markets will vary with the climate and growing season of the locality, though mid to late summer is a safe bet.

choosing the best

For basil and cilantro, look for bright, fresh leaves that are dry, not slimy. If possible, buy bunches with their root ends on. For other herbs, with no roots, look for fresh-looking, unwilted leaves. Dill will look limp compared to some herbs because it is so feathery, so check to be sure there are no dark slimy spots.

▶ When you get home Herbs that come with roots are best stored with the roots in a jar of water and a plastic bag over the leaves to keep moisture in. If the herbs come rootless, wrap them (unwashed) in damp paper towels and put in a plastic bag open at one end for air circulation. Store the herbs in the refrigerator.

facts & tips

Sprouted caraway seeds produce an herb known as caraway mint, which is often used in Vietnamese cooking.

preparing to use

Herbs that are sold with roots attached will usually need careful washing, as there will be a lot of dirt clinging to them. For whatever portion of a bunch you are using, cut off the root ends and wash them separately (if using). Wash the stalks and leaves in a salad spinner or bowl filled with water.

Some herbs are sold on the stem (basil, mint, cilantro, dill, and parsley). Generally speaking, the stems will be more bitter and sometimes less flavorful than the leaves. So either pull the leaves off the stem (as with basil and mint) before chopping, or cut off the thickest, toughest parts of the stems (as with dill, parsley, and cilantro).

For herbs that are sold just as leaves (sorrel, chives, culantro), just wash if necessary and chop or mince. Chives require some special care, however, when you're mincing: Because they are so small, a big knife will often just crush them instead of chopping them. The easiest way to get crisply cut pieces of chive is to use a pair of kitchen scissors. Scissors are also good for cutting dill, whose feathery fronds can be hard to gather up enough to chop efficiently.

serving suggestions

• Although basil is the traditional pesto herb, try making pesto with cilantro or mint instead.

• Make a vegetarian herb broth as the basis of a soup. Start with a large handful of mixed herbs (including roots if there are any) and a good amount of water. If desired, add some chopped garlic and onion (no need to sauté; simply put them in). Add some salt to bring out the herbs' flavors. Let simmer for at least an hour to infuse the stock with the herbs. The resulting broth will be fairly subtle in flavor.

• Make a mixed herb salad: Combine mint, basil, and garlic chives with a mild lettuce, such as Bibb or Boston.

• Use dill, mint, or cilantro to flavor vinegar. Just add washed sprigs to a bottle of white wine vinegar or distilled white vinegar and let sit for a week or so. You can leave the sprigs in the bottle.

• Mix any one of these green herbs, finely minced, into reduced-fat cream cheese or homemade yogurt cheese *(see page 600)* for a sandwich spread.

greens, cooking

For years, "cooking greens"—a term referring to a group of leafy green vegetables from several different plant families that are distinguished by their pungent bite and abundant nutrients—have been appreciated mainly in Southern-style cuisine. Recently, perhaps because of their substantial nutritional merits, they have become more popular. Interest in cooking greens has also been promoted by chefs (who find their assertive flavors appealing) and farmers' markets, where all manner of vegetables have found a new and appreciative audience.

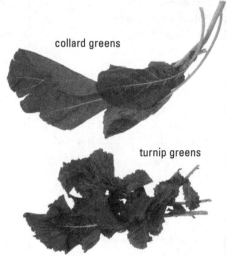

cooking greens

collard greens

turnip greens

nutritional profile

To reap the rewards from leafy greens, look for the darkest greens (and reds). Many types of intensely colored leafy plants—especially kale, collards, and others in the cabbage family—are rich in beta carotene, vitamin C, folate, and other substances that may protect against cancer, heart disease, and a host of other conditions. Cooking greens are also good sources of fiber and of various minerals, particularly iron and calcium: collards and turnip greens top the charts for calcium. (In some countries, such as China, whose populations eat primarily vegetarian diets, greens can supply their total calcium needs.) Although beet greens, spinach, and Swiss chard contain calcium, it should be noted that they also contain substances called oxalates, which prevent calcium from being properly absorbed. Still, this is no reason to throw away these greens; they are rich sources of beta carotene, which is an important health-promoting antioxidant carotenoid.

in the market

Now that greens are gaining greater recognition for their nutritional benefits, they are no longer considered a regional item and have become available throughout the country. Those listed below come from several different plant families, chief among them the cabbage family. Most of these greens can be eaten raw when young and tender, but as they mature, their strong flavors benefit from a brief cooking.

Amaranth greens See Amaranth (*page 158*).

Beet greens These are the green tops of a root vegetable, and they may be sold attached to full-sized or baby beets, or in bunches by themselves. The long-stemmed, large, green or greenish-red leaves are significantly more nutritious than the roots. Beet greens are at their best and most tender when young.

Broccoli rabe See Broccoli (*page 204*).

COLLARD GREENS
1 cup cooked

Calories	49
Protein (g)	4
Carbohydrate (g)	9
Dietary fiber (g)	5.3
Total fat (g)	0.7
Saturated fat (g)	0.1
Monounsaturated fat (g)	0.1
Polyunsaturated fat (g)	0.3
Cholesterol (mg)	0
Potassium (mg)	494
Sodium (mg)	17

KEY NUTRIENTS (%RDA/AI*)

Beta carotene	3.6 mg (32%)
Riboflavin	0.2 mg (15%)
Vitamin B$_6$	0.2 mg (14%)
Vitamin C	35 mg (38%)
Vitamin E	1.7 mg (11%)
Folate	177 mcg (44%)
Calcium	226 mg (19%)
Iron	0.9 mg (11%)

*For more detailed information on RDA and AI, see page 88.

Chinese cabbages This is a loose term that includes such greens as bok choy and napa cabbage. (*See "Chinese Cabbages," page 211.*)

Collards A cruciferous vegetable with anticancer potential, collards, along with kale, are among the oldest members of the cabbage family to be cultivated. Their large, smooth leaves, deep green in color, don't form a head, but grow outward from a central axis. Each leaf is attached to a long, heavy stalk (which is inedible). Collards are one of the milder greens; the flavor is somewhere between cabbage and kale.

Dandelion greens Whether wild or cultivated, these greens come from the common lawn weed, which is a member of the sunflower family. The leaves—pale green with saw-toothed edges—are picked before the yellow flower develops, and they have a faintly bitter taste, similar to chicory. The dandelion greens sold in markets have been cultivated for eating and are longer and more tender than wild greens; before picking wild dandelion leaves from lawns or meadows, be sure that the area has not been treated with weed killer or fungicides, and that it is not close to a heavily traveled road, where exhaust pollutants are likely to have tainted it.

Escarole See Endive & Chicory (*page 283*).

Kale See Kale (*page 365*).

Malabar spinach (vine spinach, climbing spinach) Malabar spinach is not actually a member of the spinach family. It is one of many cooking greens that are called spinach because their flavor vaguely resembles the earthiness of spinach. Malabar spinach comes from a tropical vine native to Southeast Asia. There are two principal varieties: those with green vines and those with red. Though it tastes like spinach, it actually exudes a substance that is similar to that of okra, which makes it difficult for some to warm up to, but it's a good choice for adding thickness to soups and stews.

Mustard greens Yet another cabbage-family member, mustard greens physically resemble a more delicate version of kale, but they have a stronger bite. They are the leafy part of the plant from which we get mustard seed. The

THE GREENS VERSUS THE ROOTS

While turnips and beets are nutritious vegetables, their green tops are even better sources of vitamins and minerals (with the exception of the B vitamin folate in beets, which is in higher concentration in the root than in the tops). The values are based on a 1-cup serving of cooked roots or greens and are expressed as a percentage of the RDA or AI (*see page 88*).

	Beta carotene	Vitamin C	Folate	Calcium	Iron
Beets	0%	7%	34%	2%	17%
Beet greens	40%	40%	5%	14%	34%
Turnips	0%	20%	4%	3%	4%
Turnip greens	43%	44%	42%	16%	14%

leaves, which are light green (sometimes with a bronze tinge) and slightly ruffled, taste best when they are 6 to 12 inches long and have no seeds: Seeds are a sign of overmaturity. In some markets, you may also find Asian mustard greens, which are a milder variety.

Purslane This fleshy-leafed green is used in salads as well as cooked, especially for Hispanic dishes; it's also popular in various Mediterranean cuisines. Purslane is one of a small number of foods notably high in alpha–linolenic acid (ALA), an essential fatty acid associated with lowered risk of fatal heart attack.

Spinach See Spinach (*page 539*).

Stinging nettle Commonly used in Europe as a cooking green, nettle is easily recognized by its serrated leaves (they look like they've been cut out with pinking shears). The stinging nettle is a herbaceous plant related to hops, marijuana, mulberries, and elms. Small fluid-filled hairs on the leaf surface and stem contain formic acid, which can cause a stinging or burning sensation and/or a rash. Cooking or soaking the green, however, eliminates the stinging effect.

Swiss chard See Swiss Chard (*page 565*).

Turnip greens The leafy tops from turnips are one of the sharpest-tasting greens, and like mustard greens, they are generally too assertive (and tough) for eating raw. Don't expect to find them with turnip roots attached: Most varieties grown for their tops don't develop full-grown roots. If you find roots with their tops attached, the greens are perfectly edible, but they may be too bitter and tough to eat unless they are quite young.

▶ **Availability** Though some of the greens discussed here have seasonal peaks, they are available year round, except Swiss chard, which is available from April through November.

> ## vitamin K
>
> Vitamin K is best known for its crucial role in bone health and blood clotting. However, anyone taking anticoagulant drugs such as warfarin (Coumadin), which decrease blood clotting by inhibiting the action of vitamin K, should avoid large servings of certain cooking greens. The greens with significantly high levels of vitamin K are: kale, Swiss chard, turnip greens, and mustard greens. Other vegetables high in vitamin K are broccoli and Brussels sprouts.

COMPARING GREENS	Calories	Beta carotene (mg)	Vitamin C (mg)	Folate (mcg)	Calcium (mg)	Iron (mg)
Beet greens	39	4.4	36	21	164	2.7
Bok choy	20	2.6	44	69	158	1.8
Collards	49	3.6	35	177	226	0.9
Dandelion greens	35	7.4	19	13	147	1.9
Kale	36	5.8	53	17	94	1.2
Malabar spinach	10	0.3	3	50	55	0.7
Mustard greens	21	2.6	35	103	104	1.0
Spinach	41	8.8	18	263	245	6.4
Swiss chard	35	3.3	32	15	102	4.0
Turnip greens	29	4.8	40	170	197	1.2

COMPARING GREENS **1 cup cooked**

choosing the best

Greens should be kept in a chilled display case or on ice in the market, as they will wilt and become bitter if left in a warm environment. Whatever the type of green, it is best to choose smaller-leaved plants for their tenderness and mild flavor, especially if the greens are to be eaten raw; coarse, oversized leaves are likely to be tough. Look for a fresh green color—leaves should not be yellowed or browned—and purchase only moist, crisp, unwilted greens, unblemished by tiny holes, which indicate insect damage.

When buying greens with edible stems, select those with fine stems. Make sure that dandelion greens have their roots attached. Check that mustard greens are free of seed stems.

▶ **When you get home** Wrap unwashed greens in damp paper towels, then place them in a plastic bag; store them in the refrigerator crisper. Sturdy greens, such as collards, are better keepers than delicate ones like spinach. Some greens, such as kale, develop a stronger flavor the longer they are stored; use them within a day or two of purchase.

preparing to use

Whether serving them raw or cooked, wash greens before using, as they are likely to have sand or dirt clinging to them. Trim off any roots, separate the leaves, and swish them around in a large bowl of cool water; do not soak. Lift out the leaves, letting the sand and grit settle; repeat if necessary.

Pinch off tough or inedible stems, and also the midribs (the part of the stem that extends into the leaf) if they are thick and tough. You can easily stem tender greens by folding each leaf in half, vein-side out, and pulling up on the stem as you hold the folded leaf closed. Tougher stems, such as those on kale leaves, may need to be trimmed off with a paring knife.

For stinging nettles, take care not to touch the hairs on the tops of the leaves and stems. Anyone with sensitive skin should use gloves when handling nettles.

serving suggestions

• Use collards, beet greens, or kale in place of spinach in a Greek spinach pie recipe.

• Steam whole greens, finely chop, and mix with ground turkey breast (about 3 parts turkey to 1 part greens). Form the mixture into burgers.

• Stir finely shredded greens into brown rice for the last 15 minutes of cooking. Remove from the heat and let sit covered for another 5 or 10 minutes. Stir in minced sun-dried tomatoes and toasted sunflower seeds.

• Make a greens and beans soup: Sauté onions and garlic in a small amount of olive oil. Add 1 or 2 cups of carrot juice thinned with some water. Add lots of mixed greens and let them cook down. Then add canned crushed tomatoes and cooked beans. Add enough water to reach a soupy consistency.

greens, salad

As people have become more nutrition-conscious, salads have gained in favor as an essential part of a healthy meal. Luckily, we have moved well past the iceberg lettuce salad of yesteryear. Today a multitude of different salad greens are preferred, including more interesting lettuces (*see Lettuce, page 380*) and greens from other botanical families. If iceberg is the only type of salad green you eat, you are choosing the least nutritious member of a group of nutritional champions. Any other lettuce or leafy green vegetable would be a better choice.

nutritional profile

As a general rule, the darker green the leaves, the more nutritious the salad green. Watercress, for example, has almost 10 times as much beta carotene, four times the calcium, and six times the vitamin C of iceberg lettuce. And insoluble fiber, which helps to satisfy the appetite as well as promote good intestinal function, is particularly plentiful in darkly pigmented salad greens.

Indeed, most of the nonlettuce greens listed here are higher in nutrients and phytochemicals than the basic types of lettuce. Arugula and watercress, two nonlettuce greens in the cruciferous vegetable family, are packed with beneficial plant chemicals that may help to defend against cancer.

Generally speaking, the darker the green the more beta carotene; but chicory and dandelion greens top the chart for this healthful carotenoid, with 2 cups of either one providing well over 60 percent of the RDA. Small amounts of the B vitamin folate are found in many salad greens, with chicory providing a particularly impressive amount (100 percent of the daily requirement in 2 cups). By varying the greens in your salads, you can enhance the nutritional content as well as vary the taste and texture.

in the market

In addition to all manner of lettuces, there are a host of greens that are delicious in salads. The following greens, each of which has a distinct flavor, can be used alone or mixed with lettuce to heighten the flavor of a salad as well as increase its nutritional content: Some of them contain significantly more vitamins and minerals than lettuce.

Arugula (rocket, roquette) This green used to be sold only in Italian markets, but is now widely available. Arugula consists of small, flat leaves on long stems—it resembles dandelion greens—and is often displayed with the roots attached. It has a distinct peppery taste and aroma; the more mature the green, the stronger and more mustardlike the taste. In fact, arugula grown during the summer can have a very sharp flavor, so taste it to determine how much you want to use.

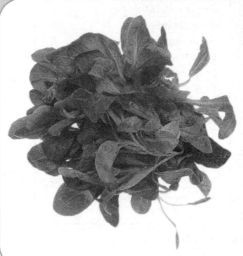

mâche

MACHE / 2 cups	
Calories	24
Protein (g)	2
Carbohydrate (g)	4
Dietary fiber (g)	1.7
Total fat (g)	0.5
Saturated fat (g)	--
Monounsaturated fat (g)	--
Polyunsaturated fat (g)	--
Cholesterol (mg)	0
Potassium (mg)	514
Sodium (mg)	5

KEY NUTRIENTS (%RDA/AI*)	
Beta carotene	4.8 mg (43%)
Vitamin B$_6$	0.3 mg (18%)
Vitamin C	43 mg (48%)

*For more detailed information on RDA and AI, see page 88.

Baby greens As a result of the mesclun craze that began a decade or so ago, lots of markets are now selling baby versions of a variety of greens, but not as a mixture (*see mesclun, below*). The most popular one is baby spinach, which are leaves usually no longer than 3 or 4 inches with thin, tender, edible stems. They are almost always sold prewashed and in bulk.

Belgian endive See Endive & Chicory (*page 282*).

Chicory See Endive & Chicory (*page 282*).

Curly endive See Endive & Chicory (*page 283*)

Dandelion greens Young dandelion greens are the best for salads because they are tender and less bitter. Dandelion greens are also good cooked (*see page 354*).

Escarole See Endive & Chicory (*page 283*).

Lamb's-quarters Also called pigfoot or wild spinach, this green (technically a weed) is a wild relative of Amaranth (*page 158*). Like domesticated amaranth, lamb's-quarters are packed with nutrients.

Mâche This expensive and delicate green, which is extremely perishable and therefore not widely available, has several names: lamb's lettuce, field salad, and corn salad. The leaves are fingerlike and velvety, with a mild taste. Mâche is usually sold in small bunches with its roots attached. It is high in beta carotene.

Mesclun The word mesclun comes from an old Provençal word meaning mixture, which is what it is, a mixture of different salad greens. A typical mesclun mix is young spring greens sold prewashed and in bulk. However, since the concept has gotten so popular, some markets sell mixtures of torn-up lettuces instead of baby greens. The greens used in mesclun can vary and some markets put together specific blends (such as Italian, mild, and spicy).

WATERCRESS / 2 cups	
Calories	8
Protein (g)	2
Carbohydrate (g)	1
Dietary fiber (g)	1.0
Total fat (g)	0.1
Saturated fat (g)	0
Monounsaturated fat (g)	0
Polyunsaturated fat (g)	0
Cholesterol (mg)	0
Potassium (mg)	224
Sodium (mg)	28

KEY NUTRIENTS (%RDA/AI*)	
Beta carotene	1.9 mg (17%)
Vitamin C	29 mg (32%)

For more detailed information on RDA and AI, see page 88.

COMPARING SALAD GREENS 2 cups raw						
	Calories	Beta carotene (mg)	Vitamin C (mg)	Folate (mcg)	Calcium (mg)	Iron (mg)
Arugula	10	0.6	6	39	64	0.6
Chicory	83	8.6	86	396	360	3.2
Dandelion greens	50	9.2	39	30	206	3.4
Escarole	17	1.2	6	142	52	0.8
Looseleaf lettuce	20	1.3	20	56	76	1.6
Mâche	24	4.8	43	15	43	2.4
Radicchio	18	0	6	48	15	0.5
Romaine lettuce	16	1.7	27	152	40	1.2
Spinach	13	2.4	17	116	59	1.6
Watercress	8	1.9	29	6	82	0.1

Mizuna These Japanese greens look like elongated chrysanthemum leaves. They are tender and, because they belong to the mustard family, have a peppery flavor.

Nasturtiums The flowers of the colorful nasturtium plant are often added to salads (*see "Edible Flowers," page 360*), but the leaves, too, make a great flavor addition. They are spicy tasting.

Purslane Purslane belongs to a large family of plants, many of which would be recognized by home gardeners as portulaca. With over 500 species, purslane has been an evolutionary success, in part due to the fact that a single plant can produce up to 52,300 seeds (which can then patiently survive for up to 30 years before germinating). The young leaves are good in salads, but the larger fleshy leaves are good cooked.

Spinach See Spinach (*page 539*).

Radicchio See Radicchio (*page 499*).

Radish greens Most markets sells radishes with their tops on. If they are in good condition, don't throw them away. They have a bright peppery flavor (like radishes) and can be used the way you would watercress.

Tatsoi The young leaves of this cabbage relative look like little spoons, hence its other name, spoon cabbage. Tatsoi tastes mildly peppery and sweet, with only the faintest hint of cabbage flavor.

Watercress See Watercress (*page 588*).

choosing the best

Above all, salad greens should be fresh and crisp. It is easy to spot wilted greens; watch out for limp, withered leaves that have brown or yellow edges, or dark or slimy spots. Once greens have passed their prime, there is no way to restore them to crisp freshness. Even delicate greens, such as arugula, should be crisp, especially the stems. The leaves should be dark green, never yellow.

▶ **When you get home** Most greens keep best wrapped in damp paper towels and then placed in a plastic bag in the refrigerator crisper. Greens sold with their roots intact keep best if you wrap the roots in damp paper towels, then place the whole bunch in a plastic bag. Delicate greens, such as arugula and mâche, are very perishable: Buy only enough for immediate use, or keep them for no more than a day or two.

Don't store greens near fruits, such as apples or bananas, which give off ethylene gas as they ripen. Otherwise, the greens will develop brown spots and decay rapidly. For appetizingly crisp greens—and to minimize last-minute preparation at mealtime—wash and dry them, then layer the leaves in clean paper towels and place in a plastic bag. Refrigerate in the crisper drawer until serving time, but not for more than a few hours, for optimal nutrient retention.

serving suggestions

One of the most important things to learn in making healthful salads is to not drown crisp, fresh greens in a sea of high-fat dressing. There are some simple salad dressings you can make that have little to no fat:

• Use what is essentially a Bloody Mary mixture and add a touch of oil to smooth out the flavors.

• Make a Thai-style salad dressing of soy sauce, lime juice, and enough brown sugar to offset the acid of the lime juice.

• For a low-fat Caesar dressing, combine fat-free mayonnaise with fat-free sour cream and thin with a touch of soy sauce and fat-free milk. The dressing should be thin enough to coat the greens lightly. Sprinkle the salad with some grated Parmesan.

• Combine apple juice concentrate with mustard.

• Stir chopped fresh basil, garlic, and black pepper into fat-free yogurt.

preparing to use

Even if greens look clean, they should be washed—and in some cases, trimmed—before you put them in the salad bowl.

Since grit tends to collect at the stem end of greens that come in heads, especially loose heads, it's important to twist off the stem and separate the leaves before washing them. To wash small-leaved greens on stems, such as watercress and arugula, cut off the roots, hold the greens by the stems, and swish them around in a large bowl of cool water. Lift out the leaves, letting the sand and grit settle, then empty and refill the bowl and repeat the process.

A salad spinner greatly simplifies the preparation of greens by drying them quickly and thoroughly—and dry leaves are a must if the dressing is to adhere properly to the greens.

You can either tear greens into bite-sized pieces by hand or cut them with a knife; each method has its proponents. Kitchen shears are useful for snipping leaves, too. As long as you use a stainless steel blade (carbon steel can cause blackening and alter the flavor) and serve the salad soon after it's prepared, it's safe to cut most greens. However, delicate leaves, such as mâche and arugula, are more appealing when torn (or left whole).

edible flowers

As a garnish or a salad ingredient, fresh flowers bring color, fragrance, and flavor to a meal. Some, like squash or zucchini blossoms, are large enough to be stuffed and cooked, while others—such as violets or pansies—simply add eye appeal and sweet scents to festive desserts or platters. Not all flowers are edible; those that are must be acquired from safe sources. If you're going to serve them as food, do not pick flowers from a pesticide-sprayed backyard or exhaust-choked roadside, or buy them from a florist. A gourmet shop or your own unsprayed garden are safe places to get edible flowers. Some farmstands or farmers' markets may offer them, too, and there are also mail-order sources for edible flowers.

Even though the flowers listed here are edible, it's advisable to make them a relatively minor component of the meal—such as a salad garnish. Some flowers (like certain herbs) can have a laxative effect if eaten in quantity.

The more common edible flowers include daisies, nasturtiums (which taste like watercress), geraniums, lavender, marigolds, pansies, roses, and violets. Herb flowers, such as oregano, thyme, and borage, taste much like the herbs themselves. Blossoms from fruit trees—apple, peach, plum, orange, and lemon—are also fragrant and delicately flavorful.

hazelnuts

Hazelnuts are sweet, acorn-shaped nuts that are often mistakenly referred to as filberts (which are actually a cultivated type of European hazelnut that is slightly larger than the American hazelnut). The hazelnut has a long, fuzzy outer husk that opens as the nut ripens, revealing a hard, smooth shell. Believed to have originated in Asia, the hazelnut is one of the oldest agricultural food crops, providing a high-quality protein and sustenance to humans for thousands of years. Ancient Chinese manuscripts dating back 5,000 years refer to the hazelnut as a sacred food bestowed directly on us by the heavens; and the ancient Greeks and Romans valued hazelnuts for their medicinal properties.

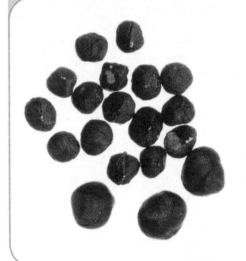

hazelnuts

nutritional profile

While ancient lore has it that hazelnuts held the cure for everything from baldness to gastrointestinal illnesses, modern research is informing us that nuts, in general, if consumed in moderation, may accord cardiovascular benefits. The monounsaturated fats in nuts are believed to lower LDL ("bad") cholesterol levels. Hazelnuts are also a source of plant sterols, substances believed to reduce the risk of heart disease and some cancers. These nuts supply good amounts of vitamins and minerals, including thiamin, vitamin B_6, iron, and magnesium; and, when compared with other nuts, they have a high vitamin E profile.

in the market

Hazelnuts are available in-shell and shelled; chopped, ground, or whole; roasted (brown skin removed) or unroasted (with skin). Hazelnuts impart a sweet, rich flavor and texture to numerous foods and are added to many products, including cookies, candies, ice cream, breakfast cereals, biscotti, tortes, chocolates, coffee, bread, liqueurs, and spreads.

other hazelnut products

Hazelnut butter This creamy, smooth spread (resembling peanut butter) is made from roasted hazelnuts and, like peanut butter, can be eaten on its own or added to recipes for a full, sweet flavor.

Hazelnut meal & flour See Flour, Nonwheat (*page 327*).

Hazelnut oil See Nut Oils (*page 299*).

Hazelnut paste This sweetened mixture of ground hazelnuts and sugar is used as a confectionery paste in hazelnut marzipan, icings, bakery fillings, ice cream, and cookies.

HAZELNUTS / 1 ounce	
Calories	179
Protein (g)	0
Carbohydrate (g)	4
Dietary fiber (g)	1.7
Total fat (g)	18
Saturated fat (g)	1.3
Monounsaturated fat (g)	14
Polyunsaturated fat (g)	1.7
Cholesterol (mg)	0
Potassium (mg)	126
Sodium (mg)	1

KEY NUTRIENTS (%RDA/AI*)	
Thiamin	0.1 mg (12%)
Vitamin B$_6$	0.2 mg (10%)
Vitamin E	6.8 mg (45%)
Iron	0.9 mg (12%)
Magnesium	81 mg (19%)

*For more detailed information on RDA and AI, see page 88.

choosing the best

If purchasing hazelnuts in the shell, look for shells that are full and heavy. Old nuts will start to dry in the shell, making them lighter. If purchasing shelled nuts, look for skins that are tight and nuts that are plump. Shop at a store with a brisk turnover to get the freshest nuts possible.

▶ **When you get home** Fresh hazelnuts are delicate and perishable. Shelled hazelnuts, in particular, should be eaten as soon as possible and kept at room temperature, away from heat and humidity. Shelled hazelnuts may be kept in the refrigerator or freezer for up to 4 months. Unshelled hazelnuts may be stored in a dry, cool place for up to 1 month.

preparing to use

The dark skin of hazelnuts is slightly bitter and can be removed by toasting the nuts in a 350° oven for 10 to 15 minutes until the skins begin to crack (this will happen to some but not all of the nuts, so don't worry and don't wait for all of them to crack). Transfer the hot nuts to a kitchen towel and vigorously rub to remove most of the skin. Some skin will remain; that's fine. Let the nuts cool before proceeding with the recipe.

If you're baking a cake or cookies, and your recipe calls for ground nuts, place them in a food processor with a little of the flour in the recipe and process; this way they'll grind without becoming oily and pasty.

serving suggestions

- Add chopped hazelnuts to salads.
- Roll goat cheese in crushed hazelnuts and serve a slice for dessert along with red grapes.
- Coat fish in a mixture of bread crumbs and crushed hazelnuts before sautéing.
- Stir coarsely chopped toasted hazelnuts into frozen yogurt.
- Add chopped hazelnuts to vegetable sautés.
- Dress salads with a light coating of hazelnut oil.
- Scatter slightly crushed toasted hazelnuts over grilled pineapple slices for dessert.
- Add hazelnuts to pilafs, risottos, and other rice dishes.

horseradish

Horseradish is a member of the cabbage family, which includes its milder and gentler cousins, cauliflower, kale, the common radish, and Brussels sprouts. Its root (gnarled and somewhat unattractive in appearance) has been cultivated and prized from the earliest times, though its exact place of origin is unknown. The Bible cites horseradish as one of the five bitter herbs (along with coriander, horehound, lettuce, and nettle), and it is served traditionally at Passover seder. Used by the ancient Greeks and the Egyptians for its medicinal value, horseradish was also considered to be an aphrodisiac and a universal cure-all for a host of ailments, including intestinal worms, coughs, gout, scurvy, food poisoning, tuberculosis, colic, and rheumatism.

Luckily for us, during the Middle Ages people, in Europe started to view horseradish as a food instead of a medicine, and by the end of the 17th century, horseradish's piquant but pleasant flavor served as a standard counterpoint to beef, fish, and oysters.

Horseradish has a highly complex flavor, a combination of biting hot and intense, with a beguiling undercurrent of sweetness. Its strong bite comes from a natural chemical, allyl isothiocynate, as well as other volatile oils. When the root is cut or grated, horseradish's natural chemicals are acted on by enzymes, thus developing its characteristic pungent odor and flavor.

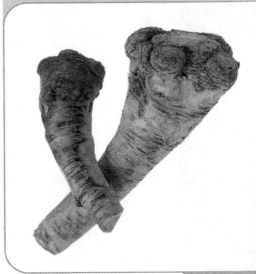

fresh horseradish

nutritional profile

Horseradish is a cruciferous vegetable, and as such may have cancer-fighting potential. Though it contains some vitamin C, horseradish is eaten in such small quantities that this is of no particular consequence.

in the market

Fresh horseradish Scruffy and gnarled, these roots vary in size from 6 to 12 inches long and 1 to 3 inches in diameter.

Prepared horseradish This horseradish, which has been grated and mixed with vinegar, comes in bottles. You can find both *white* and *red* prepared horseradish (the red is colored and flavored with beet juice).

Wasabi This is the pungent, nose-clearing green paste that accompanies sushi or sashimi in Japanese restaurants. Though wasabi is often sold (in the form of powders or pastes in the supermarket) as Japanese horseradish, what you are actually getting is Western-style horseradish that has been tinted green to resemble real wasabi. The main reason for this is that real wasabi—which is botanically related to horseradish (it is a cruciferous vegetable), but not of the same genus—is an extremely difficult, and ultimately expensive, plant to grow. Most real wasabi is still only available in Japan, but there are

PREPARED HORSERADISH 1 tablespoon	
Calories	7
Protein (g)	0
Carbohydrate (g)	2
Dietary fiber (g)	0.5
Total fat (g)	0.1
Saturated fat (g)	0
Monounsaturated fat (g)	0
Polyunsaturated fat (g)	0.1
Cholesterol (mg)	0
Potassium (mg)	37
Sodium (mg)	47

some American growers actually tackling the challenge of growing the fussy plant in this country.

choosing the best

When shopping for fresh horseradish, look for roots that are plump, not dried or withered (however, the skin may be wrinkled). Depending upon the time of year, the horseradish may have its green tops or not. Whether or not the tops are attached is not a measure of freshness.

Fresh wasabi, not generally available in local markets, can be purchased through mail–order sources. The roots should be firm and the leaves, if any, should be bright green.

▶ **When you get home** Fresh wasabi should be wrapped in damp paper towels and kept refrigerated. It can be refrigerated for about 30 days, but should be rinsed in cold water once a week to keep it at its best. Keep fresh horseradish, unwrapped, in the crisper drawer of the refrigerator.

preparing to use

Fresh horseradish should be peeled before grating. Once peeled, grate on the finest holes of a box grater.

Fresh wasabi should be gently scrubbed before grating; peeling is optional. Grate wasabi on the finest holes of a grater. Once grated, it's suggested that you crush it with the back of a knife to release more flavor. After crushing, let wasabi stand 5 minutes before using to allow the flavors and heat to develop.

serving suggestions

- Grate fresh horseradish and sprinkle on meat, seafood, or vegetables.

- Add horseradish to your favorite guacamole recipe.

- For a quick sauce, stir horseradish into reduced-fat sour cream or yogurt.

- Stir horseradish into meat or poultry stews.

- Add horseradish to tuna or chicken salads.

- Stir horseradish into mashed potatoes.

- Combine horseradish with low-fat mayonnaise and use as a sandwich spread.

- Combine horseradish with diced apples and nuts for an interesting relish.

- Jazz up ketchup with a healthy amount of prepared horseradish.

- Stir wasabi into your favorite barbecue sauce.

- Combine soy sauce with wasabi powder or paste and use as a dipping sauce for fish.

- Grate horseradish or wasabi into applesauce and use as an accompaniment for roasted or grilled meat or poultry.

- Add horseradish to mint, currant, or apple jelly to serve alongside lamb or other meat.

kale

Originating in the eastern Mediterranean, kale is one of the oldest forms of cabbage. A bit too bitter to be eaten raw, it is a "cooking green"—a term referring to a group of leafy green vegetables from several different plant families that are distinguished by their piquant, peppery flavor and plentiful nutrients (*see Greens, Cooking, page 353*). Like other cooking greens, in this country kale has been mostly a feature of Southern-style cuisine (though it has been used in Europe for years).

Kale is easy to grow, is quite tolerant of cold temperatures, and is especially sweet following a light frost. Unfortunately, for the most part, it is considered a decoration, not a vegetable. On buffet tables, the deep-green, frilly leaves are hardy enough to last without wilting and are used to decorate the serving area. And "flowering" varieties of kale are a common autumn feature of public garden areas in colder parts of the country, because they are the closest thing you can get to a colorful flower in the cold weather.

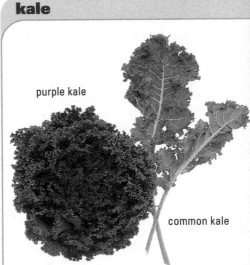

kale

purple kale

common kale

nutritional profile

This member of the cabbage family is a cruciferous vegetable and as such has a rich supply of nutrients. Kale supplies fiber, vitamin C, vitamin B_6, and beta carotene.

In addition to beta carotene, kale has handsome amounts of the carotenoids lutein and zeaxanthin. Research shows that lutein and zeaxanthin may reduce risk of age-related macular degeneration as well as cataracts by protecting the eyes from free-radical damage.

Kale also has some calcium—about 94 milligrams of the bone-nourishing mineral in 1 cup of cooked kale. Although this is only 8 percent of the RDA, if you eat 2 cups of kale you can double the calcium and still consume only 72 calories. In addition, while many greens contain compounds called oxalates, which prevent calcium from being properly absorbed, kale has lower amounts of oxalic acid, making its calcium more available.

in the market

Kale resembles collards, except that its leaves are curly at the edges. In addition, it has a stronger flavor and a coarser texture. When cooked, it doesn't shrink as much as other greens. The most common variety is deep green, but other kales are yellow-green, white, red, or purple, with either flat or ruffled leaves. The colored varieties—sometimes called salad Savoy—are most often grown for ornamental purposes, but they are edible.

Black (dinosaur kale, Tuscan kale, cavallo nero) This Italian variety of kale has crinkly leaves that resemble Savoy cabbage and a sweet, slightly spicy flavor.

KALE / 1 cup cooked	
Calories	36
Protein (g)	3
Carbohydrate (g)	7
Dietary fiber (g)	2.6
Total fat (g)	0.5
Saturated fat (g)	0.1
Monounsaturated fat (g)	0
Polyunsaturated fat (g)	0.3
Cholesterol (mg)	0
Potassium (mg)	296
Sodium (mg)	30

KEY NUTRIENTS (%RDA/AI*)		
Beta carotene	5.8 mg	(52%)
Vitamin B_6	0.2 mg	(11%)
Vitamin C	53 mg	(59%)
Iron	1.2 mg	(15%)

*For more detailed information on RDA and AI, see page 88.

➤ phytochemicals in
kale

It's well known that cruciferous vegetables such as kale are rich in compounds that have the potential to fight cancer, including antioxidants. Sulforaphane is one of these potent substances that neutralize cancer-causing chemicals. And indole phytochemicals in this cooking green may protect against breast cancer by making estrogen less potent.

serving suggestions

- Add shredded kale to minestrone, potato chowder, or vegetable soup.

- Stir sautéed kale into mashed potatoes.

- Shred kale and sauté in garlic and oil. Add canned white beans and toss with freshly cooked pasta.

- Use kale leaves instead of cabbage leaves in a stuffed cabbage recipe.

- Top a pizza with sliced steamed kale.

- Add kale to grain or rice pilafs.

- Stir kale into stuffings for poultry, meat, or seafood.

- Add shredded kale to stir-fries.

- Braise kale in a flavorful vegetable or chicken broth and serve as an accompaniment to grilled meat.

Common This is the type most commonly found in supermarkets. It has large, frilly-edged leaves and long stems. Kale grows in a loose head, but is often sold as loose leaves bound together. The color can range from pale to deep green with a slightly bluish hue.

Purple (ornamental kale, salad Savoy) Frilly and fluffy, ranging in color from pink to purple to magenta, this colorful variety is used on buffet tables for displays. It forms a rosette, which looks like an opened-up flower. While its leaves are somewhat coarse, it is edible.

Red Russian (Ragged Jack) This type of kale is sold as individual leaves like common kale. The leaves are bluish-green with a red rib. They do not have the deeply frilly edges of common kale and look just like overgrown oak leaves. Russian kale is more tender and sweeter than common kale.

White This variety of kale forms a rosette head like purple kale, but its frilly leaves are white. The flavor is strong and cabbagelike.

choosing the best

Choose smaller-leaved specimens for tenderness and mild flavor, especially if the greens are to be eaten raw; coarse, oversized leaves are likely to be tough. Look for a fresh green color—leaves should not be yellowed or browned—and purchase only moist, crisp, unwilted kale, unblemished by tiny holes, which indicate insect damage. Kale stems are edible, so check to be sure that this part of the plant is also in good condition.

➤ **When you get home** Kale develops a stronger flavor the longer it is stored, so use it within a day or two of purchase. Wrap the unwashed kale in damp paper towels, then store in a plastic bag, in the refrigerator crisper.

preparing to use

Kale that you buy at the supermarket is usually pretty sturdy (and the stems may be too tough to eat), but kale from a farmers' market—or your own garden—is likely to be more tender, even tender enough to use raw in a salad.

Whether serving it raw or cooked, you should wash kale before using, as the leaves and stems are likely to have sand or dirt clinging to them. Separate the leaves and swish them around in a large basin of cool water; do not soak. Lift out the leaves, letting the sand and grit settle; repeat if necessary.

If the stems are thin and tender, you can just trim them and cook along with the leaves. If they're somewhat thicker, but still tender, cut them off, chop them, and cook them along with the leaves, but add the chopped stems to the pot a little earlier to give them a head start. If the stems are really tough, remove them, along with the midribs (the part of the stem that extends into the leaf). You can easily stem kale by folding each leaf in half, vein-side out, and pulling up on the stem as you hold the folded leaf closed. If the stems are very tough, you may need to trim them off with a paring knife.

kiwifruit

Kiwifruit was introduced to New Zealand from China around 1906 and though it isn't related to the green gooseberry, New Zealanders called this unusual fruit "Chinese gooseberry," probably because both berries have pale green flesh. Later, as New Zealand became a primary kiwifruit-producing nation, and as foreign demand for the fruit increased, they renamed the fruit after their national bird, the kiwi. Over the years, the kiwifruit has emerged from the status of an exotic delicacy to a highly popular fruit that is widely consumed (and grown) in the United States.

Kiwifruit is somewhat deceptively plain in appearance. Beneath its fuzzy brown surface you'll find brilliant pale green flesh speckled with a ring of tiny edible black seeds. Delicate, tart, sweet, and complex in flavor, kiwifruit is a berry that can be delightfully refreshing when eaten on its own and it also serves as a colorful garnish for a variety of dishes.

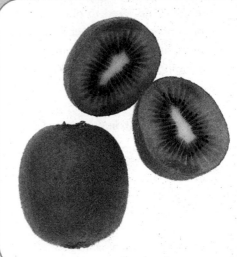

hayward kiwi

nutritional profile

While many types of fruit tend to be high in only one or two nutrients, kiwifruit is brimming with a wide complement of healthy substances. It is an outstanding source of vitamin C, dietary fiber, and potassium. Kiwifruit also supplies a good amount of folate and magnesium.

The carotenoid lutein, which is associated with a reduced risk of cataracts and macular degeneration, is another nutritional benefit. In addition, the antioxidant vitamin E is found in kiwifruit—and unlike many other foods (such as vegetable oils and nuts) that contain vitamin E, this vitamin E source is low in fat and calories.

in the market

Though other types of kiwifruit are now available in some specialty markets, far and away the commonest type of kiwifruit is the green Hayward (though it will only be labeled "kiwifruit").

Gold Gold kiwis have smooth bronze skin and a pointed cap at one end. Inside, the flesh is mustard-colored. The texture, when firm-ripe, is similar to a green kiwi, but when fully ripe becomes almost custardlike. The flavor is multilayered and complex, blending lemon, strawberry, and banana.

Hardy This is one of several varieties of kiwifruit designed to withstand colder temperatures. Once only available to home gardeners, these small, smooth-skinned, grape-sized kiwis are becoming more commercially available. They are sold in the market as *baby kiwis* or *grape kiwis*. Their flavor is similar to other kiwis, with an intriguing blend of tart and sweet. They can be eaten skin and all.

KIWIFRUIT / 2 medium	
Calories	93
Protein (g)	2
Carbohydrate (g)	23
Dietary fiber (g)	5.0
Total fat (g)	0.7
Saturated fat (g)	0
Monounsaturated fat (g)	0.1
Polyunsaturated fat (g)	0.4
Cholesterol (mg)	0
Potassium (mg)	505
Sodium (mg)	8

KEY NUTRIENTS (%RDA/AI*)	
Vitamin C	150 mg (166%)
Vitamin E	1.7 mg (11%)
Folate	58 mcg (14%)
Magnesium	46 mg (11%)

*For more detailed information on RDA and AI, see page 88.

➤ phytochemicals in kiwifruit

Kiwifruit juice has shown promise in blocking detrimental changes in cells that can lead to cancer. The phytochemicals responsible for this beneficial activity have not yet been clearly established. However, kiwifruit juice is a rich source of phenolic compounds—phytochemicals believed to play a role in preventing cancer. Phenolic compounds are also potent antioxidants, helping to disarm cell-damaging free radicals. Kiwifruit also contains chlorogenic acid, a substance that behaves as an antioxidant and may have the potential to help suppress tumor growth.

serving suggestions

• Use kiwifruit in a salad in place of (or with) tomatoes.

• Peel and dice kiwifruit and use to top frozen yogurt or sorbet.

• Puree peeled kiwifruit with another fruit juice such as mango or pineapple along with yogurt for a smoothie.

• Top a creamy rice pudding with diced kiwifruit.

• Prepare a green and gold kiwifruit salsa.

• Toss halved baby kiwifruit and bite-sized mozzarella balls (bocconcini) in a balsamic vinaigrette.

Hayward There are over 50 species of fruit that belong to kiwifruit's genus, but by far the most common variety of kiwifruit is the Hayward, which is green-fleshed and covered with brown fuzz. Although there are other fuzzy-skinned varieties (such as *Bruno, Blake,* and *Chico Early*), Hayward is the kiwifruit that most people are familiar with.

Kolomikta A type of kiwifruit designed to withstand colder temperatures, this variety, which is smaller than the Hayward, is just beginning to have a commercial presence. It's worth keeping an eye out for it, though, because ounce for ounce, kolomikta kiwifruit's vitamin C content is 10 times higher than that of Hayward kiwis.

choosing the best

When buying green or gold kiwifruit, choose plump, fragrant specimens that yield to gentle pressure. Unripe fruit has a hard core and a tart, astringent taste. If only firm kiwis are available, ripen them for a few days before eating them. Baby kiwifruit should be purchased firm and eaten that way.

➤ When you get home To ripen green and gold kiwis, place them in a paper bag with an apple, banana, or pear, and let stand a day or two at room temperature.

preparing to use

It is possible to eat kiwifruit skin and all, although with the fuzzy-skinned, green variety you should rub off the peachlike fuzz. The skin is quite thin, like the skin of a Bosc pear, and is full of nutrients and fiber. If you prefer, you can peel kiwifruit with a vegetable peeler or sharp paring knife; peeling is easier if the ends of the fruit are cut off first.

An enzyme in kiwis, called actinidin, breaks down protein, which can be a problem when combining kiwi with other foods. For example, it prevents gelatin from setting; if you want to add kiwis to gelatin, you should first briefly cook them, which deactivates the enzyme. Similarly, kiwis must be cooked before adding them to dishes containing dairy products—unless the dish will be consumed right away (such as a smoothie).

On the other hand, actinidin's protein-eating actions can be used to advantage for tenderizing meat: Puree fresh kiwis and use the puree as a marinade for beef, poultry, or pork. Or, simply cut the fruit in half, rub it over the meat, and let stand about 30 minutes before cooking.

gold kiwifruit

kohlrabi

A delicately flavored member of the cabbage family, kohlrabi gets its name from the German words *kohl*, which means cabbage, and *rabi* for turnip, hence its nickname "cabbage turnip." The kohlrabi is a swollen stem (not a root) from which spring large leaves. The origin of this tasty, crisp vegetable is currently unknown; however, plant historians estimate that it goes back to at least the Roman Empire.

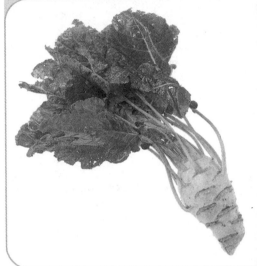

kohlrabi

nutritional profile

A rich source of vitamin C, kohlrabi is low in calories and provides fiber, vitamin B_6, and a substantial amount of potassium. In addition, this crisp, sweet-tasting vegetable supplies a good amount of vitamin E, which is unusual considering that vitamin E is mostly found in high-fat foods.

in the market

There are both *green* and *purple* varieties of kohlrabi. Purple kohlrabi tends to have a slightly spicier flavor. Both the bulb and the leaves of the kohlrabi are edible. The bulbs are sweeter and crisper than turnips, to which they have been compared. The leaves have a kale-collard taste.

choosing the best

Whether buying green or purple kohlrabi, look for crisp bulbs, without any bruises or blemishes. Leaves, if there are any intact, should be green and crisp, not wilted. While, in general, it is best to select small or medium-sized kohlrabi (less than 3 inches in diameter), there is a variety of kohlrabi that grows to be as much as 8 inches in diameter and is still very sweet and tender.

preparing to use

The tough skin of kohlrabi should be peeled before slicing, shredding, or cutting it into chunks.

KOHLRABI / 1 cup cooked	
Calories	48
Protein (g)	3
Carbohydrate (g)	11
Dietary fiber (g)	1.8
Total fat (g)	0.2
Saturated fat (g)	0
Monounsaturated fat (g)	0
Polyunsaturated fat (g)	0.1
Cholesterol (mg)	0
Potassium (mg)	561
Sodium (mg)	35

KEY NUTRIENTS (%RDA/AI*)	
Vitamin B_6	0.3 mg (15%)
Vitamin C	89 mg (99%)
Vitamin E	2.8 mg (18%)

*For more detailed information on RDA and AI, see page 88.

serving suggestions

• Make a coleslaw with kohlrabi instead of cabbage.

• Serve raw kohlrabi as part of a platter of crudités.

• Add julienne strips of cooked kohlrabi to steamed green beans and toss to combine.

• Make a gratin of sliced potatoes and kohlrabi.

• Cook kohlrabi with garlic and an apple and mash the way you would mashed potatoes.

• Add thin slices of raw kohlrabi to sandwiches.

lamb

While Americans display a fairly hearty appetite for beef, they have shown much less enthusiasm for lamb. Annually, we consume, on average, a pound of lamb per person, a fraction of our beef consumption. Yet sheep are the most numerous livestock in the world, and lamb or mutton (the flesh of mature sheep) is the principal meat in parts of Europe, North Africa, the Middle East, and India. Dishes featuring lamb range from roasted whole leg of lamb seasoned with assertive herbs—a specialty in Italy and southern France—to Greek moussaka (a ground-lamb dish), to savory kebabs, curries, and stews prepared in countries as disparate as Iraq, India, and Ireland. In these countries, as well as in New Zealand (where average per capita consumption of lamb and goat averages more than 60 pounds a year), people have taken full advantage of lamb's robust taste.

As with beef, modern breeding methods have improved lamb's taste and texture. In ages past, the meat from sheep was relatively tough and stringy, because the animals were bred for wool as well as for meat, and because they were often on the move from pasture to pasture, which made them exceptionally lean. In the 18th century, English breeders produced animals that were chunky and compact, yielding plenty of meat. Most of the lamb sold in American markets today comes from descendants of these English breeds, which are raised either for wool or for meat. As a result, lamb has become consistently more flavorful and tender.

nutritional profile

The meat is also leaner, thanks to breeding and to the extensive trimming of the external fat—on average only ¼ inch or less is left on retail lamb. Like beef, lamb is graded for quality. The same category names are used—Prime and Choice (and Good rather than Select)—but these terms do not indicate the same differences in fat content as they do in beef. The majority of lamb to reach the market is Choice or Prime, which is nutritionally comparable to these categories of beef: Many corresponding cuts contain the same amount of internal fat and offer similarly significant levels of riboflavin, vitamin B_{12}, niacin, iron, and zinc.

in the market

In the United States, meat that is labeled "lamb" comes from sheep that are less than a year old. Most of our lamb, in fact, is from animals that go to market at 5 to 7 months of age. You may sometimes encounter meat labeled "yearling mutton," which comes from an animal between one and two years old; it is more strongly flavored than lamb. Meat from animals older than two years is classified as "mutton," which is seldom sold in the United States.

The cut of lamb is the best indicator of fat content, as well as to the tenderness of the meat. Lamb has fewer retail cuts than beef. In general, leaner

LAMB, LEG 3 ounces cooked	
Calories	164
Protein (g)	7
Carbohydrate (g)	0
Dietary fiber (g)	0
Total fat (g)	6.6
Saturated fat (g)	2.4
Monounsaturated fat (g)	2.9
Polyunsaturated fat (g)	0.4
Cholesterol (mg)	76
Sodium (mg)	58

KEY NUTRIENTS (%RDA/AI*)	
Riboflavin	0.2 mg (14%)
Vitamin B_{12}	2.2 mcg (37%)
Niacin	5.4 mg (34%)
Iron	1.7 mg (10%)
Zinc	4.2 mg (38%)

*For more detailed information on RDA and AI, see page 88.

cuts, such as the foreshank and parts of the leg, are less tender than cuts from areas where the muscles are little used, such as the loin and rib. However, because lambs are smaller, younger animals than beef cattle, even lean cuts are more tender than corresponding cuts of beef.

Primal cuts—the divisions of lamb made by wholesalers—are given below, since they are used consistently throughout the country and are indicative of fat content. The most common names for retail cuts, which are used to identify the smaller cuts of meat sold in supermarkets and butcher shops, are also included, along with the preferred cooking methods.

Breast and foreshank Whole breast can be purchased unboned, or boned and rolled; it is usually roasted or braised, often with a stuffing. However, the meat is fatty and not as tender as the other cuts. This section includes *spareribs* and *riblets* (single-ribbed strips), both relatively inexpensive cuts that contain more bone than meat; they can be grilled or braised. The *foreshank*, which is connected to the breast, is a lean, stringy cut—only 29 percent of its calories come from fat. It is usually tenderized by cooking in liquid for long periods. Shank meat is also ground and cubed for stewing.

Leg The most popular cut of lamb, the leg can be roasted whole, or boned and either rolled (for roasting) or butterflied (for broiling or grilling). It is subdivided into two basic parts: the sirloin (or butt), which is well marbled, and the shank, or lower half, which is much leaner. Cuts from the sirloin include *sirloin roast* and *sirloin chops*. *Leg steaks* from the center leg are suitable for broiling or grilling. The *hind shank* is among the leanest cuts of lamb, with only 180 calories (33 percent of which come from fat) per 3 ounces.

facts & tips

The term "spring lamb" is sometimes applied to meat that is marketed during the spring and summer months. In decades past, these were the primary months fresh lamb was available, but modern breeding techniques have ensured that lamb is plentiful throughout the year. Consequently, the expression no longer has any practical meaning.

COMPARING LAMB CUTS **3 ounces cooked**

As a general rule of thumb, 4 ounces of raw boneless lamb will yield 3 ounces of cooked lamb. For 3 ounces of cooked lamb from a bone-in cut, you would start with about 8 ounces of raw. Most retail cuts of lamb will be trimmed to ¼ inch or ⅛ inch of fat. Before cooking, you should trim all remaining visible fat. The numbers below are for lamb whose external fat has been fully trimmed. The cuts are organized by percentage of calories from fat, with lowest at the top and highest at the bottom.

	Calories	Fat (g)	% Calories from Fat	Saturated Fat (g)	Cholesterol (mg)
Foreshank	160	5.1	29	1.9	89
Shank	154	5.7	33	2.1	75
Leg	164	6.6	36	2.4	76
Arm	165	8	44	3.1	74
Loin	173	8.4	44	3.2	75
Shoulder	175	9.3	48	3.5	75
Blade	179	9.9	50	3.7	75
Rib	199	11.4	52	4.1	75
Ground (20% fat)	243	16.9	63	6.9	83

serving suggestions

- Rub loin or shoulder chops with a spice mixture, such as cumin, coriander, and oregano. Broil and serve with a fat-free salsa.

- Brush butterflied leg of lamb with mint jelly and lemon juice before grilling, roasting, or broiling.

- Make lamb skewers, using a high proportion of vegetables to meat, and serve with a yogurt-parsley sauce.

- Make a lamb meatloaf using 3 parts lamb to 1 part lean ground turkey breast.

Sometimes called *shank half roast,* it can be roasted or braised. The shank meat can also be cut up for stews or pounded for cube steak.

Loin This section, considered the choicest part of the lamb, yields an excellent roast. When both sides of the loin are used, the result is a *saddle of lamb.* More frequently, the section is divided into *loin chops,* which have about 216 calories per 3 ounces, 40 percent of them fat calories. Chops can be braised, broiled, grilled, or baked.

Rib A *whole rib,* also known as a *rack,* can be purchased for roasting, but it is heavily marbled meat with a thick outer layer of fat. In fact, over 50 percent of its calories come from fat, even after trimming. *Rib chops* can be trimmed of more of their fat to yield tender, juicy meat.

Shoulder The hardest-working muscle has a good deal of fat, in addition to many bones. Sold whole with the bone intact, it is tastiest braised or stewed. Or, it can be sold boned as *rolled boneless shoulder roast* (which can also be braised). *Shoulder lamb chops* (which may be subdivided into blade chops and arm chops) are less expensive than rib or loin chops, and are somewhat leaner: The calories in arm chops are only about 40 percent fat. Shoulder chops can be cooked like other chops, or they can be cut up and used for stews or kebabs. Meat from the *neck,* which is taken from the front of the shoulder, is also good for stewing, or it can be boned and ground.

Ground lamb Usually made from shank and neck meat, as well as other trimmings, ground lamb may contain a good deal of fat. You can reduce the fat content by buying a shoulder cut and asking the butcher to trim and grind it (or do so yourself). Use ground lamb as you would ground beef.

choosing the best

Prepackaged lamb sold in supermarkets is ordinarily dated for freshness, so be sure to check the label. Other signs of freshness are firm, pinkish red meat (lamb darkens with age); bones that are reddish at the joint (and also moist); and fat that is creamy white. When buying from a butcher, ask that the external fat be trimmed.

preparing to use

While most retail cuts are sold trimmed of most external fat, some cuts, such as the leg or shoulder, may be sold with some of the fat intact. Trim it carefully before cooking: Too much fat is not only unhealthy, but can also give cooked lamb a strong flavor. Do the same for cubes of lamb used for stewing or kebabs.

Some lamb cuts may also retain pieces of the fell, a papery membrane that covers surface fat. Butchers often leave the fell intact on large cuts, since it helps the meat retain its shape and natural juices. Any fell on small cuts should be removed, as it can distort the shape of the meat during cooking.

leeks

Originally from the Mediterranean region and Asia, leeks have been culti- vated for several millennia. Ancient Roman armies took the leek as far north and west as Wales, where inhabitants eventually embraced the vegetable as their national emblem. In 640 A.D., Saint David entreated his Welsh coun- trymen to wear leeks in their hats to distinguish themselves from the enemy during the battle between King Cadwallader of Wales and the Saxons. And to this day, in Wales, an emblem of the leek is worn on March 1, Saint David's Day, a Welsh national holiday.

A member of the *Allium* genus, the leek is related to garlic, onions, and shallots. In fact, leeks resemble oversized scallions, with a slightly bulbous root end, a thick white stalk, and long, thick, flat green leaves. Leeks have a sweet, delicate flavor and a pleasing, crunchy texture when cooked, which makes them an excellent side dish as well as a flavorful addition to many recipes. Nothing is wasted with leeks as both the bulb and leaves are used in cooking. Once considered the "poor man's asparagus," the leek is a highly versatile vegetable that is gradually beginning to garner some of the same deserved recognition in the United States as it has in Europe.

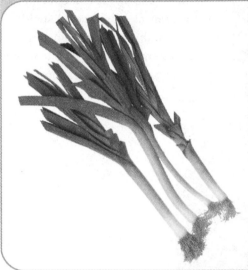

leeks

nutritional profile

Leeks are low in calories, with only about 32 calories per cup cooked and are a good source of fiber and iron.

in the market

There are several commercially grown varieties available, all similar. There are also these specialty leeks:

Baby leeks These are a small variety of leeks that look exactly like scal- lions. They are mildly oniony.

Ramps Ramps are wild leeks. In the spring, the ramp plant sprouts flat, pointed leaves that look just like those of a young leek. But these early leaves die and the plant moves on to put up a stalk and flower. The stage at which the ramps are harvested and sold as food is during this narrow window of opportunity between the first set of leaves and the flowering plant, making it a highly seasonal specialty. The flavor of ramps is quite pungent, like a combi- nation of garlic and onion.

▶ Availability Regular leeks are available year round, but ramps are quite seasonal (and often regional). They are one of the first sure signs of spring in the South. Elsewhere you may be able to find them from March through early June.

LEEKS / 1 cup cooked	
Calories	32
Protein (g)	1
Carbohydrate (g)	8
Dietary fiber (g)	1.0
Total fat (g)	0.2
Saturated fat (g)	0
Monounsaturated fat (g)	0
Polyunsaturated fat (g)	0.1
Cholesterol (mg)	0
Potassium (mg)	91
Sodium (mg)	10

KEY NUTRIENTS (%RDA/AI*)

Iron	1.1 mg (14%)

For more detailed information on RDA and AI, see page 88.

choosing the best

Leeks are usually displayed in bunches of three or four; sometimes they are sold separately. The leaf tops should be fresh and green, while the white root end should show a firmly attached fringe of rootlets and several inches of unblemished skin, which will give very slightly to pressure. Avoid leeks with obvious signs of age or mishandling, such as wilted or torn greens or bulbs that have their rootlets cut off.

▶ **When you get home** Don't trim leeks until you are ready to cook them.

> ➤ *phytochemicals in*
> leeks
>
> Like other members of the *Allium* family (onions, shallots), leeks are a rich source of a phytochemical called diallyl sulfide. It is suggested that this substance may raise levels of protective enzymes that help to inactivate and eliminate cancer-causing agents.

preparing to use

Leeks often require careful cleaning, since soil and grit can collect in between the layers of the broad overlapping leaves.

Remove any withered or toughened outer leaves. Trim off the darkest portion of the green tops (the whole leek is edible, but the darker green portions have a stronger, less pleasant flavor). Trim the rootlets at the base.

If cooking leeks whole, insert a knife about 1 inch below where the bulb just starts to turn green and slice lengthwise toward the top, where the leaves are. Then roll the leek a quarter turn and make a second lengthwise slit parallel to the first. Fan the leaves apart and wash under cool running water. The place where dirt collects on a leek is the place where the leek rose above the soil it was grown in. You can tell where this is, because that's where the leek starts to turn green (where sunlight caused the plant to produce chlorophyll).

If the leeks need to be chopped for a recipe, this cleaning process is considerably easier. Cut the leeks as directed in the recipe and place the leeks in a bowl of lukewarm water. Swish the leeks around in the water and scoop them out. The dirt should sink to the bottom of the bowl.

serving suggestions

• Cook sliced leeks with your favorite potatoes and then mash the two together.

• Steam whole leeks and top with fresh herbs and a lemon vinaigrette. Serve warm or at room temperature.

• Sauté sliced leeks with a little bit of olive oil and vinegar and use as a pizza topping.

• Cook sliced leeks along with green peas for a side dish.

• Braise whole leeks in a mixture of wine and chicken broth seasoned with black pepper and tarragon. Cook until meltingly soft.

• Trim off the darkest part of the leaves, wash well, and brush whole leeks with olive oil. Cook on a grill or roast in a 450° oven.

lemons & limes

Lemons and limes probably originated on the Indian subcontinent, and depictions of lemons were found in 2nd- and 3rd-century Roman mosaics. It seems likely that both lemons and limes were popularized in Europe at the time of the Crusades, and Columbus may have brought the seeds of both fruits to the New World on one of his voyages. Citrus fruits, including lemons and limes, were established in what is now Florida by the 16th century.

In the 18th century, the British navy ordered ships going on long journeys to carry limes for their crews—hence the nickname "limeys" for British sailors. The limes were used to prevent scurvy (a disease caused by vitamin C deficiency) even though, at the time, it was not understood exactly how the fruit prevented scurvy. During the California Gold Rush, scurvy was so rampant and fresh produce so scarce, that miners were willing to pay a dollar for a lemon (to put this into perspective, that would be a $20 lemon today). But it wasn't until vitamin C was discovered in 1932 that scientists understood that it was this vitamin, not the fresh fruit itself, that protected against the disease.

Because they are tropical plants, lemons and limes grown in warm regions in the United States. The commercial lemon and lime industry is centered principally in Florida and southern California (where citrus cultivation was established in the 1850s in response to the Gold Rush opportunities). Florida claims the bulk of the lime production and California has most of the lemon production.

nutritional profile

These tart, flavorful fruits contain some potassium and are rich in vitamin C. Just 2 tablespoons of lemon juice provides a little over 15 percent of the RDA. Lime juice contains less vitamin C than lemon juice, with 2 tablespoons providing just 10 percent of the RDA. Along with supplying substantial amounts of vitamin C, the health benefits of these fruits also rest in their fiber and phytochemicals.

in the market

There are two basic types of lemons and limes—acidic and sweet—but only acidic types are grown commercially. (The sweet types are grown by home gardeners as ornamental fruit.) Although there are some specialty lemons and limes that are identified in the marketplace (for example, Key limes or Meyer

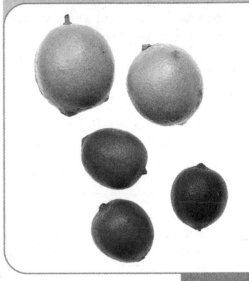

lemons & limes

LEMON JUICE ¼ cup	
Calories	15
Protein (g)	0
Carbohydrate (g)	5
Dietary fiber (g)	0.2
Total fat (g)	0
Saturated fat (g)	0
Monounsaturated fat (g)	0
Polyunsaturated fat (g)	0
Cholesterol (mg)	0
Potassium (mg)	76
Sodium (mg)	1

KEY NUTRIENTS (%RDA/AI*)

Vitamin C	28 mg (31%)

For more detailed information on RDA and AI, see page 88.

lemons), the rest of the lemons and limes sold do not specify variety—even though there are some varietal differences in size, shape, and thickness of peel, though not in flavor.

Kaffir limes These round, nubbly-skinned limes have very little juice, and what there is is bitter. They are used in Thai cooking for their zest and especially their leaves, which are fragrant with volatile oils.

Key limes (Mexican limes) These are smaller, rounder, and yellower than Tahiti limes (*see below*), with a higher acid content. They are best known as an ingredient in Key lime pie. Though Key limes were once a commercial crop in Florida, these days the majority of these limes in the marketplace—found almost exclusively in the form of juice or concentrate—is grown outside of the United States.

Lemons Most common everyday lemons are either *Eurekas* or *Lisbons*, though no market actually labels their lemons as anything but "lemons." Eureka lemons are distinguished by a short neck at the stem end; Lisbons have no distinct neck, but the blossom end tapers to a pointed nipple. Eurekas may have a few seeds and a somewhat pitted skin, while Lisbons are commonly seedless, with smoother skin. Both types have medium-thick skins and are abundantly juicy. Florida-grown lemons are likely to be Lisbon-type fruits called *Bearss* (not a misspelling, but the name of the California grower who developed the variety).

Limequats A cross between limes and kumquats, limequats are small, round, and yellowish with an acidic lime flavor.

Meyer lemons The Meyer lemon, named for Frank N. Meyer, who first imported the fruit from China in 1908, is a cross between a lemon and either an orange or a mandarin. Its orange-yellow flesh is sweeter than a lemon's, and it has a thin, smooth skin. More widely available in California (where they're the most popular variety for home growing), they can sometimes be found in specialty food stores. At one time, they carried a virus that had the potential to damage other citrus crops, so their sale was restricted. A new virus-free strain has been developed, making them somewhat easier to find.

Rangpur limes Tart, acidic, and very juicy, these fruits resemble oranges or tangerines (their flesh is decidedly orange). They are probably a cross between a lemon and a mandarin orange, but because they have a limelike aroma, they have been dubbed limes.

Tahiti limes Most of the limes in the supermarket are a Tahitian strain (they are believed to have originated on that island), which comes in two similar varieties: *Persian limes*, which are oval, egg-sized fruits cultivated in Florida; and a *Bearss* variety, which is a smaller, seedless California-grown lime. Both are greenish-yellow when fully mature, but are sold at their earlier, deep-green stage for better flavor.

→ phytochemicals in lemons & limes

The peels of lemons and limes are rich in limonene phytochemicals, which seep into the juice and may confer anticancer benefits, possibly by blocking abnormal cell growth and detoxifying cancer promoters.

LIME JUICE
¼ cup

Calories	17
Protein (g)	0
Carbohydrate (g)	6
Dietary fiber (g)	0.3
Total fat (g)	0.1
Saturated fat (g)	0
Monounsaturated fat (g)	0
Polyunsaturated fat (g)	0
Cholesterol (mg)	0
Potassium (mg)	67
Sodium (mg)	1

KEY NUTRIENTS (%RDA/AI*)
Vitamin C	18 mg (20%)

For more detailed information on RDA and AI, see page 88.

choosing the best

These fruits should be firm, glossy, and bright—beautiful enough to be treated as ornaments for your kitchen. Lemons should be bright yellow, not greenish, and limes should be dark green. (Limes turn from green to yellow as they ripen, but it's the immature fruits that have the desirably tart juice; yellowish limes have an insipid flavor.) Meyer lemons should be firm and plump, have even-colored yellow-orange skin without bruises or soft spots.

A very coarse exterior may indicate an excessively thick skin, which in turn may mean less flesh and juice (large lemons are likely to be thick-skinned); heavy fruits with fine-grained skin are juiciest. Avoid both hard, shriveled lemons and limes as well as spongy, soft ones.

▶ **When you get home** If you are planning to use lemons quickly, you can leave them in a basket at room temperature; they will keep for about 2 weeks without refrigeration. Limes are more perishable and should be refrigerated immediately. Both lemons and limes stored in a plastic bag in the refrigerator crisper will keep for up to 6 weeks. If you have extra lemons or limes on hand and want to save them before they spoil, squeeze the juice into an ice-cube tray, then transfer the frozen juice cubes to a plastic bag.

preparing to use

To get the most juice from a lemon or lime, the fruit should be at room temperature or warmer; if need be, place it in hot water or a low oven for a few minutes to warm it, or microwave it for 30 seconds. Then roll the fruit under your palm on the countertop until it feels softened.

There are lots of gadgets for juicing citrus fruits—juicers onto which you press the fruit, reamers you twist into the fruit—but it's simplest to halve the fruit and squeeze it in your hand, using your fingers to hold back the seeds (though this is not necessary with limes, which are seedless).

If you don't need all the juice at once, you can pierce the fruit with a toothpick and squeeze the juice from the opening. "Reseal" the fruit by reinserting the toothpick.

Recipes often call for lemon or lime zest—the flavorful colored part of the peel. Scrub the fruit, then use the fine side of a hand grater, a special zesting tool, a sharp paring knife, or a vegetable peeler to remove the zest. When grating or paring the zest from a lemon or lime, be careful not to remove any of the bitter white pith along with it. To have lemon or lime zest on hand, save the shells after squeezing fresh lemon juice, then wrap and freeze the shells. Grate zest as you need it from the still frozen shells.

A large lemon will yield about 3 to 4 tablespoons of juice and 2 to 3 teaspoons of zest; a large lime will provide 2 to 3 tablespoons of juice and 1 to 2 teaspoons of zest.

lentils

The lentil was an important crop in ancient Greece (where it had medicinal as well as culinary applications), but its use dates back to prehistoric times. Lentils are inexpensive, nutritious, and relatively quick-cooking (beans may take several hours; lentils take only 30 to 45 minutes). They have a distinctive, somewhat peppery flavor.

nutritional profile

Low in fat and high in protein and dietary fiber, these tiny, disk-shaped legumes supply complex carbohydrates and good amounts of thiamin, vitamin B_6, iron, zinc, and potassium. But they are particularly rich in the B vitamin folate—½ cup of cooked lentils provides almost half the daily requirement.

in the market

Lentils grow just one or two to a pod and come in many colors. A wide variety of lentils are used in Europe, the Middle East, India, and Africa; but in the United States, red, brown, and green lentils are the most common. Brown and green lentils still have their hulls on and thus hold their shape well after cooking. Red lentils, which are often sold hulled, cook more quickly and work best in purees and other dishes where softness is an advantage. Hulled lentils, it should be noted, have less dietary fiber than unhulled.

Black (beluga lentils) Tiny and jet-black, these lentils glisten once cooked, making them look like beluga caviar. Rich in flavor, they can be used in recipes calling for brown, green, or French lentils.

Brown (small Chinese, Persian) These small, plump russet-brown disks have an earthy flavor. They are not as flat as most lentils (tending toward the spherical) and are not hulled.

French (lentilles du Puy) Imported from France and also grown domestically, these are much smaller than brown or green lentils. Their color is a deep green going almost to black. Their cooked texture is somewhat firm and their flavor is slightly peppery. They are found mostly in gourmet stores.

Green This is the type of lentil you find in the supermarket, though the bags are simply labeled "lentils," and most people would be surprised to learn that these brownish-beige lentils are called "green." (And, just to confuse matters more, they are sometimes referred to as brown lentils.) They hold their shape well when cooked.

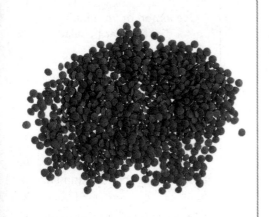

green lentils

LENTILS / ½ cup cooked	
Calories	115
Protein (g)	9
Carbohydrate (g)	20
Dietary fiber (g)	7.8
Total fat (g)	0.4
Saturated fat (g)	0.1
Monounsaturated fat (g)	0.1
Polyunsaturated fat (g)	0.2
Cholesterol (mg)	0
Potassium (mg)	365
Sodium (mg)	2

KEY NUTRIENTS (%RDA/AI*)	
Thiamin	0.2 mg (14%)
Vitamin B_6	0.2 mg (10%)
Folate	179 mcg (45%)
Iron	3.3 mg (41%)
Zinc	1.3 mg (11%)

*For more detailed information on RDA and AI, see page 88.

Ivory white These are black lentils that have been hulled. They also come split.

Red Small salmon-colored disks, these lentils usually come hulled; but in Indian markets you can also find them in the hull or hulled and split. In their hulled form, they cook much faster than most lentils.

choosing the best

Look for undamaged boxes or bags of uniformly sized lentils that aren't cracked or broken.

▶ **When you get home** Don't mix a new supply of lentils with older lentils. Older lentils (which are more dried out) take longer to cook, so if you mix the two together, they will cook unevenly.

preparing to use

There's very little preparation needed for lentils. Unlike dried beans, these dried legumes do not need to be presoaked. All you need to do is to pick them over to remove any shriveled lentils or hulls. If you buy lentils in bulk, or from an ethnic grocery, you should also be on the lookout for twigs or pebbles. Rinse lentils in the hull; hulled lentils don't really need to be rinsed.

---

other lentil products

Lentil flour See Flour, Non-wheat (*page 325*).

Lentil pasta See Pasta, Non-wheat (*page 443*).

---

serving suggestions

• Toss cooked lentils in vinaigrette while still warm (so they'll absorb more flavor). Serve on a bed of spinach with crumbled feta or goat cheese on top.

• Add cooked lentils to tomato sauce and toss with cooked pasta.

• Cook red lentils in a highly spiced broth; then puree and serve as a dip for vegetables or pita chips.

• Season mashed lentils with some bottled salsa. Put the lentil puree, chopped tomatoes, and a little shredded cheese in flour tortillas and roll up.

• Serve a puree of lentils in place of mashed potatoes.

• Lentils and nuts have a natural affinity: Serve a lentil pilaf with toasted walnuts and apples.

lettuce

red leaf lettuce

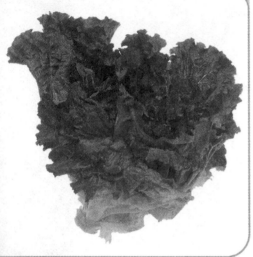

One of the world's most popular edible plants, lettuce not only serves as the basis for most salads, but it also adds texture and color to sandwiches, and quite possibly, is eaten more frequently than any other vegetable. The texture and flavor of each type of lettuce ranges from crisp to velvety and mild to assertive and peppery.

The ancient Egyptians grew lettuce some 4,500 years ago in the Nile Valley, and lettuce plants appear in hieroglyphics. The Greek father of medicine, Hippocrates, wrote about the medicinal properties of lettuce in 430 B.C. The Romans—for whom romaine lettuce is named—grew many varieties and believed in its curative properties. The vegetable eventually came to be widely appreciated throughout Asia and Europe. Christopher Columbus introduced lettuce to the New World on his second voyage.

Although compared with other salad greens (*see Greens, Salad, page 357*), most lettuces are nutritional lightweights, they do serve as a perfect salad backdrop for such heavy hitters as tomatoes, bell peppers, corn, avocado, broccoli, beets, carrots, and onions.

nutritional profile

Lettuce supplies good amounts of vitamin C and the B vitamin folate. In general, however, compared with many other leafy green vegetables, lettuce offers minimal nutritional value, with iceberg lettuce at the bottom of the list.

Some types of lettuce also supply beta carotene: A good rule of thumb in determining the beta carotene content is to select lettuce with the darkest leaves. And because the general nutritional content is also reflected in the depth of color in the leaves, it is no surprise that romaine lettuce contains more folate, iron, and potassium than do the types of lettuce with pale leaves.

in the market

In the United States, an 1885 agricultural report listed no fewer than 87 varieties of lettuce. Today, there are four basic types of lettuce (butterhead, iceberg, red and green looseleaf, and romaine). You are likely to find all of these in the produce sections of most supermarkets.

Butterhead This type includes Boston and Bibb lettuces, which are characterized by a loose head and grass-green leaves; both have a soft "buttery" texture and a sweet, mild flavor. A head of *Boston lettuce* resembles a flowering rose. *Bibb lettuce*—also called limestone—forms a smaller, cup-shaped head.

Iceberg More accurately called crisphead, this familiar pale green lettuce forms a tight, cabbagelike head. Its texture is crisp and its flavor very mild.

ROMAINE LETTUCE 2 cups	
Calories	16
Protein (g)	2
Carbohydrate (g)	3
Dietary fiber (g)	1.9
Total fat (g)	0.2
Saturated fat (g)	0
Monounsaturated fat (g)	0
Polyunsaturated fat (g)	0.1
Cholesterol (mg)	0
Potassium (mg)	325
Sodium (mg)	9

KEY NUTRIENTS (%RDA/AI*)	
Beta carotene	1.7 mg (16%)
Vitamin C	27 mg (30%)
Folate	152 mcg (38%)
Iron	1.2 mg (15%)

*For more detailed information on RDA and AI, see page 88.

Although it is not the nutritional powerhouse that other, darker-green lettuces are, it is actually not as nutrition-free as most people assume (2 cups of iceberg provide more than 10 percent of the RDA for the B vitamin folate). There are also few substitutes in the lettuce world when you want a very crisp lettuce, as for chopped salads.

Looseleaf This type of lettuce comprises a number of varieties that don't form heads, but consist of large, loosely packed leaves joined at a stem. The leaves are either green or shaded to deep red at the edges, and may be ruffled or smooth. Their degree of crispness is midway between romaine and butterhead, their taste is mild and delicate. *Red leaf* and *green leaf* are popular varieties. *Oak leaf*, both *red* and *green*, forms smaller heads, with flatter leaves shaped like big, floppy oak leaves. For home gardeners, looseleaf lettuce has an advantage over other types: If you pick leaves individually instead of pulling the whole head from the ground, the leaves will continue to replace themselves throughout the season.

Romaine Also called cos, this lettuce has long, deep green leaves that form a loaf-shaped head. Some varieties develop a closed head, others are more open. The main ingredient in Caesar salads, romaine has a crisp texture and a strong, but not bitter, taste.

Stem lettuce A thick edible stem, 6 to 8 inches long, is what distinguishes stem lettuce from other types. It is widely grown in China (it is also known as Chinese lettuce), but the only variety available in the United States is called *celtuce.* Stem lettuce has a mild flavor that is sometimes described as "nutty cucumber." Stem lettuce is good in salads, but can also be cooked like a vegetable.

choosing the best

Above all, lettuce should be fresh and crisp. It is easy to spot wilted greens; watch out for limp, withered leaves that have brown or yellow edges, or dark or slimy spots. Once greens have passed their prime, there is no way to restore them to crisp freshness. Lettuce should be displayed under refrigeration, or on ice; as it is quite perishable.

Try to choose lettuce with healthy outer leaves; these are likely to be the most nutritious part of the green, containing much more beta carotene and vitamin C than the pale inner leaves. Unfortunately, the outer leaves are usu-

LOOSELEAF LETTUCE 2 cups	
Calories	20
Protein (g)	2
Carbohydrate (g)	4
Dietary fiber (g)	2.1
Total fat (g)	0.3
Saturated fat (g)	0
Monounsaturated fat (g)	0
Polyunsaturated fat (g)	0.2
Cholesterol (mg)	0
Potassium (mg)	296
Sodium (mg)	10

KEY NUTRIENTS (%RDA/AI*)	
Beta carotene	1.3 mg (12%)
Vitamin C	20 mg (22%)
Folate	56 mcg (14%)
Iron	1.6 mg (20%)

*For more detailed information on RDA and AI, see page 88.

COMPARING LETTUCE 2 cups					
	Calories	Beta carotene (mg)	Vitamin C (mg)	Folate (mcg)	Iron (mg)
Boston	15	0.7	9	82	0.3
Iceberg	13	0.2	4	62	0.6
Looseleaf	20	1.3	20	56	1.6
Romaine	16	1.8	27	152	1.2

ally the most damaged part of the head; but from a nutritional standpoint, it's best to salvage as many as you can.

Any type of head lettuce should be symmetrically shaped. Choose a head with its dark green outer leaves intact and that's healthy looking. Avoid overly large heads of romaine, which may have tough, fibrous leaves.

Iceberg lettuce should be compact and firm, yet springy: Very hard heads may be overmature and bitter. The stem end of a head of iceberg lettuce may look brown; this discoloration is the natural result of harvesting and does not indicate damage. If the head is not wrapped, sniff the stem end: It should smell slightly sweet, not bitter.

▶ **When you get home** If you don't plan on using the lettuce right away, store unwashed greens in perforated plastic bags (if you've bought them in plastic bags, poke a few holes in the bag to allow air to circulate, and leave the bag open). Soft-leaved lettuces do not keep as well as firm greens, such as romaine or iceberg lettuce. Iceberg should keep for up to 2 weeks, romaine for about 10 days, and butterhead and leaf lettuces for about 4 days.

Don't store lettuce near fruits like apples or bananas, which give off ethylene gas as they ripen. Otherwise, the lettuce will develop brown spots and decay rapidly. For appetizingly crisp lettuce—and to minimize last-minute preparation at mealtime—wash and dry the leaves, then layer them in clean paper towels and place in a plastic bag. Refrigerate in the crisper drawer until serving time, but not for more than a few hours, for optimal nutrient retention. If you buy a cellophane-wrapped head of iceberg lettuce, leave it in the wrapper until you are ready to use it.

preparing to use

Wash all lettuce in cool water shortly before using, then dry well. A salad spinner is a good investment if you eat a lot of lettuce and salads.

---

serving suggestions

• Use soft lettuce leaves as wrappers for chicken, fish, meat, or vegetable salads.

• Serve braised lettuce as a vegetable, rather than a salad. Sauté in a small amount of olive oil, cover, and braise the lettuce in its own liquid or add a little broth.

• Wrap soft lettuce leaves around whole fish and bake. The lettuce keeps the fish moist and absorbs some of the flavor as well.

• Make a chopped salad with iceberg lettuce. Use it 2 parts to 1 with another darker green (such as watercress or arugula). Toss with diced tomato, minced onion, minced carrot, tarragon, and white wine vinaigrette.

lobster & crayfish

Two of the most popular members of the crustacean family are lobsters and crayfish (which look like tiny lobsters). American lobsters can be found in saltwater along the East Coast, from Newfoundland to the Carolinas. Crayfish (also known as crawfish or crawdads in the South) are found wild in freshwater lakes, streams, and rivers in Southern states as well as in the Pacific Northwest. They are also farmed in many states.

The king of shellfish, the American lobster is a peculiar, hard-shelled creature with a jointed body and five pairs of legs, the foremost of which is a set of heavy claws. The claws—as well as the tail and body cavity—contain a sweet, firm, succulent meat that is considered a delicacy by many. Although lobsters come in a variety of colors, including light yellow, greenish-brown, blue, grey, and pale orange, when they are cooked, they turn a vivid red (hence the expression "red as a lobster").

Until the end of the 19th century, lobster was so plentiful that it was used for fish bait. Today, due to overfishing, the supply of lobsters has dwindled greatly. In the Northeast, attempts are now being made to sustain lobster survival and ensure adequate egg production through strict monitoring of harvests.

Because most crayfish are aquafarmed, there is no danger of an inadequate supply (in spite of a heavy demand in Louisiana where crayfish are a mainstay of Creole and Cajun cuisine). Like lobsters, these tiny reddish-brown creatures turn bright red when cooked and are typically shelled and eaten with the fingers. Sweet and succulent, crayfish meat tastes somewhat like that of lobster, although it is not as dense and rich. Most of the meat is in the tail, with tiny amounts also found in the body and claws.

nutritional profile

A generous source of vitamin B_{12} and the antioxidant mineral selenium, both lobster and crayfish also supply a good deal of zinc. Because these vitamin- and mineral-rich shellfish also provide protein, they are a healthy, low-fat alternative to meat. Unlike most other shellfish, lobster and crayfish are relatively high in dietary cholesterol (61 milligrams and 117 milligrams respectively for a 3-ounce serving). However, both have only small amounts of artery-clogging saturated fat.

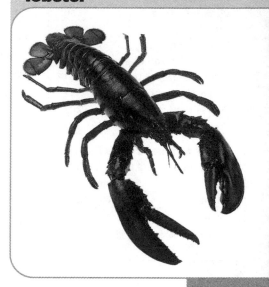

lobster

LOBSTER / 3 ounces cooked	
Calories	83
Protein (g)	17
Carbohydrate (g)	1
Dietary fiber (g)	0
Total fat (g)	0.5
Saturated fat (g)	0.1
Monounsaturated fat (g)	0.1
Polyunsaturated fat (g)	0.1
Cholesterol (mg)	61
Potassium (mg)	299
Sodium (mg)	323

KEY NUTRIENTS (%RDA/AI*)	
Vitamin B_{12}	2.7 mcg (110%)
Selenium	36 mcg (66%
Zinc	2.5 mg (23%)

For more detailed information on RDA and AI, see page 88.

CRAYFISH 3 ounces cooked	
Calories	74
Protein (g)	15
Carbohydrate (g)	0
Dietary fiber (g)	0
Total fat (g)	1.1
Saturated fat (g)	0.2
Monounsaturated fat (g)	0.2
Polyunsaturated fat (g)	0.4
Cholesterol (mg)	117
Potassium (mg)	202
Sodium (mg)	83

KEY NUTRIENTS (%RDA/AI*)	
Vitamin B_{12}	2.6 mcg (110%)
Iron	0.9 mg (12%)
Selenium	29 mcg (53%)
Zinc	1.3 mg (11%)

*For more detailed information on RDA and AI, see page 88.

in the market

American lobsters *(Homarus americanus)* The finest American lobsters (also known as Northern lobsters) come from Maine. Most of these slow-growing crustaceans are marketed at a weight of 1 to 3 pounds (the smallest are called "chicken" lobsters, the largest, "jumbo" lobsters). However, lobsters weighing 10 pounds or more can be found at some fish markets and restaurants; surprisingly, their meat is no less tender than that of smaller specimens. Lobsters are sold live, fresh-cooked, and frozen.

Rock lobsters (spiny lobsters) Because these creatures have no claws, the meat (which is coarser than that of American lobsters) is all in the tail. Rock lobsters are grouped as either warm- or cold-water varieties, depending on where they're caught. The domestic supply is from warm waters, mainly off the Florida coast. Frozen, cooked, cold-water rock lobster tails (usually from Australia, New Zealand, or South Africa) are also widely sold in American supermarkets. These are considered firmer and better-tasting than the warm-water tails. Rock lobsters are often mistakenly called saltwater crayfish; they are not the same species, however.

Crayfish The term crayfish covers the two species found in the United States; however, they are so closely related that they look almost identical. Those from Louisiana and the Mississippi bayou are slimmer and smaller than those from northern California, Washington, and Oregon. Crayfish typically weigh from 2 to 8 ounces and are harvested when they are about 5 inches long. Farmed varieties are not considered quite as tasty as wild crayfish. Both the wild and farmed varieties are sold live or fresh-frozen; their tail meat is also sold cooked and frozen in fine seafood shops.

▶ Availability Lobster is available year round, but the bulk of the catch is harvested in October and November, since lobsters molt in June and July.

The peak season for wild Southern crayfish is February to May; farmed Southern crayfish are available from January to June. The season for Northwest crayfish is May through October.

Both lobster and crayfish are sold by mail order throughout the year.

choosing the best

Live lobsters and crayfish should be very active and move their legs wildly when touched. A lively lobster will tuck its tail under its body when lifted.

When trying to decide how much live lobster to buy for a crowd, you can figure that about a third of its weight is edible. You should allow at least a 1¼- to 1½-pound lobster for each person. Choose lobsters that feel heavy for their size. As far as crayfish go, it takes about 7 pounds of whole crayfish to provide a pound of meat. You can estimate about 16 crayfish per person.

Cooked lobster or crayfish should smell very fresh (with no trace of ammonia or a "fishy" smell) and should have bright orange-red shells. Be especially wary when buying cooked lobster tails, as dealers sometimes cook lobsters that have died, rather than killing them for cooking. If the lobster was

facts & tips

Lobsters of any size can be sweet, firm, and tender. If you want to save money, however, those missing both claws, called "culls," and those with one claw, called "bullets," are often cheaper.

alive when it went into the pot, the tail will be tightly curled. Fresh-cooked seafood should not be displayed alongside raw fish or shellfish, because bacteria can migrate from the raw to the cooked.

▶ **When you get home** It's best to cook and eat live lobsters and crayfish the same day they are purchased. If you need to keep them alive for a few hours before cooking, store them in the coldest part of the refrigerator, covered with a damp towel. Remove them only when ready to cook. Fresh-cooked lobster or crayfish will keep for 2 to 3 days in the refrigerator.

preparing to use

If you plan to boil live lobsters, you can simply drop them headfirst into boiling water. If you plan to cook them by another method, such as broiling or grilling, they need to be killed first. If you want the fish seller to perform this task for you, be sure to make your purchase shortly before you plan to cook the shellfish; or you can do it at home using a heavy chef's knife.

To kill a lobster for broiling or grilling, place it belly-down and insert a knife tip at the junction of the body and tail shells. Cut the body in half lengthwise, remove the stomach and black intestinal vein, and crack the claws. Rinse the lobster well.

To prepare crayfish for boiling, first rinse under cold water, then remove the entrails as follows: The end of the tail has five tiny flaps that overlap and create a fan. Take the middle flap between your thumb and forefinger, twist it sharply clockwise, and pull. Doing so will draw the entrails right out, leaving the crayfish clean and ready to cook.

When it comes to cooking both lobster and crayfish, the trick is to heat them sufficiently to destroy harmful organisms, but not so long as to destroy the texture of the meat. This requires careful monitoring, as lobster can become toughened and crayfish can turn mushy with just a few seconds of overcooking.

serving suggestions

Instead of melted butter as a dipping sauce for lobster, try one of the following:

• A low-oil lemon vinaigrette (use only 1 part oil to 1 part lemon juice).

• A sauce of yogurt, minced fresh basil, black pepper, and lemon or lime juice.

• A dipping sauce of rice vinegar and shredded fresh ginger.

• A hot dipping sauce made by sautéing minced garlic in a bit of sesame oil, then stirring in soy sauce and cider vinegar.

say no to tomalley

Have you ever wondered what that green stuff is nestled in the body of a lobster? Surprisingly, it's the lobster's liver, which is often referred to as the "tomalley." The tomalley, for the uninitiated, is held in high regard and is considered a special treat by many lobster aficionados. The one caveat here, however, is that because it is the lobster's liver (which filters toxins from the system), the tomalley may harbor dangerously high concentrations of PCBs and other potentially harmful agents.

Even if you are a member of the gastronomic tomalley appreciators club, it is prudent to discard this green delicacy and enjoy other interesting parts of the lobster (such as the roe in the female), which is perfectly safe to eat.

mackerel

Mackerel is the common name for members of the family *Scombridae*, which includes many species of open-sea fishes, including the bonito and tuna. All of the mackerel family are swift swimmers, traveling in schools that feed mostly on herring and squid. They tend to migrate between shallow and deep waters. What we consider mackerel, however, is a small member of this larger family known as the Boston, common, or Atlantic mackerel; it is found in cold waters off Europe and North America.

Most of the commercial catch of mackerel is canned and offers a tasty alternative to canned sardines, tuna, or salmon. Fresh mackerel is also available, although it is certainly less common than such fish as flounder or halibut.

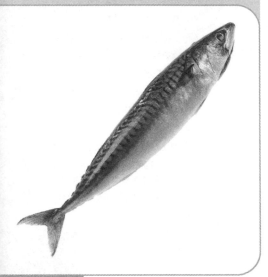

boston mackerel

nutritional profile

An oily fish related to tuna, mackerel has outer layers of red meat and lighter interior meat. The proportion of red meat and light meat varies with the species, as does the percentage of fat. However, all types of mackerel are higher-fat fish, rich in the healthful polyunsaturated fats known as long-chain omega-3s. According to the USDA, mackerel is among the top fish on the list for omega-3 content: Just 3 ounces of cooked Boston mackerel contains 1.1 grams of omega-3 fatty acids.

Growing evidence suggests these beneficial fats may protect against fatal heart attacks by making blood less likely to clot and by guarding against dangerous, sometimes fatal, abnormal heart rhythms. In addition, omega-3s appear to lower levels of triglycerides, the major type of fat that circulates in the blood. There's promising research showing that the benefits of omega-3 fatty acids may extend beyond heart health; these nourishing fats may relieve inflammation associated with such autoimmune diseases as rheumatoid arthritis and psoriasis.

Like tuna, mackerel is also an important source of protein and B vitamins, particularly vitamin B_{12}: A 3-ounce serving provides nearly 700 percent of the RDA. And mackerel offers tremendous amounts of selenium, an antioxidant mineral that helps to protect our cells against damaging free radicals.

in the market

Boston (Atlantic, common) With their brilliant blue-and-green coloring and their distinctly patterned backs, Boston mackerel are easily identified if buying them whole, or dressed. Averaging 1½ pounds and ranging from 10 to 18 inches, these have somewhat darker flesh than Spanish or jack mackerel, and a slightly stronger, oilier flavor.

Jack Generally ranging in weight from 8 to 16 ounces, the flesh of raw jack mackerel is creamy-tan. Once cooked the color is white, and the texture is soft, moist, and flaky. Like Spanish mackerel, jack have a sweet, mild flavor. Jack mackerel is commonly canned.

King (kingfish) Similar in taste to Atlantic and Pacific mackerel, king mackerel has a firm texture and a rich, savory flavor.

Pacific (chub, blue) These are similar both in flavor and texture to Boston mackerel. Chub mackerels have spots or broken wavy lines on their bodies and grow to about 20 inches.

Spanish These dark-greenish fish with silver shading and golden-yellow spots are similar in taste and texture to king mackerel. Their average weight is about 2 pounds. Like king mackerels, these are relatively light-fleshed and mild-flavored, and have less fat than other mackerels (two-thirds less than Boston mackerel).

choosing the best

Because of its high oil content, fresh mackerel is very perishable, so shop for it with particular care. This fish is marketed dressed or in fillets.

When shopping for whole mackerel, choose those with shiny, smooth skin and clear eyes. Like all fish, they should not have a fishy odor, but a pleasant smell of the sea. When buying mackerel fillets, the flesh should be firm and moist looking.

▶ **When you get home** The most important thing about storing mackerel is to do it briefly—it's best to eat the fish the same day you buy it, or no more than 24 hours after purchase. Keep the fish well inside the refrigerator—away from the door, where the temperature fluctuates each time the door is opened. (*For more information on storing fresh fish, see page 320.*)

BOSTON MACKEREL 3 ounces cooked	
Calories	223
Protein (g)	20
Carbohydrate (g)	0
Dietary fiber (g)	0
Total fat (g)	15
Saturated fat (g)	3.6
Monounsaturated fat (g)	6.0
Polyunsaturated fat (g)	3.7
Cholesterol (mg)	64
Potassium (mg)	341
Sodium (mg)	71

KEY NUTRIENTS (%RDA/AI*)	
Riboflavin	0.4 mg (27%)
Niacin	5.8 mg (36%)
Vitamin B$_6$	0.4 mg (23%)
Vitamin B$_{12}$	16 mcg (673%)
Vitamin E	1.6mg (10%)
Iron	1.3 mg (17%)
Magnesium	83 mg (20%)
Selenium	44 mcg (80%)

For more detailed information on RDA and AI, see page 88.

serving suggestions

- Marinate mackerel fillets in a soy-ginger sauce and broil or grill.

- Bake whole, dressed mackerel or fillets on a bed of parboiled Yukon gold potatoes.

- Rub mackerel fillets with a spice mixture of curry, cumin, coriander, and salt. Broil or grill.

- Top grilled or broiled mackerel with a tomato salsa.

- Make mackerel burgers or patties the way you would tuna or salmon burgers.

- Substitute cooked mackerel for tuna in your favorite tuna salad.

mangoes

An ancient fruit, mangoes are native to the Indian subcontinent where they've been cultivated for thousands of years. From there they spread throughout the tropical and subtropical world. Today mangoes are the most widely consumed fruit in the world, and in Latin America and the Caribbean, they are as common as the apple is in North America.

Though mangoes have become a supermarket staple in this country (nearby Mexico is the largest producer in the world of this luscious fruit), many Americans still view them as an ethnic oddity. However, a first taste of the fruit's delicious, juicy orange flesh should make a fan out of anyone. The flavor of mangoes is matchless, resembling a mix of peach and pineapple, only sweeter than either. The fruits are distantly related to poison ivy and poison oak (and cashews and pistachios), and for this reason some people may have a sensitivity to the mango's skin.

nutritional profile

Rich in nutrients, mangoes are full of flavor and low in calories (half a mango has less than 70 calories). Fragrant and juicy, they supply an ample amount of soluble fiber, including pectin, which helps to reduce the amount of cholesterol circulating in the blood. Their vibrant orange flesh indicates that mangoes are an excellent source of beta carotene as well as small amounts of another carotenoid, beta cryptoxanthin. Furthermore, their vitamin C content is commanding, with one average-sized mango supplying over 60 percent of the RDA. Mangoes are also one of a handful of low-fat sources of vitamin E.

in the market

Mangoes come in hundreds of varieties and a range of shapes and sizes, from plum-sized fruits to those weighing 4 pounds or more. The varieties grown commercially, however, are round, oval, or kidney-shaped, and are about the size of a large avocado or small melon. Though there are differences in color according to variety, most mangoes start off green and develop patches of gold, yellow, or red as they ripen.

In the market, mangoes aren't usually identified by their varietal names, but it's worth asking the produce manager what's available in order to take advantage of the differences in taste and texture. The most common mango available is the Tommy Atkins mango, followed by the less common varieties, such as Keitt, Kent, or Haden.

Ataulfo This Indonesian mango is small, flat, and slightly kidney-shaped. Its most distinguishing characteristic is that it turns completely yellow when ripe. It is also a variety that is just about fiber-free.

Haden This is a symmetrically oval mango, and usually weighs a pound or less. The flesh is moderately fibrous.

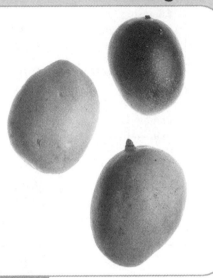

mangoes

MANGO / 1 medium	
Calories	135
Protein (g)	1
Carbohydrate (g)	35
Dietary fiber (g)	3.7
Total fat (g)	0.6
Saturated fat (g)	0.1
Monounsaturated fat (g)	0.2
Polyunsaturated fat (g)	0.1
Cholesterol (mg)	0
Potassium (mg)	323
Sodium (mg)	4

KEY NUTRIENTS (%RDA/AI*)	
Beta carotene	4.8 mg (44%)
Thiamin	0.1 mg (10%)
Vitamin B$_6$	0.3 mg (16%)
Vitamin C	57 mg (64%)
Vitamin E	2.3 mg (15%)

*For more detailed information on RDA and AI, see page 88.

Keitt This is one of the largest mangoes available. It commonly weighs in at 1½ pounds, but it can grow as large as 3 pounds. Unlike other mangoes that can have yellow and red patches when ripe, Keitts stay mostly green with just a blush of red.

Kent This largish mango can weigh up to 1½ pounds. It is a gratifying fruit to cut into, because its flesh is close to fiber-free (you can cut the flesh quite close to the pit and get a lot of fruit).

Tommy Atkins The most common variety, Tommy Atkins are symmetrical, oval-shaped fruits that are more fibrous than most other mangoes. Their fruit flavor is on the mild side.

choosing the best

The size of a mango depends on the variety; it is not an indicator of quality or ripeness. A perfectly ripe mango will have an intense, flowery fragrance and will yield slightly when touched; it should not smell fermented or have overtones of turpentine. For the most common types available, the skin should show a blush of either yellow-orange or red, which will increase in area as the fruit ripens. (A Keitt mango may remain totally green with just the slightest trace of yellow even when fully ripe, so check for softness and fragrance instead of color.) A completely greenish-gray skin indicates a mango that will not ripen properly. Black speckles on the skin are characteristic of this fruit as it ripens, but an overabundance of black spots on a ripe mango may indicate damage to the flesh beneath. A loose or shriveled skin is also a sign of a mango past its prime.

▶ **When you get home** Leave underripe mangoes at cool room temperature for a few days to soften and sweeten—very warm temperatures can cause an off-flavor to develop. Place two mangoes in a paper bag to speed ripening. Ripe fruits will keep in a plastic bag in the refrigerator for 2 to 3 days.

preparing to use

A mango is somewhat tricky to pit and slice. Hold the fruit standing on one of its ends. Make a slice vertically down one side of the pit, creating a near-half (depending on the variety, you will be able to get more or less close to the pit; the fibrous varieties will be the hardest to slice). Repeat on the other side of the pit (a band of fruit will remain around the pit). Use a paring knife to score the flesh of each half into cubes, being careful not to slice through the skin; then turn the fruit inside-out so the cut-side pops outward, and slice the cubes off the skin. Cut away the band of fruit left around the pit, then peel off the skin.

serving suggestions

- Dice mangoes and serve over waffles or pancakes.

- Combine cubed mango with yogurt or buttermilk and ice cubes, and blend to make a smoothie.

- Puree cubed mango in a blender or food processor and use as a dessert sauce over other fruits, rice pudding, or angel food cake.

- Cook cubes of mango with raisins, some brown sugar and vinegar, and perhaps some cayenne, for a quick, fresh chutney.

- Slightly underripe mangoes are suitable for cooking. They can be treated like apples or peaches, and used to make a baked crisp or brown Betty.

- Combine diced mango, red bell pepper, onion, and a squeeze of lime juice for a quick salsa.

- Add diced mango to chicken or seafood salads.

melons

Although it doesn't seem as though a honeydew melon and a Hubbard squash have much in common, the two belong to the same botanical family. Melons, squash, and cucumbers are members of the *Cucurbitaceae*, or gourd family; they all grow on vines. Except for watermelons, all melons resemble winter squash in structure—they have a thick flesh with a central seed-filled cavity. (Watermelon bears more resemblance to a cucumber, with its seeds dispersed in a radial pattern throughout its flesh.) The principal difference between melons and squash is the way they are used. While squash are treated as vegetables, melons are considered fruits—sweet and juicy.

Most melons originated in the Near East, and from there spread throughout Europe. The ancient Egyptians enjoyed muskmelons (which is what we call cantaloupes in this country), as did the ancient Romans; it was during the era of the Roman Empire that melons were introduced into Europe. But melons were not well known in northern Europe until the 15th century, when they became hugely popular at the French royal court. Melon seeds were carried to America by Columbus, and later Spanish explorers cultivated muskmelons in what is now California.

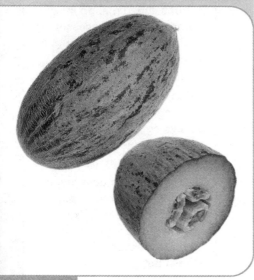

santa claus melon

nutritional profile

Melons rank somewhere between summer and winter squash: They resemble summer squash in their high water content and low calorie count, but approach winter squash in their nutrient value. Melons are a good source of potassium, vitamin C, and some of the B vitamins. Soluble pectin fiber provided by many melons may contribute to healthy cholesterol levels.

Like pumpkin or butternut squash, orange-fleshed varieties of melons contain beta carotene, but melons are also good sources of other carotenoids. For example, watermelon is a good source of lycopene (a red pigment also present in tomatoes) and honeydew melon is a good source of zeaxanthin, a carotenoid though to help shield delicate eye tissue from damaging ultraviolet radiation, among other functions.

in the market

Although cantaloupe, watermelon, and honeydew are the best-known melons, your supermarket or local farmstand may have other varieties for sale.

Ambrosia This melon looks like a cantaloupe, but has a brighter orange flesh.

Camouflage (frog skin melon) This melon has a colorful, patterned skin. Its flesh is similar to that of honeydew.

Cantaloupe See Cantaloupe (*page 214*).

HONEYDEW / 1 cup	
Calories	62
Protein (g)	1
Carbohydrate (g)	16
Dietary fiber (g)	1.1
Total fat (g)	0.2
Saturated fat (g)	0
Monounsaturated fat (g)	0
Polyunsaturated fat (g)	0.1
Cholesterol (mg)	0
Potassium (mg)	480
Sodium (mg)	18

KEY NUTRIENTS (%RDA/AI*)	
Thiamin	0.1 mg (11%)
Vitamin C	44 mg (49%)

*For more detailed information on RDA and AI, see page 88.

Casaba Pale yellow when ripe, this large melon has deep wrinkles that gather at the stem end. The flesh is white and sweet. Skin color is the best clue to ripeness when choosing a whole casaba. Unlike most other melons, it has no aroma.

Charentais This French melon has pale orange flesh and a smooth greenish-white skin with green stripes running from stem to blossom end.

Crenshaw A cross between a casaba and a Persian melon, the oblong crenshaw—which can weigh up to 10 pounds—has a buttercup-yellow rind and dense salmon-colored flesh. The flavor is both sweet and spicy.

Galia This is a cross between a honeydew and a cantaloupe. The skin is netted like a cantaloupe, but the flesh is green, like a honeydew.

Honeydew This large melon—averaging 5 to 6 pounds—has a creamy-white or yellow-green rind that ripens to creamy-yellow. The flesh is pale green, although there is a variety of honeydew that has orange flesh and a salmon-colored rind. A ripe honeydew is the sweetest of all the melons.

Horned melon These spiked melons have a bright orange to golden-yellow skin and a jellylike flesh. They are occasionally marketed as *kiwanos,* which is actually a registered trademark of the horned melons grown in New Zealand. The flavor is only vaguely sweet with a hint of cucumber. The horned melon is actually one of those members of the squash/melon family whose flavor falls somewhere between sweet fruit and savory vegetable.

Juan Canary As the name suggests, this melon is canary-yellow when ripe. It is oblong in shape and has white flesh tinged with pink around the seed cavity.

Korean melon (yellow melon) These long melons look like small spaghetti squash. They have firm, almost crispy, flesh with an aromatic cantaloupe flavor.

Ogen melon The flesh of this cantaloupe-shaped melon is green; the slightly rough skin is yellow.

Persian melon This melon resembles cantaloupe, except that it is slightly larger, the rind is greener, and the netting on the rind is finer.

Santa Claus melon Also called Christmas melon (because it peaks in December), this late-season variety resembles a small watermelon with green and gold stripes. About a foot long, it has crisp flesh, but is not as sweet as other melons.

Sharlyn A sweet melon with a netted greenish-orange rind and white flesh, Sharlyn tastes like a cross between cantaloupe and honeydew.

---

serving suggestions

• Serve melon with a dash of something acidic as a counterpoint to its sweetness. Fresh lemon or lime juice is nice, but try it with a bit of balsamic vinegar.

• Melons make a good addition to smoothies.

• Cube melon and toss with cucumber cubes, sliced red onion, and halved cherry tomatoes for a refreshing salad.

• Add cubes of melon to curries or stews.

• Toss diced melon with fresh lime juice, cumin, chopped scallion, and chopped cilantro and serve as a salsa.

• Puree melon pieces in a blender or food processor with white wine or orange juice. Season to taste, chill thoroughly, and serve in hollowed-out melon shells.

Sprite melon This grapefruit-sized hybrid melon was developed in Japan, but is cultivated in this country. It has pale skin and crisp, ivory-colored flesh.

Uzbek melon Originally from Russia, this white-fleshed melon can grow up to 2 feet long.

Watermelon See Watermelon (*page 590*).

choosing the best

Since melons have no starch reserves to convert to sugar, they will not ripen further once they have left the vine. Growers pick melons when they are ripe but still firm, to protect them during shipping. Invariably, some melons are picked too early, so it is important to know the characteristics of a ripe melon.

Unless a melon is cut, the only clue to ripeness is the condition of the rind. Furthermore, since each melon has its own characteristics, there are only a few general rules that apply to all melons. They should be regularly shaped—symmetrically round, oval, or oblong—and free of cracks, soft spots, or dark bruises. While ripe melons may be firm, slight softness is a good sign, though melons should not be spongy or "soggy." Look for a clean, smooth break at the stem end, rather than a broken bit of stem; casabas and watermelons, however, may show bits of stem. A full, fruity fragrance is a clue to the maturity of most melons, but there may be no sweet odor if the melons have been chilled, and some melons have no aroma even when ripe. Traditional methods such as thumping and shaking are not accurate indicators of ripeness.

▶ **When you get home** You can improve the eating quality of firm, uncut melons by leaving them at room temperature for 2 to 4 days; the fruit will not become sweeter, but it will turn softer and juicier. If during that time the fruit has not reached its peak ripeness, it was picked when immature and will not be worth eating. Once ripened (or cut), melons should be refrigerated and used within about 2 days. Enclose them in plastic bags to protect other produce in the refrigerator from the ethylene gas that melons give off. Ripe melons are also very fragrant, and the aroma of a cut melon can penetrate other foods.

preparing to use

With the exception of watermelon, the preparation is the same for all melons. Simply cut the melon open and remove the seeds and strings. It can be served in many attractive ways: cut into halves, quarters, wedges, or cubes; or the flesh can be scooped out with a melon baller.

CRENSHAW / 1 cup	
Calories	44
Protein (g)	2
Carbohydrate (g)	11
Dietary fiber (g)	1.4
Total fat (g)	0.2
Saturated fat (g)	0
Monounsaturated fat (g)	0
Polyunsaturated fat (g)	0.1
Cholesterol (mg)	0
Potassium (mg)	357
Sodium (mg)	20
KEY NUTRIENTS (%RDA/AI*)	
Vitamin B$_6$	0.2 mg (12%)
Vitamin C	27 mg (30%)

For more detailed information on RDA and AI, see page 88.

milk & cream

Milk, the foundation for all other dairy products, is in itself an exceptional food. Like meat, milk provides high-quality protein. Yet unlike the protein in meat, the protein in fat-free, low-fat, and reduced-fat milk does not come packaged with fat. Moreover, milk is particularly high in the amino acid lysine, which makes milk an ideal complement to cereals, breads, and other grain products, because they are lacking this this essential amino acid.

Today the words "pasteurized" and "homogenized" are so commonly seen on milk cartons that most people probably think these two processes are required by federal law. In fact, pasteurization—heating milk to destroy disease-causing bacteria, as well as yeasts and molds—is required for Grade A milk sold in interstate commerce; however, within each state or locality, compliance is voluntary. Most parts of the country do comply with the pasteurization guidelines set by the U.S. Public Health Service and the FDA, so that 99 percent of all milk sent to market is pasteurized. Not only does pasteurization ensure the safety of the milk supply, it also increases its shelf-life. At the same time, it doesn't significantly affect the nutritional value of milk.

Homogenization, which distributes the milkfat evenly through the milk, is another process we take for granted. It was developed around 1900, but until the 1950s it was common for milk to arrive at stores and households unhomogenized, with a layer of cream at the top of each bottle. You could skim off the cream and use it separately, or shake the bottle to remix the cream with the milk.

Today, almost all fluid milk is homogenized by forcing it through a small opening under high pressure. This breaks down the fat into particles so tiny they remain emulsified in the milk rather than floating to the top.

Milk's high-fat cousin cream continues to be the product separated from unhomogenized milk. Available both sweet and sour, all cream products are pasteurized or ultrapasteurized and may also contain milk, concentrated milk, dry whole milk, nonfat milk, concentrated nonfat milk, or nonfat dry milk. Also included may be emulsifiers, stabilizers, nutritive sweeteners, flavorings, and other optional ingredients.

nutritional profile

Milk is a nutrient-dense food, which means that in relation to its calories it provides an abundance of important nutrients. Rich in high-quality protein, milk is also the leading source of the bone-nourishing mineral calcium in the

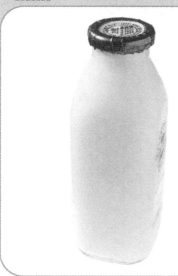

milk

LOW-FAT MILK (1%) 1 cup	
Calories	102
Protein (g)	8
Carbohydrate (g)	12
Dietary fiber (g)	0
Total fat (g)	2.6
Saturated fat (g)	1.6
Monounsaturated fat (g)	0.8
Polyunsaturated fat (g)	0.1
Cholesterol (mg)	10
Potassium (mg)	380
Sodium (mg)	123

KEY NUTRIENTS (%RDA/AI*)	
Vitamin A	144 mcg (16%)
Riboflavin	0.4 mg (31%)
Vitamin B$_{12}$	0.9 mcg (37%)
Vitamin D	98 IU (24%)
Calcium	300 mg (25%)
Selenium	5.4 mcg (10%)

*For more detailed information on RDA and AI, see page 88.

American diet. In addition, it supplies vitamins A and D, riboflavin, and vitamin B_{12}, as well as good amounts of potassium and the amino acid lysine.

Almost all milk sold commercially in the United States has vitamins A and D added. Vitamin A is a fat-soluble vitamin that is largely lost when milk fat is removed; and vitamin D is added to milk because a deficiency of vitamin D can interfere with the body's ability to absorb calcium. Fortifying milk with vitamin D assists in the prevention of osteoporosis.

While Americans have cut down on drinking whole milk, they have increased their consumption of fat-free and reduced-fat milk, which contain all the nutrients of whole milk without the extra fat. The nutrient content of flavored milks, such as chocolate milk, is similar to that of the corresponding unflavored milk, though flavored milks do have higher amounts of carbohy-

lactose intolerance

Despite all of milk's benefits, there are some children and many adults who are unable to drink milk or eat dairy products without symptoms of gas, bloating, diarrhea, and cramps. Known as lactose intolerance (or the inability to digest the lactose, or milk sugar, in milk), this problem affects 5 to 10 percent of Americans of northern European origin; it is also common among Blacks, Asians, Jews, some Mediterranean and Hispanic peoples, and Native Americans.

Lactose consists of two chemically combined sugars, glucose and galactose. The problem of digesting dairy products occurs in people who have a deficiency of lactase, an intestinal enzyme that breaks lactose into these two sugars to render them absorbable. Humans produce peak amounts of lactase in infancy, when milk is necessary for survival; thereafter, the supply begins to diminish.

Despite this problem, millions of people like milk and other dairy products, and want to continue enjoying them throughout their lives. It has been found that most lactose-intolerant people can eat at least some dairy products as part of a meal but not alone; many can even drink a full glass of milk with a meal.

Cultured dairy products, such as yogurt and buttermilk, are easier for lactose-intolerant people to digest. And because most of the lactose is removed during cheese-making, cheese is rarely a problem. Lactose is present, however, in fluid, evaporated, condensed, and powdered milk, whether the product is whole milk or fat-free milk.

Today, lactose-free and lactose-reduced milk treated with lactase are sold in many supermarkets. Lactase is also available in a liquid form that must be added to dairy products at least 24 hours before eating them.

If you think you can't digest lactose, talk to your doctor to see if you are really lactose intolerant.

drates and calories due to the addition of sucrose and other nutritive sweeteners *(see "Chocolate Milk: A Healthy Alternative?" page 402)*.

Not surprisingly, health-conscious Americans have also cut back on their
use of full-fat sweet and sour cream products, preferring to use reduced-fat
versions of these products, sparingly, instead.

in the market

milk

Buying milk is no longer a question of telling the milkman to leave one bottle or two. Not only is the milkman almost a thing of the past, your local
supermarket may carry 10 or more different types of fresh milk, as well as
canned and dried forms. Although most milk is sold fresh for immediate consumption, some forms of dairy products are processed and packaged so they
can be kept on the shelf for future use.

Milk solids (consisting of milk's protein, carbohydrates, minerals, vitamins,
and sometimes fat—everything but the water) may be added to standardize
the milk-solids content of milk from different sources. These solids add protein to any type of milk, and lend opacity, body, and flavor to low-fat and fat-
free milk. Milk is graded according to its quality and intended use. All the
fluid milk we buy in the stores is Grade A. Grade B and C milks are processed
into cheese and other dairy products.

COMPARING MILK & CREAM

The comparisons here are not cup for cup, but rather are a more realistic comparison of serving sizes. The
serving size for milk is 1 cup. The serving size for evaporated milk is ½ cup, because if it were reconstituted to
whole milk, it would have roughly another ½ cup of water added to it. Because condensed milk is sweetened, a
serving would be about 2 tablespoons. The serving size for cream is 1 tablespoon, the amount in an individual
portion of coffee cream. With heavy cream, 1 tablespoon translates to 2 tablespoons of whipped cream.

	Calories	Fat (g)	% Calories from Fat	Saturated Fat (g)	Cholesterol (mg)	Calcium (mg)
Heavy cream (1 tablespoon)	51	5.5	97	3.4	20	9.5
Light cream (1 tablespoon)	29	2.9	90	1.8	10	10
Half-and-half (1 tablespoon)	20	1.7	77	1.1	6	15
Whole milk, 3.3% (1 cup)	150	8.2	49	5.1	33	290
Reduced-fat milk, 2% (1 cup)	121	4.7	35	2.9	79	298
Low-fat milk, 1% (1 cup)	102	2.6	23	1.6	10	300
Fat-free milk (1 cup)	86	0.4	4	0.3	5	301
Nonfat dry milk (reconstituted to 1 cup)	109	0	0	0	5	284
Buttermilk (1 cup)	99	2.2	20	1.3	9	284
Evaporated milk, whole (½ cup)	169	9.5	51	5.8	37	329
Evaporated milk, fat-free (½ cup)	100	0.3	3	0.2	5	371
Condensed milk (2 tablespoons)	123	3.3	24	2.1	13	109

Whole milk By federal law, whole milk must contain at least 3.25 percent milkfat and 8.25 percent nonfat solids by weight—which means it derives about 50 percent of its calories from fat. Because of this relatively high fat content, whole milk is best used only for infants and young children up to age 2, and not by older children or adults.

Reduced-fat milk (2%) This type of milk contains 2 percent milkfat by weight and not less than 8.25 percent nonfat solids. It's important to keep in mind that while "2% milk" refers to the milkfat percentage by weight, much of milk's weight is water. Once you subtract the water from this type of milk, you're left with a product that contains 20 percent fat by weight; in fact, such milk actually derives 35 percent of its calories from fat. Drinking reduced-fat milk is a good way to wean yourself from whole milk at first, but it is still too high in fat to be a permanent choice, unless your diet is otherwise very low in fat.

Low-fat milk (1%, light) This designation covers milk that contains from 0.5 to 1.5 percent milkfat. However, these low percentages (and the "low-fat" designation itself) are deceptive. In truth, low-fat milk gets 23 percent of its calories from fat.

Fat-free milk (skim, nonfat) This type of milk has as much fat as possible removed: It may not contain more than 0.5 percent milkfat by weight, and usually contains less than half a gram of fat per cup, deriving just 5 percent of its calories from fat. Fat-free milk has about half the calories of whole milk. It is the best choice for most adults, and is the only type of milk that should be consumed by people on strict low-fat diets. Today some dairies are taking some of the natural water out of their fat-free milk, or adding back

antibiotics and BST in milk

Does milk contain drug residues? Antibiotic drugs given to cows can and do pass into milk, and millions of samples are tested each year to detect residues. Some surveys have turned up signs of drugs that are illegal in dairy cows—though often the levels are so low as to be barely detectable. The Federal Drug Administration (FDA) has taken corrective steps. But some investigators believe that FDA rules are not tough enough and insist that milk should be free of all antibiotic residues. A fair goal—yet even FDA critics conclude that you're better off drinking milk than not drinking it, and that the U.S. milk supply is safe.

With that in mind, it is also important to be aware that in 1993, the FDA approved supplementing dairy cows with a genetically produced hormone protein known as bovine somatotropin (BST) in an effort to increase the cows' milk production by up to 25 percent. Scientists assert that the composition of milk from BST-injected cows is not altered and has no biological effect on humans, although many opponents are not convinced. There is no mandatory labeling for milk from BST-supplemented cows. However, some products are voluntarily labeled as "farmer certified to not come from BST-supplemented cows."

In a major report issued in 1999, the FDA confirmed that milk that comes from cows treated with BST is safe. In fact, tests of the milk from treated and untreated cows could not determine which was which.

in some nonfat dry milk, to give the milk a more appealing appearance and a mouth feel that is closer to reduced-fat (2%) milk.

Organic milk If a milk product is labeled "organic," it usually implies that it has come from cows fed and raised without the use of pesticides, synthetic fertilizers, antibiotics, and hormones. This may not necessarily be true, however, since federal regulations defining standards for the production, handling, and processing of "organic" products are not always followed. Therefore it's best to look for organic milk that is certified under a program overseen in your state. Also keep in mind that organic milk may cost twice as much as regular, and it offers no health advantages over regular milk, including hormone-treated milk.

Raw milk Usually only available in health-food stores or at farmstands, this type of milk has not been pasteurized. Advocates say it's better nutritionally because the vitamins and natural enzymes have not been destroyed by heat. But while the dairies that are certified to sell raw milk have rigid hygiene standards and their herds are inspected regularly, the milk is still not pasteurized and therefore carries some potential risk of disease.

specialty milks

In addition to catering to the need for milk with varying fat contents, dairies supply specialty milk in response to particular health concerns and taste preferences. For instance, the widespread recognition of lactose intolerance in the American population has brought lactose-reduced and lactose-free milk to the dairy case; and the growing awareness of osteoporosis has prompted the development of calcium-fortified milk. Buttermilk, though not as popular a drink as it once was, is now a low-fat product that has many cooking uses.

Acidophilus milk This type of milk (usually low-fat or fat-free) has the same nutritional value as the milk from which it is made. It differs from regular milk in that the bacterium *Lactobacillus acidophilus* has been added to it. (Unlike acidophilus yogurt, however, acidophilus milk isn't fermented.) Some people believe that acidophilus milk is good for digestive upset, or can help combat lactose intolerance. However, a study undertaken by the Mayo Clinic failed to find that acidophilus milk is useful in the treatment of irritable bowel syndrome; neither did this type of milk forestall the digestive problems caused by an inability to digest lactose.

Another benefit attributed to acidophilus milk is that it can help restore beneficial bacteria to the intestines after taking antibiotics (it's believed that *L. acidophilus* is normally present in the intestines); this could be true, but even the National Dairy Council, which would like to see the public consume

---

milk & kids

Most pediatricians recommend that children ages 4 to 8 get 800 milligrams of calcium a day, or the equivalent of 2 to 3 glasses (8 ounces each) of low-fat milk. Adolescents and young adults, ages 9 to 18, whose bones are growing very fast, need 1,300 milligrams, or about 4 or 5 glasses of low-fat milk. This can be consumed in the form of yogurt or other dairy products as well. (However, milk is still the most efficient source for calcium, because other dairy products are generally not fortified with vitamin D, which enhances calcium absorption.)

Whole milk is the best—and only—choice for children under the age of 2; low-fat milk products aren't good for babies and toddlers because their rapidly growing bodies need the fat that milk provides. After age 2, however, switch your children to low-fat milk and dairy products to help foster a lifetime habit of low-fat eating.

more milk products of every kind, says there is no evidence that acidophilus milk will provide any permanent digestive benefits. Still, acidophilus milk can't hurt you, and if you like the taste there is no reason not to drink it.

Buttermilk Originally a by-product of buttermaking, buttermilk is now made by culturing milk—usually fat-free or low-fat—with a lactic-acid culture. Because of culturing, some buttermilk may have a lower lactose content and therefore may be better tolerated by lactose-intolerant people. Sometimes a small amount of butter is added for a smoother flavor and texture, but generally buttermilk gets just 20 percent of its calories from fat. A small amount of salt may also be added. Buttermilk isn't usually fortified with vitamins A and D.

Calcium-enriched milk You can pack even more calcium into a glass of milk with this low-fat milk, which is fortified with 500 milligrams of added calcium per cup.

Lactose-free milk This milk is 100 percent lactose-reduced.

other "milks"

Almond milk This nondairy beverage is made by crushing almonds, steeping them in water, then straining and pressing them to extract their liquid. Like rice milk, manufacturers generally add vitamins and minerals, such as vitamin D and calcium. Almond milk is also high in vitamin E. It can be found in health-food stores, packed in aseptic containers.

Coconut milk Canned coconut milk is available in regular and light forms, as well as coconut cream. This milk is made by heating coconut meat with water, then steeping, straining, and pressing it to extract the liquid. Regular coconut milk and coconut cream have higher proportions of coconut fat to water, resulting in richer products (and more fat), than light coconut milk. Coconut cream should not be confused with sweetened "cream of coconut," which is mainly used in drinks and desserts.

Goat's milk Goat's milk contains most of the same nutrients as cow's milk, though goat's milk is slightly higher in calcium and is deficient in vitamin B_{12} and folate. Moreover, goat's milk is higher in fat, and is rarely sold in low-fat or fat-free versions. Because goat's milk has a higher percentage of small fat globules—which in theory are more easily broken down by digestive enzymes—some people think it is more digestible than cow's milk. But homogenization reduces the size of the fat globules in cow's milk, too. Goat's milk contains lactose in the same amounts as cow's milk, so it is not the answer for people with lactose intolerance. Just be sure the goat's milk you buy is pasteurized. In some states it is legal to sell raw goat's milk at farmstands, in spite of the high risk of bacterial contamination.

Rice milk Rice milk is an acceptable alternative for those who don't want to drink cow's milk. Rice milk is made from water and brown rice and has few nutrients, but manufacturers add oils, salt, flavorings, and usually vitamins and minerals, such as calcium. Rice milk is sometimes also fortified with the cultures found in yogurt. Thus, depending on the additives in the brand you buy, rice milk may have a similar nutritional profile to cow's milk, though rice milk usually has less protein—and no cholesterol. Check the label to see if it has vitamin D and calcium comparable to cow's milk (which has about 300 milligrams of calcium and 100 IU of vitamin D per cup). Rice milk should not be given to infants, since it lacks essential nutrients. If your infant is allergic to breast milk or formula, get professional advice.

Soymilk See Soyfoods (*page 535*).

Lactose-reduced milk This milk has about 70 percent less lactose than regular milk does. The enzyme lactase is added to this milk to help lactose-intolerant people digest it more easily. Its flavor is slightly sweet, but it has virtually the same nutrient values as low-fat milk.

Low-sodium whole milk Although salt is not added to milk, dairy products are naturally fairly high in sodium. Low-sodium milk has been treated to replace about 95 percent of its natural sodium with potassium. Its sodium content is about 6 milligrams per cup, compared with 120 milligrams per cup in regular whole milk. The treatment almost doubles the milk's potassium content (from 370 to 617 milligrams per cup).

milk in other forms

Because they can last on the pantry shelf for months, canned, dried, or aseptically cartoned milks are useful for those times when you suddenly run out of milk and it's inconvenient to go to the store. However, some of these products have special qualities that make them unique cooking ingredients as well, so they needn't be used only as temporary replacements for fresh milk. For example:

Dry milk powder To make nonfat dry milk powder (whole milk powder is mostly used in food manufacturing), the water is partially evaporated from fluid milk, then the milk is sprayed in a drying chamber to further dehydrate it. You reconstitute the resulting powder by adding water, usually in a proportion of about 1 cup of water to 3 tablespoons of powdered milk. Instant nonfat dry milk, which consists of large, flakelike particles, dissolves quickly and smoothly. Nonfat dry milk can also be used in recipes—or stirred into liquid milk—to add protein and calcium with minimal calories and no fat. A tablespoon of nonfat dry milk contains 94 milligrams of calcium, 27 calories, and no fat, and has added vitamin A and D.

Evaporated milk This kitchen-cabinet standby is made by removing about 60 percent of the water in milk. The milk is then homogenized, fortified with vitamin D and sometimes vitamin A, canned, and heat-sterilized. Since the cans may be stored at room temperature, this milk product is convenient to keep on hand for cooking and for emergencies. To use evaporated milk in place of fresh milk, reconstitute it with an equal amount of cold water

COMPARING SOUR CREAMS **2 tablespoons**				
	Calories	Fat (g)	% Calories from Fat	Saturated Fat (g)	Cholesterol (mg)
Full-fat	62	6.0	87	3.7	13
Reduced-fat	41	3.6	79	2.2	12
Low-fat	40	2.5	56	2.0	10
Fat-free	25	0	0	0	0

(or use it undiluted in recipes that so specify). Evaporated milk comes in whole, reduced-fat, and fat-free forms. Nutritionally, fat-free is preferred—it contains less than a gram of fat per cup compared to 18 grams of fat in a cup of whole—and it is a versatile ingredient for low-fat cooking. Undiluted, it is as thick as heavy cream and can be substituted for cream in soups and sauces; if it is very well chilled, you can even whip it (*see box at left*).

Sweetened condensed milk This is a canned concentrate of whole milk to which sugar has been added to prevent spoilage. It comes in whole and fat-free forms.

Ultra-high temperature (UHT) or **ultrapasteurized milk** This type of dairy product is processed at temperatures higher than those used in regular pasteurization, thereby lengthening shelf-life. In fact, UHT milk, packed in cartons (like juice boxes) that are presterilized and aseptically sealed, can be stored at room temperature for about 6 months.

cream

Half-and-half (cereal cream) A mixture of milk and cream, half-and-half must have a milkfat content at least 10.5 percent and no more than 18 percent by weight.

Light cream (coffee cream, table cream) This cream must have at least 18 percent and no more than 30 percent milkfat by weight.

Whipping cream (**light whipping cream**) Whipping cream must contain at least 30 percent and no more than 36 percent milkfat by weight.

Heavy cream This cream has 36 percent or more milkfat by weight. It should not be confused with whipping cream although it can, of course, be whipped. It is occasionally labeled, "heavy whipping cream."

sour creams

Most sour creams are made by culturing cream and/or milk with lactic acid bacteria. Sometimes the enzyme rennet and/or nonfat milk solids are added for more body.

Full-fat sour cream In order to be labeled full-fat, sour cream must contain at least 18 percent milkfat by weight.

Reduced-fat sour cream Reduced-fat sour cream must have one-third less fat than full-fat sour cream.

Light sour cream Made from cultured half-and-half, light sour cream has 40 percent less fat than full-fat sour cream.

Fat-free (nonfat) sour cream Made from cultured fat-free milk, fat-free sour cream must have less than 1 percent total fat.

low-fat whipped cream

A tablespoonful of whipped cream is not such a dietary disaster—if you can really limit yourself to one spoonful. If you can't, try whipped evaporated fat-free milk, chilled very thoroughly. For best results, pour the undiluted milk into a shallow pan and place it in the freezer until ice crystals form at the edges. Use a chilled bowl and beaters to whip the milk, and serve it within an hour.

To make it further ahead and to stabilize the whipped milk so it does not deflate, add a little unflavored gelatin, using 1½ teaspoons of gelatin per cup of evaporated milk: Warm ⅓ cup of the milk slightly and dissolve the gelatin in it. Chill the mixture, then add it to the remaining ⅔ cup of chilled milk and whip; add a little confectioner's sugar and vanilla, if desired.

You can also make whipped cream from nonfat dry milk that has been reconstituted with ice water.

other cultured milks

Crème fraîche A number of specialty markets also sell a cultured pasteurized cream product called crème fraîche. It has a slightly tangy, nutty flavor and a velvety rich texture. Read the label for nutritional information, since this is generally a high-fat product.

Yogurt See Yogurt (*page 598*).

choosing the best

The milk products in your local supermarket or convenience store will nearly always be marked with a "sell by" date. Generally, the date is determined by the producer, although in some areas it may be regulated by a local authority. A common standard for setting an expiration date is 8 to 12 days from the time the milk is pasteurized.

Since the lower part of a refrigerated display case is colder than the top, select a carton from the bottom of the display if possible. Try not to buy more milk than you need; a larger size is no bargain if it goes bad before you finish it. If you're not sure you'll be able to use a full half-gallon, you're better off buying two quarts and leaving the second carton unopened until needed. Opening milk and exposing it to warm air activates bacteria, causing the milk to spoil more quickly, even if it is re-refrigerated.

It's hard to find milk in glass bottles these days, but translucent plastic jugs are very common. Some studies suggest that milk in translucent plastic containers is more susceptible to significant losses of riboflavin and vitamin A from the effect of the fluorescent lights in supermarkets. Low-fat and fat-free milks are particularly sensitive to light. Cardboard containers, however, seem to protect against the light.

► **When you get home** All fresh dairy products should be promptly refrigerated, otherwise they will turn sour within a matter of hours. Dairy products last longer and taste better when kept cold—at 45° or below. If the temperature of milk is allowed to reach 50°, the shelf life is halved. (A 20-minute trip by car on a hot day can raise the temperature of milk by as much as 10°.)

And because you don't know if the store kept the milk you bought under constant refrigeration (who knows if it sat on a loading dock in the sun?), sniff the opened container for any sign of sourness before tasting. Even cultured products like buttermilk should smell fresh, not bitter or sharp.

Milk containers should be kept closed or covered, as milk readily picks up flavors and aromas from other foods. It's best to leave fresh milk in its original container, and protect it from exposure to strong light, since light can reduce its riboflavin content and cause off-flavors.

love that latte

If your main source of milk is caffè latte, you'll be glad to know that its nutrients survive steaming. The protein and calcium are not affected by steaming, nor are other minerals. Even the vitamins survive: Milk heated for 10 minutes retains 80 to 100 percent of its B vitamins, according to the FDA.

Do be sure your latte is made with low-fat or fat-free milk, however, and try to get additional calcium from other sources. And don't be concerned about the caffeine: It does not significantly interfere with calcium absorption or adversely affect bone density, according to the most recent studies.

If you prefer to serve milk or cream in a pitcher or creamer rather than from the carton, pour just the amount you need into the serving container, and don't return any leftover milk or cream to the carton. Cover and store any that's left over separately, since it will spoil sooner.

Canned evaporated or condensed milk can be stored at room temperature for a year. Invert the cans every 2 months. Once opened, the milk should be transferred to a clean, opaque container, covered tightly, and refrigerated; the milk should keep for 3 to 5 days.

Aseptically packaged UHT milk has a shelf-life of about 6 months at room temperature. For the best flavor, refrigerate it in the sealed package to thoroughly chill it before serving.

Unopened packages of nonfat dry milk should be stored in a cool, dry place. Reseal opened packages, as moisture will make powdered milk lumpy and eventually cause it to spoil. Discard nonfat dry milk if it smells scorched or rancid.

Freezing of milk is not recommended. It causes undesirable changes in the milk's texture and appearance. Microwaving milk is not recommended to extend its shelf-life or as a means of pasteurization.

preparing to use

Fluid milk is ready to use as it comes from the carton; nonfat dry milk needs to be mixed with water. For richer-tasting milk (and more concentrated nutrients), use ½ cup less water than the package instructions specify for each 1-quart envelope of dry milk. For best flavor and texture, mix the milk in a blender, and prepare it far enough in advance to allow for thorough chilling before you serve it.

chocolate milk: a healthful alternative?

Many children—and adults, too—have trouble drinking as much milk as they should: Milk flavored with chocolate syrup or sweetened cocoa may be more appealing, but people naturally worry about the nutritional value of chocolate milk. There's no cause for concern, however. Low-fat (1%) chocolate milk is relatively low in fat: 1 cup contains 3 grams of fat (about 17 percent of the calories). The chocolate syrup used to flavor the milk is loaded with sugar, but it's low in fat—less than 1 gram per 2-tablespoon serving. And the amounts of calcium and other nutrients remain about the same. (Still, because of the sugar, chocolate milk has about twice as many calories as plain milk.)

It is commonly believed that the chocolate in chocolate milk "binds" calcium and makes it difficult for the body to absorb this mineral. Chocolate does contain oxalic acid (a chemical found in many plants), which can combine chemically with calcium to form calcium oxalate—a compound thought to make the calcium unusable. But milk contains a lot of calcium, while the amount of chocolate typically added to milk contains only a little oxalic acid; hence there's plenty of "free" calcium left over. Only about 2 percent of the calcium in low-fat chocolate milk is "tied up" as calcium oxalate. One study found that cocoa does not inhibit calcium absorption to any significant degree.

millet

An easily cultivated, fast-growing grain, millet was an important food in Europe in the Middle Ages, but it was supplanted by other grains, such as barley. However, it has long been a staple in North Africa, where it probably originated, and it is widely consumed in India, China, and Japan as well. In India, finely ground millet is made into a flatbread called *roti*. (Millet has no gluten and so cannot be used for raised breads.) In the United States, millet is known principally as feed for birds and poultry.

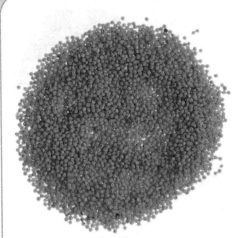

millet

nutritional profile

It is certainly worth giving this ancient grain a try—it's easy to use, and it supplies a rich assortment of vitamins and minerals, including thiamin, riboflavin, niacin, vitamin B$_6$, folate, iron, magnesium, and zinc. Millet is low in fat and a good source of plant protein and fiber.

in the market

Flour or **meal** See Flour, Nonwheat (*page 324*).

Cracked millet Millet in its hulled and cracked form is occasionally sold as couscous (though the packaged couscous available in North America is most often made from semolina, which is the milled endosperm of hard wheat).

Pearl millet The outer layer of millet is indigestible, so millet is always hulled (pearled). The tiny, pale yellow or reddish-orange beads of millet can be cooked like any other grain.

Puffed millet This is millet that has been puffed under pressure. Use it as a breakfast cereal.

choosing the best

While some supermarkets carry millet, it is easier to find in health-food stores. When shopping for whole-grain millet, look for a bright, golden color. Don't buy millet from feed or pet stores as it still has the indigestible outer hull intact. Look for grains that are plump, not broken, and uniform in size and color.

serving suggestions

• Cook millet in milk with a pinch of spice. Stir in chopped apples and serve as a hot cereal.

• Cook millet and mix while warm with a tart vinaigrette and chopped cucumbers and tomatoes.

• Sweeten cooked millet with honey and almond extract. Stir in dried fruits and toasted almonds and serve as a dessert pudding.

• Use cooked millet instead of bulgur in tabbouleh.

MILLET / ½ cup cooked	
Calories	286
Protein (g)	8
Carbohydrate (g)	57
Dietary fiber (g)	3.1
Total fat (g)	2.4
Saturated fat (g)	0.4
Monounsaturated fat (g)	0.4
Polyunsaturated fat (g)	1.2
Cholesterol (mg)	0
Potassium (mg)	149
Sodium (mg)	5

KEY NUTRIENTS (%RDA/AI*)	
Thiamin	0.3 mg (21%)
Riboflavin	0.2 mg (15%)
Niacin	3.2 mg (20%)
Vitamin B$_6$	0.3 mg (15%)
Folate	46 mcg (11%)
Iron	1.5 mg (19%)
Magnesium	106 mg (25%)
Zinc	2.2 mg (20%)

*For more detailed information on RDA and AI, see page 88.

mushrooms

The mushroom's distinctiveness stems in part from the fact that it isn't truly a vegetable but a fungus—a plant that hasn't any roots or leaves, that doesn't flower or bear seeds, and that doesn't need light to grow (although some do need light to fruit). Instead mushrooms proliferate in the dark and reproduce by releasing billions of spores. There are about 38,000 varieties of mushrooms, some of them edible, others highly toxic. *(See "Mushroom Safety," page 406.)*

Mushrooms have a long and esteemed history. The Chinese used them for medicine, and the Egyptian pharaohs were so enamored of them that they decreed them a royal food. The French, however, took the passion for mushrooms to a new level, being the first to cultivate them in caves, beginning in the 17th century. By the late 1800s, mushrooms were being grown on a commercial scale in other European countries, as well as in the United States, where farmers in Pennsylvania eventually developed new methods for growing them indoors.

While some mushrooms are still cultivated in caves or cellars, today most are grown year round in specially designed buildings in which all aspects of the environment—light, temperature, humidity, and ventilation—can be controlled. As a result, cultivated versions of wild mushrooms, which were once considered an expensive delicacy, are now affordable and widely available.

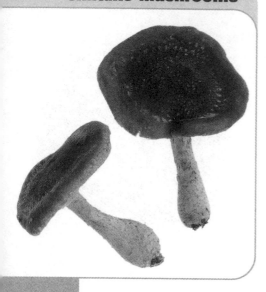

shiitake mushrooms

nutritional profile

Because they lack the brighter colors of so many other vegetables, mushrooms are not usually thought of as a nutritionally beneficial food. In truth, mushrooms actually do supply some key nutrients: The B vitamins niacin and riboflavin (as well as some B_6 and folate), and iron, potassium, and selenium. Mushrooms are also low in calories (a cup of raw mushrooms has about 20) and are a good source of dietary fiber (particularly cholesterol-lowering beta glucan) as well.

in the market

Not so long ago, button mushrooms dominated the marketplace, but today you'll find dozens of different mushrooms—both cultivated and wild, fresh and dried—in greengrocers, gourmet stores, ethnic markets, and farmers' markets. Many mushrooms are also available by mail order.

The following are some of the more popular mushroom varieties. Some can be quite expensive, but even just a few wonderful specimens can transform a dish.

Black trumpets (black chanterelles) See chanterelles (*opposite page*).

Button mushrooms (white mushrooms) For many years, these mild-flavored, smooth, round-capped mushrooms were the only ones grown

SHIITAKE MUSHROOMS 1 ounce dried	
Calories	84
Protein (g)	3
Carbohydrate (g)	21
Dietary fiber (g)	3.2
Total fat (g)	0.3
Saturated fat (g)	0.1
Monounsaturated fat (g)	0.1
Polyunsaturated fat (g)	0
Cholesterol (mg)	0
Potassium (mg)	435
Sodium (mg)	4

KEY NUTRIENTS (%RDA/AI*)	
Riboflavin	0.4 mg (28%)
Niacin	4.0 mg (25%)
Vitamin B_6	0.3 mg (16%)
Folate	46 mcg (12%)
Selenium	39 mcg (70%)
Zinc	2.2 mg (20%)

*For more detailed information on RDA and AI, see page 88.

commercially in the United States. In fact, they still make up most of the domestically cultivated crop. These mushrooms can be found in several different colors—white, off-white, and brown (called cremini)—but they all belong to a single species, *Agaricus bisporus*. They range in diameter from ½ inch (the real "buttons") to 3 inches (called "jumbos") and are often sold prepackaged. Their mild flavor intensifies and improves when cooked.

Cèpes (boletes, ceps, porcini) These mushrooms are distinguished by a stout stem and a spongy surface (rather than gills) underneath the brown caps, which range in diameter from 1 to 10 inches. Found in Washington State and Oregon, and imported from France and Italy during the summer and fall, they are expensive, but their earthy, woodsy flavor is well worth the cost. Cèpes are also available dried.

Chanterelles (egg mushrooms, girolles, pfifferings) The name chanterelle covers an entire family of trumpet-shaped mushrooms with frilly caps that range in color from white and yellow-gold to black. In France, *black chanterelles* are known by the misleading name *trompettes de la mort* ("trumpets of death"), though they are not poisonous. Chanterelles aren't cultivated, but are gathered wild, mainly in the Pacific Northwest (where specimens larger than a foot wide and heavier than 2 pounds are not uncommon); they are also imported. Chanterelles vary in flavor from pleasantly flowery or fruity to nutty. Dried chanterelles can be quite rubbery when cooked.

Chicken-of-the-woods (sulfur mushrooms) This large fan-shaped mushroom gets its name from its meaty, almost chickenlike, texture and flavor. The top of the mushroom is a deep red-orange, while the underside is yellow. Though it can grow to 16 inches across, only the younger, smaller mushrooms are worth eating.

Cremini (crimini) Also called brown or Italian brown mushrooms, cremini are actually a variety of button mushroom *(opposite page)* with a more intense flavor. Mature, full-grown cremini are marketed as portobellos *(page 406)*.

Enoki (enokitake, enoki-daki) Native to Japan (the name means "snow puff" in Japanese), ivory-colored enoki are used in many Asian dishes. They have tiny caps and look like a cluster of long-legged sprouts joined in a clump at the base. Their mild, almost sweet taste and crisp texture is best appreciated when they are served raw, or very lightly cooked.

Hen-of-the-woods See maitake *(page 406)*.

Huitlacoche (cuitlacoche, corn smut, maize mushrooms, Mexican truffles) Pronounced wee-tlah-KOH-cheh, this fungus grows primarily on sweet corn in damp weather. The infected kernels become swollen and oddly shaped, turning black inside and silvery gray outside. Long considered a delicacy in Mexico, huitlacoche can be purchased fresh or frozen by mail order or canned in some Hispanic markets. Whether fresh or canned, the fungus exudes a black juice when cooked and has an inky, wild mushroomy taste that many find indescribable. Do not purchase fresh huitlacoche if the fungus looks dry and powdery; it's too old.

BUTTON MUSHROOMS
1 cup sliced raw

Calories	18
Protein (g)	2
Carbohydrate (g)	3
Dietary fiber (g)	0.8
Total fat (g)	0.3
Saturated fat (g)	0
Monounsaturated fat (g)	0
Polyunsaturated fat (g)	0.1
Cholesterol (mg)	0
Potassium (mg)	259
Sodium (mg)	3

KEY NUTRIENTS (%RDA/AI*)

Riboflavin	0.3 mg (24%)
Niacin	2.9 mg (18%)
Iron	0.9 mg (11%)
Selenium	8.6 mcg (16%)

For more detailed information on RDA and AI, see page 88.

Maitake (hen-of-the-woods) This Japanese mushroom, which resembles the body of a small hen, is now commonly cultivated in the United States. Maitakes have a distinctive aroma and a rich, woodsy taste. They are also available dried.

Morels One of the highest-priced varieties because they are usually harvested in the wild (though they are grown commercially in Michigan), morels are small, dark brown mushrooms with conical, spongy caps. They have an especially intense, earthy flavor, which some describe as nutty or smoky. The morel's honeycombed surface (which requires special attention to clean) makes it ideal for absorbing sauces, and its hollow cap is perfect for stuffing. They are also available dried.

Oyster mushrooms (pleurotus, tree oysters, phoenix, sovereigns) These mushrooms come in a range of colors, including off-white, pink, yellow, and gray-brown. Oyster mushrooms grow in tight clusters and are incredibly tender (in fact, they melt in your mouth). They have an elusive flavor that some say is reminiscent of oysters. They are also available dried.

Porcini The Italian name for cèpes (*page 405*).

Portobellos (Romas) Originally imported from Italy, but now widely grown in the United States, tan/brown portobellos are actually fully mature cremini mushrooms. As large as 4 to 5 inches in diameter, these hearty, rather meaty-flavored mushrooms are sold with and without their fibrous stems, and unlike many other mushrooms, their black gills are completely exposed. They are especially well-suited to grilling or roasting.

Reishi Widely prized in Asia, where they are believed to be an immune-booster, bitter-flavored reishi can be found both fresh and dried in Asian markets and by mail order. Try these mushrooms in Chinese soups.

Shiitake (golden oak, forest, black forest, Chinese black) Grown for hundreds of years only in Japan, China, and Korea, shiitake mushrooms are now cultivated in a number of U.S. states. The caps have a leathery feel and a pronounced mushroomy taste, with a slightly peppery finish. Sev-

mushroom safety

It may be tempting to eat mushrooms you have picked yourself in the wild. But beware: They could be highly toxic, and even deadly. Indeed, some wild mushrooms bear such a striking resemblance to edible mushrooms that they occasionally fool even the most experienced mushroomer. Most victims of life-threatening mushroom poisoning in North America are those who mistake Death Caps (*Amanita phalloides*) for edible Paddy Straw (*Volvariella volvacea*) mushrooms. It's best to leave foraging for wild mushrooms to the experts and gather your own from the market instead.

eral packaged commercial brands are available in supermarkets and gourmet stores. Dried shiitakes are often sold in Asian and other markets as "Chinese black mushrooms."

Straw mushrooms (paddy straws) These are the classic little mushrooms used by Chinese restaurants in stir-fries. They are almost always sold canned, but can be purchased fresh or dried by mail order and in some gourmet markets. It's worth keeping an eye out for dried straw mushrooms, because they have a far more intense flavor than the canned.

Truffles Grown completely underground on the roots of oak trees, truffles are the ultimate edible fungi, with a uniquely intense earthy flavor and aroma. Scarce and exceptionally difficult to cultivate and harvest (they require a trained pig or dog to sniff them out), these delicacies cost a small fortune (prices fluctuate with the year, but can easily run to more than $400 a pound). *Black truffles* usually come from Perigord in southwestern France; *white truffles* are gathered around Alba, Italy. White (and some black) truffles are also being grown in Oregon. Fresh truffles (both black and white) are only available from late December to March. They are also available in cans and jars at some gourmet shops.

White mushrooms See button mushrooms (*page 404*).

Wood ears (cloud ears, tree ears, black fungus) This short-stemmed mushroom grows wild on the trunks of walnut, elder, and beech trees. Once sold only in dried form in Asian markets, fresh wood ears are now more widely available. They have fitted caps that vary greatly in size and may have a damp, jellylike appearance (this is normal). The mushroom's slightly gelatinous, almost crunchy, texture provides an interesting contrast in stir-fries, noodle and grain dishes, soups, and stews.

Yellow foots (yellow chanterelles) This variety of chanterelles (*page 405*) is less meaty and flavorful than some of the other chanterelles.

▶ Availability Button, shiitake, oyster, and enoki mushrooms are available all year, while other specialty varieties are on the market more sporadically, with supplies best in summer and fall. Pennsylvania grows much of the domestic crop; California, Oregon, Washington State, Florida, and Michigan are also leading suppliers. Dried mushrooms, naturally, are available year round. (Some, like the wood ear, are mainly sold in Asian markets.)

choosing the best

For common cultivated mushrooms (button, cremini) Choose those that have a firm texture and even color; reject any that appear slimy, bruised, or pitted. Also look for mushrooms with closed "veils"—the area where the cap meets the stem: A wide-open veil indicates that the mushroom has aged and will have a shorter storage life. If you're not fussy about appearance, slightly older mushrooms (which actually have a richer flavor) may be bought for immediate use. To minimize waste in recipes that call for caps only, choose mushrooms with short stems.

---

serving suggestions

• Fill cooked portobello mushrooms with diced tomatoes and a topping of shredded mozzarella for portobello "pizzas."

• Try an assortment of sautéed mushrooms in your favorite spinach salad.

• Grill large mushrooms and toss in a vinaigrette.

• Stuff large white mushrooms with chopped turkey bacon, broccoli, and goat cheese. Bake until heated through.

• Substitute raw enoki mushrooms for sprouts in salads and sandwiches.

• Add sautéed mushrooms to tomato sauces for pasta, meat, or poultry.

• Add finely chopped raw mushrooms to turkey burger and meatloaf mixtures to provide extra moisture.

• Toss cooked mushrooms into potato salads.

• Use dried mushrooms in vegetarian chilis to give them a meaty flavor.

For fresh specialty mushrooms Certain mushrooms, such as oysters, portobellos, and cèpes, naturally have open caps (or do not have separate caps or gills). Particularly if gathered in the wild, these mushrooms will not have the clean, uniform appearance of cultivated mushrooms. They should, however, be firm and meaty, as well as dry to the touch but not withered. Even uncooked, they should have a pleasant, earthy fragrance.

▶ **When you get home** It is important to conserve just the right amount of moisture when storing mushrooms. If left completely uncovered, they will dry out; if enclosed in moisture-proof wrapping, they will become soggy and begin to decay. A good compromise is to place mushrooms purchased in bulk in a loosely closed paper bag or in a shallow glass dish covered with a kitchen towel or a lightly moistened paper towel. Leave prepackaged mushrooms in their unopened package. Don't wash or trim mushrooms before storing them.

Keep mushrooms on the refrigerator shelf—not in the refrigerator crisper, which tends to be humid—for only a few days. Unopened, prepackaged mushrooms will keep for up to a week. If the mushrooms begin to darken (and their caps open) with age, they can still be used for cooking and flavoring foods.

Dried mushrooms will keep almost indefinitely if wrapped in plastic or placed in a tightly closed jar and stored in the refrigerator or freezer. They can also be stored in a cool, dark place for up to 6 months.

preparing to use

Since all mushrooms are very absorbent, try to minimize their contact with water when cleaning them. You can simply trim off any obviously tough or dirt-encrusted ends and wipe the main part of the mushroom clean using a dry paper towel or a damp sponge or cloth. Or you can also use a new soft-bristled paintbrush, or a special mushroom brush available at shops that sell kitchen gadgets. If absolutely necessary, place the mushrooms in a colander and rinse them very quickly under cold running water.

After cleaning, trim off the spongy tip of each mushroom stem and discard; then break or cut off the stems if the recipe requires it. Do not discard the stems; if you cannot use them immediately chop them, then wrap and freeze them for later use in a stock or soup. Shiitake mushrooms are the exception: Their stems are generally too tough and fibrous to eat. You can use the stems, however, to flavor stock.

You can also pulverize dried mushrooms in a food processor or blender, then use the powder to flavor and thicken sauces and stews: Before processing the dried mushrooms, place them in a sieve with a fairly coarse mesh and shake to strain out any dirt or grit.

mussels

These slender blue-black bivalves are found on both the Atlantic and Pacific coasts; in their natural state, they attach themselves to surf-washed rocks and spend half the time submerged and half the time in the air as the tide comes and goes.

nutritional profile

Low in fat, rich in protein, mussels supply an exceptional amount of vitamin B_{12}. They are also a rich source of iron and selenium. Other nutrients in mussels include thiamin, riboflavin, niacin, folate, magnesium, potassium, zinc, and omega-3 fatty acids.

in the market

Because mussels are severely affected by pollutants, they are now being commercially farmed in "safe" waters.

Blue The most abundant of dozens of mussel species, these are found along the Atlantic and Pacific coasts. Beneath their thin shells lies sweet tender flesh.

Greenshell Originally known as New Zealand green-lipped mussels, this imported variety sports a bright green shell and is considerably larger than blue mussels.

▶ Availability Mussels are available year round; but in late spring, when mussels spawn, they tend to be of inferior quality.

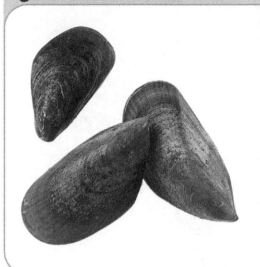

greenshell mussels

choosing the best

Mussel shells should be tightly closed, or should close tightly when the shell is tapped; don't buy any with open or cracked shells. Freshly shucked mussels should smell perfectly fresh, with no trace of ammonia or a "fishy" smell.

▶ When you get home When you buy mussels, it is imperative to keep them alive—or cold—until you are ready to cook and serve them. Store them in the refrigerator (if possible at 32° to 35°), covered with wet kitchen towels. Don't put them in an airtight container or submerge them in fresh water, or they will die. Cold mussels should keep (in a live state) for 4 to 7 days. Be sure to remove any that die (look for open shells) during that period so they do not contaminate the rest. Shucked mussels should be kept in tightly covered containers, immersed in their liquor, for a day or two.

preparing to use

To prepare mussels for cooking (they are most commonly cooked in their shells), scrub the shells (with a stiff brush, if necessary). Pull the stringy "beards"—the fibrous dark tufts protruding from the shells—out of the mussels. Scrape any tough encrustation from the shells with a sturdy knife. Rinse under cold running water.

MUSSELS / 3 ounces cooked	
Calories	146
Protein (g)	20
Carbohydrate (g)	6
Dietary fiber (g)	0
Total fat (g)	3.8
Saturated fat (g)	0.7
Monounsaturated fat (g)	0.9
Polyunsaturated fat (g)	1.0
Cholesterol (mg)	48
Potassium (mg)	228
Sodium (mg)	314

KEY NUTRIENTS (%RDA/AI*)	
Thiamin	0.3 mg (21%)
Riboflavin	0.4 mg (27%)
Niacin	2.6 mg (16%)
Vitamin B_{12}	20 mcg (851%)
Folate	64 mcg (16%)
Iron	5.7 mg (71%)
Selenium	76 mcg (139%)
Zinc	2.3 mg (21%)

*For more detailed information on RDA and AI, see page 88.

nectarines

The name nectarine most likely comes from the Greek *nektar*, the drink of choice for most of the Greek gods. It is believed that the nectarine goes back over 3,000 years to China and possibly Egypt. Nectarines made their way from the Middle East to Europe, including Spain; this is of note, because nectarines were introduced in this country by Spanish missionaries in California.

The history of the nectarine is so closely intertwined with that of its close cousin, the peach, that details of its history remain rather obscure. Botanically, the nectarine is classified as a subspecies of the peach, but it is more accurate to describe each fruit as a genetic variant of the other, akin to first cousins. In fact, so close is their association, that, though rare, it is possible to find nectarines and peaches growing on the same tree.

Nectarines are drupes (or stone fruits) that belong to the rose family. Juicy, fragrant, and quite luscious, nectarines are (unlike peaches) smooth-skinned and fuzzless. Judging from historical references, early nectarine varieties were small and white-fleshed, with skins that could be green, red, or yellow. Modern crossbreeding techniques—in which nectarine varieties are crossbred with one another as well as with peaches—have yielded larger, peachlike nectarines with gold or red skin and yellow or white flesh.

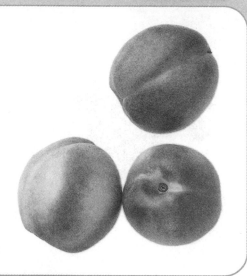

nectarines

NECTARINE / 1 medium	
Calories	67
Protein (g)	1
Carbohydrate (g)	16
Dietary fiber (g)	2.2
Total fat (g)	0.6
Saturated fat (g)	0.1
Monounsaturated fat (g)	0.2
Polyunsaturated fat (g)	0.3
Cholesterol (mg)	0
Potassium (mg)	288
Sodium (mg)	0

nutritional profile

Sweeter and darker-fleshed peaches, nectarines are low in calories and are a good source of potassium and fiber. Two antioxidant carotenoids, beta carotene and beta cryptoxanthin, bestow a vivid golden-yellow hue to nectarine flesh.

in the market

There are more than 150 nectarine varieties that differ slightly in size, shape, taste, texture, and skin coloring (which ranges from golden yellow with a red blush to almost entirely red). The fruit may be clingstone or freestone (a classification indicating how tightly the flesh clings to the pit). No single variety is superior in all respects, but the most popular varieties—among them *Fantasia, Rose Diamond, Summer Grand, Royal Giant,* and *May Grand*—are all equally desirable. A few of the more unusual varieties are:

Blanca del Jalon This variety of nectarine has flesh that is greenish-white and is sweet and juicy.

Honeydew nectarine This fruit cross between a honeydew melon and a nectarine is the size of an apricot, has the texture of a nectarine, and the pale green flesh and taste of a honeydew melon.

Mango nectarine This fruit has the shape and feel of a nectarine but the flavor of both nectarine and mango. It ripens from green to bright yellow.

White nectarine While most nectarines have yellow flesh, the white nectarine has cream-colored flesh and red skin. White nectarines are low in acid, very sweet, and quite fragrant. Some varieties are *Sweet Home* and *Bright Pearl.*

▶ Availability Domestic nectarines are available throughout the summer. Some nectarines are imported in winter and early spring, but these generally aren't as sweet because they are picked at an earlier stage (to withstand shipping). Once a mature nectarine is picked, it won't get much sweeter; it does, however, become juicier and softer when kept at room temperature.

choosing the best

Select bright, well-rounded nectarines with shades of deep yellow under a red blush. Ripe fruit should yield to gentle pressure, particularly along the seam, and should have a sweet fragrance. If you select brightly colored fruits that are firm or moderately hard, they will ripen within 2 or 3 days at room temperature. Avoid fruits that are rock hard or greenish—signs that the fruit was picked too soon and won't ripen properly. Also pass up fruits that are mushy or have shriveled skins, both signs of decay. Sometimes the skin of a nectarine may look stained, as though the blush has spread out in an irregular pattern under the skin, but this doesn't affect taste or texture. Moreover, a rosy blush doesn't indicate the degree of ripeness, but is simply a characteristic of the variety.

▶ When you get home Allow hard nectarines to ripen by storing them for 2 to 3 days at room temperature in a loosely closed paper bag, away from sunlight. Once the fruit gives slightly to gentle pressure, it's ready to eat. You can keep it fresh for another 3 to 5 days by storing it in the refrigerator crisper.

preparing to use

Since the flesh of a fresh nectarine darkens when exposed to air, don't slice it until you are ready to use the fruit. You can preserve its color temporarily by dipping the slices in a cup of water to which you've already added a tablespoon of lemon juice, or by simply tossing them with lemon juice.

serving suggestions

• Add diced nectarines to rice pudding.

• Add thick wedges of nectarines to stir-fries.

• Use sliced or chopped nectarines, raw or cooked, as a topping for waffles, pancakes, or French toast.

• When sautéing chicken breasts, add nectarine slices to the pan for the last few minutes of cooking, then spoon the fruit over the chicken at serving time.

• Add diced nectarines to a traditional Greek salad.

• Thinly slice nectarines and add to a turkey and cheese sandwich.

• Toss sliced nectarines with pasta, cherry tomatoes, and chopped basil for a summer pasta salad.

• Grill nectarine halves and offer them as an accompaniment to barbecued meat or poultry, or serve them for dessert.

nuts

All through human history societies have benefited from the rich nutritional profile of nuts. They served as an alternative to meat and fish and were especially vital during periods of famine when hunting and fishing were hindered by weather conditions or when prey was scarce. And in some parts of the world where meat is forbidden, nuts are still a staple food, just as they were in ancient times. Nomadic people first gathered nuts growing in the wild, and around 10,000 B.C. settled populations began to cultivate nut trees.

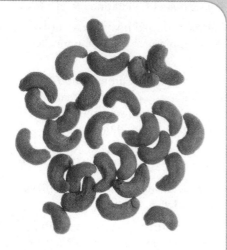

cashews

Highly varied in shape, size, texture, and flavor, nuts grow all over the world and are marketed in a variety of forms. Most nuts can be eaten as is from the tree, and others are dried to preserve them (a process that helps to improve flavor). While we tend to regard nuts as a snack food, they are actually much more nourishing than most snacks and are an important source of a wide range of nutrients. Nuts are also versatile cooking ingredients, and for centuries they have been processed into butterlike pastes, ground into nutritious flours, pressed for fragrant cooking oils, and pulverized with water to produce beverages that resemble milk.

nutritional profile

In recent history, nuts were considered high-fat villains, but they are now emerging as nutritional heroes. Nuts are a nourishing, concentrated source of plant protein, heart-healthy monounsaturated fatty acids, and a vast array of vitamins and minerals. Since nuts are intended to feed the new plants they are meant to propagate, they are full of nutrients required for the early growth of the new nut tree.

Though the amino acid content of nuts isn't perfect, it nevertheless provides a high-quality plant protein. And while their fat content is rather high, very little of it is saturated. Instead, nuts are high in monounsaturated and polyunsaturated fats, which help lower blood cholesterol, especially when substituted for foods high in saturated fat, such as meat or cheese. The fat content varies from nut to nut, with chestnuts having the least fat and macadamias containing the most (though 70 percent of it is monounsaturated).

Each nut has its own nutritional virtues, which is just another reason to eat a variety of these valuable foods. For example, walnuts stand out for their heart-healthy alpha-linolenic acid (ALA) content; Brazil nuts provide an exceptional amount of the antioxidant mineral selenium; and almonds offer excellent protein and vitamin E with less fat than other nuts.

in the market

Nuts are marketed in a variety of forms—with or without shells; whole, chopped, and slivered; raw, dry-roasted, and oil-roasted; salted, sugared, spiced, or plain; packaged or loose. Most nuts are also pressed to make oils (*see Nut Oils, page 299*) and are made into butters and flours.

Commercial "roasting" of shelled nuts is actually a form of deep-frying, and the fat used is often highly saturated coconut oil. The process can add about 10 calories per ounce of nuts (and a bit more fat—saturated fat, if coconut oil is used). Roasted nuts are usually heavily salted, too, although you can find unsalted roasted cashews and peanuts. Nuts can be roasted or toasted at home without fat.

Dry-roasted nuts are not cooked in oil, but they are only marginally lower in calories and fat than oil-roasted nuts. In fact, when you round off the fractional differences in fat and calorie counts, oil-roasted and dry-roasted nuts are about the same. Like regular roasted nuts, dry-roasted nuts may be salted or contain other ingredients, such as corn syrup, sugar, starch, monosodium glutamate (MSG), and preservatives.

Acorns Once a staple in the Native American diet, acorns are still gathered in the wild, but they are not cultivated. Acorns from red oaks need to be shelled and soaked in several changes of water to remove bitter tannins. Acorns from white oaks are less bitter and don't need to be soaked. In either case, acorns should be roasted. Their flavor is similar to hazelnuts.

Almonds See Almonds (*page 156*).

Beechnuts The beech tree is a member of the acorn and chestnut family and produces reddish burrs that house two small triangular nuts. They are similar in taste to walnuts.

Brazil nuts See Brazil Nuts (*page 202*).

COMPARING NUTS 1 ounce

The values below are for shelled, unroasted nuts except for those marked with an asterisk. For a frame of reference, 1 ounce of most nuts, chopped, is about ¼ cup.

	Calories	Protein (g)	Total Fat (g)	% Calories from Saturated/ Monounsaturated/Polyunsaturated	Vitamin E (mg)	Iron (mg)	Magnesium (mg)
Almonds	167	6	15	7/48/16	7.0	1.0	84
Brazil nuts	186	4	19	21/29/31	2.2	1.0	64
Cashews*	163	4	13	14/40/12	2.1	1.7	74
Chestnuts	70	1	0.6	2/3/3	0.2	0.3	9
Coconut	100	1	9.5	71/3/1	0.2	0.7	9
Hazelnuts	179	4	18	6/65/8	6.8	0.9	81
Macadamias	199	2	21	13/70/2	0.1	0.7	33
Peanuts*	166	7	14	10/35/22	2.2	0.6	50
Pecans	189	2	19	7/53/21	0.9	0.6	36
Pine nuts	160	7	14	12/28/31	1.0	2.6	66
Pistachios	172	4	15	9/50/11	1.5	0.9	37
Walnuts, black	172	7	16	8/17/51	0.7	0.9	57
Walnuts, English	182	4	18	7/19/51	5.6	0.7	48

*dry-roasted

serving suggestions

- Finely chop nuts and add to breading for fish or poultry.

- Toss hot cooked pasta with chopped nuts and nut oil.

- Stir nuts into rice pilafs.

- Grind nuts to a paste to make your own nut butter.

- Add nuts to stuffings for poultry.

- Make a sandwich spread with reduced-fat cream cheese (Neufchâtel) and coarsely chopped nuts.

- Make a smoothie with bananas, frozen yogurt, and peanut or other nut butter.

- Drizzle apple slices with honey and sprinkle with chopped toasted nuts.

- Stir nut butter into soups or stews to help thicken and give body.

- Scatter a few chopped nuts instead of croutons over a bowl of soup.

Butternuts See Walnuts (*page 586*).

Cashews These nuts are the seeds of a tree that is native to Africa and South America. Today, most cashews are imported from India. The kidney-shaped nuts grow in a double shell that hangs off the ends of small pear-shaped fruits called cashew apples. (Though the cashew apple is what is called a pseudofruit, it is actually a swollen stalk. The cashew apple is usually discarded when the cashew is harvested, but in some countries it is saved and made into a liquor.) Cashews are always sold shelled because their shells contain a caustic oil (the cashew is related to poison ivy); in fact, the nuts must be carefully extracted to avoid contamination with this oil. In the United States, these flavorful nuts are more popular for snacking than for cooking, yet they make a particularly delicious nut butter. They are sold raw (unroasted), roasted, or dry-roasted. Cashews are a good source of iron, magnesium, zinc, and vitamin E. They're lower in total fat than most nuts and seeds, but are relatively high in saturated fat.

Chestnuts See Chestnuts (*page 236*).

Coconuts See "Coconuts" (*page 416*).

Coquito nuts These small, marble-shaped nuts, known as mini coconuts grow on the Chilean palm *Jubaea chilensis*. They are woodlike on the outside and white on the inside, and are sweet, crunchy, and similar in taste and texture to coconut.

Gingko nuts The Maiden Hair tree produces a round, reddish-orange fruit, resembling a wild plum. When ripe, the fruit opens to reveal a silvery shell containing a single nut, which is surrounded by inedible tissue. The fruit itself releases foul-smelling butyric acid, but the nut is much prized, especially by the Chinese. Once shelled, gingko nuts must be blanched or soaked in water to remove the surrounding soft tissue before eating. They are also available canned.

Hazelnuts See Hazelnuts (*page 361*).

Hican These are a cross between the hickory nut and pecan with a round, thin shell like the pecan. Hicans have a sweet, buttery flavor.

Hickory nuts There are several varieties of hickories, some producing sweet nuts, others producing bitter nuts. (Pecans are a type of hickory nut.) Of the sweet variety, the shagbark and the shellbark are the most well known. *Shagbark hickory nuts* are thin-skinned and easy to shell. *Shellbark hickory nuts* are larger than shagbark with thicker shells. Both are similar in flavor to pecans and have a limited commercial production. The bitter hickory nut is used to flavor hickory-smoked cured meats.

Macadamia nuts These "gourmet" nuts were named for Dr. John Macadam, an Australian who reputedly discovered that they were deliciously edible. Indigenous to Australia and now one of the best-known products of Hawaii, macadamias have a sweet, delicate taste and creamy, rich texture. However, they contain more fat and calories than any other nut. On the plus side, macadamias supply some iron, magnesium, and thiamin. Most commonly eaten as a dessert nut, macadamias are nearly always sold shelled, as their shiny round shells are very thick, requiring some 300 pounds of pressure to crack them. They are harvested five or six times a year, but the demand still exceeds the supply; consequently, they're usually quite expensive.

Peanuts Peanuts are actually a type of legume, but are commonly used as nuts. See Peanuts (*page 452*).

Pecans See Pecans (*page 464*).

Pine nuts Pignoli, pine nuts, piñon nuts, pinyon nuts, Indian nuts—these are all names for the seeds of various types of nut pine trees, which grow in several areas of the world. The seeds come from pinecones and range in size from that of an orange seed to more than 2 inches in length (from South American nut pines). To harvest the nuts, the pinecones are dried to free the nuts, then the nutshells are cracked to release the kernels. Because of the intricacy of harvesting pine nuts, they are quite expensive. Slender ivory-colored pignoli are an important cooking ingredient in the Mediterranean region, while the pinyons of the American Southwest have been a staple of the Native American larder since ancient times. In general, European species of pine nuts are richer in protein and lower in fat than the American varieties, but American pine nuts offer more vitamins and minerals. Pine nuts are available from Europe (Italian pignoli are the most widely sold) as well as Russia and China. Imported pine nuts are usually sold shelled; American pine nuts, or pinyons, are sold both ways, in-shell and shelled.

Pistachio nuts See Pistachios (*page 475*).

Walnuts See Walnuts (*page 586*).

▶ **Availability** Most shelled nuts, sold in vacuum-sealed cans or jars, or in cellophane bags, can be found in supermarkets year round. Fresh tree nuts in the shell (such as walnuts, pecans, and hazelnuts) are more seasonal—supplies are best in the fall and early winter.

choosing the best

Whether you choose nuts in the shell or shelled is mostly a matter of convenience. Nuts keep better in their shells, but they do require cracking before you can eat or cook with them. Most nuts in their shells and some shelled nuts, are sold raw, that is, unroasted. Raw nuts have the advantage of no added fat, but their flavor is rather bland compared with that of roasted nuts, and once shelled they do not keep as well.

When buying packaged nuts, look for a freshness date on the jar, can, or bag. The kernels, if visible, should be plump and uniform in size. If you buy

---

heart-healthy nuts

Perhaps the most famous study to give nuts a boost was the one of Seventh-Day Adventists from 1997: It found that people who ate nuts at least five times a week cut their risk of a heart attack in half, compared with those who ate nuts less than once a week. This was followed by other studies, such as two large ones involving only women, which also found that nut eaters had a lower risk of heart disease, even when researchers controlled for other variables that affect the risk. Other studies have also suggested that nuts may help lower blood cholesterol levels.

There are plenty of substances in nuts that may explain these heart-healthy results including monounsaturated and polyunsaturated fatty acids, vitamin E, folate, magnesium, copper, potassium, and fiber, as well as plant sterols. And while it's still too early to say for sure that nuts can substantially lower the risk of heart disease, when substituted for high saturated-fat foods, nuts can offer a commanding range of nutritional quality.

shelled nuts at a candy store, health–food store, or other bulk source, be sure that they're crisp and fresh, not limp or rubbery, musty, or rancid smelling.

When selecting nuts with shells from a basket or bin, choose those with undamaged shells; look out for cracks, scars, or tiny wormholes. Nuts should feel heavy, and the kernel should not rattle when the nutshell is shaken; if it does, the kernel may be withered and dry.

▶ **When you get home** The high fat content of nuts makes them prone to rancidity; heat, light, and humidity will speed spoilage. Raw unshelled nuts, however, keep very well—6 months to a year if stored in a cool, dry place.

Shelled nuts will keep for 3 to 4 months at room temperature in a cool, dry place. Keep them in their original package or, once the package is opened, transfer them to plastic bags or freezer containers. For longer storage,

coconuts

The coconut is the seed of a fruit (like most tree nuts, such as almonds and walnuts), but we rarely see the fruit in which it grows. More familiar is the egg-shaped, hairy shell of the nut itself. Coconuts grow on the tropical coconut palm, and most of the coconuts sold in the United States come from Central America and Puerto Rico. Unlike most nuts, the coconut shell does not contain an inner kernel; instead, the shell itself is lined with a layer of rich white "meat," and the hollow at the center of the coconut is filled with a watery, slightly sweet liquid that can be used as a beverage.

Another characteristic that distinguishes coconuts from other nuts is that nearly all of its substantial fat content is saturated. Coconut oil, used in many processed foods in this country, is the most highly saturated of all vegetable oils. Moreover, coconut has no redeeming vitamin or mineral assets (though it has some dietary fiber). Therefore, it is best to eat the nut in very small quantities.

You can buy whole coconuts and crack them yourself, or choose from several types of processed coconut: shredded and dried (which comes sweetened or unsweetened, and sometimes toasted) or

pressed for its milk (see "Other Milks," page 398). When buying a whole coconut, choose one with a firm shell. Heft and shake it to see if it is heavy and full of liquid, which are signs of freshness. A whole, unbroken coconut will keep for a month or two at room temperature. Tightly wrap a cracked or opened coconut and use the meat within a week.

Macapuno coconut This small coconut from the Philippines does not have a coconut-milk-filled cavity as other coconuts do. Instead, it is solid in the center. The coconut is harvested when the flesh is soft. It is sold in jars, as long shreds.

Young coconuts (jelly coconuts) These are coconuts picked at the stage before their flesh hardens to the coconut meat we are familiar with. The flesh of a young coconut is soft enough to be eaten with a spoon.

COCONUT / ¼ cup shredded fresh

Calories	71
Protein (g)	1
Carbohydrate (g)	3
Dietary fiber (g)	1.8
Total fat (g)	6.7
Saturated fat (g)	5.9
Monounsaturated fat (g)	0.3
Polyunsaturated fat (g)	0.1
Cholesterol (mg)	0
Potassium (mg)	71
Sodium (mg)	4

keep them in the refrigerator or freezer. If they are properly wrapped, freezing will not significantly affect the texture or flavor of nuts, and they need not be thawed for cooking purposes. Nuts for eating should be thawed at room temperature and then toasted or freshened in the oven before serving.

preparing to use

Usually the only preparation necessary for nuts in the shell is to shell them. For those that have hard shells, use a nutcracker or a small hammer.

If shelled nuts seem a little soft (but do not smell rancid), they can be freshened by spreading them on a baking sheet and heating them in a very low oven (150°) for a few minutes.

Chop nuts with a good-sized chef's knife on a large cutting board. For efficient chopping, spread the nuts on the board. Start by gently cutting the nuts into smaller pieces so they don't go flying. Then, when they have been very coarsely chopped, hold down the tip of the knife blade with one hand and raise and lower the knife, moving it fanwise across the nuts until they are more finely chopped. A curved chopper used in a wooden bowl works well, too.

When chopping nuts in a food processor or blender, process a small amount at a time and pulse the machine on and off; don't overprocess the nuts, as this will release their oils and turn them into paste.

If you need very finely chopped nuts, as for certain cakes or other desserts, there are special hand-cranked nut grinders with sharp, rotating blades. The blades actually shave the nuts into small flakes instead of chopping them. This keeps the resulting mixture light and fluffy instead of heavy and oily.

Some recipes may call for blanched nuts. When applied to nuts, this term refers not to a brief cooking in boiling water, but to the process used to remove the papery skin from the kernel. Nuts can be blanched in several different ways. Oven-toasting hazelnuts will enable you to remove their skins. Other shelled nuts can be blanched in boiling water. Drop the nuts into the boiling water and boil for 30 seconds. Drain, and when the nuts are cool enough to handle, slip off the skins, or rub them off with a kitchen towel. To dry them, spread the nuts on a paper towel or toast them briefly in a 250° oven.

Toasting nuts before using them browns and crisps them and helps to bring out their rich flavor. Nuts can be toasted in a variety of ways.

On the stovetop: Place shelled nuts in a heavy skillet and toast over medium heat until crisp and fragrant. *In the oven:* Place them in a pan and toast them at 350° until crisp and fragrant (timing varies depending upon the nut, so check after 5 minutes to prevent burning.) *In the microwave:* Place the nuts on a paper towel or paper plate and microwave until crisp.

nut milks

Nut milks are used by those who are avoiding dairy milk for reasons that range from lactose intolerance to a vegan diet. There are several commercial nut milks, most notably almond milk and coconut milk (*see "Other Milks," page 398*). However, you can also make your own. Grind nuts in a food processor, add water to cover, and let stand for 30 minutes. Strain, pushing on the solids to extract as much liquid as possible. Use the liquid as an alternative to dairy milk in puddings, cakes, and breads.

oats

Oats have probably been cultivated since the 1st century A.D. With the exception of a few countries such as Scotland, where the grain has long been a staple food for humans, oats have been used primarily for animal fodder. Brought to the New World by English colonists, oats were planted in Massachusetts in the mid-1600s, and were first packaged in the United States for wide distribution in 1852. Over the years, however, the grain has gained very little in popularity with consumers; even today, only about 5 percent of the world's oat crop is used as food for humans (mostly as oatmeal, and in only a few countries, including the United States, Canada, and Scotland).

Interest in the grain peaked in the late 1980s, when highly publicized studies showed that oats—especially oat bran—can lower blood cholesterol. Encouraged by press reports and food manufacturers, many people came to believe that oats were a magic bullet against cholesterol. When other studies found the anticholesterol effect of a daily serving or two of the grain to be modest, there was a backlash against oats. Since then, however, researchers have learned more about this and other potential health benefits of oats.

nutritional profile

Oats are hard to beat for nutritional impact. As a whole grain, they are a prime source of the complex carbohydrates that help to sustain energy. They contain about 50 percent more protein than bulgur wheat, and twice as much as brown rice. They offer impressive levels of thiamin, iron, and selenium, and respectable quantities of magnesium and zinc.

But it is the high soluble-fiber content of oats that captures the attention of many nutritionists. Oats are particularly rich in this form of fiber, which has been credited with helping to lower blood cholesterol levels. A cup of cooked oatmeal has 4 grams of fiber—16 percent of the total amount of fiber you should eat each day—and about half of that is soluble fiber. In 1997 the FDA allowed the labels on oat products to bear the statement that this soluble fiber, when part of a diet low in saturated fat and cholesterol, "may reduce the risk of heart disease." Some oat products sport the check mark of the American Heart Association. Oats are the best source (along with barley) of a particular type of soluble fiber called beta glucan. This seems to play a special role in lowering total blood cholesterol and LDL ("bad") cholesterol—especially the small dense LDL particles that are most likely to endanger coronary arteries, according to research.

The fiber in oats has other benefits besides lowering cholesterol. Research suggests that oat fiber may also help control blood sugar and improve insulin

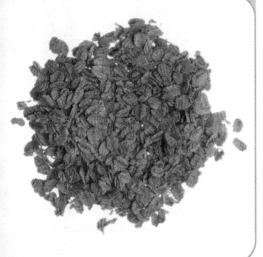

rolled oats

OATS / 1 cup cooked	
Calories	145
Protein (g)	6
Carbohydrate (g)	25
Dietary fiber (g)	4.0
Total fat (g)	2.3
Saturated fat (g)	0.4
Monounsaturated fat (g)	0.8
Polyunsaturated fat (g)	0.9
Cholesterol (mg)	0
Potassium (mg)	131
Sodium (mg)	2

KEY NUTRIENTS (%RDA/AI*)	
Thiamin	0.3 mg (21%)
Iron	1.6 mg (20%)
Magnesium	56 mg (13%)
Selenium	19 mcg (34%)
Zinc	1.1 mg (10%)

*For more detailed information on RDA and AI, see page 88.

sensitivity and thus be a boon for people with insulin resist-ance or diabetes. But no one knows how much of it you have to eat to get a significant effect. Oat fiber may also help to reduce high blood pressure. Oats may also help to promote weight loss because they are digested slowly, leading to a gradual, steady supply of blood sugar (glucose), which keeps hunger in check.

in the market

Bran This outer layer of the grain, lighter and finer than wheat bran, is high in fiber and nutrients. It can be eaten as a cereal.

Flour See Flour, Nonwheat (*page 325*).

Groats These nutty-tasting whole grains can be eaten as cereal, but are more commonly served as a main or side dish. They can be used as a stuffing for vegetables or poultry or to thicken soups and sauces. They are typically found in health-food and specialty food stores.

Rolled These are the familiar forms of oats sold in the supermarket. The grains are heated and pressed flat with steel rollers to shorten the cooking time. There are three types of rolled oats: *Old-fashioned* (the whole grain is rolled), *quick-cooking* (the grains are sliced before rolling), and *instant* (the grains are precooked, dried, and then rolled very thin). Instant oatmeal is often packaged with extra ingredients, such as salt, sugar, and flavorings.

Steel-cut Usually imported from Ireland or Scotland, this form of the grain is made by thinly slicing the oats lengthwise. Commonly eaten as a breakfast cereal, steel-cut oats have a dense, chewy texture and take longer to cook than rolled oats. You can also add them to soups and stews.

choosing the best

Because oats have a slightly higher fat content than other whole grains, they can turn rancid more quickly. Buy them in small quantities. When buying oats from bulk bins, make sure they smell fresh and are free from chaff or other debris. Try to be sure the store has a fast turnover.

▶ **When you get home** Keep oats in airtight containers. Store oat prod-ucts at room temperature (or in the refrigerator in hot weather) for up to a month. In the freezer oat products can be kept for 2 to 3 months.

➤ *phytochemicals in* oats

Oats contain phytochemicals that may help reduce the risk of heart disease along with other benefits. Biochemists in Canada (where most North American oats are grown) have identified many of them, including saponins and antioxidants. Some of these antioxidants resemble vitamin E and seem to work in tan-dem with it, helping to maintain proper blood flow. Preliminary research has found that, like vitamin E, these compounds can counter the vessel-constricting effect of a high-fat meal in susceptible people. Of course, neither eating oats nor taking vitamin pills can undo all the damaging effects of high-fat meals.

---

serving suggestions

• Add oats to burger and meatloaf mixtures.

• Use oat groats instead of rice in a pilaf recipe.

• Add oats to soups and stews. The finer cuts will help thicken the liquid. The coarser and whole-grain types will add texture.

• Use steel-cut oats instead of rice in a rice pudding.

• Finely grind oats and use for one-fourth of the flour in a pie crust recipe.

• Coat fish or chicken with toasted, coarsely chopped oats before panfrying.

okra

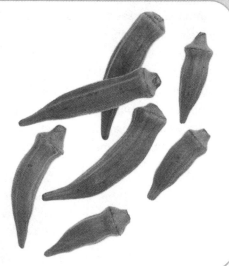

okra

Okra is a tropical plant that originated in Ethiopia and made its way in the 1700s to Louisiana (courtesy of the slave trade). Today, this small, fuzzy, green pod is best known as a key ingredient in the thick Louisiana stew called gumbo. The name of the stew actually comes from the word *gombo*, which in West African dialect means okra.

Okra is one of those love-it-or-hate-it vegetables. Cooked sliced okra exudes a slimy juice that is a combination of tongue-twisting chemical substances (acetylated acidic polysaccharide and galacturonic acid). It is this mucilaginous quality that makes some people give okra a wide berth, but that causes others to seek it out, especially for its ability to add a thickness to stews like gumbo. Okra's flavor and texture are unique, resting between that of eggplant and asparagus.

nutritional profile

This unusual vegetable has much to offer nutritionally. It is a good source of B vitamins, vitamin C, magnesium, potassium, and fiber, as well as the carotenoids lutein and zeaxanthin. It is particularly rich in soluble fiber, which may help to lower LDL ("bad") cholesterol levels.

in the market

You can find okra in varying shades of green or white and in chunky or slender shapes, with either a ribbed or smooth surface. Varieties with green, ribbed pods are the most common.

▶ **Availability** Fresh okra can be difficult to find outside areas where it is a culinary tradition (the South). However, frozen okra—both whole pods and sliced—is available in supermarkets in other parts of the country.

choosing the best

Small, young pods—no more than about 3 inches long—are the most tender; as the vegetable matures, it becomes fibrous and tough. Choose pods that are clean and fresh (overmature ones will look dull and dry), and that snap crisply when broken in half; avoid okra pods that are hard, brownish, or blackened.

▶ **When you get home** Don't wash okra until just before you cook it; moisture will cause the pods to become slimy. Store untrimmed, uncut okra in a paper or plastic bag in the refrigerator crisper.

preparing to use

If the pods are very fuzzy, rub them with a vegetable brush to remove some of the "fur." If you are cooking whole okra, trim the barest slice from the stem end and tip, without piercing the internal capsule; prepared this way, the juices won't be released and the okra won't become gummy. If you're slicing okra, however, you can trim the stem end more deeply.

OKRA / 1 cup cooked	
Calories	51
Protein (g)	3
Carbohydrate (g)	12
Dietary fiber (g)	4.0
Total fat (g)	0.3
Saturated fat (g)	0.1
Monounsaturated fat (g)	0
Polyunsaturated fat (g)	0.1
Cholesterol (mg)	0
Potassium (mg)	515
Sodium (mg)	8

KEY NUTRIENTS (%RDA/AI*)	
Thiamin	0.2 mg (18%)
Vitamin B6	0.3 mg (18%)
Vitamin C	26 mg (29%)
Folate	73 mcg (18%)
Magnesium	91 mg (22%)

*For more detailed information on RDA and AI, see page 88.

olives & olive oil

Olives are fruits that are enjoyed worldwide. They are grown primarily in Mediterranean countries, and in some parts of the United States, Australia, and New Zealand. Believed to have originated in Asia Minor, the olive tree is among the oldest known cultivated trees in the world. The allure of olives can be attributed to their texture, aroma, and a beguiling complexity in flavor that varies from sour to bitter to piquant to sweet. The delicate oil from the tiny olive fruit has been a principal source of dietary fat in the Mediterranean region for thousands of years.

nutritional profile

A large percentage of the caloric content of olives and olive oil is monounsaturated fatty acids, which research shows may help to lower LDL ("bad") cholesterol levels when they replace saturated fat in the diet. It is also thought that monounsaturated fatty acids (as well as minor constituents in olive oil) are less susceptible to LDL oxidation in coronary arteries. Both olives and olive oil also contain the antioxidant vitamin E.

The lower rates of certain chronic diseases in Mediterranean countries may possibly be attributed to a diet that includes fewer than 30 to 40 percent calories from fat—with the primary fat consumed being the monounsaturated fats in olive oil.

It's important to note, however, that olives bring quite a bit of sodium along with their heart-healthy monounsaturated fats.

in the market

olives

Olives come in two main colors: green and black. The color of an olive is actually determined by its degree of ripeness. Green olives are unripe and black olives are fully ripe. (There are also colors in between, including red and purple, which are color changes the olives go through on their trip from unripe to ripe.) The notable exception to this is that some canned "black" olives processed in this country are picked green and then processed (by soaking in an alkaline solution and oxidizing via exposure to air) to turn them black.

Olives are also categorized according to processing method. Because all fresh olives are very sharp and bitter in flavor, they need to be processed to make them edible. The processing removes an acrid, bitter-tasting compound

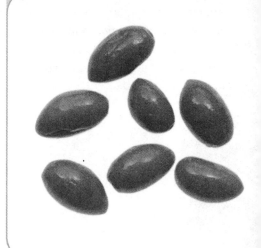

picholine olives

CALIFORNIA BLACK OLIVES 6 super colossal	
Calories	74
Protein (g)	1
Carbohydrate (g)	5
Dietary fiber (g)	2.3
Total fat (g)	6.3
Saturated fat (g)	0.8
Monounsaturated fat (g)	4.6
Polyunsaturated fat (g)	0.5
Cholesterol (mg)	0
Potassium (mg)	8
Sodium (mg)	819

KEY NUTRIENTS (%RDA/AI*)	
Vitamin E	2.7 mg (18%)
Iron	3.0 mg (38%)

*For more detailed information on RDA and AI, see page 88.

called oleuropin, present in olive skin. The different processing techniques include: oil-curing (soaking in oil for several months), water-curing (rinsing and resoaking in water for many months), brine-curing (soaking in brine for 1 to 6 months), and dry-curing (storing in salt for 1 or more months). Each of these methods leaches out the oleuropin.

The permutations of olive style (variety of olive, where it grew, ripeness, and processing method) are myriad. Like wines and cheeses, regional styles account for hundreds of different olives. Until recently, this country had just a handful of olives available, and they often were identified by nothing more sophisticated than "black" and "green." But times have changed, and most specialty food stores (and supermarkets) now carry a wide array of olives. The following is a list of a few that are more readily available. In spite of the increased complexity of olive names, there are still quite a few olives that are identified by more generic terms like "Greek black."

Agrinion These are huge, dull green, brine-cured Greek olives with a sour taste and very soft flesh that is easily torn from the pit.

Alphonso These large Chilean olives are cured unconventionally in wine or vinegar, giving them a dark purple color, tender flesh, and a slightly tart, bitter flavor. They are easy to pit.

Arbequina Becoming more available in the United States, these tiny green Spanish olives have a meaty, smoky flavor. They are hard to pit.

Bella di Cerignola These large, bright green, brine-cured olives come from the Adriatic coast of southern Italy. They are mild and sweet with dense flesh. They are hard to pit.

California Sicilian-style These large, dull green, brine-cured, sometimes cracked olives have a crisp bite. They are hard to pit.

French oil-cured Small, sleek, and wrinkled black, these olives have a strong, intense flavor. They are easy to pit.

Gaeta These are small, wrinkled, salt-cured black olives from Italy. They have a strong flavor and are often hard to pit.

Greek black These are large, dark brown to purple, brine-cured olives with soft pulp and a gentle flavor. They are easy to pit. "Greek black" is sometimes the generic label for Kalamata olives.

Greek green These are plump, juicy, pale green, brine-cured olives with an acrid edge. They are easy to pit.

Kalamata (or Calamata) These dark purple, brine-cured olives from Greece have a strong aftertaste. They are often sold packed in vinegar and are a familiar supermarket olive. They are easy to pit.

Ligurian Similar to Niçoise olives, these small, black Italian olives are brine-cured. They are hard to pit.

> ➤ *phytochemicals in*
> olive oil

Olive oil is an important source of two important polyphenol phytochemicals called hydroxytyrosol and oleuropein. These substances are under investigation for their antioxidant properties and their potential to help protect against breast cancer, clogged arteries, and high blood pressure.

OLIVE OIL / 1 tablespoon	
Calories	119
Protein (g)	0
Carbohydrate (g)	0
Dietary fiber (g)	0
Total fat (g)	14
Saturated fat (g)	1.8
Monounsaturated fat (g)	10
Polyunsaturated fat (g)	1.1
Cholesterol (mg)	0
Potassium (mg)	0
Sodium (mg)	0

KEY NUTRIENTS (%RDA/AI*)

Vitamin E	1.7 mg (11%)

For more detailed information on RDA and AI, see page 88.

Manzanilla These popular, small to medium, brine-cured Spanish green olives have crisp flesh and a smoky flavor. They are easy to pit, though they are often sold pitted and stuffed with pimientos or almonds.

Moroccan oil-cured These oil-cured, shriveled, black olives from Morocco have a slightly bitter, smoky flavor. They are easy to pit.

Niçoise Salt-cured, small, dark brownish-purple French olives, Niçoise have a tart, sharp flavor with faint buttery undertones. Their large pit is often hard to remove.

Nyon These black, slightly wrinkled olives from France are salt-cured. They are easy to pit.

Picholine Small, pointy, pale green, brine-cured olives from France, picholines have a sweet, slightly acidic flavor and a crunchy texture. In this country they are usually packed in citric acid. They are hard to pit.

Sevillano (or Queen) This huge, green, bland, brine-cured variety is grown in California and Spain. They are hard to pit.

Sicilian green These large, pale, greenish-brown, brine-cured olives from Sicily have a dense flesh and sour taste. They are easy to pit.

olive oil

Pressed from tree-ripened olives, the flavor and color of olive oil can vary widely depending on the types of olives used and the region they come from. There are hundreds of different types of olive trees, and most olive oils are blends of several varieties. In addition to the varietal differences, the oil derived from olives also depends on the ripeness of the fruit. When olives ripen (in the fall and winter), the olives change from green to dark purple. Olives harvested early will produce a richer, fruitier oil, and olives that are picked later on in the season produce a milder oil with a less robust flavor and character.

The cost of olive oil is determined by any given year's crop and weather conditions. And, despite innumerable efforts to develop mechanized harvesting methods, olives for the best olive oils are often harvested by hand, a cost that is passed on to the consumer.

Extra-virgin This is olive oil from the first pressing of the olives; it has a low acid content and a delicate flavor. Industry standards stipulate that extra-virgin olive oil must be free of acidity (expressed as oleic acid of not more than 1 gram per 100 grams, or 1%). But in addition to this quantitative analysis, extra-virgin olive oil is also put through a more subjective test by a panel of experts who taste and smell the olive oil and then rate it on a 9-point scale: The oil must score 6.5 or higher to receive the "extra-virgin" designation.

Virgin Virgin olive oil has a higher acid content than extra-virgin (with acidity of between 1% and 3%). Virgin olive oil comes from the second pressing of the olive pulp that remains after the first pressing (for extra-virgin oil).

Fino This is a blend of extra-virgin and virgin oils.

---

serving suggestions

• Chop olives and sprinkle them over pizza or pasta.

• Make an olive paste by pureeing olives with a little citrus zest, olive oil, and fennel seed.

• Add chopped olives to salsas.

• Stir chopped olives into fat-free or reduced-fat cream cheese (Neufchâtel) for a sandwich spread.

• Add olives to stuffings for vegetables, poultry, or fish.

• Top grilled bread with a mixture of chopped tomatoes and olives for an Italian-style appetizer.

• Add chopped olives to pilafs or baked rice dishes.

Refined If a virgin olive oil does not qualify for the virgin designation (as defined by its acidity level and other factors), the oil is then refined to correct the flavors and lower the acidity. The result is a fairly bland, middle-of-the-road oil that is often blended with other, stronger oils.

Pure This is one of the cheapest olive oils available. It is a blend of virgin olive oil and refined olive oil. These olive oils tend to have little flavor and are best used for sautéing rather than for salads.

Cold-pressed This designation indicates that an olive oil has been pressed without the application of any heat. Cold-pressed oils are full and rich tasting with much of the original olive's flavor maintained in the oil. "First cold press" on the label of an olive oil indicates that it is of superior quality (being not only cold-pressed, but also the first pressing), and there is usually a lofty price tag to prove the point.

Extra-light This is olive oil that has been refined to produce a lighter color and flavor. It does not mean that the olive oil is lower in fat (the calories and fat content for extra-light are the same as for any olive oil). The labeling for this category of olive oil is difficult to pin down, because there are no guidelines governing the terms used. Some labels say "light," some say "mild-flavored," some say "extra-light," and some use a combination of these terms. Extra-light olive oil is ideal when an olive oil flavor would be intrusive (baking, for example).

choosing the best

If you are looking for a specific olive, it might be necessary to shop in a large supermarket or specialty food store. If buying in bulk, the containers should be clean and smell of olives. Avoid any olives that have mold or appear dried up. The liquid in jars of olives should be clear, not cloudy.

Purchase olive oil from a store that rotates its stock and that keeps the olive oil out of direct sunlight and in a relatively cool area. If you purchase your oil from a specialty food store it might be worthwhile to look for one from a specific olive. Like olives themselves, the oil that each olive produces is somewhat different. Some oils are actually labeled with the name of the olive that's been pressed to extract the oil.

preparing to use

Some olives are easier to pit than others. If a recipe calls for pitted olives, choose a soft-fleshed variety and press it firmly with the flat side of a chef's knife. This will crack the flesh and expose the pit, making it easy to remove.

onions & scallions

A peerless staple and a universal food, the onion has played a key role throughout culinary history. There is some evidence that onions were consumed in prehistoric times and were widely eaten in ancient Egypt, Greece, and Rome. Onions have historically been valued for their mystical significance and healing properties; and in many cultures they were also a symbol of eternity. In the 17th century, Europeans consumed onions as a breakfast "health" food.

Onions and their relatives—which include shallots, garlic, scallions, and leeks—are known botanically as alliums. There are more than 500 alliums, and all of the edible species are bulbing plants that have a characteristic pungent smell or taste, which is produced once their layers of skin are cut.

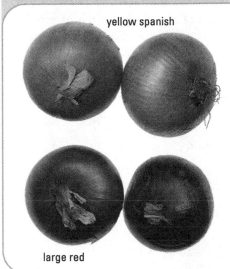

onions

yellow spanish

large red

nutritional profile

Onions are low in calories and fat, and in most nutrients, but are a moderate source of fiber, vitamin C, vitamin B_6, potassium, and some promising phytochemicals. Shallots have some vitamin B_6 and iron.

Nutritionally, young onions with green tops (like scallions or spring onions) have a distinct advantage over other onions: Their green tops, which can be enjoyed along with the white part, provide beta carotene, while the bulb provides a respectable amount of vitamin C.

in the market

Onions (their botanical name is *Allium cepa*) come in an impressive array of sizes, colors, and shapes. Because onions are easily crossbred, growers are continually developing new varieties and hybrids. The ubiquitous medium-sized yellow globe onions, which are available year round, encompass many different varieties, with subtle differences in taste or texture. (The globe shape is popular with consumers, so growers have emphasized it.) Whatever names are bestowed upon onions, though, they fall into two general categories: storage onions and spring/summer onions.

storage onions

These have firm flesh, dry, crackly outer skins, and pungent flavors. Grown in northern areas of the United States, they are harvested in late summer and early fall. After a brief period of drying out (a process known as "curing"), they are stored for several months. In stores, these onions may simply be

YELLOW ONION / 1 large	
Calories	65
Protein (g)	2
Carbohydrate (g)	15
Dietary fiber (g)	3.1
Total fat (g)	0.3
Saturated fat (g)	0
Monounsaturated fat (g)	0
Polyunsaturated fat (g)	0.1
Cholesterol (mg)	0
Potassium (mg)	267
Sodium (mg)	5

KEY NUTRIENTS (%RDA/AI*)	
Vitamin B_6	0.2 mg (12%)
Vitamin C	11 mg (12%)

*For more detailed information on RDA and AI, see page 88.

labeled by color—yellow, red, or white. There are no nutritional differences among these types.

Bermuda onions This large storage onion is sweet and mildly flavored.

Boiling onions These are very small onions that are picked when they are 1 to 1½ inches in diameter. They can be red, white, or yellow, though in supermarkets they are usually white.

Cipolline These squat, disk-shaped onions were originally from Italy but are now being grown in the United States. They are bittersweet and tender and can be used like pearl onions. They can be yellow or red.

Pearl onions These are actually pearl-shaped bulbs from a number of different onion varieties. They are so densely planted that they attain a size of only an inch or less in diameter. While pearl onions were once only available as white onions, they are now available in white, gold, and dark red or purple varieties.

Red (globe) onions A somewhat sweet type of storage onion, these are good in salads and lend color to sandwiches.

Spanish onions These are a variety of very large storage onion, distinguished by their mild flavor; the skin color can range from yellow to purple.

White onions Most often sold as small boiling onions (*see above*), there are also large versions of these onions. Their skin is thinner and more papery than other onion types, and they tend to spoil a little more easily.

Yellow (globe) onions These are storage onions and come in a variety of sizes. They are the commonest onions on the market and the type that most people think of when they think of onions.

spring/summer onions

The category of spring/summer onions includes so-called "sweet" onions as well as members of the onion family that are sold in the early shoot stage (the prime example being scallions). Unlike storage onions, spring/summer onions are not stored, but are shipped almost immediately after harvesting. All of the "sweet" onions have a very high water and sugar content, which means that they spoil more quickly and will not hold up as well as storage onions do. Quite juicy and in some cases mild enough to be eaten raw, sweet onions are grown primarily from fall to spring in warm-weather states, such as Texas, Georgia, Arizona, and Hawaii. Some are designated by names referring to their growing areas, such as Vidalia (from Georgia), and others are known by their varietal name, such as Granex and Grano. Most sweet onions have a characteristically flattened shape.

AmeriSweet These large, round, globed-shaped sweet onions have a thick, deeply colored skin.

Green onions This term is used by most people interchangeably with scallions (*opposite page*), but there is actually a minor technical difference,

---

> **▶ phytochemicals in**
> **onions & scallions**
>
> Onions (and other members of the *Allium* genus) are a rich source of a phytochemical called diallyl sulfide, which research suggests may raise levels of protective enzymes that help to inactivate and eliminate agents that can cause cancer.

Strictly speaking, scallions are bulbless, while green onions are harvested at the miniature bulb stage. But from a consumer's viewpoint, the two types are nearly identical.

Imperial sweets These onions hail from California's Imperial Valley.

Italian bottle onions These red-skinned, bottle-shaped "heirloom" Italian onions are sometimes sold as *torpedo onions.*

Maui sweets Grown in volcanic soil in Hawaii, and first introduced on the mainland by tourists returning from vacation, the Mauis are sweet and make good slicing onions.

Oso sweets These come from South America and are said to contain 50 percent more sugar than Vidalias.

Scallions Though they look like skinny leeks (an onion relative), scallions are true onions—just very immature ones. Scallions are pulled from the ground while their tops are still green and before a significant bulb has formed. In some countries, such as China, scallions are the most popular form of onion.

Spring onions In addition to being a category of onion, this is also a market term for green onions. They are very small onion bulbs with their green tops on.

Texas 1015 This sweet onion derives its name from its ideal planting date, 10/15. A type of Grano, it can grow to softball-size. Horticulturist Leonard Pike from Texas A & M University isolated the tear-causing chemical pyruvate and decreased the amount in these sweet onions. Its nickname is the "million-dollar baby," because of the money spent to develop it.

Vidalia Perhaps the best-known of the sweet onions, these are grown in 20 counties in Georgia. Although you can often identify these onions by their distinctive shape (somewhat flat on the stem end and rounded on the bottom), you will find that Vidalias and many of the other specialty sweet onions are stamped with a label telling you just what they are.

Walla Walla These large, round, sweet onions are named for the city in Washington where they are grown. In order to claim the name Walla Walla, they must be grown within a specific area in the Walla Walla valley.

▶ Availability Storage onions and scallions can be found year round, but sweet onions are in greatest supply from late spring through the summer.

choosing the best

Consider how you plan to use the onions. As a rule, the large, mild "sweet" onions are good for eating raw or for cooked dishes in which you want a subtle flavor. The crisp, assertive character of storage onions makes them better suited for dishes that require long cooking, since they can hold their flavor. An onion's flavor is not only determined by its variety, but also by the local soil and climatic conditions where it grew. Consequently, onions with the same appearance can taste considerably different, depending on where

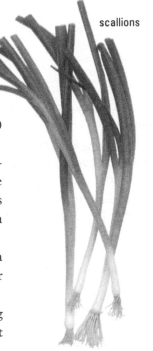

scallions

SCALLIONS / ½ cup chopped	
Calories	16
Protein (g)	1
Carbohydrate (g)	4
Dietary fiber (g)	1.3
Total fat (g)	0.1
Saturated fat (g)	0
Monounsaturated fat (g)	0
Polyunsaturated fat (g)	0
Cholesterol (mg)	0
Potassium (mg)	138
Sodium (mg)	8

KEY NUTRIENTS (%RDA/AI*)

Vitamin C	9 mg (10%)

For more detailed information on RDA and AI, see page 88.

and when they were grown. But you may have to experiment, particularly when it comes to choosing the mildest onions.

Many shoppers prefer a particular color, though color is not a reliable guide to flavor or texture. (White onions tend to be more pungent than yellows or reds, but this rule of thumb may not be true in your area.) Size is another consideration: For raw onion slices in salads and sandwiches, select large onions. They are also a more efficient choice for peeling and chopping. For cooking whole or in wedges, choose small- to medium-sized onions.

Most onions are sold loose by the pound, though globe and pearl onions also come in mesh bags. (Pearls are frequently packaged in small boxes.) Whatever type you choose, look for ones that feel dry and solid all over, with no soft spots (a sign of rot) or sprouts. The neck should be tightly closed, and the outer skin should have a crackly feel and a shiny appearance. Onions should smell mild, even those that are pungent when you cut into them; a strong odor is a sign of decay. Also avoid onions with green areas, which can taste unpleasant, or with dark patches, which may indicate a mold.

As for scallions, look for green, crisp tops and clean bottoms. As a rule, the more slender the bottoms, the sweeter the scallions.

▶ **When you get home** Whole onions should be kept in a cool, dry, open space, away from bright light (which can turn their flavor bitter). They do best in an area that allows plenty of air to circulate around them; either spread them out in a single layer or hang them in a basket. Onions will absorb moisture, causing them to spoil more quickly, so don't store them under a sink (which can be damp) or place them near potatoes, which give off moisture and produce a gas that causes onions to spoil more quickly. Storage onions can last 3 to 4 weeks under these conditions, sweet onions about half as long. (Though humid weather will shorten storage time.)

You can extend the life of onions, particularly sweet varieties, by storing them unwrapped in the refrigerator crisper.

Compared to storage onions, scallions and spring onions are quite perishable: Store them in the refrigerator in a tightly closed plastic bag and use them within 3 days; otherwise, the tops will begin to wilt.

preparing to use

Chopping or slicing an onion brings its sulfur-containing amino acids into contact with enzymes to form volatile compounds, one of which strikes the tongue, while another irritates the eyes, apparently by turning into sulfuric acid. The older an allium is, the stronger these compounds become. Fortu-

---

serving suggestions

• Fold finely chopped sweet onions into a meatloaf mixture.

• Toss whole scallions with Mexican spices, such as cumin and coriander, and a touch of oil, then grill them.

• Cook thinly sliced onions briefly with some balsamic vinegar (no oil) and use as a pizza topping.

• Thread chunks of sweet onions on skewers, brush with a little olive oil, and grill them.

• Hollow out large red or yellow onions, stuff them with a rice or grain mixtures, and bake in a seasoned broth.

• Cook sliced onions until they are caramelized and meltingly tender, and use as a sauce for pasta.

• Make an old-fashioned Irish dish called "champ": Mash potatoes and scallions—in a roughly 3-to-1 ratio—with milk until the mixture is uniformly green and savory.

• Braise spring onions (or plump scallions) like leeks and serve as a side dish.

nately for our taste buds, cooking produces further chemical changes that render these compounds much milder. In addition, some of the compounds in onions appear to be converted into a substance that is 50 to 70 times sweeter than table sugar.

Onions can be sliced, chopped, diced, or grated, but first they must be peeled. To make this task easier, trim off the tops and bottoms; then halve the onions and peel away the paper skin and any silvery membrane. To lessen eye irritation, hold the onions under cold running water as you peel; this trick carries away the sulfur compounds before they can reach your eyes. Chilling the onions beforehand may also help. With small boiling onions, cut an "X" in the root end of each to keep the onion intact once you slip off the skin.

For scallions, first cut away any wilted parts from the green ends and trim off the rootlets from the bulb end. Both the white and green portions can be used as seasonings or salad ingredients, sliced or chopped according to the size you need.

shallots

A small, mild-tasting member of the *Allium* genus, the shallot resembles both the onion and garlic (and its taste falls somewhere between the two). The shallot bulb is wrapped in a delicate, onionlike coppery skin, and it is divided into small, segmented cloves like garlic. However, unlike garlic, the cloves are not enclosed by a sheath and as a result are easier to separate. Shallots can be found in both yellow and red varieties.

The guidelines for buying and storing garlic also apply to shallots—select those that are firm, dry, and free of sprouts; store them (for up to a month) in a cool, well-ventilated space. They will also keep in the refrigerator in a tightly closed jar. Shallots are grown domestically, but some shallots are imported from France. Use shallots with, or in place of, onions to impart a subtle savory flavor.

Like other onions, shallots are a good source of vitamin B_6, though you would have to eat about ¼ cup cooked (not impossible) to get more than 10 percent of the RDA for this vitamin.

SHALLOTS
3 tablespoons chopped

Calories	22
Protein (g)	1
Carbohydrate (g)	5
Dietary fiber (g)	0.2
Total fat (g)	0
Saturated fat (g)	0
Monounsaturated fat (g)	0
Polyunsaturated fat (g)	0
Cholesterol (mg)	0
Potassium (mg)	100
Sodium (mg)	4

oranges & tangerines

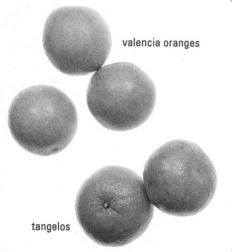

oranges & tangerines

valencia oranges

tangelos

ORANGE / 1 medium	
Calories	64
Protein (g)	1
Carbohydrate (g)	16
Dietary fiber (g)	3.4
Total fat (g)	0.1
Saturated fat (g)	0
Monounsaturated fat (g)	0
Polyunsaturated fat (g)	0
Cholesterol (mg)	0
Potassium (mg)	249
Sodium (mg)	1

KEY NUTRIENTS (%RDA/AI*)	
Thiamin	0.1 mg (10%)
Vitamin C	80 mg (89%)
Folate	47 mcg (12%)

For more detailed information on RDA and AI, see page 88.

Because of their prevalence and their popularity, we tend to take oranges for granted, but at one time they were an expensive delicacy and rarely found in cooler climates. Oranges are semitropical and, like other citrus fruits (including tangerines and tangelos), they probably originated in Southeast Asia. Columbus brought orange seeds and seedlings with him to the New World, and by the 1820s, when Florida became a U.S. territory, there were thriving orange groves in St. Augustine. By 1910, Florida was on its way to achieving its current status as the number-one citrus-growing state.

In the 1940s, frozen orange-juice concentrate was developed, which led to oranges becoming the main fruit crop in the United States. Today, Florida produces a large percentage of the country's oranges, and about 90 percent of the crop is processed into juice. California and Arizona are the other two states where oranges are cultivated. Their oranges, however, have thicker skins than Florida fruits, a characteristic that helps to protect them against the drier climates of the West.

What we call tangerines are actually a subclass of the mandarin orange species. Native to China, the name mandarin is thought to have come from the noble Mandarins who wore bright yellow robes. It is believed that the fruits were then introduced to Europe via Tangiers, hence the name tangerine, or "native of Tangiers." Christopher Columbus is also responsible for the advent of tangerines (as well as oranges and many other foods) to the New World.

nutritional profile

Americans consume most of their oranges in the form of juice, 1 cup of which provides 91 percent of the suggested intake for vitamin C. Nevertheless, the whole fruit offers more nutritional advantages. For example, a whole orange compared with a glass of juice, provides about the same amount of vitamin C with the added benefit of more than 3 grams of fiber. While oranges (and their juice) are the primary source of vitamin C for most Americans, oranges also provide generous amounts of the B vitamin folate as well as potassium and some thiamin.

Tangerines are also highly nutritious and contain the carotenoids beta cryptoxanthin, lutein, zeaxanthin, and beta carotene. Tangerines provide a good amount of vitamin C (an average-sized tangerine supplies about 26 milligrams, or 29 percent of the RDA), thiamin, and some heart-healthy soluble pectin fiber.

in the market

oranges

There are two types of oranges, sweet and sour. The majority of oranges grown commercially in the United States are the sweet type.

Blood The blood-red color of their flesh and juice gives these sweet, juicy oranges their name. Blood oranges are small- to medium-sized fruits, with smooth or pitted skin that is sometimes tinged with red. The red color comes from anthocyanin pigments (which also provide color to raspberries and other dark berries) and may account for the raspberry flavors ascribed to blood oranges. Originally a Mediterranean import, blood oranges are now grown in this country. There are three main varieties available here, two grown in this country—*Tarocco* and *Moro*—and a third, *Sanguinelli,* imported from Spain.

Cara Cara These oranges are navels with a reddish-pink flesh. Like other reddish-fleshed oranges (such as blood oranges), there are overtones of raspberries in their flavor.

Hamlin One of the earliest-maturing oranges, Hamlins are grown primarily in Florida. These small, thin-skinned oranges are practically seedless, with rather pulpy flesh; they are better for juicing than for eating.

Jaffa These oranges are imported from Israel. They are similar to Valencias, but have a sweeter flavor.

Navel These large, thick-skinned oranges are easily identified by the "belly-button" scar located at their blossom end. Navels are seedless, almost effortlessly peeled, and easily segmented—qualities that, along with their sweet-tart flavor, make them excellent eating oranges. They can be used for juice, but they should be squeezed as needed because the juice turns bitter over time, even when it is refrigerated.

Pineapple Similar to Hamlins in appearance, these oranges—named for their aromatic quality—are seedy but very flavorful and juicy; though best for juicing, they are good for eating if you don't mind the seeds.

Seville This sour orange is the type used to make marmalade. It is not sold for eating out of hand, because it has a thick skin and a sour flavor. The thick skin, however, is what makes it desirable for marmalade.

Valencia These are the most widely grown oranges, accounting for about half the crop produced each year. Medium- to large-sized, Valencias have a smooth, thin skin and an oval or round shape. They are dual-purpose oranges, because they can either be eaten whole or squeezed for juice. Florida Valencias, which are available in the middle of the orange season, are considered the best juice oranges.

ORANGE JUICE / 1 cup	
Calories	110
Protein (g)	2
Carbohydrate (g)	25
Dietary fiber (g)	0.5
Total fat (g)	0.7
Saturated fat (g)	0.1
Monounsaturated fat (g)	0.1
Polyunsaturated fat (g)	0.2
Cholesterol (mg)	0
Potassium (mg)	473
Sodium (mg)	3

KEY NUTRIENTS (%RDA/AI*)	
Thiamin	0.3 mg (23%)
Vitamin C	82 mg (91%)
Folate	45 mcg (11%)

For more detailed information on RDA and AI, see page 88.

tangerines & mandarins

Mandarin oranges (*Citrus reticulata*) are a class of oranges with loose, easily peeled "zipper" skin, with red undertones. The carpels, or segments, of mandarins separate more easily than those of oranges. Though the term tangerine is an alternative name for all mandarins, it is also a subgroup of mandarins. Those mandarins and tangerines you are most likely to find in the market are:

Clementine Also called Algerian tangerines, these small, sweet-tasting fruits are seedless. The membranes covering the carpels are thinner than in other tangerines, and the texture of the fruit is very delicate.

Dancy This is the leading tangerine on the market. It rarely appears by its varietal name and is usually just labeled "tangerine."

Delite These mandarins originated in Morocco, but are now grown in California, too. They are virtually seedless and low in acid.

Satsuma This is another subgroup of mandarin oranges that originated in Japan. They are sweet, juicy, and nearly seedless.

tangors & tangelos

There are dozens of orange and mandarin interspecifics—that is, deliberate or accidental crosses between sweet oranges, mandarins, tangerines, and grapefruits or pomelos. (One well-known interspecific was a cross between the pomelo and a sweet orange. The result was the grapefruit.) Tangors are a cross between a tangerine and an orange; and tangelos are a cross between tangerines and pomelos.

Minneola This popular tangelo variety has a distinct knoblike projection on the stem end. Although they are closer to tangerines than to grapefruits in flavor, minneolas have a taste all their own.

TANGERINE / 1 medium	
Calories	37
Protein (g)	1
Carbohydrate (g)	9
Dietary fiber (g)	1.9
Total fat (g)	0.2
Saturated fat (g)	0
Monounsaturated fat (g)	0
Polyunsaturated fat (g)	0
Cholesterol (mg)	0
Potassium (mg)	132
Sodium (mg)	1

KEY NUTRIENTS (%RDA/AI*)

Vitamin C	26 mg (29%)

For more detailed information on RDA and AI, see page 88.

preserving vitamin C

The vitamin C in orange juice is relatively stable. According to a study by the USDA, orange juice retains about 90 percent of its vitamin C after a week under typical home refrigerator conditions, and over 66 percent after 2 weeks. Still, improper handling can significantly decrease the vitamin C content of orange juice. To get the most vitamin C from your orange juice, follow these steps:

• Check the freshness date, if the juice has one.

• Keep orange juice cold.

• Store juice made from frozen concentrate in glass jars with screw tops rather than in plastic jugs or uncovered pitchers.

• If not drinking fresh-squeezed juice immediately, store it in the refrigerator in a glass container with a screw top; it will keep for up to 24 hours without suffering any serious loss of vitamin C. Remember, though, that the flavor of fresh-squeezed juice will change if it's stored for any length of time.

Murcott (honey tangerine) This tangor has deep orange flesh, with a skin that is more green than orange. They are very sweet.

Temple Sometimes also called Royal mandarins, these tangors resemble overgrown tangerines and have many seeds. They are very sweet and juicy, and their flavor is similar to that of an orange.

▶ Availability Although oranges, mandarins, and tangerines are at their peak in the winter, imports have made seasonality for the main varieties a nonissue. The more unusual varieties, on the other hand, may still have small windows of availability. For example, blood oranges are still mostly available from December through mid-spring. And Cara Cara oranges are available for only 1 to 2 months, starting in December.

choosing the best

Choose oranges that are firm, heavy for their size (they will be juiciest), and evenly shaped. The skin should be smooth rather than deeply pitted, although juice oranges are generally smoother than navels. Thin-skinned oranges are juicier than thick-skinned specimens, and small- to medium-sized fruits are sweeter than the largest oranges. There's no need to worry about ripeness— oranges are always picked when they are ripe.

Skin color is not a good guide to quality: Some oranges are artificially colored, while others may show traces of green although they are ripe. Superficial brown streaks will not affect the flavor or texture of the fruit, but oranges that have serious bruises or soft spots, or feel spongy, should be avoided.

Mandarins and tangerines, with their loose-fitting skins, will feel soft and puffy compared to oranges, but should be heavy for their size; otherwise, they are likely to be pithy and dry. Choose fruits with glossy, deep orange skins, but disregard small green patches near the stems.

preparing to use

Halve unpeeled oranges crosswise for juicing, or halve them either crosswise or lengthwise and then cut each half into thirds, for a juicy snack to be eaten from the peel. For garnishing, halve an orange lengthwise, then cut each half crosswise into slices.

Navel oranges, tangerines, and mandarins peel easily if you insert your finger into the opening and pull back the peel. To peel other types of oranges, cut a disk of peel from the top, then cut slices of peel lengthwise from top to bottom. Finally, cut the remaining peel from the bottom. Or, peel spiral-fashion (as you would an apple) after removing a slice from the top. Separate the orange segments by cutting between the membrane and flesh with a sharp knife. Work over a bowl to catch the juices.

To prepare mandarins or tangerines for use in fruit salad or cooked dishes, peel the fruit, separate the segments, and then pull off the membrane from each segment, if desired. Remove and discard the seeds, which may be many or few depending on the variety.

If you need orange zest—the flavorful colored part of the peel—use the fine side of a hand grater, a special zesting tool, a sharp paring knife, or a vegetable peeler to remove the zest from a scrubbed orange. Try not to scrape any of the bitter white pith from the fruit along with the colored part of the peel. Check that the oranges you use for zest are not artificially colored or waxed.

Two to four medium-sized oranges will yield about 1 cup of juice; one medium-sized orange will yield about 4 teaspoons of grated zest.

orange oranges

The color of an orange depends on the climate where it was grown. In tropical climates, like Florida's—where the days and nights are warm—fully mature oranges can remain slightly green. In more temperate areas, like California, where the days are warm and the nights cool, oranges turn their familiar orange color. Thus, Florida oranges are more likely than California oranges to be tinged with green on the outside.

Two other factors can contribute to the color of an orange peel. The first is a phenomenon known as "regreening." Chlorophyll is produced by an orange tree to feed its blossoms. Since the tree can bear both blossoms and fruit at the same time, sometimes the already mature fruit receives some of this chlorophyll, which gives its skin a greenish tinge. Such oranges are extra-ripe and often sweeter.

The second factor is that some orange producers use a harmless vegetable dye to enhance the appearance of mature green oranges. (By law, however, growers are not allowed to give the oranges a better color than they would develop naturally.) According to FDA regulations, oranges treated in this manner must be stamped "Color Added" on the containers they are shipped in or must have a sign affixed to the crate declaring this fact. Only oranges that are produced in Florida are dyed in this manner, however; California and Arizona state laws prohibit adding color to citrus fruits.

Whatever the color of the skin, only fully developed oranges are picked. Growers do not depend solely on the color of the skin to judge ripeness, but harvest fruit based on characteristics such as the ratio of juice solids to acid content of the juice. The point at which an orange is considered mature is regulated by state laws and strictly enforced.

oysters

Long valued as a culinary delicacy, the oyster is a shellfish that is harvested wild from natural beds or, more often, from cultivated grounds. Within its rough, hinged outer shells rests the soft, edible body, which can vary widely in taste and texture. In the United States today dozens of different types of oysters are available.

While it's easy to understand why the famous 18th-century satirist Jonathan Swift wrote, "He was a bold man that first ate an oyster," this remarkable food has nevertheless been touted widely (and wrongly) over the centuries for everything from improving vitality to enhancing one's sex life. The Romans purportedly fed wine and pastries to oysters to fatten them up before bacchanals. Colonial settlers were said to eat them by the gross (144) rather than by the dozen because they were so widely available (oysters commonly grew to 6 to 8 inches back then).

In recent decades, coastal development and pollution along U.S. shores, as well as overharvesting, have greatly reduced the number of natural oyster beds. However, thanks to national seeding programs and commercial farming, oysters are still in abundance. Although there are health risks associated with eating raw oysters (*see the safety information on pages 119–122*), many people continue to eat this succulent shellfish on the half-shell, in addition to sautéed, baked, grilled, or broiled.

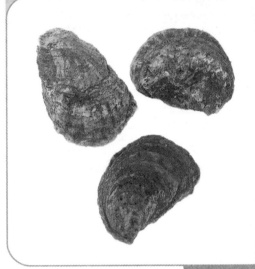

oysters

nutritional profile

Oysters supply a rich compendium of nutrients, including thiamin, riboflavin, niacin, vitamins C, D, and E, iron, magnesium, and selenium. They also contain an extraordinary amount of vitamin B_{12}, which plays a critical role in the production of DNA and RNA, the genetic material in cells. In addition, these plump, mineral-rich bivalves provide a good amount of zinc, a key component in a healthy immune system. Oysters are also a good source of protein. And while they contain dietary cholesterol, they are low in saturated fat, which has a greater impact on blood cholesterol. Small amounts of heart-healthy omega-3 fatty acids can also be found in oysters.

in the market

Because most oysters sold today are commercially cultivated, a wide selection is often available both live and shucked. Although there are just four common species of oyster, there are dozens of different varieties. To distinguish them in the marketplace, they are typically named for their place of origin. Since oysters take on the flavor of the water they're grown in, there are as many differences in flavor as there are oysters. In general, however, oysters from the Pacific Northwest tend to be mild, meaty, crisp, and sweet. Those from California have slightly stronger flavors. Varieties from the Gulf and the Southeast

OYSTERS 6 medium, cooked	
Calories	245
Protein (g)	28
Carbohydrate (g)	15
Dietary fiber (g)	0
Total fat (g)	6.9
Saturated fat (g)	1.5
Monounsaturated fat (g)	1.1
Polyunsaturated fat (g)	2.7
Cholesterol (mg)	150
Potassium (mg)	453
Sodium (mg)	318

KEY NUTRIENTS (%RDA/AI*)	
Thiamin	0.2 mg (16%)
Riboflavin	0.7 mg (51%)
Niacin	5.4 mg (34%)
Vitamin B$_{12}$	43 mcg (1,800%)
Vitamin C	19 mg (21%)
Vitamin D	937 IU (234%)
Vitamin E	2.7 mg (18%)
Iron	14 mg (173%)
Magnesium	66 mg (16%)
Selenium	231 mcg (420%)
Zinc	50 mg (453%)

*For more detailed information on RDA and AI, see page 88.

are usually softer, with an earthier flavor. And those from the Mid-Atlantic and Northeast are quite crisp and distinctively salty. Some varieties even have a fruity or slightly nutty finish.

Shucked oysters are typically graded and sold according to size, usually in 8-ounce, 12-ounce, pint, or gallon containers in their own clear liquor. The largest shucked oysters are called selects, while the smaller ones are standards. Ask your seafood seller where the oysters are from if the label doesn't specify.

The following are the four most common oyster species, along with some of the more popular varieties:

Eastern (or Atlantic) Eastern oysters, which account for most of the American oyster supply, are found in coastal waters from the Canadian Maritimes to the Gulf of Mexico. Generically known as *Blue Points,* Eastern oysters are also often named for their place of origin. Among the most popular are *Alabama Gulf* (from Bayou La Batre and Mobile Bay), *Chesapeake Bay* (from Maryland and Virginia), *Malpeque* (from Prince Edward Island), and *Wellfleet* (from Cape Cod, Massachusetts).

European flat These oysters, originally found in European waters, are cultivated in the United States as well. The most common are *Belon,* raised in Maine, New Hampshire, and along the West Coast. While American Belons are the same species as the famed Belon oysters from the Belon River in Brittany in northern France, their lemony, metallic taste is very different than that of their prized French cousins. Another European flat variety cultivated in the United States is the *Westcott.*

Olympia The Olympia is the only oyster indigenous to the West Coast and is considered a rare delicacy. Olympias are tiny, about the size of a quarter to a half dollar in diameter. The majority of Olympias on the market are farmed in Washington's Puget Sound.

Pacific Formerly know as Japanese oysters, Pacific oysters are found in the waters of the Pacific Ocean. Common Pacific oyster varieties grown off the U.S. coast include: *Hamma-hamma, Penn Cove,* and *Quilcene* (all from Washington State); and *Kumamoto* (from California and Washington).

▶ Availability Oysters are generally at their peak in late fall and winter, but thanks to improved management, processing, and preservation, consumers can get fine oysters year round. (*See "What About the R Months?" opposite page.*)

choosing the best

Sold live, oysters should smell briny-fresh, and look bright and clean. The shells should be tightly closed (so that you can't pull them apart), or should close tightly when tapped; never buy oysters with open shells.

When purchasing freshly shucked oysters, look for the processor's permit number on the sealed container and check the "sell by" date. Allow one-third to one-half pint of shucked oysters per serving.

▶ **When you get home** It is imperative to keep oysters alive until you are ready to cook and/or serve them. Live oysters can be stored in the refrigerator, covered with wet kitchen towels or paper towels. Don't put them in an airtight container or submerge them in fresh water, or they will die. The key is to keep them truly cold: if possible, at 32° to 35°. Within that range, oysters should keep (in a live state) for about 4 to 7 days. Be sure to remove any that die (look for open shells) during that period, so they do not contaminate the remaining oysters.

Shucked oysters should be kept in tightly covered containers, immersed in their liquor; preserved this way, they should keep for up to a week.

You can freeze shucked raw oysters in their liquor in airtight containers. They should keep for about 2 months if the freezer is set at 0° or colder. Be sure to thaw frozen oysters in the refrigerator, not at room temperature.

preparing to use

Unless you have experience in shucking live oysters, it's safer and faster to have this service performed by the fish seller. If that isn't possible, or you want to store the oysters unshucked, then do it yourself.

First discard any oysters with open shells—they have died and are not fit to eat. To prepare the remainder, scrub the shells (with a stiff brush, if necessary) and rinse under cold running water. Scrape any tough encrustations from the shells with a sturdy knife.

Shucking oysters is easier if you have the right tools: An oyster knife has a very short, strong blade and a guard to protect your fingers. It's not uncommon for the knife to slip while you're applying pressure to open a shell, so wear a pair of work gloves to protect your hands.

To shuck an oyster, place it on top of a folded cloth (or hold it in a gloved hand) with the deeper shell downward. Hold it firmly as you insert the oyster knife between the two halves of the shell and twist the knife to pry the halves apart. Work the blade around to the hinge. Holding the opened oyster over a bowl to catch the juices, cut the muscle that holds the shell together, then remove the top half. Slip the knife under the oyster to free it. Strain the oyster liquor before using it in recipes, to remove any broken bits of shell.

what about the R months?

You've probably heard the old saw, "Eat oysters only in months whose name includes the letter R (the cold months)." This rule no doubt originated in the days before refrigeration, when oysters could quickly spoil in hot weather. Moreover, because oysters typically spawn in the warm summer months (usually May through August), they can be watery and less succulent during this time. Today, the R rule no longer holds true. With modern shipping and storage methods preventing spoilage, and oyster farming rendering some types of oysters sterile (so they don't spawn at all), these tasty creatures are wholesome and delicious 12 months a year.

serving suggestions

• Oven-broil crumb-coated shucked oysters—a good alternative to frying them.

• Poach shucked oysters in fish stock, or a mixture of water and lemon juice or wine (flavor the liquid with herbs, if you like).

• Top oysters on the half shell with barbecue sauce and grill in the shell over high heat.

• Add precooked shucked oysters to an omelet.

• Bake oysters on the half shell topped with pesto or another favorite sauce.

• Stir shucked oysters into a risotto during the last few minutes of cooking.

papaya

Although this fruit has emerged from its status as an exotic import, the romance and lure of the tropics is still part of the papaya's appeal. Today, papayas are found in most supermarkets, which is fortunate for the consumer.

The papaya is a melonlike fruit with yellow-orange flesh enclosed in skin that ranges in color from green to orange to rose. At the papaya's center is an oblong cavity containing dozens of small glistening black seeds. The papaya is sometimes referred to as a papaw, but that is a misnomer, as the papaw is a separate fruit that belongs to an unrelated botanical family and has a different taste and texture.

Exactly where the papaya originated is unknown. It is probably native to the Americas, but it has been introduced into other continents and grows profusely throughout the world's tropical regions. The papaya can grow from seed to a 20-foot, fruit-bearing tree in about 18 months. The fruit grows in groups at the top of the tree and can weigh from half a pound to 20 pounds each. The fruit can be round, pear-shaped, or elongated like a banana, depending upon the particular strain.

nutritional profile

Sweet and refreshing, and an excellent source of vitamin C, papaya also provides fiber, folate, vitamin E, potassium, and the carotenoids beta cryptoxanthin and beta carotene.

in the market

The papayas that most frequently appear on the market are the Solo varieties grown in Hawaii. Papayas from Mexico—another major producer and exporter—are not as common, though you may be able to find them in Hispanic markets.

Babáco This papaya hybrid is a native of Ecuador. It is 8 to 12 inches long and 4 inches in diameter; it is pentagonal in cross-section. The skin is entirely edible, and turns from green to yellow as it ripens. This fragrant fruit is extremely juicy and has hints of pineapple. Choose the yellowest fruits that are still firm, as these will be the sweetest. Add babácos to fruit salads and desserts only at the last minute, because they have more papain than regular papayas and will quickly turn other ingredients mushy.

Mexican These are large papayas—reaching lengths of 2 feet and weighing 10 pounds or more. They are not as sweet as the more common Solo papayas. *Mexican red* papayas have mellow-flavored, rose-colored flesh. *Mexican yellow* papayas can grow up to 10 pounds.

Solo These fruits are pear-shaped, about 6 inches long, and weigh from 1 to 2 pounds each. They have green-yellow skin and their flesh can be bright

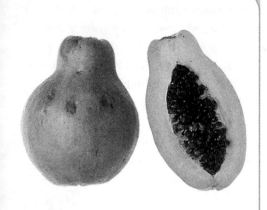
solo papayas

PAPAYA / 1 cup cubes	
Calories	55
Protein (g)	1
Carbohydrate (g)	14
Dietary fiber (g)	2.5
Total fat (g)	0.2
Saturated fat (g)	0.1
Monounsaturated fat (g)	0.1
Polyunsaturated fat (g)	0
Cholesterol (mg)	0
Potassium (mg)	360
Sodium (mg)	4

KEY NUTRIENTS (%RDA/AI*)	
Vitamin C	87 mg (96%)
Vitamin E	1.6 mg (10%)
Folate	53 mcg (13%)

*For more detailed information on RDA and AI, see page 88.

golden or pinkish. *Sunrise Solo*, developed at the University of Hawaii, has a unique reddish-pink color and a flavor reminiscent of strawberries. *Strawberry Sunrise* is another Solo from Hawaii. It has reddish-orange to pink flesh and is very sweet and flavorful.

choosing the best

Papayas are picked when firm-ripe to help them survive long-distance shipping; those in the market are likely to be partially ripe. Papayas turn from green to yellow-orange as they ripen, so you should choose fruits that are at least half yellow; the color change begins at the bottom and progresses toward the stem end. Papayas that are completely green with no tinge of yellow have been picked too soon and may never ripen properly.

Fully ripe papayas are three-quarters to totally yellow or yellow-orange; they will give slightly when pressed gently between your palms, but should not be soft and mushy at the stem end. The skin should be smooth, unbruised, and unshriveled; but slight, superficial blemishes may be disregarded. Uncut papayas have no aroma; cut papayas should smell fragrant and sweet, not harsh or fermented.

▶ **When you get home** A papaya that is one-quarter to one-third yellow will ripen in 2 to 4 days if left at room temperature; place it in a paper bag with a banana for faster ripening. Transfer ripe papayas to a plastic bag and store in the refrigerator. They will keep for up to a week, but the delicate flavor fades with time, so use them within a day or two, if possible.

preparing to use

Wash the papaya, then cut it in half lengthwise and scoop out the seeds. Save the seeds for a crunchy topping for a salad, if desired (*for more on using papaya seeds, see Seeds, page 524*). Peel the papaya with a paring knife or vegetable peeler and cut the flesh into wedges, slices, or dice.

Don't use unripe papaya in gelatin molds, as the papain it contains (*see "Papain," at right*) will prevent the mixture from gelling. Also, if adding papaya to other dishes, add it at the end so that the papain will not make the other ingredients mushy.

---

serving suggestions

• Serve wedges of papaya with thin slices of smoked turkey for an appetizer.

• Serve sliced papaya for dessert with wedges of lemon or lime.

• Make a chicken or seafood salad and add chunks of papaya just before serving.

• Top frozen yogurt with diced papaya.

• Puree papaya and stir in a bit of lime juice. Serve on waffles or pancakes.

• Cut half-ripe papayas lengthwise and remove the seeds. Sprinkle the cavities with cinnamon and nutmeg and bake as you would apples.

• Unripe (green) papaya can be treated more like a vegetable than a fruit: Add chunks of green papaya to stews.

---

papain

Papaya contains an enzyme called papain that breaks down protein, thus making the fruit a good meat tenderizer. Only unripe papayas and the leaves of the papaya tree have papain; ripe papaya holds very little. Cooks in the Caribbean islands wrap meats in papaya leaves before baking or grilling, and they also marinate stew meats and poultry with chunks of unripe papaya before cooking to tenderize the meat. Papain is also extracted from papaya, dried to a powder, and sold as a meat tenderizer. Simply sprinkling the powder on the surface of the meat, however, will not produce the desired effect; the meat must be pierced all over with a fork or skewer to allow the tenderizer to penetrate it.

parsnips

A root vegetable, the parsnip is a member of the *Umbelliferae* family whose members include carrots, celery, chervil, fennel, and parsley. Parsnips are grown for their delicate tasting, carrotlike roots, which can grow up to 20 inches long and 3 to 4 inches across at the top. The smaller parsnips are preferable and more delicate in flavor than the larger ones. Parsnips' flavor is best in winter, when they are most abundant. Planted in the spring, they take a full three to four months to mature. Then, they are left in the ground until a hard frost occurs in late fall, which initiates the conversion of the starches in the vegetable to sugars, giving parsnips their pleasantly sweet, nutty flavor. In fact, parsnips are one of the few vegetables that actually benefits from an early frost.

Parsnips served as a good source of starch for 4,000 years. They were cultivated during Roman times and were enjoyed for dessert with honey and fruit and in little cakes. Their popularity continued through the Renaissance and well into the 18th century, when they were widely used in savory dishes such as stews, soups, and purees, but also in puddings and bread. However, the parsnip's status as a culinary star in Europe was challenged at that point when the nutritional benefits of potatoes became widely known. The poor parsnip never recovered its popularity. And although it has been in this country since the 17th century, it has never gained any prominence on American tables.

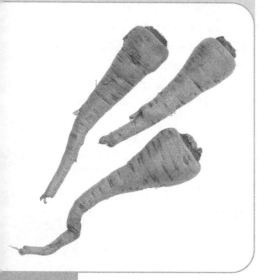

parsnips

nutritional profile

Low in calories, parsnips are rich in fiber, especially the soluble fiber pectin, which may lower LDL ("bad") cholesterol levels, thus helping to prevent heart disease. Good amounts of vitamin C and the B vitamin folate are found in this subtle, sweet-flavored root vegetable, along with respectable amounts of thiamin, vitamin E, iron, and magnesium.

in the market

Parsnips range in color from pale yellow to off-white. Although they can grow up to 20 inches long, they are most tender when about 8 inches— roughly the size of a large carrot. There are many common varieties, among them the *All-American,* the most popular, which is distinguished by its broad shoulders (tops), white flesh, and tender core.

choosing the best

Very large parsnips are likely to be overmature and have tough, woody cores. The characteristic "broad-shouldered" shape is not a sign of overmaturity, but the wide top should taper smoothly to a slender tip. Parsnips should be firm and fairly smooth; an abundance of hairlike rootlets is undesirable. Soft or

PARSNIPS / 1 cup cooked	
Calories	126
Protein (g)	2
Carbohydrate (g)	30
Dietary fiber (g)	6.2
Total fat (g)	0.5
Saturated fat (g)	0.1
Monounsaturated fat (g)	0.2
Polyunsaturated fat (g)	0.1
Cholesterol (mg)	0
Potassium (mg)	573
Sodium (mg)	16

KEY NUTRIENTS (%RDA/AI*)	
Thiamin	0.1 mg (11%)
Vitamin C	20 mg (23%)
Vitamin E	1.6 mg (10%)
Folate	90 mcg (23%)
Iron	0.9 mg (11%)
Magnesium	45 mg (11%)

*For more detailed information on RDA and AI, see page 88.

withered parsnips are likely to be fibrous. Irregularly shaped parsnips are acceptable, but wasteful, as you'll have to trim away a good deal while preparing the vegetables for cooking. Parsnips with moist spots should also be avoided.

Most parsnips are sold "clip-topped," but if the leafy tops are still attached, they should look fresh and green. When buying parsnips in a 1-pound plastic bag (many are sold this way), be sure to take a close look at the vegetables through the wrapping; the bag may have fine white lines printed on it in an effort to enhance the appearance of the parsnips.

Sometimes you'll find parsnips sold in a package of soup greens (a "soup bunch"), along with a carrot, turnip, some celery tops, or other greens. If you're buying a parsnip for flavoring stock, it needn't be in prime condition.

preparing to use

Unlike carrots, parsnips are almost always eaten cooked, as they tend to be quite fibrous. (Be careful not to overcook them, however; their flavor is sweetest when just tender. Brief cooking also helps to preserve nutrients.) Just before cooking, cut off the root and leaf ends; trim any major rootlets or knobs. Peel the parsnips before or after cooking, depending on how you plan to prepare them:

If you're going to cut them into chunks for a stew, or if you simply want to shorten the cooking time, peel them first, as thinly as possible using a paring knife or vegetable peeler. Then cut the parsnips as you wish: Halve them crosswise and then quarter each half lengthwise; dice them; or cut them into "coins" or julienne strips.

If you're going to puree parsnips, peel them after cooking. This technique helps to preserve their color and flavor, and also saves nutrients since you'll be able to remove a thinner layer of peel. Make a lengthwise cut through the skin down one side, then pull the peel off with your fingers. Halve the cooked parsnips lengthwise; if you find a fibrous, woody core, pry it out with the tip of a sharp paring knife.

If the tops of the parsnips are much thicker than the bottoms, halve the vegetables crosswise and cook the top halves for a few minutes before adding the bottom halves. Then the slender tips will not cook through before the bulbous tops do.

Whenever you cook parsnips in liquid, save the flavorful liquid for making a sauce or adding to a stock or soup; the liquid contains any nutrients that may have leached out in cooking.

---

serving suggestions

• Toss cut-up parsnips, carrots, and turnips with some olive oil. Roast until tender.

• Cook parsnips with potatoes and mash the two together.

• Steam sliced parsnips and toss, while still hot, with olive oil, lemon juice, and minced fresh mint and parsley. Serve warm or chilled as a salad.

• Add diced parsnips to vegetable soups and stews.

---

poisonous parsnips?

The folklore and myths surrounding parsnips has generated some misconceptions about this root vegetable. One false notion attests that parsnips left in the ground over the winter are poisonous, which is ironic considering that parsnip growers leave the roots in the ground on purpose to enhance their flavor. It's probably not a good idea, however, to try to forage in the woods for wild parsnips, which are not only unpalatable but contain furanocoumarins, natural plant chemicals that once absorbed by the skin and exposed to solar UV light can cause painful blistering (photodermatitis).

pasta, nonwheat

When people think of pasta, what comes to mind is Italian pasta, made from wheat (*see Pasta, Wheat, page 445*). However, as with flours, pastas can be made from a variety of grains, roots, legumes, and tubers. Many of these nonwheat pastas are staples in Asian and Indian cooking. Others have been developed for people who have gluten allergies or wheat sensitivity. Since many of these pastas do not include semolina, farina, durum flour, or eggs, they don't conform to government standards for macaroni or noodles and so may be labeled "alimentary paste" or "imitation noodles." The FDA has begun to allow manufacturers of Asian noodles to label their products "Asian noodles."

nutritional profile

Pastas made from plants other than wheat are excellent alternatives for people who are allergic to wheat or to gluten (the protein formed when wheat flour is made into batter or dough). These pastas also have their own nutritional pluses aside from their lack of gluten: Depending upon the source, some types of nonwheat pasta will be rich in protein (such as brown rice pasta), while others will be low in calories (buckwheat noodles). Each type offers its own nutritional and culinary merits.

in the market

Many of the Western-style nonwheat pastas have been created for the health-food market for people who have problems with gluten. However, not all nonwheat pastas are entirely wheat-free, so make sure to read the label. While these nonwheat pastas can be substituted for wheat pastas, be aware that they each cook up differently and have different textures.

For the Asian-style pastas, many different countries (and regions within those countries) have the exact same type of noodle, but call them different things. We have listed a number of the more common names you might encounter in an Asian market (since most Asian markets sell products from multiple Asian cultures).

bean & legume pastas

Cellophane noodles Chinese: *fen si, fun sie*; Japanese: *sarifun, harusame*; Korean: *dang myun*; Vietnamese: *bun tau*. Made from mung bean flour, these semi-translucent noodles turn clear when cooked and often are called *glass noodles* or *bean thread noodles.* They can be quickly stir-fried or braised with

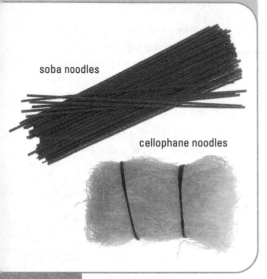

nonwheat pastas

soba noodles

cellophane noodles

BUCKWHEAT NOODLES 1 cup cooked	
Calories	113
Protein (g)	6
Carbohydrate (g)	24
Dietary fiber (g)	1.3
Total fat (g)	0.1
Saturated fat (g)	0
Monounsaturated fat (g)	0
Polyunsaturated fat (g)	0
Cholesterol (mg)	0
Potassium (mg)	40
Sodium (mg)	68

other ingredients. The noodles are nearly pure starch, containing almost no protein, vitamins, or minerals.

Lentil pasta Made from ground lentils, this pasta has a meaty, rich, slightly peppery lentil flavor.

grain pastas

Amaranth pasta Light brown in color and resembling whole-wheat pasta, amaranth pasta has the bite and consistency of regular pasta.

Barley pasta This slightly nutty-tasting pasta is made from barley flour.

Buckwheat noodles Chinese: *qiao mian*; Japanese: *soba*; Korean: *naeng myun*. These flat, gray Asian noodles are made from buckwheat and wheat flour, or just buckwheat flour. They are rich in protein. They may be served hot (usually in a broth) or chilled, accompanied by a dipping sauce. In Japan, soba noodles are eaten for lunch or as a snack, and are essential to a traditional dish prepared at New Year's.

Buckwheat pasta While buckwheat flour is used in Asian noodles, it is also used to make a popular Italian pasta called *pizzocheri*. It has a rich, nutty flavor and a chewy texture.

Corn pasta Corn pasta has about half the protein of regular pasta, but otherwise is nutritionally comparable; it is a good alternative for people allergic to wheat.

Milo pasta Milo, also known as grain sorghum, produces a pasta with a slightly sweet, interesting flavor.

Millet pasta Millet is ground into a flour and used to make pasta, most often small macaroni.

Oat pasta Oat flour makes a satisfying pasta, most often in small macaroni shapes.

Quinoa pasta Quinoa is ground into a flour to make pasta the color of whole-wheat pasta but with the consistency of regular pasta.

Rice noodles Chinese: *sha he fen, sa ho fun, gan he fen, gon ho fun*; Vietnamese: *bun, banh pho, banh hoi*. Dried Asian rice noodles, which are usually sold coiled in bags, are either thread-thin or spaghettilike. The thinner form is usually sold as *rice vermicelli*; the thicker form is called *rice sticks*. Typically, they are boiled or stir-fried for use in salads or soups. *Fresh rice noodles,* a standard feature of the Chinese brunch called dim sum, are sold in wide sheets for making dumplinglike dishes, or cut into ¾-inch-wide ribbons. They are precooked and are ready to eat once boiling water is poured over them. Like cellophane noodles, rice noodles are almost pure starch and are thus low in protein.

Rice papers (rice wrappers) These round translucent sheets of dried rice noodle are used in Vietnamese cooking as a wrapper for food. They do not need to be cooked; they are softened in warm water until flexible and then wrapped around various fillings.

CORN PASTA 1 cup cooked	
Calories	187
Protein (g)	4
Carbohydrate (g)	42
Dietary fiber (g)	7.1
Total fat (g)	1.1
Saturated fat (g)	0.2
Monounsaturated fat (g)	0.3
Polyunsaturated fat (g)	0.5
Cholesterol (mg)	0
Potassium (mg)	46
Sodium (mg)	0
KEY NUTRIENTS (%RDA/AI*)	
Magnesium	54 mg (13%)

For more detailed information on RDA and AI, see page 88.

Rice pasta Both white and brown rice are used to make rice pasta. These pastas tend to be fairly tender and may not hold up well when served with heavy sauces.

Teff pasta Generally made from a combination of teff flour (*see page 326*) and another grain, it can be used like regular pasta.

root & tuber pastas

Cassava pasta Made from the starchy tropical tuber known as cassava, this very white pasta tastes similar to wheat pasta. It does not expand a great deal when cooked.

Jerusalem artichoke pasta This pasta is made from a combination of Jerusalem artichoke flour and wheat flour.

Malanga pasta A starchy tropical tuber, malanga is used to make a pasta that closely resembles wheat pasta.

Potato pasta Made from potato flour, sometimes with the addition of rice flour, this pasta is fairly sturdy and holds up well with rich sauces.

White sweet potato pasta Made from white sweet potato starch, this pasta has a slightly sweet flavor.

Yam pasta Like white sweet potato pasta, this has a slightly sweet flavor.

▶ Availability Dried and fresh Asian noodles can be found in Asian markets. For other nonwheat pastas, your best bet is a health-food store.

choosing the best

Look for packages of dried pasta that are tightly sealed with whole, rather than broken-up pasta shapes. If you can, check packages for small bugs. Shop where the shelves are replenished frequently and the store does a brisk business. For fresh pastas, packages should be well-sealed and the pasta should not look dry around the edges.

▶ When you get home Store dried pasta in airtight containers in your pantry. Dried pastas will keep for several months. Store fresh pastas for a day or two in the refrigerator or for 3 months in the freezer, tightly wrapped. Fresh rice noodles become stiff when cold, so they are often sold at room temperature and will keep for a day or two.

preparing to use

Most nonwheat pastas require no more preparation than regular wheat pastas. There are some Asian noodles, however, that are a little different. The flavor and texture of dried rice noodles benefit from soaking before use in recipes. Soak the noodles for 15 or 20 minutes in hot water, then quickly rinse them to wash away excess starch. Cellophane noodles require 10 to 30 minutes of presoaking. Once soaked, cellophane noodles and rice noodles need to be only briefly heated before serving.

---

serving suggestions

• Make stuffed rice wrappers: Soften rice papers in warm water, then fold around cooked vegetables, shrimp, or chicken. Make a soy-ginger dipping sauce.

• Soak cellophane noodles until soft and silky and add to salads, or soak just until chewy and use in stir-fries or sautés.

• Serve chili over corn pasta instead of with corn bread.

• Toss cold cooked buckwheat noodles with slivers of cooked duck breast, scallions, and cooked green beans. Dress with a light sherry wine vinaigrette.

• Use potato pasta instead of potato gnocchi.

• Use yam pasta in a sweet noodle dessert such as kugel.

pasta, wheat

Many of the names given to types of pasta are Italian, but the Italians hardly have a monopoly on this food. Although the origin of pasta hasn't been established, the evidence indicates that various forms developed independently in many cultures. The Chinese may have eaten noodles as early as 5000 B.C. And it is widely believed that Marco Polo brought pasta to Italy from the Far East in 1295. But if he did, it was probably to compare it to the pasta already there, since the Etruscans, who occupied part of what is now Italy, were making pasta as early as 400 B.C. The history of pasta in the United States is much clearer. Thomas Jefferson was the first to bring it to this country (in the late 1700s) after tasting some during a visit to Naples while he was the American ambassador to France. The first pasta factory in the United States opened in 1848 in Brooklyn, New York, but pasta remained a relatively uncommon food until the late 19th century, when Italian immigrants introduced the dried wheat pastas that have since become the most popular types of pasta in this country.

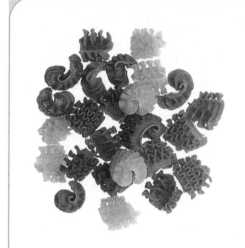

tri-color radiatore

nutritional profile

Rich in complex carbohydrates and protein, and low in fat, pasta is a highly nutritious food. Enriched wheat pastas (the bulk of commercially available pastas) also offer good levels of thiamin, riboflavin, niacin, folate, iron, and selenium.

Pasta is made from a mixture of water and flour or semolina (which is a type of flour made from durum, a hard spring wheat with a high protein content and golden color). The more semolina a pasta contains, the more protein it provides, though the protein from pasta is incomplete. When eggs are added to pasta, the pasta will then provide fat and dietary cholesterol, as well as other nutrients found in eggs.

Pasta also contains gluten, a protein formed when water and wheat flour are mixed (gluten is what gives bread dough its elasticity). People with celiac disease may be allergic to wheat and wheat products and anyone on a gluten-restricted diet should avoid wheat pasta.

Since 1998, all refined grain products in the United States have been fortified with folic acid. For instance, 1 cup of cooked pasta contains about 100 micrograms of folic acid, which is 25 percent of the recommended daily intake. And studies show that the folic acid used to fortify foods (as well as that in supplements) is actually better absorbed by the body than the vitamin naturally found in foods.

Many people regard pasta as a fattening food, which is a recurring myth. There's no evidence that eating carbohydrate-rich foods stimulates the appetite or leads to more (or easier) fat storage and weight gain, as some car-

ENRICHED SPAGHETTI 1 cup cooked	
Calories	197
Protein (g)	7
Carbohydrate (g)	40
Dietary fiber (g)	2.4
Total fat (g)	0.9
Saturated fat (g)	0.1
Monounsaturated fat (g)	0.1
Polyunsaturated fat (g)	0.4
Cholesterol (mg)	0
Potassium (mg)	43
Sodium (mg)	1

KEY NUTRIENTS (%RDA/AI*)	
Thiamin	0.3 mg (24%)
Riboflavin	0.1 mg (11%)
Niacin	2.3 mg (15%)
Folate	98 mcg (25%)
Iron	2.0 mg (24%)
Selenium	30 mcg (54%)

*For detailed information on RDA and AI, see page 88.

EGG NOODLES 1 cup cooked	
Calories	213
Protein (g)	8
Carbohydrate (g)	40
Dietary fiber (g)	1.8
Total fat (g)	2.4
Saturated fat (g)	0.5
Monounsaturated fat (g)	0.7
Polyunsaturated fat (g)	0.7
Cholesterol (mg)	53
Potassium (mg)	45
Sodium (mg)	11

KEY NUTRIENTS (%RDA/AI*)	
Thiamin	0.3 mg (25%)
Riboflavin	0.1 mg (10%)
Niacin	2.4 mg (15%)
Folate	102 mcg (26%)
Iron	2.5 mg (32%)
Selenium	35 mcg (63%)

*For more detailed information on RDA and AI, see page 88.

bohydrate-bashers claim. However, if you drown your pasta in heavy meat sauces, or cream- or cheese-based sauces, then it is indeed a fattening food.

in the market

The pastas that we associate with Italy—among them spaghetti (from *spago*, or "strand"), rigatoni (from *rigati*, meaning "grooved"), vermicelli ("little worms"), and linguine ("little tongues")—are most commonly made from semolina. This high-protein flour is milled from the endosperm (the starchy portion of a wheat kernel that remains after you strip it of its hull, bran, and germ) of durum wheat and yields high-quality pasta with a golden color, mellow flavor, and sturdy texture. Durum wheat is the hardest of all the wheats, meaning that it's highest in protein. Wheat doughs, when kneaded, develop gluten—a tough, elastic protein substance formed from other proteins in the wheat—and the harder a wheat is, the more gluten it will have. Dough made from semolina is high in gluten, which gives it the resiliency and strength to stand up to the mechanical pasta-making process and to hold its shape during cooking.

Despite the various Italian names used to identify most of the shapes popular in the United States, the FDA legally defines all dried pasta as either macaroni or noodles.

the shape of pasta

Commercial pasta is produced by mixing enriched semolina and sometimes other hard-wheat flours with a small amount of water to form a stiff dough, which is mechanically kneaded to form gluten—a type of protein that gives the pasta dough its form and strength. The dough is then forced through dies—metal plates that have variously shaped holes drilled into them.

Long, solid pastas, such as spaghetti or linguine, are pushed through dies with round or oval holes. Hollow pastas are extruded through dies with pins in the center of the holes. Elbow macaroni is shaped by a die with a notched pin, which forces the dough to pass through more quickly on one side, causing the pasta rods to curve.

The die also affects the pasta's texture and appearance. Teflon-lined dies, popular in the United States, produce a smooth, polished pasta with a high-yellow color. Imported pastas usually go through brass dies, which yield a rougher texture and whiter color. (Egg noodles, on the other hand, are rolled by machine into thin sheets that are mechanically sliced to the desired length and width.) Once the pasta is shaped, mechanical knives cut it into the appropriate lengths. The pasta is then carefully dried on racks or, for short pastas such as elbow macaroni, on conveyor belts.

Macaroni This designation is applied to an array of pasta shapes and sizes, whether they're strands (like spaghetti), tubes (like elbow macaroni, penne, and cannelloni), or shells (conchiglie), to mention just a few. Macaroni must be primarily composed of semolina, farina, and/or flour milled from durum wheat; these three components can be used separately or in any combination, along with water. Optional ingredients, such as egg whites, salt, or flavorings, are permitted. Some types of macaroni—spaghetti and vermicelli, for example—must also conform to certain size designations.

Noodles In addition to the guidelines set for macaroni, noodles must also contain no less than 5.5 percent egg by weight. As a result, noodles have some fat and cholesterol. (Some manufacturers make noodles from egg whites, which have neither cholesterol nor fat.) The protein content of macaroni and noodles is about the same. Although the egg in noodles adds protein, most of these noodles are prepared by combining semolina with softer wheats, such as farina, which have less protein than semolina. There are also Italian-style pastas that are made with egg (fettuccine is a classic example), but that do not qualify under these guidelines as "noodles."

Other than the official definitions imposed by labeling laws, the principal difference for Western-style pastas of any culinary importance is the difference between fresh and dried.

dried pasta

Most dried pastas are made from 100 percent semolina, but some manufacturers market versions that combine semolina with other wheat flours, such as farina, which is the coarsely ground endosperm of a wheat that is not as hard as durum. (Farina is a prime ingredient in many breakfast cereals.) When cooked, these combined-wheat pastas are whiter and softer than 100-percent semolina pasta.

Pasta makers use molds or dies to fashion the many different shapes that range from plain spaghetti to intricate cartwheels (rotelle) and bowties (farfalle). Most Western pastas are classified according to whether they are long or short; round, tubular, or flat; smooth or ridged; solid or hollow. While some names for the various shapes are fairly standard, others are not, particularly in Italy, where one shape can come in several different sizes and have several different names.

fresh pasta

Made from durum or other types of wheat flour, water, and, usually, whole eggs, fresh pasta has a higher moisture content and softer consistency than dried. It is used mainly for dumplings, such as ravioli and tortellini, but also for spaghetti, fettuccine, and other shapes that

---

facts & tips

Most supermarkets routinely stock 20 to 30 pasta shapes, which may seem like more than enough. But the Italians have created over 600 pasta shapes, and 150 of them are available in the United States, mostly in specialty and gourmet food shops.

---

serving suggestions

Try these ideas for healthful, low-fat pasta sauces:

• Puree low-fat cottage cheese with garlic and fresh herbs and toss with hot pasta.

• Prepare your favorite meat sauce with ground turkey rather than beef.

• For a light sauce, simmer flavorful dried mushrooms in broth and use cornstarch to thicken.

• For a Mexican take on pasta, look for a low-sodium salsa, add some corn and cilantro, and toss with pasta.

• For a low-fat pesto, puree fresh basil with garlic, a few walnuts, and broth instead of lots of olive oil. Add a small amount of grated Parmesan for flavor and body.

• In the summer, a fresh, uncooked tomato sauce is always satisfying. Just toss hot, cooked pasta with chopped ripe tomatoes, herbs, and a little fruity olive oil. Add finely chopped vegetables if you like. Serve hot or at room temperature.

are sold dried. Fresh pasta colored with vegetable purees is also available. When made with whole eggs, fresh pasta is slightly higher in fat than dried pasta and contains 56 milligrams of cholesterol per 6-ounce cooked serving. In addition, if it is stuffed with cheese or meat, as with ravioli or tortellini, fresh pasta can be high in fat and cholesterol; if it is stuffed with vegetables or seafood, the fat content is likely to be lower, though these stuffings may also include cheese.

other wheat pastas

In addition to the well-known Western-style pastas and noodles, there are a number of other forms of wheat-based pastas available:

Asian wheat noodles *See box below.*

facts & tips

A tablespoon of grated Parmesan cheese adds flavor to pasta, and only 29 calories and 2 grams of fat. It's fairly high in sodium, however, with a tablespoon providing just over 100 milligrams.

asian wheat noodles

Like their American counterparts, Asian wheat noodles are made with or without egg and are available fresh and dried. What they are called in the market will vary considerably depending on the country they're from. We have included some of the more common names.

Egg noodles In Chinese, these are called *dan mian* or *don mein*. These versatile noodles are added to soups, boiled and topped with meat or sesame sauce, or eaten cold with a dressing of sesame oil, soy sauce, and vinegar. The noodles are also sold as fresh sheets of dough used for making wontons and egg rolls.

Chinese wheat noodles These noodles (called *gan mian* or *sun mian*) come in a variety of shapes, thicknesses, and colors, and are sold both fresh and dried. Their nutritional value is close to that of Western-style wheat pasta, except that the sodium content may be higher. Chinese wheat noodles are used in lo mein and chow mein dishes. (Don't confuse these chow mein noodles with the crispy "chow mein noodles" that come in cans and that are found at many supermarkets. The canned noodles are deep-fried and contain about 14 grams of fat per cup.)

Ramen These Japanese noodles are often packaged as an instant soup. They are instant because they are precooked by steaming and then dried by deep-frying, leaving them with a residue of about 18 percent oil by weight (and over 5 grams of fat per serving).

Somen Similar in shape to vermicelli, this Japanese wheat noodle is most often eaten cold, but is sometimes served in soups. There is also a type of somen called *tamago somen* that is made with egg yolks.

Udon Thick and chewy, these Japanese wheat noodles are usually served in broth. Udon are sold both fresh and dried.

Couscous Popular in North Africa, couscous is made from semolina that has been precooked and then dried. It is different from both Western and Asian pastas; the tiny grains resemble rice or grits more than they do noodles. Couscous is not enriched, and so contains fewer B vitamins and iron than macaroni or noodles. There are quick-cooking ("instant") couscouses available that simply require steeping in boiling broth or water. There is also a larger couscous (the size of a small pea) called *toasted Israeli couscous,* which requires longer cooking.

Flavored pastas Some pastas are made with vegetable powders (such as spinach, tomatoes, or beets), which add more color than flavor. Other pastas are flavored with such seasonings as saffron, lemon, garlic, or pepper. These additives do not affect the nutrition in any significant way.

High-protein pasta Enriched with soy flour, wheat germ, yeast, or dairy products, this type of pasta contains 20 to 100 percent more protein than standard pasta. Although it tastes like regular pasta, it may cook up stickier and will be chewier.

Whole-wheat pasta Whole-wheat pasta has a distinctive robust taste and a chewy texture that take getting used to. Since this type of pasta is made from whole-wheat flour or whole-wheat durum flour, it is naturally higher in nutrients than *unenriched* semolina pasta. However, since semolina pasta is enriched, whole-wheat pasta is actually lower in B vitamins and iron than semolina pasta. But whole-wheat pasta is still a good source of these nutrients, and contains about two-thirds more fiber that semolina. Moreover, whole-wheat pasta is significantly higher in the antioxidant mineral selenium.

WHOLE-WHEAT PASTA 1 cup cooked	
Calories	174
Protein (g)	8
Carbohydrate (g)	37
Dietary fiber (g)	3.9
Total fat (g)	0.8
Saturated fat (g)	0.1
Monounsaturated fat (g)	0.1
Polyunsaturated fat (g)	0.3
Cholesterol (mg)	0
Potassium (mg)	62
Sodium (mg)	4

KEY NUTRIENTS (%RDA/AI*)	
Thiamin	0.2 mg (13%)
Iron	1.5 mg (19%)
Magnesium	42 mg (10%)
Selenium	36 mcg (66%)

For more detailed information on RDA and AI, see page 88.

choosing the best

It is difficult to tell when a particular batch of dried pasta was made (though some packages are stamped with a "sell by" date). Luckily, dried pasta keeps almost indefinitely, so "freshness" isn't a particular concern. Just be sure that the package is intact and hasn't been exposed to water, and that the pasta inside is not broken.

Fresh pasta is perishable, however, and should be displayed in a refrigerated case or in a freezer. Buy it from a store with a high turnover; if it is packaged, check the "sell by" date. Keep in mind, too, that a pound of fresh pasta won't serve as many people as a pound of dried (since the fresh absorbs much less water during cooking).

▶ **When you get home** Store dried pasta in a cool, dry place and it will keep for many months. As an extra precaution, remove the pasta from its original package and place it in an airtight container.

Store fresh pasta tightly wrapped in plastic wrap; it will keep for a week in the refrigerator or a month in the freezer. Fresh Asian noodles will keep for a day or two under refrigeration, or for 3 months in the freezer, if tightly wrapped.

peaches

Peaches were first cultivated in China thousands of years ago. In China, the peach is considered the most sacred symbolic plant of the Taoist religion, and it is still customarily served at birthday celebrations as a symbol of hope for longevity. The Romans brought the peach to Europe, and it was introduced to the New World by Spanish explorers in the 16th century.

Eventually, early settlers and Native Americans distributed the peach up and down the eastern seaboard, establishing the fruit so firmly in the United States that some botanists in the mid-1700s assumed that the peach was native to America. Commercial growing began in the early 1800s, and soon Georgia became known as the Peach State because of its famous peach, the Elberta.

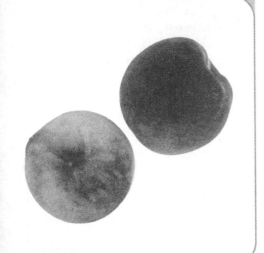

peaches

nutritional profile

Peaches have moderate amounts of fiber, including pectin, which can lower cholesterol. Though the amount of vitamin E in a single peach is only 7 percent of the RDA, it is worth noting, since it's rare to find this vitamin in a low-fat food.

in the market

Like plums and nectarines, to which they are related, peaches are primarily classified as either freestone or clingstone; a few varieties fall in between and are referred to as semi-freestone. Nearly all the varieties that are sold fresh are freestone—the flesh slips easily off the pit. Freestone peaches are softer and juicier than clingstone varieties, which are generally used for canned fruit.

For many years Elberta, a Georgia peach, was the country's quintessential peach. But peaches are now grown in every state, with about 30 states responsible for the bulk of the commercial crop. Older standards, such as *Elberta, Hale,* and *Rio Oso Gem,* which can have a tender, "melting" texture, are much more likely to be found at either farmers' markets or roadside fruit stands than in supermarkets.

Dozens of new varieties have been developed since the Elberta's heyday; these are larger and firmer, but the differences among them are relatively minor. Though some have white flesh, growers seem to have emphasized the yellow-fleshed varieties. The following are a number of unusual peaches you may encounter in the supermarket:

Babcock This aromatic white peach has a slight blush on its almost fuzzless skin. The flesh is tender, very juicy, and sweet.

Donut peaches A relatively new variety, these peaches are descendants of Chinese flat white peaches. Sweet and juicy, these easily recognizable peaches are shaped like a flat donut with rounded sides that draw in toward the small center pit.

PEACH / 1 medium	
Calories	42
Protein (g)	1
Carbohydrate (g)	11
Dietary fiber (g)	2.0
Total fat (g)	0.1
Saturated fat (g)	0
Monounsaturated fat (g)	0
Polyunsaturated fat (g)	0
Cholesterol (mg)	0
Potassium (mg)	193
Sodium (mg)	0

Elegant Lady This freestone is large and firm when ripe. It has bright red skin and sweet, juicy flesh.

Indian peaches This freestone variety is distinguished by its pinkish-gold, velvety skin and marbleized, delicately sweet flesh.

Ryan Sun This peach has very sweet and juicy yellow flesh. The skin has a bright red blush.

choosing the best

When you buy local peaches in summer, you'll undoubtedly find softer, sweeter, more fragrant fruit than you'll ever encounter in your supermarket during other seasons. (Peaches don't get any sweeter after they have been harvested, though fruit will become softer and juicier as it matures.)

Whenever you buy peaches, look for skins that show a background color of yellow or warm cream—the amount of pink or red "blush" on their cheeks depends on the variety, and is not a reliable indicator of ripeness. Undertones of green, however, mean that the peaches were picked too soon and will not be sweet. Look for plump, medium- to large-sized peaches with unwrinkled skins.

Avoid the rock-hard fruits and choose those that yield slightly to pressure along the seam, even if they may otherwise be fairly firm. Peaches such as these will soften if kept at room temperature for a few days. (To hasten ripening, place peaches in a brown bag with an apple and let sit at room temperature.) Once peaches are picked, their sweetness will not increase, so choose fruits that are fragrant.

For immediate eating pleasure (especially when buying locally grown peaches), choose soft, perfume-y fruit. Watch out for dark-colored, mushy, bruised peaches that are overripe and beginning to spoil. Tan circles or spots on the skin are early signs of decay.

▶ **When you get home** Once peaches ripen, store them in the refrigerator crisper if you are not going to eat them within a day. They should keep for 3 to 5 days.

preparing to use

Serve peaches chilled or at room temperature, as you prefer. Wash them before eating or cooking. To halve a freestone peach, cut it along the seam right down to the pit, and then twist the halves apart. Lift out the pit with the tip of a paring knife. For a clingstone, cut the flesh into quarters or wedges by making cuts into the fruit toward the pit, then lifting each section off the pit.

To peel peaches, place them in a pot of boiling water; remove them after about a minute and cool in a bowl of ice water. Then pull or rub off the peel, using your fingers or a paring knife. Peeled or cut peaches will turn brown if exposed to air, so rub peeled fruit with lemon or orange juice or dip slices into the citrus juice.

serving suggestions

- Combine sliced peaches, yogurt or buttermilk, and ice in a blender and puree.

- Sauté peaches with ginger and a touch of garlic and serve with meat or poultry.

- Add peaches to a home-made barbecue sauce.

- Finely chop peaches and fold into a spicy ketchup for a quick relish.

- Add diced peaches to pancakes as they cook.

- Make baked peaches instead of baked apples.

- For a quick dessert, top flour tortillas with sliced peaches and a sprinkling of ground cinnamon and sugar, and bake.

- Cook peaches in peach or mango nectar until tender and serve as a sauce for frozen yogurt.

facts & tips

You may remember the fuzzy beard that was present on the skin of peaches not so long ago. Today's peaches have no fuzz, but it's not because growers have developed "fuzzless" varieties. Most people don't like the fuzz, so commercially grown peaches are mechanically brushed after harvest to remove most of it. You may still find fuzzy peaches at farmers' markets and roadside stands.

peanuts

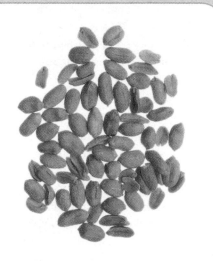

peanuts

One of the most popular and familiar nuts in the United States, peanuts are actually not true nuts, but rather the shell-enclosed seeds of a leguminous plant that's related to peas and beans. The peanut pods grow below the ground, and both the shell and kernel are soft until the peanuts are dried. While their physical structure and nutritional benefits resemble that of other legumes, their culinary use is similar to that of nuts.

Peanuts are thought to have originated in South America. Archeological evidence shows that ancient Incan graves contained jars filled with peanuts, probably left with the dead to provide nourishment during their long journey to the afterlife. In the 1500s peanuts migrated to Africa with Spanish and Portuguese explorers. They were introduced to Colonial America by African slaves in the 18th century. Known as groundnuts, goobers, or ground peas in those days, peanuts were generally regarded as food for livestock and the poor. With the outbreak of the Civil War, however, consumption of peanuts increased as soldiers on both sides turned to this food for nourishment.

By the late 19th century, peanuts were being sold freshly roasted by street vendors and at baseball games, fairs, and circuses. Peanut butter had also been developed by this time *(see "A Peanut Butter Primer," page 455)*. The peanut didn't come into its own horticulturally, however, until botanist George Washington Carver began researching peanuts, sweet potatoes, and soybeans as rotation crops for cotton in 1903. His work at Tuskegee Institute in Alabama led him to eventually develop hundreds of different uses for peanuts (including shoe polish and shaving cream), and he came to be known as the father of the peanut industry.

Peanut production rose rapidly during and after the World Wars, and today some 3.4 billion pounds of peanuts are produced in the United States each year (about 50 percent going into peanut butter).

nutritional profile

Packed with nutritional benefits, peanuts supply an impressive amount of plant protein as well as vitamin E, folate, niacin, and magnesium. They also provide a good amount of fiber, and are low in saturated fat and rich in beneficial fats. Peanuts also contain cholesterol-lowering plant sterols.

Research indicates that diets high in mono- and polyunsaturated fats and low in saturated fat can be heart-healthy. While peanut butter is rich in fat, it is highly monounsaturated, a type of fat that doesn't boost blood cholesterol. In fact, a study in the *American Journal of Clinical Nutrition* found that a diet that included peanuts and peanut butter could actually reduce total blood

PEANUTS 1 ounce dry-roasted	
Calories	166
Protein (g)	7
Carbohydrate (g)	6
Dietary fiber (g)	2.3
Total fat (g)	14
Saturated fat (g)	2.0
Monounsaturated fat (g)	7.0
Polyunsaturated fat (g)	4.5
Cholesterol (mg)	0
Potassium (mg)	187
Sodium (mg)	2

KEY NUTRIENTS (%RDA/AI*)	
Thiamin	0.1 mg (10%)
Niacin	3.8 mg (24%)
Vitamin E	2.2 mg (15%)
Folate	41 mcg (10%)
Magnesium	50 mg (12%)

*For more detailed information on RDA and AI, see page 88.

cholesterol by 10 percent and LDL ("bad") cholesterol and triglycerides (blood fats) by more than 13 percent. Surprisingly, a diet that derived 36 percent of its calories from fat but that included lots of peanuts and peanut butter (with their healthful fats) had an even better effect on blood cholesterol than a low-fat diet. Peanut oil, too, contains heart-healthy monounsaturated and polyunsaturated fats.

It is important to keep in mind that although peanuts and peanut butter have a favorable fats profile, they are still high in calories and should be eaten in moderation.

in the market

In the United States, peanuts are mostly eaten dried or roasted, as a snack, in candies, or in the form of peanut butter. They are also pressed for their oil (*see Nut Oils, page 299*) and ground into a high-protein, partially defatted flour (*see Flour, Nonwheat, page 324*). In the South, raw (unroasted) peanuts are particularly popular. These are often eaten right out of the shell, or they can be oven-roasted or boiled in the shell and then eaten. At certain times of the year green peanuts (or peanuts fresh from the field) are available; because they spoil quickly, they are often sold boiled. Peanuts also come oil-roasted, dry-roasted, and blanched.

Four major types of peanuts are grown in the United States:

Runners Introduced in the 1970s, and known for their uniform, medium-sized kernel, these peanuts now dominate the industry, but with more than half of those grown being made into peanut butter, peanut candies, and snack nuts. Runners are mainly produced in Georgia, Alabama, Florida, Texas, and Oklahoma.

Spanish peanuts Small round nuts with a reddish-brown skin, Spanish peanuts are the smallest of the four types. Because they have a higher oil content than the others, they are primarily used in peanut oil, as well as in candies, salted peanuts, and peanut butter. They are primarily grown in Oklahoma and Texas, and account for only a small part of U.S. production.

> ### → phytochemicals in peanuts
>
> A protective flavonoid in peanuts called resveratrol may possibly exert a beneficial effect on blood cholesterol and may also have cardioprotective anticlotting actions. Peanut butter contains small amounts of resveratrol, according to laboratory studies.

COMPARING PEANUTS 1 ounce

All the values below are for 1 ounce of peanuts out of the shell, which is just shy of ¼ cup. There is clearly no difference in the amount of fat from one roasting method to another.

	Calories	Fat (g)	% Calories from Fat	Saturated Fat (g)
Oil-roasted peanuts	165	14	76	2.0
Dry-roasted peanuts	166	14	76	2.0
Unroasted peanuts	161	14	78	1.9

Valencia These peanuts, grown almost exclusively in New Mexico, typically have three or more small dark-red to bright-red kernels in a long pod. Very sweet, they are usually roasted and sold in the shell. They are also excellent for fresh use as boiled peanuts.

Virginia peanuts (cocktail nuts) Grown in North Carolina as well as Virginia, these peanuts have large plump pods that contain two large crunchy kernels. They are the type most familiar to consumers and are especially popular at sporting events. When shelled, they are sold as snack peanuts.

choosing the best

When buying packaged peanuts, look for the "sell by" date on the jar, can, or bag. The kernels, if visible, should be plump and uniform in size, crisp and fresh, not limp or rubbery, musty, or rancid smelling.

When selecting in-shell peanuts from a basket or bin, choose those with undamaged shells; look out for cracks, scars, or tiny wormholes.

▶ **When you get home** The high fat content of peanuts makes them susceptible to rancidity; heat, light, and humidity will speed spoilage. But when stored in a cool, dry place, raw unshelled peanuts keep for about 6 months. Shelled peanuts should be refrigerated once the vacuum-sealed package is opened. Transfer peanuts from non-recloseable packages to plastic bags or freezer containers. Shelled peanuts will keep for up to a year in the freezer. If they are properly wrapped, freezing will not significantly affect their texture or flavor, and they need not be thawed for cooking purposes. Nuts for eating should be thawed at room temperature and then toasted or freshened in the oven briefly before serving.

preparing to use

Peanuts have soft shells that are easy to crack with your fingers. You can eat the peanuts with or without the skins. If you want to remove the skins from shelled raw peanuts, you can freeze the peanuts for several hours or overnight, then slip the skins off with your fingers. Or you can roast shelled raw peanuts in a 350° oven for 3 to 5 minutes; cool slightly, then rub between your fingers to remove the skins.

If you purchase shelled peanuts and they seem a little soft (but do not smell rancid), they can be freshened by spreading them on a baking sheet and heating in a very low oven (150°) for a few minutes.

You can chop peanuts by hand or in a food processor or blender. If you chop them by hand, use a good-sized chef's knife on a large cutting board. For efficient chopping, spread the nuts on the board; hold down the tip of the knife blade with one hand and raise and lower the knife, moving it fanwise

a peanut butter primer

Peanut butter first made its appearance in the United States in 1890. It was then that an un-named physician in St. Louis supposedly began grinding peanuts in a hand-cranked meat grinder to use as a nutritious protein substitute for people with poor teeth who couldn't chew meat. A few years later, Dr. John Harvey Kellogg also began experimenting with peanut butter as a vegetarian source of protein for his patients at the renowned Battle Creek Sanitarium in Michigan.

In 1904, peanut butter was introduced to the world at the Universal Exposition in St. Louis by a man named C. H. Sumner. It is said that Sumner sold a remarkable $705.11 worth of the treat at his concession stand there. It was not until 1922, however, that peanut butter became commercially available. In that year, J. L. Rosefield, owner of the Rosefield Packing Company in Alameda, California, received a patent for a shelf-stable peanut butter that would stay fresh for up to a year because the oil didn't separate. Rosefield was also the first to develop crunchy-style peanut butter (sometime around 1934), by adding chopped peanuts to his creamy peanut butter.

Today, approximately half of all edible peanuts cultivated in the United States are used to make peanut butter. By FDA regulation, any product labeled "peanut butter" must consist of at least 90 percent peanuts with no more than 10 percent by weight of seasonings and stabilizing ingredients. These optional ingredients may include salt, sugars, and partially hydrogenated vegetable oil. They cannot include lard or other animal fats, artificial flavorings, artificial sweeteners, chemical preservatives, or colors. Peanut butters labeled "natural" can use only peanuts and oil (usually peanut oil). The oil separates to the top of the jar and must be stirred in to blend with the peanut butter.

Similar peanut butter products that don't adhere to the 90 percent/10 percent rule must be labeled "peanut spread." Many of these are reduced-fat products (25 percent less fat than regular) that use maltodextrin (a type of corn starch) to replace some of the fat from peanuts. Some reduced-fat products also contain soy protein and mineral supplements. Because there are so many different peanut butter and spread products available today—some containing jelly, honey, chocolate, apples, cinnamon, or other ingredients—read the nutrition labels carefully.

When buying peanut butter be sure to look for the "sell by" date on the jar. You can store peanut butter that contains preservatives at room temperature for 2 to 3 months, or it can be refrigerated. Avoid excessive heat, which can cause the oil to separate, or excessive cold, which can change the texture. Freezing peanut butter is not recommended. The best guide to judging freshness is to simply smell and taste the peanut butter. Because it has no preservatives, natural peanut butter must be refrigerated.

Some people prefer to make their own peanut butter at home. Simply process the peanuts of your choice in a food processor until the butter is as chunky or smooth as you like. Add a little oil and/or salt, if you wish. Because homemade peanut butter does not contain preservatives, it should be kept in the refrigerator.

PEANUT BUTTER / 1 tablespoon

Calories	95
Protein (g)	4
Carbohydrate (g)	3
Dietary fiber (g)	0.9
Total fat (g)	8.2
Saturated fat (g)	1.7
Monounsaturated fat (g)	3.9
Polyunsaturated fat (g)	2.2
Cholesterol (mg)	0
Potassium (mg)	107
Sodium (mg)	75

KEY NUTRIENTS (%RDA/AI*)

Niacin	2.1 mg (13%)
Vitamin E	1.6 mg (11%)

*For more detailed information on RDA and AI, see page 88.

across the nuts. A curved chopper used in a wooden bowl works well too, as does an inexpensive mechanical nut chopper. When chopping peanuts in a food processor or blender, process a small amount at a time and pulse the machine on and off; don't overprocess the nuts, as this will release their oils and turn them into peanut butter.

facts & tips

The shells, skins, and kernels of peanuts have been used over the years to make a variety of nonfood products. The shells may be found in wallboard, fireplace logs, and kitty litter. The skins are sometimes used in paper making. And the nuts themselves may be used as an ingredient in detergents, salves, metal polish, bleach, ink, axle grease, shaving cream, face creams, soap, linoleum, rubber, cosmetics, paint, explosives, shampoo, and some medicines.

peanuts & aflatoxin

Peanuts can be a source of aflatoxin, a group of toxins produced by certain strains of mold, usually in very humid conditions. Studies in Africa and Southeast Asia (where aflatoxin contamination is common), along with lab studies, have suggested that it may be linked to liver disease, including cancer. Peanuts and corn, as well as other nuts and grains, are most susceptible to these strains of mold.

Although it is impossible to produce a peanut crop completely free of aflatoxin, you need not worry that the peanuts and peanut butter you buy are unsafe. The FDA has set a maximum permissible level for aflatoxin of 20 parts per billion, and the USDA inspects peanut shipments for any sign of the mold; they will ban any crop with detectable contamination. In addition, most American food processors have established rigorous programs to monitor the presence of aflatoxin, and peanut products generally fall considerably below the allowable 20 parts per billion.

Thus, commercial peanut butter and commercially packaged roasted and dry-roasted-peanuts are likely to be safe. Another protective factor: Any added salt helps to prevent the mold from forming. However, you should take the following precautions when buying and using peanuts and freshly ground peanut butter:

• Look carefully at the peanuts you buy whether they're in or out of the shell. Discard any that are discolored, shriveled, or show signs of mold.

• Peanut butter that is ground in a store may not be as safe as commercial brands. Peanuts that sit around after they have passed inspection may pick up mold if not stored properly. In addition, freshly ground peanut butter won't contain any added salt, so it should be refrigerated as soon as possible to slow rancidity.

• If peanut butter from any source becomes moldy, don't just skim off the mold. Throw the whole container out.

pears

Members of the *Rosaceae* family and related to apples and quince, pears were first cultivated some 3,000 years ago. The delicate, sweet flavor of pears was valued by the ancient Greeks. Indeed, Homer is said to have made reference to the pear in his writing, calling it "the gift of the gods." Over the centuries the fruit made its way across Europe, and was introduced to North America in the 1700s by early settlers who planted cuttings from European stock. Pears are now grown in temperate regions all over the world (so enthusiastically that to date some 5,000 varieties have been developed).

Today, in the United States, the pear is almost as popular as the apple, and can be enjoyed fresh, canned, and cooked. The fruit is seldom tree-ripened (if left to ripen on the tree, the flesh will become mealy): Growers pick pears when they are mature but still green and firm, allowing them to ripen in the marketplace and at home. As pears ripen, their starch converts to sugar and their flesh gets sweeter, juicier, and more succulent, with an almost melting texture that led Europeans to nickname some of the varieties "butter fruit."

bosc pears

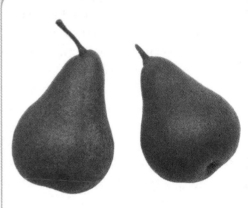

nutritional profile

Pears have a high sugar content, which makes them slightly higher in calories than some other fruits. Still, juicy and tender pears offer a very good amount of dietary fiber, including soluble pectin.

in the market

While there are countless pear varieties, only a handful are available in most areas of the country. Most pears are fall to winter fruits, with the exception being Bartletts, which appear in summer. A number of varieties are imported when their domestic counterparts are out of season. Each type has a distinct shape and color, with subtle differences in flavor and texture.

Asian pears (nashi, apple pears) Asian pears are the oldest cultivated pears known, originating in China, possibly as early as 1100 B.C. They remain a favorite in Asian cuisine. Almost perfectly round, with pale yellow-green to russet skin, these pears look like a cross between an apple and a pear, although they are not a hybrid. The firm, aromatic pulp can range from juicy to slightly dry in texture, and from semisweet to bland in flavor. Unlike other pear varieties, most Asian pears are sold ready to eat, and they store very well even when ripe.

Anjou The most abundant (and least expensive) of the winter pears, the Anjou is oval-shaped, and somewhat stubby, with smooth yellow-green skin and creamy flesh. It has a slightly blander taste than that of a Bosc or Bartlett. Anjous make a succulent fresh dessert pear and are firm enough for baking or poaching.

BARTLETT PEAR / 1 medium	
Calories	98
Protein (g)	1
Carbohydrate (g)	25
Dietary fiber (g)	4.0
Total fat (g)	0.7
Saturated fat (g)	0
Monounsaturated fat (g)	0.1
Polyunsaturated fat (g)	0.2
Cholesterol (mg)	0
Potassium (mg)	208
Sodium (mg)	0

Bartlett Accounting for approximately 75 percent of commercial production, the Bartlett is a summer pear and the most popular variety. It is also the principal pear for canning and is also sold dried. Of medium size and juicy, a ripening Bartlett turns from dark green to golden-yellow (often with a rosy blush). Growers have also developed a red-skinned variety, which tastes the same as the yellow.

Bosc This aromatic, juicy-sweet, and finely textured pear has a long, tapering neck and rough reddish-brown skin. It holds its shape well when baked or poached.

Clapp (Clapps favorite) Sweet and juicy, this pear has very white flesh and a deep red blush over approximately 50 percent of its smooth greenish-yellow skin. There is also a completely red type available. Clapps are well-suited for eating raw, or for baking or poaching.

Comice This squat pear has the reputation of being the sweetest and most flavorful. Too delicate for cooking, it makes a fine fresh dessert pear. It is likely to be the type included in gift boxes and fruit baskets. Its dull greenish-yellow skin may show slight blemishes and discolorations (which do not affect the flavor).

Forelle A little larger than the Seckel, this small, bell-shaped pear is too small for cooking and is ideal for snacking. It has golden-yellow skin and freckles, called "lenticles," that turn bright red during ripening. Forelles are very sweet, with flesh that is slightly firmer than that of most other pears. Believed to have originated in Saxony, the name means "trout" in German, and indeed this pear's brilliant red lenticles do resemble the colors of a rainbow trout.

Seckel (sugar pear) This small chubby pear is the smallest of the commercially grown varieties. It has a grainy texture and a delicious spicy flavor. Typically brownish-yellow, it can sometimes have speckling (russeting).

other pear products

Dried pears Diced dried pears often come in dried fruit mixtures, but you can find dried pear halves in health-food stores and stores that specialize in dried fruit and nuts.

Pear nectar This juice (with pulpy solids in it) is sold canned or bottled in many markets. Its high sugar content makes it higher in calories than most fruit juices (150 calories per cup, compared to 116 in apple juice and 110 in orange juice). Often fortified with vitamin C, a cup supplies over two-thirds of the RDA; unfortified brands contain very little of this vitamin, however.

choosing the best

In general, pears should look relatively unblemished and well-colored, but in some varieties full color will not develop until the fruit ripens. Bartletts turn golden-yellow but may or may not develop their characteristic blush even when they're ready to serve; Anjous stay green-yellow when fully ripe. Russeting—a brown network or speckling on the skin—is common on many types of pears and may indicate superior flavor.

Since they are always picked unripe, pears are a "plan ahead" fruit; they will usually be quite hard in the market and need additional ripening at home to soften and attain their best flavor. Some stores offer ripe or near-ripe pears, but unless these are individually wrapped and displayed just one or two deep, they are likely to be bruised by their own weight or by customer "testing." If you find ripe, undamaged pears, handle them carefully until you get them safely home. Ripe pears will give to gentle pressure at the stem end, depending on the particular variety: Crisp Bosc pears and firm Anjous never get as soft or as fragrant as Bartlett or Comice pears. Watch out for pears that are soft at the blossom end (the bottom), shriveled at the stem end, or that show nicks or dark, soft spots. Small surface blemishes can be ignored.

▶ **When you get home** You can handle the ripening of pears in two ways: Ripen them at room temperature first, then refrigerate them for no longer than a day or two before eating them. Or, refrigerate the pears until you're ready to ripen them—the cold will slow, but not stop, the ripening process. Remove the pears from the refrigerator several days before you plan to eat them, and let them ripen at room temperature.

To speed ripening, place the pears in a paper or perforated plastic bag, turning them occasionally to ensure more even ripening. The process will take from 3 to 7 days. Never store pears—either in or out of the refrigerator—in sealed plastic bags; the lack of oxygen will cause the fruit to brown at the core. Check the fruit often and refrigerate it (or eat it) as soon as it yields to gentle pressure.

preparing to use

When eaten raw with their skins, pears need only to be washed (and sliced, if you like). For other purposes, you can peel the pears with a paring knife or vegetable peeler, if desired, then either core the pears with an apple corer from either end, or halve the fruit lengthwise and scoop out the core with a teaspoon or a melon baller. Coat the peeled or cut pears with lemon juice to keep them from darkening.

serving suggestions

- Spread a thin layer of Roquefort or Stilton on fresh pear halves.

- Add sliced pears to watercress or endive salads and top with a crumbling of toasted pecans.

- Stuff whole, cored pears with diced dried pears, brown sugar, and cinnamon. Bake as you would an apple. Serve the baked pears with a dollop of low-fat yogurt.

- For a savory main-dish accompaniment, halve pears lengthwise, core, sprinkle with Parmesan, and bake until firm-tender.

- Fill the hollows of halved, cored pears with a mixture of low-fat cream cheese and chopped figs.

- Cook pears until very thick to make pear butter.

- Add pear puree or diced pears to sauces for duck or pork.

- Sprinkle peeled, cored, and halved pears with sugar, drizzle lemon juice over them, and bake until soft and syrupy.

- Add diced dried pears to breads, muffins, and cookies.

peas, dried

Though peas belong to the same family as beans and lentils, they are set apart by common usage rather than by a botanical distinction. The peas represented here are of several different species, but they share one thing in common (which also sets them apart from beans and lentils): They are all spherical. Most peas that are sold fresh are also available in their dried form. Dried peas are sometimes also called field peas and include split peas (green and yellow), black-eyed peas, pigeon peas, and chick-peas.

nutritional profile

Dried peas, which are legumes, are highly nutritious. A low-fat food, and a good source of both soluble and insoluble fiber, dried peas also provide potassium, iron, thiamin, and folate as well as complex carbohydrates, and a moderate amount of protein.

in the market

Generally speaking, the peas that are grown to be sold fresh are not the same as those that are cultivated for their mature seeds, which are subsequently dried. Among other things, the mature seeds are higher in starch, which makes them suitable for hearty dishes and long cooking.

Black-eyed peas (cowpeas, black-eyed beans) Marked by a single black spot on their skin, these kidney-shaped, creamy-white legumes have a pealike flavor and firm, resilient texture.

Chick-peas See Chick-peas (*page 237*).

Green peas Dried green peas come whole as well as split (*below*). The whole peas taste like split green peas, but they take quite a bit longer to cook because they have their skins on (which also gives them more fiber).

Pigeon peas (gunga peas, no-eyed peas) These yellowish-gray peas are about the size of a green pea, but are generally sold split.

Split peas Once peas are dried and their skins removed, they split apart naturally. *Green split peas* are favored in the United States and Great Britain, while *yellow split peas,* which have a more pronounced nutlike flavor, are preferred in Scandinavia and other regions of northern Europe. Neither type requires presoaking, and both cook quickly.

preparing to use

As with dried beans, some dried peas need to be soaked before cooking. This is not necessary with any of the peas that are skinned and split, as they will cook fairly quickly. But peas with their skins still on (like whole green peas and chick-peas) should be soaked in water for several hours or overnight to shorten their cooking time.

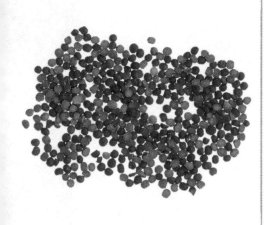

green split peas

GREEN SPLIT PEAS ½ cup cooked	
Calories	116
Protein (g)	8
Carbohydrate (g)	21
Dietary fiber (g)	8.1
Total fat (g)	0.4
Saturated fat (g)	0.1
Monounsaturated fat (g)	0.1
Polyunsaturated fat (g)	0.2
Cholesterol (mg)	0
Potassium (mg)	355
Sodium (mg)	2

KEY NUTRIENTS (%RDA/AI*)	
Thiamin	0.2 mg (16%)
Folate	64 mcg (16%)
Iron	1.3 mg (16%)

*For more detailed information on RDA and AI, see page 88.

peas, fresh

Peas are legumes: plants that bear pods enclosing fleshy seeds. Only a handful of legumes are sold in their fresh form (*see Beans, Fresh, page 183*), but peas—in particular green peas, snow peas, and sugar snaps—are more commonly sold and cooked as fresh vegetables.

Peas in their dried form (*see Peas, Dried, opposite page*) have been used as a food since ancient times—archaeologists found them in Egyptian tombs—but it was not until the 16th century that tender varieties were developed to be eaten fresh. In the 17th century, Louis XIV and his courtiers discovered the delights of eating young fresh peas. And Gregor Mendel, an Austrian botanist, used peas as the basis for his famous plant breeding experiments in the latter half of the 19th century; his work with pea plants is considered the foundation of modern genetics.

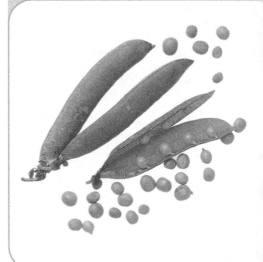

green peas

nutritional profile

Like most legumes, peas are a low-fat, high-fiber food. They are a good source of plant protein, though the protein is incomplete because peas lack certain essential amino acids. Green peas, compared with snow peas, provide more nutrients, particularly riboflavin, niacin, and zinc. Snow peas, on the other hand, provide more than three times the amount of vitamin C as green peas, and also supply a good amount of vitamin E, folate, lutein & zeaxanthin.

in the market

Today, only about 5 percent of all peas grown come to the market fresh; more than half the crop is canned or frozen. Frozen peas retain their flavor and nutrients better than canned and are low in sodium. If just thawed and not cooked, frozen peas can be substituted for fresh peas in salads and other uncooked dishes.

Of those that do make it to the market fresh, there are two main types: edible-pod peas—such as snow peas and sugar snap peas—as well as the more common podded peas that need to be "shelled."

edible-pod peas

Snow peas (Chinese pea pods) These edible-pod peas have light green flat pods with small, immature-looking peas (they are picked before the seeds have developed in the pod). Probably developed in Holland in the 16th century, snow peas are most familiar today as a component of stir-fries.

Snow pea shoots These are the very young beginnings of a snow pea plant. The shoot includes the young, tender vine and leaves, as well as the baby tendrils that the vining plant puts out to climb over the ground or up a trellis. They are very sweet and flavorful, and a favorite in Chinese stir-fries.

GREEN PEAS / 1 cup cooked

Calories	134
Protein (g)	9
Carbohydrate (g)	25
Dietary fiber (g)	8.8
Total fat (g)	0.4
Saturated fat (g)	0.1
Monounsaturated fat (g)	0
Polyunsaturated fat (g)	0.2
Cholesterol (mg)	0
Potassium (mg)	434
Sodium (mg)	5

KEY NUTRIENTS (%RDA/AI*)

Thiamin	0.4 mg (35%)
Riboflavin	0.2 mg (18%)
Niacin	3.2 mg (20%)
Vitamin B$_6$	0.4 mg (20%)
Vitamin C	23 mg (25%)
Folate	101 mcg (25%)
Iron	2.5 mg (31%)
Magnesium	62 mg (15%)
Zinc	1.9 mg (17%)

For more detailed information on RDA and AI, see page 88.

facts & tips

There are some pea varieties that never make it to the market fresh. They are grown specifically for canning, the best-known example being LeSueur petit pois. This is unfortunate, since canned peas are lower in nutrients and higher in sodium than either fresh or frozen peas.

Sugar snap peas These edible-pod peas (which the French call *mange-tout*, or "eat-all") were created in the 1970s as a cross between the snow and the green pea. They have plump pods filled with very sweet, tender peas.

shell peas

Black-eyed peas These peas are mostly available frozen (and dried). In the South, fresh black-eyed peas can be found in some farmers' markets.

Green peas Also known as English peas because of the many varieties developed in England, green peas possess a large, bulging, grass-green pod enclosing peas that are typically round and sweet; some homegrown varieties are more strongly flavored. The pods are not edible. Packaged green peas differ from fresh garden varieties in appearance, color, texture, and flavor. Moreover, different varieties are grown specifically for freezing.

Pigeon peas These are most often sold in their dried form, but you can occasionally find them fresh, especially if you live near any sizable Caribbean population. Gunga peas (as they are called in many parts of the Caribbean) are a staple ingredient in Jamaican cuisine.

▶ Availability Fresh green peas in the pod and sugar snaps have a somewhat limited season: Their peak is April through July, and they are least plentiful from September through December (though you can occasionally find some peas in winter). Fresh snow peas are available most of the year, especially in Chinese neighborhoods. Pea shoots are available in the beginning of the snow pea season, and since they are pretty much a local commodity, availability will vary with the locality.

choosing the best

Garden peas in the shell should be kept refrigerated; if not, half their sugar content will turn to starch within 6 hours. Low temperatures also help to preserve their texture and nutrient content. Look for firm, glossy pods with a slightly velvety feel that are filled almost to bursting; the peas should not rattle loosely in the pod. Choose medium-sized pods rather than overlarge ones. The stem, leaves, and tip should be soft and green. Toss back pods that are puffy, dull, yellowed, or heavily speckled. If possible, crack open a pod and taste a few peas for sweetness. You may find trays of preshelled peas in the market; though these will save you time and labor, such peas are likely to be mealy and not very sweet because of the rapid conversion of their sugar to starch.

Snow peas should be shiny and flat, with the tiny peas barely visible through the pod; small ones will be the sweetest and most tender. Old snow peas often appear twisted. Sugar snaps should be bright green, plump, and firm; the pod should tightly encase the small peas. Avoid limp or yellowed sugar snaps; break a pod in two if you can to see if it snaps crisply.

Pea shoots should be bright green and not limp.

▶ **When you get home** Don't shell green peas until just before you plan to cook or eat them, and don't wash them before storing.

preparing to use

To shell peas, pinch off the stem with your fingernails and pull the string down the length of the pod. Immediately, the pod will pop open, then you can push out the peas with your thumb. If the pods are clean on the outside, you need not wash the peas. (When cooking the peas, you can add three or four pods for extra flavor. Or, save the pods for flavoring chicken or vegetable stock; discard them with any other solids when the stock is strained.)

Snow peas and sugar snaps should be rinsed before use. With snow peas, simply remove the tips from both ends of the pod. Sugar snaps should have the string removed whether they are to be eaten raw or cooked. Unlike green peas, the string on a sugar snap runs around both sides of the pod. It's easiest to start at the bottom tip and pull the string up the front, then snap off the stem and pull the string down the back. Snow peas and sugar snaps, as well as shelled green peas, can be eaten raw. But if you cook them, do so briefly so that they retain their flavor and texture.

Pea shoots do not need any special preparation except for a quick rinse.

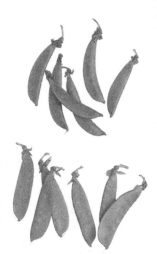

Edible-pod peas: sugar snap peas (top) and snow peas (bottom).

serving suggestions

· Use raw sugar snaps and snow peas for crudités with dips.

· Stir cooked black-eyed peas and a little grated Parmesan into cooked rice for an easy version of *risi e bisi*, a classic Italian dish.

· Toss cooked fresh pigeon peas and green peas with diced red onion, chopped cilantro, and a lemon and olive oil vinaigrette for a mixed pea salad.

· Add cooked pigeon peas to a potato or pasta salad.

· Puree cooked green peas with broth, mint, and yogurt for a quick soup.

· Toss steamed sugar snaps and grated lemon zest with an herbed olive oil.

· Mash cooked green peas along with cooked potatoes for an interesting mashed potato dish.

· Substitute thawed frozen green peas for half the avocado in a guacamole recipe (or use all peas).

SNOW PEAS / 1 cup cooked	
Calories	67
Protein (g)	5
Carbohydrate (g)	11
Dietary fiber (g)	4.5
Total fat (g)	0.4
Saturated fat (g)	0.1
Monounsaturated fat (g)	0
Polyunsaturated fat (g)	0.2
Cholesterol (mg)	0
Potassium (mg)	384
Sodium (mg)	6

KEY NUTRIENTS (%RDA/AI*)	
Thiamin	0.2 mg (17%)
Vitamin B$_6$	0.2 mg (14%)
Vitamin C	77 mg (85%)
Vitamin E	4.7 mg (31%)
Folate	47 mcg (12%)
Iron	3.2 mg (39%)
Magnesium	42 mg (10%)

*For more detailed information on RDA and AI, see page 88.

pecans

The pecan tree is a species of hickory and grows wild from Illinois to the Gulf of Mexico. An important crop tree, the pecan is grown commercially in orchards in the South and southeastern United States (this country is the world's largest producer). The pecan fruits grow in clusters, and when the pecan is mature, the fruit splits and the pecan shell drops to the ground. Inside the inch-long, smooth, beige shell rests the golden-brown, succulent pecan nut. Cultivated pecans are bred for thin ("paper") shells, which are easier to crack than the hard shells of wild pecans.

Pecans served as an important staple food for Native Americans who collected the nuts and stored them for long periods during the winter when food was scarce. Native Americans also traded pecans for goods. Purportedly, the name "pecan" is a Native American word of Algonquin origin that was used to describe "all nuts requiring a stone to crack." Pecans also provided sustenance for early settlers, and in the late 18th century, pecan orchards were planted by two high-profile Americans: Thomas Jefferson and George Washington. However, pecans weren't cultivated on a large or commercial scale until the late 19th century.

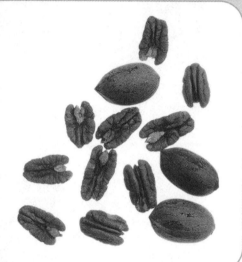

pecans

nutritional profile

Not only are pecans rich in thiamin, zinc, and fiber, they also provide heart-healthy monounsaturated and polyunsaturated fats: These fats can lower blood cholesterol, especially when substituted for foods high in saturated fat, such as meat or cheese. And research indicates that the plant sterols found in pecans can help to lower LDL ("bad") cholesterol levels. Like other nuts, it is best to try to eat small amounts on a regular basis and not overdo it: While pecans are considered a healthful food, they are nonetheless high in calories and should be consumed in moderation.

in the market

There are more than 200 varieties of pecans, but in general pecans are known in the marketplace not by their variety but by where they are grown. The names of the pecan varieties grown in any given region are likely to have some of the flavor of that region. For example, many of the pecan varieties grown in Texas (and other states) have Native American names: Choctaw, Mohawk, Shoshonee, and Pawnee. Other pecans are given names according to the developer's whimsy, such as Moneymaker, Desirable, and Kernoodle. But none of these varietal names appear as labels in the market.

Like most nuts, pecans are available shelled and unshelled. Shelled pecans come as halves or pieces. There are roasted and salted versions, too.

PECANS / 1 ounce	
Calories	189
Protein (g)	2
Carbohydrate (g)	5
Dietary fiber (g)	2.2
Total fat (g)	19
Saturated fat (g)	1.5
Monounsaturated fat (g)	12
Polyunsaturated fat (g)	4.7
Cholesterol (mg)	0
Potassium (mg)	111
Sodium (mg)	0

KEY NUTRIENTS (%RDA/AI*)	
Thiamin	0.2 mg (20%)
Zinc	1.6 mg (14%)

*For more detailed information on RDA and AI, see page 88.

▶ **Availability** Pecan halves and pieces are available all year, but pecans in the shell (only 20 percent of the crop is sold this way) can be difficult to find outside of pecan-growing regions except at holiday time, when there is a high market demand for them. Luckily, the pecan harvest coincides with this demand, beginning in late September.

choosing the best

When buying packaged nuts, look for a freshness date on the jar, can, or bag. The kernels, if visible, should be plump and uniform in size. If you buy shelled nuts at a candy store, health-food store, or other bulk source, be sure that they're crisp and fresh, not limp or rubbery, musty, or rancid.

When selecting nuts with shells from a basket or bin, choose those with undamaged shells; look out for cracks, scars, or tiny wormholes. Each nut should feel heavy, and the kernel should not rattle when the nutshell is shaken; if it does, the kernel may be withered and dry.

▶ **When you get home** Like all nuts, the high fat content of pecans makes them prone to rancidity; heat, light, and humidity will speed spoilage. Raw unshelled nuts, however, keep very well—6 months to a year when stored in a cool, dry place.

Shelled pecans should be kept in the refrigerator in airtight containers where they will be good for about 9 months. In the freezer (in sealed plastic bags) they will be good for up to 2 years. If they are properly wrapped, freezing will not significantly affect the texture or flavor of pecans, and they need not be thawed for cooking purposes. Pecans for eating should be thawed at room temperature and then toasted or freshened in the oven before serving.

preparing to use

Shelling pecans requires a nutcracker. If possible, pressure should be applied at the two ends of the shell instead of across the middle. This keeps the nutmeat from being crushed in the process. The nutmeat should come out cleanly and in one piece. The nutmeat does not need to be skinned, as some nutmeats do.

To chop pecans For large pieces, break the nutmeats by hand. For finer sizes, use a good-sized chef's knife on a large cutting board, or use a curved chopper in a wooden bowl or a mechanical nut chopper.

other pecan products

Pecan butter Like peanut butter, a ground paste of pecans.

Pecan flour See Flour, Nonwheat (*page 327*).

Pecan granules Pecan growers sell nuts in various granulations. This is like a very finely chopped nut and it is used for coating foods. It is rarely available in stores, but is available directly from growers and by mail.

Pecan meal This is a very fine granulation of chopped pecans, just short of being a flour, and is usually available only by mail order.

Pecan oil See Nut Oils (*page 299*).

serving suggestions

• Toast pecans, then chop, and sprinkle over oatmeal.

• Use pecans instead of pine nuts in a pesto recipe.

• Combine pecan granules with whole-wheat bread crumbs and use as a coating for baked fish or poultry.

• Stir a small amount of pecan butter into stews and soups.

• Stir chopped pecans and dried cranberries into homemade yogurt cheese (*page 600*) or reduced-fat cream cheese (Neufchâtel) for a sweet sandwich spread.

peppers, sweet

Peppers are not pepper: The plant that produces dried peppercorns, the spice we use as a seasoning, is native to Asia and is entirely unrelated to the shrubby plant that gives us the familiar sweet bell peppers and their many relatives. Members of the genus *Capsicum*, peppers are native to the western hemisphere and have been domesticated in its tropical regions for several thousand years.

The vegetable was given its name by Spanish explorers who had set out with Columbus on his second voyage in search of the peppercorns of India. When they landed in the New World and encountered this odd species, perhaps they thought the flavor resembled that of peppercorns, and so misnamed them. The explorers returned home with the capsicum peppers, which quickly became popular in Europe as a food, spice, and condiment. Over the next 200 years, peppers were introduced to many other parts of the world, where they were domesticated and bred for either their sweet qualities or for their fiery heat *(see Chili Peppers, page 244)*.

bell peppers

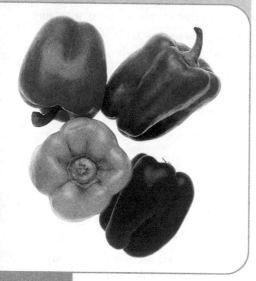

nutritional profile

All sweet peppers are packed with nutrients, such as vitamin B_6 and vitamin C, as well as dietary fiber. However, compared with other sweet peppers, yellow peppers supply slightly higher quantities of folate and iron. Moreover, both yellow and red peppers contain more than twice the amount of vitamin C found in green peppers. Red peppers are also an important source of the carotenoids beta carotene and beta cryptoxanthin, and orange peppers are a top source of the carotenoid zeaxanthin.

in the market

The most popular sweet pepper in the United States is the bell, which accounts for more than 60 percent of the domestic pepper crop. While chili peppers are primarily used to season foods, it's possible to consume sweet peppers in sufficient quantities so that they make a significant nutritional contribution to your diet.

Banana peppers These mild yellow peppers, resembling bananas in shape and color, are available fresh or pickled in jars. It's important to taste one before using it in a recipe because of its resemblance to a moderately hot twin called Hungarian wax. Both banana and Hungarian wax peppers may be labeled "yellow wax" in stores, with no indication of their heat level.

GREEN BELL PEPPER 1 large	
Calories	44
Protein (g)	2
Carbohydrate (g)	11
Dietary fiber (g)	3.0
Total fat (g)	0.3
Saturated fat (g)	0.1
Monounsaturated fat (g)	0
Polyunsaturated fat (g)	0.2
Cholesterol (mg)	0
Potassium (mg)	290
Sodium (mg)	3

KEY NUTRIENTS (%RDA/AI*)	
Vitamin B_6	0.4 mg (24%)
Vitamin C	147 mg (163%)

*For more detailed information on RDA and AI, see page 88.

Bell peppers With three to four lobes, these sweet bell-shaped peppers can be green, red, yellow, orange, purple, or brown (known as chocolate peppers), depending on the variety and the stage of ripeness. Most are picked and sold in the mature green stage—fully developed, but not ripe. As they ripen on the vine, most bell peppers turn red and become sweeter. Bell peppers have no "bite" at all, since they contain a recessive gene that eliminates capsaicin, the compound that gives peppers their hotness. Instead, they have a mild tang and a crunchy texture that makes them suitable for eating raw; their size, shape, and firmness also allow them to be stuffed whole and baked.

Cubanelle This long, tapered pepper, about 4 inches in length, is either light green or yellow. Occasionally, you will find fully mature cubanelles, which are red. Cubanelles are more flavorful than bell peppers and are perfect for sautéing.

Italian frying peppers This is a marketplace name for cubanelles and sometimes for banana peppers.

Mexi-Bells These are a cross between a bell pepper and a chili pepper. They look like small bell peppers, but have a hotter bite.

Pimientos Large and rather heart-shaped, pimientos (sometimes spelled "pimentos") are generally sold in jars, but every so often you can find them fresh—fully ripe and red—in specialty food markets. These sweet peppers are mild yet flavorful; their thick, meaty flesh makes them good candidates for roasting; in fact, the pimientos sold in jars are usually roasted and peeled. Large red bell peppers are sometimes packaged as pimientos. You can tell the difference by the shade of red; true pimientos will have an orangy cast, while bells are bright red.

choosing the best

Fresh peppers come in a wide variety of shapes, sizes, and colors, but the guidelines for choosing them are practically the same. Peppers should be well-shaped, firm, and glossy. Their skins should be taut and unwrinkled, and

RED BELL PEPPER 1 large	
Calories	44
Protein (g)	2
Carbohydrate (g)	11
Dietary fiber (g)	3.3
Total fat (g)	0.3
Saturated fat (g)	0.1
Monounsaturated fat (g)	0
Polyunsaturated fat (g)	0.2
Cholesterol (mg)	0
Potassium (mg)	290
Sodium (mg)	3

KEY NUTRIENTS (%RDA/AI*)	
Beta carotene	5.0 mg (46%)
Vitamin B$_6$	0.4 mg (24%)
Vitamin C	312 mg (346%)

For more detailed information on RDA and AI, see page 88.

serving suggestions

• Top toasted or grilled bread with an assortment of colorful roasted peppers and a drizzle of olive oil.

• Add diced fresh peppers to salsa.

• Combine pureed roasted bell peppers and garlic, and use as a topping for pasta or as a fat-free sauce for poultry or pasta.

• Add a swirl of red pepper puree to a creamy soup for both flavor and color contrast.

• Scatter Mexi-bell pepper slices over pizza.

• Stuff peppers with chili, pasta, rice, or vegetables and bake.

• Add roasted red peppers to pesto.

• Prepare a green sauce with roasted green peppers, green herbs, lime juice, and a little olive oil. Serve with grilled chicken or fish, or toss with pasta.

their stems fresh and green. Bell peppers are best when they are thick-walled and juicy, so they should feel heavy for their size. Look out for soft or sunken areas, slashes, or black spots.

If a green bell pepper shows streaks of red, it will be slightly sweeter than a totally green one; however, once picked, it won't get any redder—or sweeter.

▶ **When you get home** Store unwashed sweet peppers in a plastic bag in the refrigerator for up to a week; green peppers will keep somewhat longer than red or other ripe peppers. Check them frequently; immediately use any peppers that have developed soft spots.

Chopped peppers freeze well without blanching. Upon thawing, the peppers still retain some crispness and can be used in cooked dishes or raw in uncooked preparations.

preparing to use

Wash peppers just before you use them. If you are going to cut the peppers into strips or pieces, cut the pepper lengthwise into flat panels. Discard the stems, spongy cores, and seeds (which can have a bitter taste). If you are using the pepper whole, cut the stem end off and then discard the core and seeds. Or, for pepper halves, cut the pepper in half lengthwise (not crosswise).

Some people find pepper skin unpleasantly tough in cooked dishes; you can easily peel peppers by blanching or roasting them (*see below*). For most recipes, the various colors of bell peppers are interchangeable (keep in mind, however, that red, yellow, and orange peppers are sweeter than green peppers).

YELLOW BELL PEPPER 1 large	
Calories	50
Protein (g)	2
Carbohydrate (g)	12
Dietary fiber (g)	1.7
Total fat (g)	0.4
Saturated fat (g)	0.1
Monounsaturated fat (g)	0.1
Polyunsaturated fat (g)	0.2
Cholesterol (mg)	0
Potassium (mg)	394
Sodium (mg)	4

KEY NUTRIENTS (%RDA/AI*)	
Niacin	1.7 mg (10%)
Vitamin B$_6$	0.3 mg (18%)
Vitamin C	342 mg (380%)
Folate	48 mcg (12%)
Iron	0.9 mg (11%)

For more detailed information on RDA and AI, see page 88.

grilling & roasting tips

Sweet peppers take on wonderful smoky flavor when broiled, grilled, or fire-roasted whole over an open flame (fire-roasting works best for thin-walled peppers). Cooking peppers this way also allows you to peel them easily.

Broiling or grilling To prepare a pepper for broiling or grilling, slice it lengthwise into four or five flattish panels. Discard the stem, ribs, and seeds. Lay the pieces on the grill skin-side down, or on a broiler pan skin-side up, and cook about 4 inches from the heat until the skin is blackened. Place the peppers in a bowl, cover with a pot lid or a plate, and let the peppers "sweat" for about 15 minutes; this will loosen the skin. Then it's easy to peel off the skin with your fingers or a table knife. Cooking time: 6 to 10 minutes.

Fire-roasting To fire-roast whole peppers, cut a small slit near the stem of each one. Impale each pepper on a long-handled cooking fork and hold over the flame of a gas stove or grill, turning to char the skin evenly. Once charred, follow the same procedure for removing the skin as above.

persimmons

The persimmon, with its beautiful, orange-red glossy skin, arrives in markets just as summer is ending. Nevertheless, it hasn't become as popular in the United States as it has in Japan, where the fruit is widely cultivated and as eagerly consumed as oranges are in the West. Though there are native persimmon trees in the United States, the varieties that Americans eat were brought here from Japan in the late 19th century (and are now grown mainly in California).

There are two basic types of persimmons: astringent and nonastringent. As novice persimmon eaters often belatedly discover, the astringent persimmon has two personalities. When soft and ripe, it possesses a rich, sweet, spicy flavor that some say is like a blend of mango and papaya; others find it reminiscent of apple and orange or even pumpkin. The unripened fruit, however, is so astringent that biting into it causes the mouth to pucker. The astringency is due to the presence of tannins, a group of chemicals that occur in tea, red wine, and in a few other fruits, such as peaches and dates, before they ripen—though the quantity in a persimmon is much greater. As the fruit ripens and softens, the tannins become inert and the astringency disappears.

Nonastringent persimmons can be eaten before they soften, skin and all, without causing the mouth to pucker. They are sweet and crisp when not quite ripe and custardy when ripe.

persimmons

fuyu

hachiya

nutritional profile

Persimmons are well worth trying, not only for their exceptional flavor but also for their vitamin C content, with one large persimmon providing nearly 14 percent of the daily requirement. Carotenoid pigments in persimmons are notable as well; the vivid color of the fruit is due to alpha carotene, beta carotene, and beta cryptoxanthin (which is present in particularly high amounts).

in the market

Of the hundreds of varieties cultivated in the United States, there are only two of commercial importance, the Fuyu and the Hachiya. They can be purchased fresh or dried. Other, more obscure persimmons, may be available locally or in specialty food markets.

Chocolate persimmon Its brown-streaked flesh and faint chocolate flavor give this persimmon its name.

Fuyu This pale- to bright-orange, tomato-shaped variety makes up most of what's in the market today. Because it has no tannins, it is not astringent like the Hachiya, and can be eaten while still firm. It is crisp, sweet, and crunchy, rather like a Fuji apple. If you're wondering why you don't see more

HACHIYA PERSIMMON 1 large	
Calories	118
Protein (g)	1
Carbohydrate (g)	31
Dietary fiber (g)	6.1
Total fat (g)	0.3
Saturated fat (g)	0
Monounsaturated fat (g)	0.1
Polyunsaturated fat (g)	0.1
Cholesterol (mg)	0
Potassium (mg)	271
Sodium (mg)	2

KEY NUTRIENTS (%RDA/AI*)	
Beta carotene	2.2 mg (20%)
Vitamin B$_6$	0.2 mg (10%)
Vitamin C	13 mg (14%)

*For more detailed information on RDA and AI, see page 88.

of them in your local market, it's because they are primarily sent into ethnic markets where the demand is high. The reddish-orange *Giant Fuyu* (also known as Jumbu or Hana Fuyu) is also sometimes available.

Hachiya Shaped like an acorn and about the size of a medium peach, this persimmon has shiny, bright orange skin. It is extremely astringent until it is soft-ripe, at which point the skin dulls and it becomes incredibly sweet.

Sharon fruit Named after the valley of the river in Israel where the fruit is primarily grown, the Sharon fruit is a plump, nearly seedless persimmon that's about the size of a tomato. It has pale orange to brilliant red-orange skin. Its flavor is mild and sweet. Like the Fuyu, it doesn't have astringent tannins and can be eaten while still firm.

Tanenashi This persimmon is primarily grown in Florida. It is cone-shaped with a yellow-orange skin and, like the Hachiya, should be eaten when soft-ripe.

▶ Availability Persimmons are available (either domestic or imported) from late September through May.

choosing the best

Persimmons are usually tucked into individual egg "nests," rather like egg cartons, for shipping and store display; the fruits are very susceptible to bruising and won't survive careless handling. Persimmons reach their full color while still hard, and they are harvested and shipped in this hard, pre-ripened state.

When selecting Fuyu persimmons, look for ones that are yellow-orange in color and firm to the touch. Hachiyas should be deep orange without any green (except at the stem) or yellow showing. They may occasionally have dark spots caused by sunburn, which is fine unless the flesh is sunken at those spots. There shouldn't be any breaks in the skin, but scarring caused by rubbing against tree branches during harvesting is harmless.

Though persimmons are shipped unripe, your grocer may have some ripe ones to offer. Buy ripe fruits, if you can find them, to eat immediately, and plan to ripen firmer ones at home for later use. Ripe Hachiya persimmons should be completely soft—their thin skins virtually bursting with jellylike, juicy flesh. (In this state of ripeness, they have been compared to water balloons.) Fuyu persimmons, by contrast, are crisp when ripe.

▶ When you get home For good eating, a very firm Fuyu persimmon may need to be put aside for just a day or two. An unripe Hachiya, filled with mouth-puckering tannins, will probably need more time to soften and lose its astringency.

There is some controversy about the best way to ripen these fruits. One way is to put them in a paper bag along with an apple, which will produce ethylene gas (and hasten the ripening). Be sure to turn the fruit occasionally so it ripens evenly. For Fuyus, this may take only a couple of days; for Hachiya persimmons, the process may take a couple of weeks.

facts & tips

Appalachian folk wisdom has it that persimmon seeds can predict the type of winter to come. When you split the seed down the center and open it up carefully, you expose the small white embryo. If the leaves of the embryo lay on top of each other, it looks like a spoon and legend predicts lots of snow. If the leaves are spread a bit so that the points resemble a fork, then legend predicts a winter with a moderate amount of snow. If the leaves are particularly narrow, resembling a knife, there will be little or no snow that winter.

Another approach for Hachiya persimmons—a modified version of a technique Japanese shippers use—incorporates two ripening principles: One method involves excluding oxygen, causing the persimmons to produce aldehydes, which counteract the astringency of the tannins. The other requires exposing the persimmons to alcohol, encouraging the fruits to produce their own ethylene gas. The kitchen adaptation of this method is quite simple: Stand the fruits in a plastic food-storage container, place a few drops of liquor (brandy or rum, for instance) on each of the leaflike sepals, then cover the container tightly. The fruits will soften considerably as they turn sweeter, so don't expect to be able to slice them. Hachiyas treated in this manner may ripen in less than a week.

Freezing is also sometimes recommended as an overnight ripening method for Hachiya persimmons. But while the fruit will emerge from the freezer softened, it will not develop the sweetness that only slow ripening can produce. You may want to leave the persimmons in the freezer for several weeks to sweeten them up. Or, if you prefer, you can leave them in the freezer for several months and they should still retain their flavor.

Ripe persimmons should be placed in a plastic bag, stored in the refrigerator, and used quickly.

preparing to use

You can wash a Fuyu persimmon and eat it like an apple, either whole or cut into slices or wedges. They are easy to peel (although it's not necessary) with a paring knife. Pull off the sepals before serving, or cut off the stem end with a cone-shaped "core" of flesh. The thicker-skinned Hachiya can be messy to bite into in its soft, ripened state, and is therefore easier to handle if halved lengthwise and eaten from the skin with a spoon. Some persimmons contain a few seeds, which should not be eaten and are easily removed.

serving suggestions

- Partially freeze ripe Hachiya persimmons, peel, and puree for a quick sorbet.

- Cut Fuyu persimmons into wedges and add to savory tossed salads.

- Slice Fuyu persimmons and substitute for sliced tomato on a sandwich.

- Add sliced Fuyu persimmons to fruit for a cobbler.

- Use Hachiya puree in quick breads, muffins, or steamed puddings.

- Add dried persimmons to trail mix or granola, or cook some along with oatmeal.

- Dice dried persimmons and add to cookies or cakes.

- Make a salsa for grilled meat or poultry using diced Fuyu persimmons.

- Puree peeled Hachiya persimmons and use as a sauce for angel food cake.

oven-drying persimmons

Peel firm, ripe Fuyu persimmons and cut into to 1/8- to 1/4-inch-thick slices. Place the slices on baking sheets, in a single layer. Place in a 140° oven and leave the door slightly ajar. If possible, aim a fan at the oven so that air will circulate over the drying persimmons. Bake for about 12 hours, rotating the baking sheets occasionally. The dried fruit will be light to medium brown and feel leathery, not sticky, when done. Keep an eye on it. Let the dried fruit cool, then store airtight in a sealed plastic bag or a glass jar with a lid.

pineapple

Sweet, lush, and highly flavorful, the pineapple has long been a valued food as well as a symbol of welcome and hospitality. Its pleasing texture and lush sweetness, combined with a trace of tartness, make it a favorite fruit among many Americans.

Pineapples probably first grew wild in parts of South America and then spread to the West Indies, where Columbus encountered them (on the island of Guadaloupe) during his second voyage to that region. The Europe to which Columbus returned with his discoveries (including the exotic pineapple) was a civilization largely bereft of sweets and fresh produce, and the arrival of this remarkable fruit created quite a stir. (It is said that these same Spanish explorers introduced the custom of using carved pineapples above front doors, having seen the natives place whole pineapples or pineapple tops near the entrances to their huts as a signal of welcome.)

By 1600, European explorers had carried pineapples as far as China and the Philippines, and about 200 years later, the fruit was introduced to Hawaii. It was not until the 1880s, however, when steamships made transporting the perishable fruit viable, that commercial cultivation of pineapples began in the Hawaiian Islands. Today the state continues to be a major producer of this fruit.

Like melons, pineapples have no built-in reserves of starch that convert to sugar. This is because the starch is stored in the stem of the plant rather than in the fruit itself. It is only just before the fruit ripens completely that the starch converts to sugar and enters the fruit. For this reason, growers ripen pineapples on the plant to a point where they are almost fully ripe, with a high sugar content and plenty of juice. Once the fruit has been harvested, it won't get any sweeter, and if too ripe, the fruit may spoil before it gets to market. After harvesting, the pineapples are shipped to market as quickly as possible, arriving within two to three days.

nutritional profile

Pineapples provide thiamin, as well as a good amount of vitamin C. Just 1 cup of pineapple chunks provides 27 percent of the RDA for this vitamin, and a cup of juice provides 50 percent. Pineapple is also rich in manganese.

in the market

Today Hawaii is a just one producer of fresh and canned pineapple. The fruit is also grown in Florida and is imported fresh and/or canned from Mexico, Central America, the Far East, and a number of other places. The following varieties are the ones most commonly found in supermarkets or specialty food stores:

pineapple

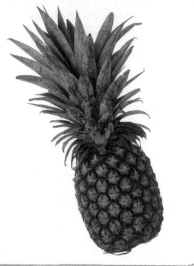

PINEAPPLE / 1 cup chunks	
Calories	76
Protein (g)	1
Carbohydrate (g)	19
Dietary fiber (g)	1.9
Total fat (g)	0.7
Saturated fat (g)	0.1
Monounsaturated fat (g)	0.1
Polyunsaturated fat (g)	0.2
Cholesterol (mg)	0
Potassium (mg)	175
Sodium (mg)	2

KEY NUTRIENTS (%RDA/AI*)	
Thiamin	0.1 mg (12%)
Vitamin C	24 mg (27%)

*For more detailed information on RDA and AI, see page 88.

Costa Rican Gold Almost like shimmering gold, Costa Rica pineapple is scrumptiously sweet and deliciously juicy. Its very low acid content makes room for its very high sugar content. The tender, bright yellow flesh is encased in an attractive very yellow shell.

Red Spanish Weighing roughly 2 to 5 pounds, this pineapple has pale yellow flesh and a squarish shape.

Smooth Cayenne This cone-shaped Hawaiian pineapple is the most popular (and is considered by many to be the best tasting). It has pale yellow to yellow flesh and weighs roughly 5 to 6 pounds. Small versions are sold as *Baby Hawaiian Pineapples.*

South African These pineapples measure roughly 5 inches high and 3 inches wide and have golden-colored skin and a bright yellow interior. They are sweet in flavor, very juicy and tender, and have a crunchy core that can be easily eaten.

Sugar Loaf This large pineapple has skin that is still green when ripe. It can grow up to 20 pounds, although the average size in the market is between 2 and 5 pounds. It's also sold under the name Baby Sugar Loaf.

choosing the best

Since you can't ripen a pineapple at home, it's important to choose one in prime condition. But most of the traditional "secrets" to selecting this fruit are, in fact, unreliable. Don't bother trying to judge the fruit by its color (it can range from green to yellow-gold depending on the variety), or by thumping it to test its "soundness," or by pulling a crown leaf to see how loose it is. Your best guide to quality is a label or tag indicating that the pineapple was jet-shipped from the grower. These pineapples are more likely

facts & tips

Pineapples do not grow on trees, as many people mistakenly think. They are the fruit of a bromeliad, rising from the center of the plant on a single spike surrounded by swordlike leaves. Though the pineapple plant is not the only bromeliad to produce edible fruit—there are several examples, such as feijoa (*page 287*)—it is certainly the most common.

serving suggestions

- Toss pineapple chunks in a blender along with plain yogurt or buttermilk and ice to make a smoothie.

- Substitute pineapple for tomato in a chunky salsa recipe.

- Grill or broil pineapple slices as they are, or sprinkled with a little brown sugar.

- Serve thinly sliced pineapple topped with a lightly sweetened and spiced yogurt or ricotta cheese.

- Add pineapple chunks to chicken or pork salad.

- Top a cheese pizza with finely diced pineapple.

- Make pineapple sauce instead of applesauce.

- Replace some of the zucchini in zucchini bread with finely chopped pineapple.

- Add pineapple wedges to meat or poultry kebabs and grill.

- Cook carrots in pineapple juice.

- Toss sliced strawberries, raspberries, pineapple wedges, and sliced bananas in pineapple juice for a dessert.

to be in prime condition (and also more expensive) than those brought in by truck or boat. Pineapples grown in Central America are often picked too green, which means they may be fibrous and not very sweet.

A large pineapple will have a greater proportion of edible flesh to rind and core, but small and medium-sized pineapples can still be delicious. The fruit should be firm and plump, as well as heavy for its size, with fresh-looking green leaves. Look out for bruises or soft spots, especially at the base. A good pineapple should be fragrant, but if the fruit is cold, the aroma may not be apparent. Never buy a pineapple with a sour or fermented smell.

▶ **When you get home** Although it will not increase in sweetness, a pineapple will get somewhat softer and juicier if it is left at room temperature for a day or two before serving. After ripening, it can be refrigerated for 3 to 5 days—no longer, or the fruit may be damaged by the cold. Refrigerate the pineapple in a plastic bag to help conserve its moisture content. Cut-up pineapple, stored in an airtight container, will keep for about a week.

enzyme action

Fresh pineapple contains an enzyme called bromelain, which digests protein. The fresh fruit is never used in gelatin molds because the bromelain would break down the protein in the gelatin and prevent it from setting. (Heating pineapple to the boiling point, however, inactivates the enzyme, so canned pineapple can be safely substituted.) Fresh pineapple should not be mixed with yogurt or cottage cheese until just before serving, or the bromelain will begin to digest the protein in these foods, too, changing their flavor and consistency.

On the plus side, this same enzyme action means you can use pineapple to tenderize meats and poultry. Include the fresh fruit (shredded, pureed, or juiced) in marinades.

preparing to use

Some stores have pineapple coring and shelling devices in their produce department to simplify the preparation of this fruit. If you take advantage of this convenience, you may lose some of the fruit you're paying for, as the device cannot be adjusted to the size of the individual fruit and may remove more flesh than necessary.

To cut pineapple into chunks, twist or cut off the leafy crown (or leave it on for a more decorative presentation). Using a large, heavy knife, halve the fruit lengthwise from bottom to top, then cut the two halves in half again to form quarters. Slice off the core from the top of each wedge-shaped quarter, then slide a knife between the flesh and rind to free the flesh. Cut the wedge of fruit as required for your recipe. Or use the pineapple rind as a serving "boat": After cutting between the flesh and rind, make crosswise cuts to divide the fruit into bite-sized pieces. Leave the pineapple pieces in place on the rind.

There are two methods for cutting round slices. It's easiest to cut off the top and bottom of the pineapple, then cut the unpeeled fruit into slices and peel and core each slice individually. Or, to peel the pineapple first, cut off the top and bottom, then stand the fruit on a cutting board and cut downward to remove the rind in wide strips; the "eyes" will remain intact. With a paring knife, follow the diagonal pattern made by the eyes, cutting spiraling grooves to remove them. Then cut the pineapple crosswise into slices and cut the core from each slice.

pistachios

Botanically related to peaches, mangoes, and cashews, pistachio nuts are thought to have originated in the Middle East, where they grew wild for thousands of years. In fact, the pistachio is one of the oldest edible nuts on the planet. During the time of King Solomon, the Queen of Sheba prized pistachio nuts and decreed that all of the pistachios produced in her domain be given to her and her court. Ancient Roman aristocrats and the emperor Vitellius considered pistachios to be a delicacy and a status food. Centuries later, medieval English cookery books reveal that pistachios were often used in various meat dishes and meat pies.

In its ripe state, the pistachio shell is partially open, revealing the nut within. This feature is unique to the pistachio and is why people in the Middle East refer to the pistachio as the "smiling pistachio" and the Chinese call it the "happy nut."

The natural color of the pistachio shell ranges from tan to yellow and various shades of green. In the 1930s, when pistachios were just becoming popular in the United States (and were being sold in vending machines), they were dyed red with vegetable dye to cover blemishes on the shell. Later on, the red dye served as a way for marketers to draw attention to the nut and to distinguish it from peanuts. Most companies no longer dye pistachios, though a few still do to appeal to traditionalists.

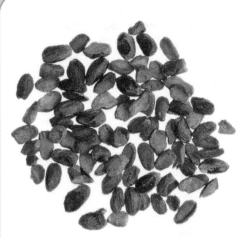

pistachios

nutritional profile

A nut whose buttery, sweet, delicate-flavored kernel is naturally green, the pistachio is rich in fiber, thiamin, vitamin E, iron, magnesium, and potassium. In addition, pistachios are an excellent source of monounsaturated fatty acids, a "good" fat that helps to reduce LDL ("bad") cholesterol levels. Compared with most nuts, the monounsaturated fat content of pistachios is high, similar to that of almonds. Plant sterols, substances believed to reduce the risk of heart disease and some cancers, are plentiful in pistachios.

in the market

Pistachios are usually marketed by the name of the country of origin rather than by variety. The western United States, Turkey, Iran, Syria, Italy, Greece, and Australia are the major growers of pistachios. The two varieties generally available in the market are the *Kerman* and the *Antep*. The Kerman is large in size with a vibrant green nut, while the Antep is smaller with a darker shell. Both types are found in supermarkets. Pistachios are available in-shell, roasted and salted, as well as shelled and unsalted.

Several producers are also marketing pistachios in and out of the shell, seasoned with hot chili peppers, lemon, and other seasonings.

PISTACHIOS / 1 ounce	
Calories	164
Protein (g)	6
Carbohydrate (g)	7
Dietary fiber (g)	3.1
Total fat (g)	14
Saturated fat (g)	1.7
Monounsaturated fat (g)	9.3
Polyunsaturated fat (g)	2.1
Cholesterol (mg)	0
Potassium (mg)	310
Sodium (mg)	2

KEY NUTRIENTS (%RDA/AI*)	
Thiamin	0.2 mg (19%)
Vitamin E	1.5 mg (10%)
Iron	1.9 mg (24%)
Magnesium	45 mg (11%)

*For more detailed information on RDA and AI, see page 88.

choosing the best

If you are buying in bulk, look for nuts whose shells are split or partially split open. This characteristic indicates ripeness. Any pistachio that is not partially open is not merely an inconvenience, but an indication that the shell contains an immature nut and should be discarded.

▶ When you get home As with most nuts, pistachios are best stored in the refrigerator or freezer to keep their oils from going rancid.

preparing to use

If you've bought pistachios in the shell and some are split, but not totally, use half of another shell to open the partially split ones.

If shelled pistachios have gotten soggy but are still good, they may be refreshed in a 200° oven for 10 to 15 minutes or until crisp.

There is no need to remove the skin from pistachios before using them.

serving suggestions

• Sprinkle chopped pistachios over poached pears for dessert.

• Fold chopped pistachios into lightly sweetened cottage cheese or part-skim ricotta and serve with fruit for dessert.

• Coat poultry or fish with a mixture of bread crumbs and finely chopped pistachios.

• Stir pistachios into stuffings for poultry.

• Steep chopped pistachios in warm milk until the milk has a pistachio flavor; discard the nuts and make a pudding with the milk.

• Substitute pistachios for pine nuts in pesto.

• Make pistachio butter: Place a handful of pistachios in a food processor or blender and puree until pasty; add salt if you like.

• Add pistachios to fruit, poultry, or vegetable salads.

• Add chopped pistachios to quick breads and muffins.

• Add pistachios to rice puddings.

plums

Anyone who likes plums has an abundance of choices—there are more than 140 varieties of this colorful fruit sold fresh in the United States. The plum is a drupe—a pitted fruit—related to the nectarine, peach, and apricot. But the plum is far more diverse than its relatives, coming in a wider range of shapes, sizes, and especially skin colors: Plums vary in color from green, pale yellow, or red, to the deepest purple-black or purple-blue. Plum shapes are also highly varied, from globular to an elongated oval or egg shape, pointed or bluntly rounded at either or at both ends. The size ranges from less than an inch to between 3 and 4 inches in diameter. The flavor varies from extremely sweet to quite tart.

Plums are native to a number of temperate regions around the world, including North America. Early settlers brought European varieties with them, forgoing wild American plums. In the late 19th century, more European varieties and new Asian plum types were cultivated and crossbred to create some of the myriad plum types now available. One of the most influential American plum breeders was the horticulturist Luther Burbank, who developed a variety called the Santa Rosa in 1907; today it accounts for a large percentage of the total domestic crop.

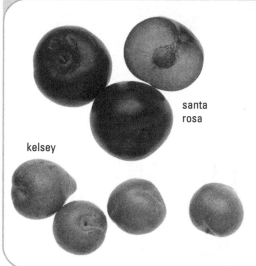

plums

santa rosa

kelsey

nutritional profile

Tasty and juicy, plums provide vitamin C and fiber. Plums are a modest source of vitamin E—though one plum has only 6 percent of the RDA, it is noteworthy, since finding vitamin E in a low-fat food is relatively rare. Dried plums (*see Prunes, page 492*) are a more concentrated source of the nutrients found in fresh plums.

in the market

About 20 varieties dominate the commercial supply of plums, and most are either Japanese or European varieties. In spite of our stronger cultural connections with Europe when it comes to food, it is actually the Japanese plum that most people would identify as the typical American plum.

Smaller, denser, and less juicy than Japanese varieties, *European-type plums* are often blue or purple, and their pits are usually freestone, meaning they separate easily from the flesh. The flesh is golden-yellow. The other main type of plums are the *Japanese plums*. (They are also known as salicina plums, after their Latin name, *Prunus salicina*.) Originally from China, these plums were introduced into Japan some 300 years ago, and were eventually brought from there to the United States. Most varieties have yellow or reddish flesh that is

PLUM / 1 large	
Calories	62
Protein (g)	1
Carbohydrate (g)	15
Dietary fiber (g)	1.7
Total fat (g)	0.7
Saturated fat (g)	0.1
Monounsaturated fat (g)	0.5
Polyunsaturated fat (g)	0.2
Cholesterol (mg)	0
Potassium (mg)	195
Sodium (mg)	0

KEY NUTRIENTS (%RDA/AI*)

Vitamin C	11 mg (12%)

*For more detailed information on RDA and AI, see page 88.

quite juicy and skin colors that range from crimson to black-red (but never purple). They are also clingstone fruits—that is, their flesh clings to the pit.

California French plums (d'Agen) These small, meaty European-style plums are descendants of the French *pruneaux d'Agen*, which are used in France to make prunes. Most of the California French plum crop is destined to be sold as dried plums, but you can occasionally find them fresh.

Casselman These smooth, red-skinned plums can be either fairly firm or slightly soft and are very sweet.

Damson This small, tart, blue-purple European-type plum is used mainly for jams and preserves.

El Dorado This dark, almost black-skinned plum has amber flesh and a sweet flavor even when firm.

Elephant Heart Distinguished by their dark, mottled skin, blood-red flesh, and heart shape, these plums are extremely sweet and juicy.

Empress These large, dark-blue plums have sweet greenish flesh and taste like prune plums.

European This small, slightly tart clingstone, is a red-skinned European-style plum.

Freedom This plum is sweet and juicy and has mottled light red skin.

Friar These are large, round, black-skinned plums with very sweet, amber flesh.

Greengage Distinguished by its deep-green skin, white dusty coating, and succulent yellow flesh, this European clingstone is very popular.

Kelsey This large heart-shaped, green-skinned freestone plum is firm and very sweet. The ripe Kelsey often has a red blush to the skin at the tip.

Laroda Similar to a Santa Rosa, these mature a little later, are slightly larger, and are very juicy and sweet.

> ➤ *phytochemicals in*
> ## plums
> The plant pigments that make plums purple are called anthocyanins. These robust phytochemicals behave as potent antioxidants.

serving suggestions

- Sauté sliced plums and serve alongside grilled meat or poultry.

- Toss sliced plums in a salad with arugula, red onion, and crisp turkey bacon.

- For a wonderful dessert, poach halved plums in red wine or port along with cinnamon, orange zest, sugar, and a touch of pepper.

- Add diced prune plums to muffins, quick breads, and pancake batter.

- Puree plums with yogurt and a little honey for a quick smoothie.

- Add diced plums to a blueberry pie recipe.

- Make a plum salsa to serve with baked tortilla chips.

- Thinly slice plums and add to a sandwich with roast turkey, romaine lettuce, and Dijon mustard on whole-grain bread.

- Make plum sauce instead of applesauce.

Mirabelle This small, round, yellow plum is sweet and full-flavored.

Nubiana This large, slightly flat, purple-black, amber-fleshed plum is similar to the El Dorado.

Plumcot This is a cross between an apricot and a plum, though it more closely resembles a plum. Some varietal names of plumcots are *Plum Parfait* and *Flavorella*.

Pluot This is another hybrid, a cross between a plumcot and a plum, so though there is apricot somewhere in the mix, this fruit looks distinctly like a plum. It is also sold as *Dinosaur Eggs.* It has purplish skin and sweet flesh that ranges in color from amber to red. This hybrid has a long-lasting flavor.

Prune plums (Italian prune plums) This deep purple plum is covered in a light dusty film that protects it from the weather. Under the purple skin, the flesh is greenish-amber and very sweet. These are tangy when firm, and sweet when mature.

Santa Rosa This very popular plum has reddish-purple skin and red-tinged amber flesh. Its taste is tangy-sweet.

▶ Availability The domestic plum season extends from May through October, with Japanese types coming on the market first and peaking in August, followed by European varieties in the fall.

choosing the best

Plums should be plump and well-colored for their variety. If the fruit yields to gentle pressure, it is ready to eat; however, you can buy plums that are fairly firm but not rock hard and let them soften at home. They will not, however, increase in sweetness. Ripe plums will be slightly soft at the stem and tip, but watch out for shriveled skin, mushy spots, or breaks in the skin.

▶ When you get home To soften hard plums, place several in a loosely closed paper bag and leave them at room temperature for a day or two; when softened, transfer them to the refrigerator. Ripe plums can be refrigerated for up to 3 days.

preparing to use

Wash plums before eating or cooking them. They'll be juiciest (and to most palates taste sweetest) at room temperature. To pit European-style plums and other freestone types, cut the fruit in half along the "seam," twist the halves apart, and lift out the pit. To slice or quarter clingstone plums, use a sharp paring knife and cut through the flesh toward the pit.

Japanese plums are most commonly eaten raw, although they can be poached. European plums are better for cooking as they are easier to pit and their firmer, drier flesh holds up well when heated.

---

facts & tips

Umeboshi plums are a sour, pickled yellow fruit that's served as a condiment in both Chinese and Japanese cuisine and used to make Chinese plum sauce. Though they are called plums, they are actually a type of Japanese apricot.

pomegranates

The pomegranate (whose name means "seeded apple" in Middle French) has appeared throughout history as a symbol of fertility, royalty, hope, and abundance. Celebrated in art, mythology, religious texts, and literature, pomegranates appear on floor mosaics in Pompeii, in Egyptian papyrii, and in the Old Testament, under the name of rimmon. In fact, the pomegranate may be the fruit that led to Adam and Eve's expulsion from the Garden of Eden. In Greek mythology, the pomegranate was a symbol of procreation and abundance (perhaps because the average pomegranate has about 800 seeds). And, according to Greek mythology, the reason we have winter is because Demeter (the goddess of the harvest) goes into mourning once a year when her daughter, Persephone, returns to live in the underworld, a life sentence imposed on her because she ate seven pomegranate seeds.

About the size of a large orange or apple, the pomegranate has a tough, dark red or brownish-red rind. Encased within a white, spongy, inedible membrane are the seeds. And surrounding the seeds is the pomegranate's juicy, translucent scarlet-red flesh. Possibly one of the reasons the pomegranate isn't as popular as it deserves is that it takes time and care to get to the seeds, but it is well worth the effort (though Persephone might disagree).

pomegranates

nutritional profile

The sweet edible flesh around the seeds provides vitamin B$_6$, vitamin C, and lots of potassium. Pomegranate juice also provides these nutrients.

POMEGRANATE / 1 medium	
Calories	105
Protein (g)	2
Carbohydrate (g)	27
Dietary fiber (g)	0.9
Total fat (g)	0.5
Saturated fat (g)	0.1
Monounsaturated fat (g)	0.1
Polyunsaturated fat (g)	0.1
Cholesterol (mg)	0
Potassium (mg)	399
Sodium (mg)	5

KEY NUTRIENTS (%RDA/AI*)	
Vitamin B$_6$	0.2 mg (10%)
Vitamin C	9 mg (10%)

*For more detailed information on RDA and AI, see page 88.

other pomegranate products

Pomegranate juice Pomegranate juice (found in health-food stores and ethnic groceries in Russian or Middle Eastern neighborhoods) comes both unsweetened and in its "cocktail" form. The unsweetened juice is quite tart; you can add a bit of honey or sugar to taste. The "cocktail" version, which is quite high in sugar, can have as little as 20 percent juice.

Pomegranate molasses This highly concentrated form of pomegranate juice (it's as thick as molasses, hence its name) is a traditional ingredient in Middle Eastern and Russian cooking. It is available in ethnic markets. Not only does it concentrate the pomegranate's healthful compounds, it's a delicious addition to foods and cooking. With a tartness that has a sweet edge, pomegranate molasses can be used the way you might use balsamic vinegar. There are also some American versions of this thick syrup from California, often sold as pomegranate essence.

in the market

In California—the principal commercial producer of pomegranates in this country—there are numerous types of pomegranates, but these varietal names are not used in the marketplace. The most common are the *Wonderful* (and an early-maturing version of it called the *Early Wonderful*) and the *Granada*.

▶ Availability One of the few fruits in this country that still has a season, domestic pomegranates are available from September through the beginning of January, with their peak in late October through November. There are occasionally imports available other times of the year.

choosing the best

Pick up the fruit to feel its weight (the seeds represent about 52 percent of the weight of the whole fruit). If it feels light for its size, select a heavier one. The skin should appear shiny, taut and thin, without cracks or splits.

▶ When you get home Store whole pomegranates in a dark, cool place for up to a month and in the refrigerator for up to 2 months.

preparing to use

Pomegranate juice is used to make jelly, juice, sauces, vinaigrettes, and marinades. The whole seeds can be sprinkled on salads, desserts, and used as a garnish for meat, poultry, or fish.

To remove the seeds, slice the crown end off and gently score the rind vertically in several places from top to bottom. Place the pomegranate in a large, deep bowl of water. Carefully break the sections apart, prying the seeds from their anchors on the pith with your fingers. Remove the thin membranes that separate the clusters of seeds (the seeds will sink and the rind and membranes will float). Skim off and discard the skin and membranes and drain the seeds into a colander. The seeds can be refrigerated for up to 3 days. To freeze them, place the seeds in an airtight container; they will keep in the freezer for about 6 months. When the seeds thaw, they will no longer be good for eating out of hand, but they will be fine for extracting the juice. In fact, the freezing process will break down the cell walls of the pulp surrounding the seeds and as they thaw, they will naturally give up their juice.

To make juice, place the pomegranate seeds in a food processor or blender and process until a juice is formed. Strain the seeds out of the juice through a fine-meshed sieve or a strainer lined with cheesecloth. If you've made pomegranate juice, it can be frozen for about 6 months in an airtight container.

Generally, a medium-sized pomegranate yields about ¾ cup of seeds or ½ cup of juice.

➤ *phytochemicals in* pomegranates

Pomegranate juice is a concentrated source of phytochemicals and may have two to three times the antioxidant power of equal quantities of green tea or red wine.

• Two antioxidant phytochemicals found in pomegranates are catechins and anthocyanins (the pigments that lend pomegranates their crimson color).

• Ellagic acid, plentiful in pomegranates, is under review for its potential to fight off carcinogenic agents.

facts & tips

Grenadine, which gets its name from the French word for pomegranate, *grenade*, is a ruby-colored syrup used to flavor drinks and desserts. Once made from pomegranate juice, sadly it is now made from sugar syrup and food coloring.

pork

Because it is the source of bacon, sausage, spareribs, hot dogs, and other high-fat products, pork has gained a bad reputation in recent decades. The pork industry has tried to counter this, fairly successfully, by promoting pork as the "other white meat." According to one definition of white/dark meat, which measures certain proteins in the meat, pork is indeed closer to chicken than to red meat (beef). But it still depends on which pork cuts and products you choose.

In fact, pork generally has become leaner over the years. Thanks to changes in the breeding and feeding of hogs, many cuts are at least 30 percent leaner than they were 20 years ago. In fact, some cuts are actually among the leanest meats: Well-trimmed tenderloin, for instance, has almost as little fat as skinless chicken breast. And the fat in pork is slightly less saturated than that in beef or lamb.

nutritional profile

Pork provides high-quality protein as well as significant amounts of thiamin, riboflavin, niacin, and selenium. It also has good amounts of vitamin B_6, vitamin B_{12}, iron, potassium, and zinc. Even so, fattier cuts of pork and pork-based meats (such as sausage, bacon, and ribs)—still the most popular fare—are hard to justify on a heart-healthy diet. And pork, like all meats and poultry, contains 20 to 25 milligrams of cholesterol per ounce, whether it's lean or fatty.

As with beef, the guidelines for including pork in your diet are to choose lean cuts (such as tenderloin and center loin or extra-lean ham), to eat small portions (3 to 4 ounces cooked), and to trim all visible fat before cooking. However, unlike beef, you can't rely on a grading system for pork to give you a clue to the fat content of the cut. Because fresh pork is consistent in quality, there is no grading system used. But, like beef, pork is inspected by the USDA for wholesomeness.

It's important to be aware that if you're trying to cut down on sodium, you need to make an effort to avoid cured pork products such as bacon, ham, and other cold cuts. Since salt and other sodium-containing substances are necessary for curing the meat, cured pork products can be exceptionally high in this mineral—just 3 ounces of cured ham, for example, can contain almost one-half of the maximum recommended daily intake of sodium. Some lower-sodium products are available, however.

in the market

Like beef, pork is divided into primal, or wholesale, cuts that refer to the part of the animal they come from. Pork is further subdivided into retail cuts, which are the ones found in the supermarket. For fresh pork, the cut determines the fat content and cooking method.

PORK TENDERLOIN 3 ounces cooked	
Calories	140
Protein (g)	24
Carbohydrate (g)	0
Dietary fiber (g)	0
Total fat (g)	4.1
Saturated fat (g)	1.4
Monounsaturated fat (g)	1.6
Polyunsaturated fat (g)	0.4
Cholesterol (mg)	67
Potassium (mg)	372
Sodium (mg)	48

KEY NUTRIENTS (%RDA/AI*)	
Thiamin	0.8 mg (67%)
Riboflavin	0.3 mg (26%)
Niacin	4.0 mg (25%)
Vitamin B_6	0.4 mg (21%)
Vitamin B_{12}	0.5 mcg (19%)
Iron	1.3 mg (16%)
Selenium	41 mcg (74%)
Zinc	2.2 mg (20%)

*For more detailed information on RDA and AI, see page 88.

Only one-third of the pork produced each year is sold fresh. The rest is cured, smoked, or processed. Curing was once a method of preserving meat so that it would be available throughout the winter. Today, pork is cured for flavor; and though the method lengthens cured pork's storage life, most cured pork must be kept refrigerated.

Fresh and cured pork are very different, therefore they are discussed separately below.

fresh pork

Leg Fresh hams come from this section of the hog. The whole leg can be sold as a ham that weighs 10 to 14 pounds. More often, it is divided into *butt half* and *shank half* (the butt half is much meatier). These cuts are sold with or without the bone. You may also find *top leg (inside roast)*. Sometimes slices are cut from the leg and sold as *pork cutlets*. The leg can be roasted or braised, and leg cutlets can be broiled, braised, or sautéed.

Loin This part of the pig supplies the largest number of fresh cuts and also the leanest, with meat that is tender and flavorful. The loin is divided into three parts: *blade loin,* nearest the shoulder; *center loin;* and *sirloin,* nearest the leg. You may also find *top loin chops* and *center loin cutlets*. The cuts from

EXTRA-LEAN HAM 3 ounces	
Calories	123
Protein (g)	18
Carbohydrate (g)	0
Dietary fiber (g)	0
Total fat (g)	4.7
Saturated fat (g)	1.5
Monounsaturated fat (g)	2.2
Polyunsaturated fat (g)	0.5
Cholesterol (mg)	45
Potassium (mg)	244
Sodium (mg)	1,023

KEY NUTRIENTS (%RDA/AI*)	
Thiamin	0.6 mg (53%)
Riboflavin	0.2 mg (13%)
Niacin	3.4 mg (21%)
Vitamin B_6	0.3 mg (20%)
Vitamin B_{12}	0.6 mcg (23%)
Iron	1.3 mg (16%)
Selenium	17 mcg (30%)
Zinc	2.5 mg (22%)

For more detailed information on RDA and AI, see page 88.

COMPARING PORK CUTS 3 ounces cooked

As a general rule of thumb, 4 ounces of raw boneless pork will yield 3 ounces of cooked pork. For 3 ounces of cooked pork from a bone-in cut, you would start with about 8 ounces raw. Most retail cuts of pork will be trimmed to ¼ inch or ⅛ inch of fat (the exception being some cured hams). Before cooking, you should trim all remaining visible fat. The values below are for pork whose external fat has been fully trimmed. The cuts are organized by percentage of calories from fat, from most to least.

	Calories	Fat (g)	% Calories from Fat	Saturated Fat (g)	Cholesterol (mg)
Country-style ribs	279	22	71	7.8	78
Spareribs	338	26	69	9.4	103
Ground pork	253	18	64	6.6	80
Ham, fresh	232	15	58	5.5	80
Shoulder chops	220	14	57	5.1	81
Boston butt, fresh	196	12	55	4.1	77
Picnic shoulder, fresh	194	11	51	3.7	81
Cured ham	151	7.7	46	2.7	50
Pork cutlets	180	8.8	44	3.1	76
Center loin chops	172	6.9	36	2.5	70
Canned ham, extra-lean	130	4.9	34	1.6	47
Cured ham, extra-lean	123	4.7	34	1.5	45
Tenderloin	140	4.1	26	1.4	67

either end are not as tender as the center loin, and thus the center loin is the most expensive. You'll find both roasts and chops with or without the bone. Thick chops—an inch or more in thickness—can be broiled, sautéed, or braised. Roasts can be roasted or braised.

The *tenderloin,* which comes from the center loin, is often sold on its own as a roast, and is also included as part of loin or sirloin chops. It is about a foot long and 2 inches in diameter at its thickest point. It's well worth the price; not only is the meat exceptionally tender, but the tenderloin is the leanest cut of fresh pork. Roast or braise the whole tenderloin; it cooks rapidly. Or slice it into medallions and sauté the slices.

The loin is also the source of the impressive *crown roast,* which is two *center rib roasts* fastened together in a circle to form a hollow that can be stuffed and then roasted. Crown roasts are usually ordered from a butcher, since the backbone must be removed or cracked and the rib ends must be trimmed. The shoulder end of the loin produces *country-style ribs,* which are not true spareribs (spareribs come from the side). Meatier and leaner than spareribs, they can be braised, broiled, or roasted.

Shoulder From this section come two large pork roasts, *Boston (or shoulder) butt* and *picnic shoulder,* which is really the foreleg of the pig. A Boston butt roast is flavorful, but contains a lot of sinew; it is best braised to dissolve this connective tissue. Picnic shoulder can be roasted or braised. You can also

specialty hams

There are many ways of curing and smoking hams, each producing different flavors. Here are some of the different types of cured ham:

Black Forest ham This is a German ham that is smoked over pine wood. It is often dipped in beef blood to produce its black surface. Some Black Forest hams are produced in the United States, but beware, they may have brine or water added.

Jamon serrano Many consider this Spanish dry-cured ham, which is produced using methods similar to those used in Italy for making Parma prosciutto, to be the finest in the world. Compared to prosciutto, it has a sweet, earthy, and less-salty flavor, and a texture that is a bit drier and smoother. Like prosciutto, serrano ham should be eaten in wafer-thin slices.

Smithfield ham State law specifies that these country hams must originate within the city limits of Smithfield, Virginia. Until 1966, they had to come from pigs fed nothing but peanuts, but that regulation was dropped because of the cost of raising peanut-fed hogs.

Prosciutto This golden-pink Italian-style ham is dry-cured and air-dried, but not smoked. It is usually eaten uncooked, often thinly sliced and served with figs or melon. When added to cooked dishes, it's added at the last minute. The most famous, called Parma, is made in Parma, Italy, and has recently become quite popular in this country. Prosciutto is also made in the United States and some is imported from Switzerland and Canada.

Southampton ham This refers to hams produced in Southampton County, Virginia, just a few miles from Smithfield. Southamptons are traditionally short shanked and a bit milder than Smithfields.

Westphalian ham From Germany's Westphalian forest, this ham is smoked with juniper berries and beechwood. It has very dark flesh and is similar to Black Forest ham.

cut these roasts into chunks (or have the butcher do it for you), then marinate them, and grill or broil them.

Side The only fresh cut from this section is *spareribs.* These are extremely fatty. They are best roasted, broiled, or braised; you can reduce the fat in spareribs if you parboil them before cooking.

cured pork: bacon

Bacon Pork belly, which comes from the side of the hog, is called bacon once it has been cured and smoked. A solution of brine and water is injected into the pork belly; a smoked flavor may also be injected, or the bacon may be smoked after it is cured. Bacon is very high in fat, saturated fat, and sodium.

Canadian bacon A leaner alternative to regular bacon, Canadian bacon is smoked and cured pork loin. (In Canada and Great Britain, it is called back bacon.) It's used in much the same way as bacon, though it resembles ham in appearance and taste.

Pancetta Pancetta is an Italian-style bacon; the whole pork belly is rolled into a sausage shape and sold either rolled or sliced.

cured pork: ham

Ham True ham is pork leg that has been cured and sometimes smoked. There are many types of ham on the market. Most hams are brine (or wet) cured, whereby the pork leg is injected with a solution of water, salt, sodium nitrite, and sugar. Some hams are dry-cured: The meat is rubbed with salt, sugar, sodium nitrate, sodium nitrite, and seasonings. These may also be called country hams. The dry-curing process draws out moisture and intensifies the color and flavor of the meat.

Most hams are sold "fully cooked," that is, they have been cooked to a high enough internal temperature to make them safe to eat. Hams that require cooking will be marked as such on the label.

The types of ham found in the market include *bone-in hams,* which contain the shank bone and are available whole or in sections; *semi-boneless hams*, which have had the shank bone removed, leaving the round leg bone; *boneless hams,* which have been rolled or molded and packed in a casing; and *canned hams,* brine-cured ham pieces that have been molded, vacuum-sealed, and fully cooked. There is also *picnic ham,* which is a cured-pork product, but is not a true ham because it comes from the shoulder, not the leg.

Ham is further divided by the percentage of protein it contains by weight. Because the curing solution can add greatly to the weight of the ham, the USDA has categorized ham in the following way: Products labeled "ham" have no added water and are at least 20.5 percent protein. "Ham with natural juices" is at least 18.5 percent protein. "Ham–added water" is at least 17 per-

---

pork safety

Don't overcook pork, unless you like it well-done. Medium is okay. Many people, worried about trichinosis, still think they have to cook chops and roasts to the consistency of shoe leather. But trichinosis in pigs has been on the decline for decades, thanks to improved production methods, and it has been virtually eliminated from pork in the United States. In any case, the parasite is destroyed at about 140°. To allow for a margin of safety, the USDA recommends cooking pork to an internal temperature of 160° (instead of 170°, or well-done), which leaves the meat juicy, with a pink blush in the middle. The leaner the meat, the more quickly it will cook.

cent protein. "Ham and water product" can contain any amount of water, but must state the percentage of added ingredients on the label.

You'll also find some hams labeled lean or extra-lean. Lean hams must contain no more than 10 percent fat by weight; extra-lean hams, no more than 5 percent.

choosing the best

Look for cuts of fresh pork that are well trimmed of fat; retailers are now trimming the external fat on pork to about ⅛ inch. The meat should be pinkish-gray to pink in color; the leg and shoulder cuts tend to be darker than the loin cuts. Pork tenderloin is deep red, however. The fat should be creamy white. The bones, if present, should be red and spongy at the ends; the whiter the bone ends, the older the animal was when it was slaughtered and the less tender the meat will be.

When choosing cured pork products, be sure to read the label. It will tell you what type of product you're getting and also give you important information about how to cook and store it.

► **When you get home** Since the fat in pork is less saturated that that of beef, it turns rancid faster. Fresh pork will keep for 2 to 3 days in the refrigerator depending on the size of the cut (smaller cuts spoil more quickly). Keep pork in its original store wrapping in the coldest part of the refrigerator. Cooked pork will keep in the refrigerator for 4 to 5 days.

Cured pork products keep much longer than fresh pork. Vacuum-packed bacon is often marked with a "sell by" date; the unopened bacon will keep for a week after this date. Once opened, it will keep for about a week if tightly wrapped. Slab bacon will keep for several weeks if tightly wrapped and

serving suggestions

Instead of making pork or ham the centerpiece of a meal, use it as one of many components in a mixed-ingredient dish, such as a soup, salad, stir-fry, or casserole.

• *For a salad:* Toss thin strips of smoked ham with chunks of cooked sweet potatoes, apples, and romaine lettuce.

• *For a soup:* Grind pork tenderloin; season with oregano, salt, pepper, and Parmesan. Shape into tiny meatballs and drop into a simmering pot of minestrone soup or chicken broth.

• *For a sandwich:* Place broiled pork cutlets on whole-grain rolls with mustard, arugula, and thinly sliced red onion.

• *For stir-fried rice:* Cut chunks of ham and sauté with strips of red bell peppers, leeks, cooked brown rice, and toasted pine nuts.

• *For a "pizza":* Scatter slivers of prosciutto over pita bread. Top with mozzarella and sliced tomatoes and bake.

• *For a casserole:* Add bits of pork and barbecue sauce to a bean dish to make your own pork and beans.

refrigerated. Canadian bacon will keep for 3 to 4 days if sliced, up to a week if in large pieces.

Cured hams keep for about a week in the refrigerator. If the ham is vacuum-packed or sealed in plastic, leave it in its wrapping. If not, rewrap it tightly in aluminum foil. Canned hams should be refrigerated; they will keep for up to 6 months if unopened. Once opened, tightly wrap the leftovers and use within a week. Some canned hams do not need refrigeration, but be sure to check the label. If in doubt, refrigerate. Dry-cured hams should be refrigerated; they'll keep for 6 months.

preparing to use

Trim all external fat from fresh pork before cooking. Be sure to wash everything that comes into contact with the raw meat in hot soapy water to guard against contamination. Cured hams that are not marked "fully cooked" must be treated like fresh pork. Even hams that are marked fully cooked may benefit from cooking to improve flavor.

The surface of country-style hams may be coated with a mold that is a normal part of the curing process. These hams must be scrubbed with a stiff-bristled brush to remove the mold and excess salt on the surface. The ham must then be soaked for several hours and then simmered before baking. Most country-style hams come with detailed directions for preparation.

about sausage

Technically, sausage can be made from any kind of chopped or ground meat—even from poultry or fish—but most of the familiar varieties are pork-based. Sausage may be stuffed into a casing or sold in bulk like ground beef.

There are four types of sausage: *fresh,* which is made from raw meat and sometimes contains grains (such as rice) or bread crumbs, must be thoroughly cooked before eating; *semi-dry,* a smoked and partially dried sausage; *dry,* which is fully dried and may be smoked or not; and *cooked,* which is ready to eat, but may be served hot. It is important that you know which type of sausage you are buying so you can prepare it correctly.

For all types of sausage, the meat is highly seasoned and sometimes smoked; it's the seasoning that gives each variety of sausage its individual flavor. For example, fresh Mexican chorizo sausage is seasoned with vinegar, garlic, cumin, and hot peppers. Another fresh sausage, Italian link, is seasoned with garlic, wine, fennel, and for the hot variety, red pepper. Polish kielbasa, a semi-dry sausage, is usually smoked and contains garlic, pepper, paprika, and other herbs.

Sausage is very high in fat, calories, and sodium. Dry and semi-dry sausages may have been cured with sodium nitrate and sodium nitrite. When you eat sausage, do so in moderation. Use it as a flavoring in dishes, rather than as the main course.

Every scrap of federally inspected meat from the animal carcass can be used in making sausage, and sometimes animal fat is added. Blood sausage is made from blood, pork fat, and seasonings. Liverwurst is made from pork liver. Mortadella, which can be made from pork or beef, is larded with fat.

Fresh sausage will keep for only a day or two in the refrigerator. Semi-dry sausages will keep for 2 to 3 weeks; dry sausages for 4 to 6 weeks. Cooked sausages will keep for a week.

potatoes

A member of the nightshade family of plants, the potato is a tuber—a swollen underground stem (not a root) that stores surplus carbohydrates to feed the leafy green plant sprouting above the soil. Left undisturbed, the potato plant will bear fruit resembling small green tomatoes. But unlike its relatives—including bell peppers, tomatoes, and eggplants—the fruit isn't edible; only the tuber is.

Though cultivated by the ancient Incas high in Peru's mountains thousands of years ago, this humble tuber was not fully accepted as an edible food in Europe until quite late, sometime in the 16th century. One reason that it took so long to become accepted was the fear that the potato was poisonous—a fear that undoubtedly stemmed from the fact that all parts of the potato plant (except for the edible tuber) are indeed indigestible and can cause illness.

The myth that the potato was an inedible poisonous plant was luckily debunked by Sir Walter Raleigh, who initiated interest in potatoes when he planted them on an estate he owned near Cork, Ireland. The Irish soon realized the value and benefits of growing and eating potatoes. However, the dependence on this food in that country became so great that when the crop failed in the 1846, it led to a famine.

The potato was introduced to the United States sometime in the mid–17th century. And although French fries (called "French fried") were introduced to the country when Thomas Jefferson served them at Monticello and at the White House during his presidency in the early 1800s, they didn't become popular until around 1900.

Today the potato is the world's most widely consumed and economically important vegetable. In this country alone, per capita consumption is about 140 pounds per person (the equivalent of one large baked potato every single day). Sadly more than 60 percent of that is in the form of fast foods or snack foods, which bring with them unhealthy fats and high levels of sodium.

nutritional profile

Only a few other foods are as wholesome as a potato. Not only does it contain complex carbohydrates, but it also supplies protein and ample vitamins and minerals such as vitamin B_6, vitamin C, potassium, and iron. And potato skin is a rich source of fiber.

in the market

Potatoes are often differentiated according to age. They may be sold soon after they are dug, or kept in cold storage for up to a year before sale. But only potatoes that are freshly harvested may be called "new." Many consumers believe that "new" simply denotes a small, round red or white potato; but true

potatoes

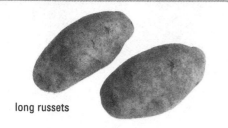

long russets

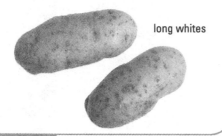

long whites

BAKING POTATO 4 ounces baked, with skin	
Calories	133
Protein (g)	3
Carbohydrate (g)	31
Dietary fiber (g)	2.9
Total fat (g)	0.1
Saturated fat (g)	0
Monounsaturated fat (g)	0
Polyunsaturated fat (g)	0.1
Cholesterol (mg)	0
Potassium (mg)	510
Sodium (mg)	10

KEY NUTRIENTS (%RDA/AI*)	
Thiamin	0.1 mg (11%)
Niacin	2.0 mg (13%)
Vitamin B_6	0.4 mg (25%)
Vitamin C	16 mg (17%)
Iron	1.7 mg (21%)

*For more detailed information on RDA and AI, see page 88.

new potatoes have thin "feathering" skins that can be brushed off with your fingers. Mature potatoes, by contrast, have thick skins, frequently with a meshlike netting on their surface. New potatoes may be as small as marbles or as large as full-sized mature potatoes. They have a high moisture and sugar content, so they cook quickly and have a delicate, sweet flavor.

However, in the supermarket, potatoes are more likely to be labeled according to their end use: baking potatoes, all-purpose potatoes, or boiling potatoes. *Baking potatoes* have a low-moisture, high-starch content, with a so-called "mealy" flesh, making them fluffier than other potatoes when baked or mashed. (They are not suited to cutting into chunks for salad, because they will fall apart when cooked.) *Boiling potatoes,* on the other hand, have high moisture and low starch and what is called "waxy flesh." These potatoes do not do well when mashed (they get gluey) and are best for potato salads because they hold their shape well when cut into chunks. *All-purpose potatoes* can be used either as baking potatoes or boiling potatoes, since their starch and sugar content are caught between that of the mealy-fleshed and the waxy-fleshed potatoes.

Moreover, potatoes can be found in dozens of shapes and skin colors, from yellow and tan to blue and purple.

Blue potatoes There are a number of blue-fleshed potatoes. They have grayish-blue skin, dark blue flesh, and a delicate flavor. Two varieties of blue potatoes are *Blue Carib* and *All Blue.* These potatoes can be a challenge to eat, not because of their taste, which is delicious, but because they turn an unpleasant gray when cooked.

Fingerlings These are the "new potato" version of long (rather than round) potatoes. They get their name from the fact that they are sold when they are about the size of a finger. Many of the larger varieties of potatoes, such as russets, long whites, and purple potatoes, can be found in their fingerling form.

Finnish yellow wax This waxy-fleshed potato has deep yellow flesh. Its rich taste and "buttery" appearance may convince you to forgo butter.

Long russets Typified by the Russet Burbank, these are the favorites among baking potatoes and are the leading variety grown. (Most *"Idaho"* baking potatoes are Russet Burbanks.) These large, oval-shaped potatoes, which can weigh up to 18 ounces each, have a hard brown skin and starchy flesh. Typical of a russet is a fine netting pattern over the skin called "russeting."

Long whites The *White Rose* is one of the better-known varieties of these all-purpose potatoes. When new, they are thin-skinned and waxy; when mature, they are starchy and weigh an average of half a pound.

Marble potatoes These are tiny (yes, marble-sized) potatoes. They are very small versions of one or another of the round red or round white potato varieties.

Purple potatoes Purple potatoes have a deep-purple skin and flesh, which fades as the potatoes cook.

Round reds These red, smooth-skinned boiling potatoes, notably the *Red LaSoda* and *Red Pontiac,* are most commonly sold "new," or small. But they are also available in larger sizes.

Round whites The *Katahdin* (the principal variety grown in Maine) and the *Kennebec* are representative of these multipurpose potatoes. They have a light tan skin and are smaller than the long whites, averaging three per pound.

Yukon gold These are yellow-fleshed all-purpose potatoes.

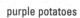

purple potatoes

choosing the best

If possible, choose individual potatoes from a bulk display. Buy a large bag (5 or 10 pounds) only if you can check the condition of the potatoes through the packaging—and if you are sure of using all of them before they spoil. Look for clean, smooth, well-shaped potatoes, free from sprouts. (A sprouting potato, though edible, has started to age and may contain increased amounts of solanine, a naturally occurring toxin.) Potatoes should feel firm, the "eyes"—the buds from which sprouts can grow—should be few and shallow, and the skins should be free of cracks, wrinkles, or dampness. Reject any with green-tinged skins, indicating improper storage (and the presence of solanine), and those with black spots, bruises, or other discolorations.

what to do about the skin

Ounce for ounce, the skin is by far the most nutritious part of the potato: The skin contains most of the iron, calcium, and fiber. However, you should not eat the skin if it has a greenish tinge. The green is chlorophyll, and although not harmful in itself, it may signal a high concentration of a toxic alkaloid called solanine. Potatoes normally contain harmless quantities of this bitter compound, small amounts of which contribute to the vegetable's characteristic flavor; it's only when exposed to light (the green tinge is called "sunburn") or extreme temperatures after harvesting that they develop larger amounts. Eating such damaged potatoes can cause cramps, diarrhea, and headache.

Potatoes that have begun to sprout also contain lots of solanine; however, the concentration in undamaged potatoes is so low that you would have to eat about 12 pounds of potatoes at one sitting to be adversely affected.

If you discover that your potatoes have turned green or have sprouted, do the following: Peel away the green areas of skin taking off at least ⅛ inch of the flesh beneath as well. To remove sprouts, dig them out with a sharp paring knife.

The USDA has established grades for potatoes, according to appearance and size. "U.S. Extra No. 1" is a premium grade, followed by "U.S. No. 1," which is the most common grade and denotes potatoes that have few defects and are at at least 1¾ inches in diameter. However, grade labeling is not required, and many potatoes are not marked.

▶ **When you get home** Few modern homes have root cellars, but a cool (45° to 50°), dark, dry place makes the best storage area, as light and warmth encourage sprouting. Don't put potatoes in the refrigerator or anywhere below 45°. Their starch will turn to sugar, giving them an undesirable sweet taste (although leaving them at room temperature for a few days allows the sugar to reconvert to starch). Keep the potatoes in a burlap, brown paper, or perforated plastic bag. Check them occasionally and remove any that have sprouted, softened, or shriveled; a bad one can adversely affect the condition of the ones remaining.

Mature potatoes will keep for up to 2 months under optimum conditions; new potatoes are more perishable and should be used within a week of purchase. Don't wash potatoes before storing, or they will spoil more quickly. And don't store onions together with potatoes: The gases given off by onions accelerate the decay of potatoes, and vice versa. Neither raw nor most cooked potatoes freeze well; however, mashed potatoes may be packed into containers and frozen.

preparing to use

Potato skin is an excellent source of fiber, so try to leave it on. But if you decide to peel it because you don't like the taste of the skin, do so carefully. Use a swivel-bladed vegetable peeler to remove the thinnest possible layer, and thus preserve the nutrients just below the skin. Better yet, simply scrub unpeeled potatoes under cold water before cooking; remove any sprouts, green spots, or deep eyes with a sharp paring knife.

Potatoes occasionally turn gray or dark after they are boiled; this color change may be caused by the conditions under which they were grown or stored. It's impossible to tell which potatoes will turn dark, but the discoloration does not affect flavor, texture, or nutritional value. Contact with aluminum or iron will also discolor potatoes, so cook them in stainless steel pots. For the same reason, raw potatoes should not be cut with a carbon steel (nonstainless) knife. If exposed to air, peeled raw potatoes will also discolor. Cook the potatoes immediately in a pot of water that has already been brought to a boil. And if you are interrupted while preparing them, place them in a bowl of cold water, then add a few drops of lemon juice or vinegar. This will help to keep the potatoes white.

---

low-fat chips & fries

Scrub and very thinly slice a baking potato (a vegetable peeler makes the thinnest slices). Lightly coat a baking sheet with nonstick cooking spray or cooking oil, place the slices in a single layer, spray or brush them lightly with oil, and sprinkle with paprika. Bake in a 400° oven for 30 minutes, turning the chips halfway through the cooking time. Reduce the oven temperature to 300° and bake for 15 to 20 minutes longer, or until the chips are crisp. For oven fries, cut the potatoes into ½-inch-thick sticks and proceed as above, but bake the potatoes in a 450° oven for 35 to 40 minutes, turning them occasionally.

---

facts & tips

Some people mistakenly think that potatoes are a fattening food, which is not true. It's the things that people usually have with potatoes—butter, sour cream, mayonnaise, gravy—that are fattening. Nutritionally, speaking, the less you add to a potato, the better. Or use it as a back-drop for healthful, low-fat toppings such as lemon juice, chopped fresh herbs, or minced sun-dried tomatoes.

prunes

The dried fruit we know as a prune has recently had its name officially changed to dried plum. Though there are several types of fresh plum that are sold in their dried form, far and away the commonest is the prune plum. The prune plum is a variety of plum with a higher sugar content, firmer flesh, smaller pit, and a higher acid content—characteristics that make for a meatier, more flavorful dried fruit.

In the transition from fresh to dried, the plums are first allowed to mature on the tree until they are fully ripe and have developed their maximum sweetness. They are then mechanically harvested and dried for 15 to 24 hours under closely monitored conditions of temperature and humidity. Because the plums lose so much water, about 3 to 4 pounds of the fresh fruit are needed to produce 1 pound of dried plums. After drying, the dried plums are sorted by size and then stored to await packing, at which point they are moisturized by hot water.

The most common variety of plum used for drying in this country is California French, also known as d'Agen. The variety is a descendant of the first prune plums brought to the United States from France (Agen is the name of a town in France also known for its delicious dried plums) in the 1850s.

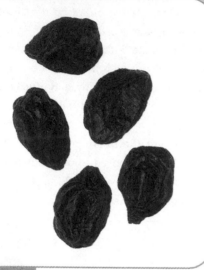

dried prune plums

nutritional profile

As with other dried fruits, the drying process concentrates the nutrients in dried plums. First and foremost, dried plums are a high-fiber food, and over half of this fiber is of the soluble type that studies have linked to lowered levels of blood cholesterol.

In addition to their well-documented high-fiber attributes, dried plums are an excellent source of carbohydrates, iron, and potassium.

If you're not fond of whole dried prune plums, an excellent substitute is prune juice, which retains a far higher proportion of the whole fruit's nutri-

DRIED PRUNE PLUMS ¼ cup	
Calories	102
Protein (g)	1
Carbohydrate (g)	27
Dietary fiber (g)	3.0
Total fat (g)	0.2
Saturated fat (g)	0
Monounsaturated fat (g)	0.1
Polyunsaturated fat (g)	0.1
Cholesterol (mg)	0
Potassium (mg)	317
Sodium (mg)	2

KEY NUTRIENTS (%RDA/AI*)

Iron	1.1 mg (13%)

For more detailed information on RDA and AI, see page 88.

other prune products

Prune juice Prune juice is made by pulverizing dried prune plums and dissolving them in hot water. Available in bottles and cans, check the label to be sure you're getting unsweetened juice.

Prune butter (lekvar) This thick paste made of pureed dried prune plums is used in baby foods, as a pastry filling, as a spread, and as a fat replacement in low-fat baked goods.

ents than the juice made from most other fruits. But prune juice is also relatively high in calories—182 calories per cup. To avoid excess calories, don't purchase brands with added sugar; prune juice is sweet enough on its own.

in the market

While there are other varieties that are cultivated and dried, the California French prune plum makes up 99 percent of the dried plums commercially produced.

Dried prune plums Today about 70 percent of the world's dried plum supply, and nearly 100 percent of domestic dried plums, come from California prune plum orchards. Dried prune plums are available both with and without pits, and chopped or diced.

Dried mirabelles The small, round, fleshy plums called mirabelles are also sold in their dried form. They are smaller than the average dried prune plum.

Sour prunes In addition to the standard-issue American dried plum, you can sometimes find sour prunes. Orangish in color, these are a staple in Middle Eastern and Greek cuisines, among others. Red plums are dried in the sun or in special kilns to produce sour prunes. Although they are called sour, their flavor is a combination of tart and sweet.

choosing the best

If you don't mind the chore of pitting them, whole unpitted dried plums are less expensive than pitted ones.

▶ **When you get home** After opening the package, reseal it as tightly as possible or transfer the dried plums to an airtight container. Store them in a cool, dry place or in the refrigerator for up to 6 months.

preparing to use

You can pit dried plums by splitting them open with your fingers, or slitting them open with a knife and pushing out the pits. Pitted dried plums are ready to use directly from the package, but be sure to check for the occasional pit in pitted dried plums; the mechanical process is not foolproof.

Cutting, chopping, or dicing dried plums can be tedious work because the knife quickly becomes sticky. To make the job easier, use kitchen scissors and either dip the blades into warm water between cuts or spray the scissors with nonstick cooking spray to keep them clean.

---

serving suggestions

• Add diced dried plums to carrots as they cook.

• Soften dried plums in red wine, port, or Marsala and serve with a dollop of sweetened nonfat yogurt for dessert.

• Add diced dried plums to chicken and pork stews.

• Poach dried plums in orange juice and use as a topping for frozen yogurt.

• Add diced dried plums to chili.

• Poach fresh plums in prune juice spiced with black pepper and allspice.

• Stuff mushrooms with a mixture of diced dried plums and bread crumbs.

---

facts & tips

Prunes (dried plums) are at the top of the list of foods that were studied for their antioxidant potential. The study was conducted at the USDA Human Nutrition Research Center on Aging at Tufts University to determine which foods may have the greatest abilities to fight off harmful free radicals. Foods with a high antioxidant potential are called high-ORAC (oxygen radical absorbance capacity)—a quality that scientists can now measure. Studies suggest that high-ORAC foods boost the antioxidant power of human blood substantially.

pumpkin

Believed to have originated in Central America, pumpkins have been culti-vated for thousands of years and were an important food source for Native Americans, who utilized as much of the pumpkin as possible: For example, they dried strips of the rinds and wove them into mats, they ate roasted pumpkin flesh, and they prized the nutritious oil-rich seeds for food as well as medicine. Not surprisingly, it was a welcome discovery for this country's early settlers, who soon learned to regard the pumpkin as an important staple—not only on Thanksgiving day, but as an everyday side dish, as a soup, and for making beer.

A type of winter squash, the pumpkin is a hard-shelled gourd that grows on a trailing vine and is related to watermelons and muskmel-ons. Its shape is round, with depressions at both stem and blossom ends. Its color ranges through various shades of green to orange. Like other winter squash (and melons) pumpkins have a hollow interior contain-ing edible seeds (*see Pumpkin Seeds, page 496*).

nutritional profile

The wealth of carotenoid pigments that make pumpkins orange may protect against chronic diseases such as heart disease and cancer, and may also ward off age-related vision loss. Mounting evidence suggests that people who eat lots of carotenoid-rich foods seem to have the healthiest eyes. Pumpkin is a top source of lutein, a carotenoid linked to a reduced risk of cataracts and macular degeneration, the leading cause of blindness or near-blindness in Americans over age 60. Tremendous quantities of the carotenoids alpha carotene and beta carotene are present in pumpkin as well. Also noteworthy in pumpkin are healthy amounts of fiber, potassium, riboflavin, vitamin C, and iron. Pumpkin is also a good low-fat source of vitamin E.

in the market

Pumpkins are available in all shapes, colors, and sizes, from the miniature to the gigantic. However, most of us, when we hear the word "pumpkin" think of Halloween jack-o'-lanterns. Though the pumpkins that are used as Hal-loween decorations can be eaten, there are better options for cooking.

Cinderella This deep orange, variegated pumpkin looks like a regular pumpkin that got squashed flat (appropriate, since it belongs to the squash family).

Jack-o'-lanterns This is not a botanical designation, but a market term than refers to pumpkins that are grown for their large cavities and thin walls, making them perfect for carving (but not as interesting for cooking).

jack-o'-lantern

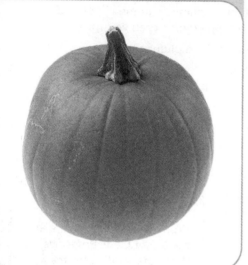

PUMPKIN 1 cup cooked mashed	
Calories	49
Protein (g)	2
Carbohydrate (g)	12
Dietary fiber (g)	2.7
Total fat (g)	0.2
Saturated fat (g)	0.1
Monounsaturated fat (g)	0
Polyunsaturated fat (g)	0
Cholesterol (mg)	0
Potassium (mg)	564
Sodium (mg)	0

KEY NUTRIENTS (%RDA/AI*)	
Beta carotene	16 mg (142%)
Riboflavin	0.2 mg (15%)
Vitamin C	12 mg (13%)
Vitamin E	2.6 mg (17%)
Iron	1.4 mg (17%)

*For more detailed information on RDA and AI, see page 88.

Japanese pumpkins These are also sold as a type of winter squash called kabocha (*see Squash, Winter, page 551*).

Mini pumpkins These minuscule versions of the real thing are cute, but more of an ornament than a vegetable. In addition to the standard pumpkin-orange color, these come in a beautiful cream-white.

Pie pumpkins There are a number of pumpkins with a very high flesh-to-seed-cavity ratio. They are intended for cooking rather than pumpkin carving. One especially flavorful pumpkin in this category is called *sugar pumpkin.*

▶ Availability Many pumpkins are destined to be turned into canned pumpkin puree. The remainder are pumpkins that are grown specifically for the Halloween market. Because of the limited market demand for fresh pumpkins, they are only available fresh in the fall (October and November).

choosing the best

If you're buying a fresh pumpkin during the limited fresh-pumpkin season, there's not much to know. Any pumpkin you buy will have been picked ripe (or it wouldn't be the requisite orange color). But check for soft spots anywhere on the pumpkin, and especially at the stem.

▶ When you get home Jack-o'-lantern pumpkins are bred to have thin walls and therefore do not store as well as other winter squash. If you buy Cinderella, Japanese, or pie pumpkins, all of which have thicker walls, they will keep as well as other winter squash.

preparing to use

Pumpkin can be eaten in chunks (as you would winter squash) or as a puree (as for pumpkin pie). Cut out the stem of the pumpkin and remove the string and seeds (save for roasting). Cut the pumpkin flesh into wedges and peel. Then cut into chunks.

---

canned pumpkin

Canned pumpkin puree is not only a convenient form of pumpkin, but also a very rich, low-fat source of all the nutrients in fresh pumpkin. Canned pumpkin puree is much denser than homemade mashed pumpkin, because it has been cooked down enough to prevent it from being too watery in a pumpkin pie. As a result it is about twice as high in calories as homemade (but still only 83 calories a cup). However, its nutrient content is impressive. One cup has 290 percent of the daily requirement for beta carotene (32 milligrams) and 43 percent of the RDA for iron. Be sure when you are looking for canned pumpkin to get the unsweetened solid-pack puree, not "pumpkin pie filling," which is pre-sweetened and pre-spiced.

---

serving suggestions

• Add chunks of pumpkin to chili.

• Thin canned pumpkin puree to a soup consistency with broth. Season with salt and a dash of cinnamon, and heat. Stir in a bit of reduced-fat sour cream and top with toasted pumpkin seeds.

• Stir pumpkin puree into tomato-based pasta sauces.

• Stir minced chipotle peppers, toasted cumin, lime juice, and minced cilantro into pumpkin puree and serve as a dip with baked tortilla chips.

pumpkin seeds

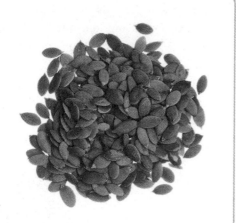

pumpkin seeds

Pumpkins not only generously yield their flesh for delicious pies and their firm rinds for jack-o'-lanterns at Halloween, but these remarkable orbs also give us seeds that can be roasted. Roasted pumpkin seeds have a rich, almost peanutlike flavor and can be eaten as snacks or added to salads, soups, and casseroles. Pumpkin seeds can also be ground and used to make sauces. A by-product of pumpkin seeds is a flavorful salad oil (*see Fats & Oils, page 298*).

nutritional profile

Pumpkin seeds are rich in vitamin E, iron, magnesium, and zinc. In addition, these tasty morsels provide both essential and unsaturated fatty acids.

in the market

Pumpkin seeds are sold in the shell, shelled, roasted, and raw. They can be found in health-food stores and some supermarkets. The shelled pumpkin seeds are often labeled *pepitas* (which just means "little seeds" in Spanish).

choosing the best

▶ **When you get home** The oil in pumpkin seeds can easily go rancid, so keep pumpkin seeds in the refrigerator or freezer.

preparing to use

You can roast your own pumpkin seeds if you have a fresh pumpkin. Remove the pumpkin seeds from inside the pumpkin and rinse them in a colander. Pull any pulp or strings from the seeds and rinse again. Blot the seeds dry and place in a bowl. Add a few drops of olive oil (maybe just a drop of sesame oil, too, for added flavor) and spread them on a cookie sheet. Sprinkle the seeds lightly with salt. Roast the seeds at 375° for about 45 minutes, or until they are golden. Cool the seeds completely and store in an airtight container.

HULLED PUMPKIN SEEDS 1 ounce	
Calories	153
Protein (g)	7
Carbohydrate (g)	5
Dietary fiber (g)	1.1
Total fat (g)	13
Saturated fat (g)	2.5
Monounsaturated fat (g)	4.0
Polyunsaturated fat (g)	6.0
Cholesterol (mg)	0
Potassium (mg)	229
Sodium (mg)	5

KEY NUTRIENTS (%RDA/AI*)	
Vitamin E	3.1 mg (21%)
Iron	4.3 mg (53%)
Magnesium	152 mg (36%)
Zinc	2.1 mg (19%)

For more detailed information on RDA and AI, see page 88.

quince

Though it resembles a pear, the quince does not share the popularity of that fruit, most likely because its flavor is somewhat astringent and its texture is rather dry. Because of its mouth-puckering flavor, quince is usually cooked. The quince is often used to make jams and jelly (it has a high pectin content) as well as in long-cooking dishes, since it retains much of its shape and texture when cooked.

While it is a neglected fruit in the United States, the quince has a long history of cultivation in the Middle East and the Mediterranean. The quince tree is thought to have originated from regions in Asia, where it still grows wild. Its fragrant flowers and musky-scented fruit were enjoyed by the Greeks and Romans, who gave a quince to a bride on her wedding day as a symbol of fertility, a ritual that continued into the Christian era.

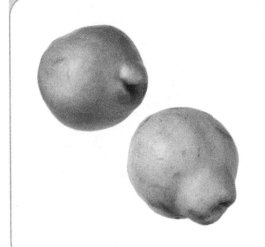
quince

nutritional profile

The aromatic quince provides substantial amounts of dietary fiber, including cholesterol-lowering pectin, and vitamin C.

in the market

There are many varieties of quince, but only a few are of commercial interest.

Aromatnaya These quince have a pineapple flavor and, if very ripe, can be eaten fresh.

Orange quince These are round and have bright colored fruit.

Pineapple quince This white-fleshed variety, when picked ripe, has a fragrance similar to pineapple.

Smyrna These are large yellow-skinned fruit that can weigh up to 3 pounds (the average quince weighs only about 4 ounces).

▶ Availability Because the demand is so small for these fruits, they are only in the market from October through March (and imports don't fill in the gaps when local crops are not available).

choosing the best

Look for quince that feel heavy for their size. They should be fragrant and free of blemishes. As quince are always cooked and most recipes call for peeling them, choose large, smooth fruit, which will be easier to peel.

preparing to use

While one variety of quince, the Aromatnaya, is said to be edible when raw, most varieties of quince must be cooked in order to be edible. Wash the fruit to remove any woolly covering, peel, and core. Save the seeds, skin, and core; tie them in cheesecloth and cook along with fruits or jams to give body.

QUINCE / 1 cup raw	
Calories	105
Protein (g)	1
Carbohydrate (g)	28
Dietary fiber (g)	3.5
Total fat (g)	0.2
Saturated fat (g)	0
Monounsaturated fat (g)	0.1
Polyunsaturated fat (g)	0.1
Cholesterol (mg)	0
Potassium (mg)	363
Sodium (mg)	7

KEY NUTRIENTS (%RDA/AI*)	
Vitamin C	28 mg (31%)
Iron	1.3 mg (16%)

*For more detailed information on RDA and AI, see page 88.

quinoa

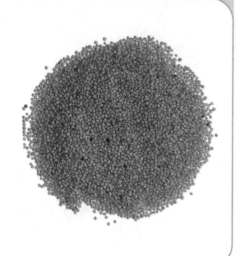

quinoa

An ancient grainlike product that has recently been "rediscovered" in this country, quinoa (pronounced keen-wah) is not a true grain (neither is buckwheat or amaranth), but it looks like one and has similar uses. It is related to leafy vegetables such as Swiss chard and spinach.

Though quinoa is a fairly recent introduction to the American larder, this native Andean crop sustained the Incas just as amaranth did the Aztecs. In a parallel sequence of events, the cultivation of quinoa, like that of amaranth, may also have been suppressed by the Spanish conquistadors. However, this valuable food plant survived in remote areas and has been cultivated continuously for over 5,000 years.

Quinoa's survival through the millennia may be attributed to the resinous, bitter coating that protects its seeds from birds and insects. This coating, called saponin, is soapy and must be removed in a strong alkaline solution to make the grain palatable (in South America the water used in this process is made into a shampoo). Most quinoa sold in this country has already been cleansed of its saponin coating.

Quinoa grains are about the same size as millet, but are flattened, with a pointed, oval shape. As quinoa cooks, the external germ, which forms a band around each grain, spirals out, forming a tiny crescent-shaped "tail." Although the grain itself is soft and creamy, the tail is crunchy, providing a unique textural complement.

nutritional profile

Quinoa's key nutritional distinguishing factor is its high level of lysine, an amino acid necessary for the synthesis of protein, making it one of the best sources of plant protein. Quinoa also provides riboflavin, vitamin E, iron, magnesium, potassium, zinc, and fiber.

in the market

Mostly the province of health-food stores, some supermarkets may carry quinoa in its whole-grain form. Quinoa is more expensive than most grains.

Flakes Quinoa grain is steamed, rolled, and flaked. This form cooks quickly and is intended to be used as a hot cereal.

Flour See Flour, Nonwheat (*page 325*).

Whole grain The most common quinoa is an ivory-white, but the whole grain can also be found in pale-yellow, red, and black.

preparing to use

Quinoa should be rinsed to remove any powdery residue of saponins. Place the grain in a fine strainer and hold it under cold running water until the water runs clear; drain well. Brown the grain in a dry skillet for 5 minutes before simmering or baking to give it a delicious roasted flavor.

QUINOA / ¼ cup raw	
Calories	159
Protein (g)	6
Carbohydrate (g)	29
Dietary fiber (g)	2.5
Total fat (g)	2.5
Saturated fat (g)	0.3
Monounsaturated fat (g)	0.7
Polyunsaturated fat (g)	1.0
Cholesterol (mg)	0
Potassium (mg)	315
Sodium (mg)	9

KEY NUTRIENTS (%RDA/AI*)	
Riboflavin	0.2 mg (13%)
Vitamin E	2.1 mg (14%)
Iron	3.9 mg (49%)
Magnesium	89 mg (21%)
Zinc	1.4 mg (13%)

*For more detailed information on RDA and AI, see page 88.

radicchio

A variety of chicory (*see Endive & Chicory, page 282*), radicchio is a salad green that has only recently begun to gain favor in this country. In Italy, on the other hand, radicchio (which means chicory in Italian) dates back to the 16th century. Radicchio's mildly bitter flavor has a subtle spicy undertone. Because its texture is quite firm but still tender, it does well both in salads and as a cooked vegetable. While most radicchio is imported from Italy, domestic growers are beginning to cultivate this salad vegetable.

nutritional profile

Radicchio has a good amount of the B vitamin folate, and is a good low-fat (almost fat-free) source of vitamin E.

in the market

Radicchio comes in a range of colors, from light green to deep purple-red. The vegetable itself goes through several stages as it matures, starting with a green head and eventually turning deep burgundy in the cold weather. Most of the varieties that we get in this country have retained their Italian place names, which is how the Italians differentiate among the various types.

Radicchio di Castelfranco This radicchio is quite loose-leafed; it looks like a butterhead lettuce rosette. The leaves are variegated pink.

Radicchio di Chioggia This cabbage-headed radicchio comes in a range of colors, from white-green to red to variegated purple-green.

Radicchio di Treviso The size of a very large endive, Treviso's elongated head looks like a purple-red Romaine lettuce.

Radicchio di Verona This looks like a miniature red cabbage, but the white of the ribs and the deep burgundy of the leaves are in stark contrast. The head is quite compact.

Zuckerhut This is what is called a "green-heading" radicchio, which means it is sold when it is green. It is a dense, elongated head like romaine lettuce.

choosing the best

The leaves of both round and elongated radicchios should be firm and the edges should not be brown.

► **When you get home** Radicchio has a relatively short storage life. Though it looks like a cabbage, its tender, fleshy leaves are less hardy and should be treated more like lettuce for storage. Heads of radicchio should be stored in well-ventilated plastic bags in the crisper drawer.

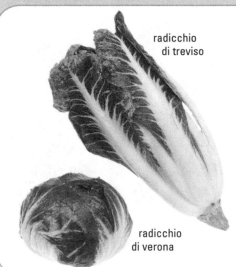

radicchio

radicchio di treviso

radicchio di verona

RADICCHIO / 2 cups	
Calories	18
Protein (g)	1
Carbohydrate (g)	4
Dietary fiber (g)	0.7
Total fat (g)	0.2
Saturated fat (g)	0.1
Monounsaturated fat (g)	0
Polyunsaturated fat (g)	0.1
Cholesterol (mg)	0
Potassium (mg)	242
Sodium (mg)	0

KEY NUTRIENTS (%RDA/AI*)	
Vitamin E	1.8 mg (12%)
Folate	48 mcg (12%)

For more detailed information on RDA and AI, see page 88.

radishes

Radishes are root vegetables that resemble beets or turnips in appearance and texture. But their flavor is distinctive, ranging from the relatively mild flavor of the familiar red globe radish to the sharp bite of the turnip-shaped black radish. Like their relatives broccoli, cabbage, and kale, radishes are cruciferous vegetables that offer cancer-protecting potential. They were first cultivated thousands of years ago in China, then in Egypt and Greece, where the vegetable was so highly regarded that gold replicas were made of it.

In the United States, radishes are usually eaten raw; however, they can be added to cooked dishes such as soups, heated and served as a vegetable, or they can be pickled. As with many other root vegetables, their green tops are edible and lend a peppery taste to salads.

nutritional profile

A good low-calorie snack, this root vegetable has less than 25 calories per cup and supplies potassium and impressive amounts of vitamin C: 29 percent of the daily requirement in 1 cup of red radish slices.

in the market

Growers classify radishes by shape—round, oval, oblong, and long—but markets label them by color—red, white, and black. Far and away the most common supermarket radishes are round red globe radishes.

Black radishes Turniplike in size and shape (about 8 inches long), these have dull-black or dark brown skin. When peeled, their flesh is white, quite pungent, and drier than other radishes. Commercially grown black radishes are usually a type called *Black Spanish,* which are available in round and long varieties.

California mammoth whites A larger variety than the white icicles (*opposite page*), these radishes have oblong-shaped roots about 8 inches long; their flesh is slightly pungent.

Chinese radishes (lo bok) These plump, elongated radishes can range in length from 12 to 20 inches. They are crisp with a sharp radish flavor.

Daikons Native to Asia, these are very large carrot-shaped radishes (up to 18 inches long and weighing 1 to 2 pounds). Also called Japanese or Oriental radishes, daikons have a juicy white flesh that is a bit hotter than that of red radishes but milder than that of black ones.

French breakfast radishes These oblong radishes are pink at the top and white at the bottom. Their flavor is slightly sweet and delicate.

Horseradish See Horseradish (*page 363*).

Korean radishes (moo) Similar to Chinese radishes and daikon, these rather large radishes have pale green skin and crisp white flesh that ranges in flavor from sweet to slightly hot.

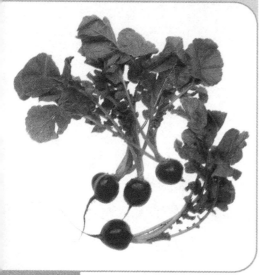

red globe radishes

RED RADISHES 1 cup slices	
Calories	23
Protein (g)	1
Carbohydrate (g)	4
Dietary fiber (g)	1.9
Total fat (g)	0.6
Saturated fat (g)	0
Monounsaturated fat (g)	0
Polyunsaturated fat (g)	0.1
Cholesterol (mg)	0
Potassium (mg)	269
Sodium (mg)	28

KEY NUTRIENTS (%RDA/AI*)	
Vitamin C	27 mg (29%)

*For more detailed information on RDA and AI, see page 88.

Purple plum radishes These large, round, reddish-purple radishes look like plums. Their texture is firm and crisp and their flavor is mild.

Radish sprouts See Sprouts (*page 543*).

Red globes Americans are probably most familiar with these small round or oval-shaped "button" red radishes. They range from about 1 to 5 inches in diameter and have solid, crisp, white flesh.

Snowballs As their name implies, these are round and white. The texture is crisp and the flavor is mild.

Wasabi See Horseradish (*page 363*).

Watermelon radishes These large, mild-flavored radishes have thin greenish skin. Just under the skin is a layer of white, and at the center is fuschia flesh, hence the name watermelon radish.

White icicles Long (up to 6 inches) and tapered, these have white flesh that is milder than that of red globe radishes.

choosing the best

Although red globe radishes can grow to as big as 5 inches in diameter, the ones you'll find in the produce bin will probably be closer to the size of a ping-pong ball—about 1 to 1½ inches in diameter. Much larger than that, red radishes are likely to be pithy. Radishes with their leaves intact are usually tied in bunches, while topped radishes are sold in plastic bags. If the leaves are attached, they should be crisp and green (they can be added to salads).

For all radishes, look for well-shaped roots that are heavy for their size (lightweight radishes may have pithy insides). If they are colored radishes, their color should be deep. The roots should be hard and solid, with a smooth, unblemished surface. Check bagged radishes to make sure they are free of mold. Long white radishes, such as daikon, should have a glossy, almost translucent, sheen.

▶ **When you get home** If you've bought radishes with their leaves attached, remove the tops unless you'll be serving them the same day (leaf-topped radishes are handsome on a crudité platter). Radishes will not keep as well with their tops left on. Place radishes in plastic bags if they are not already packaged. Both red radishes and daikons will keep for up to 2 weeks in the refrigerator. Black radishes can be stored for months if they remain dry; store them in perforated plastic bags in the refrigerator.

preparing to use

Scrub the radishes and trim off the stem end and tip. Unless you object to the skin, don't bother to peel it.

Daikons have a very thin skin that can be removed with a vegetable peeler, if you wish. Black radishes should be well scrubbed; whether you peel them or not depends on the thickness of the skin. If it is thin, leave it on; the dark color provides a striking contrast with the white flesh.

Small radishes can be served whole, raw, or cooked; larger and sharper radishes are usually cut up or grated.

---

serving suggestions

• Halve small red radishes and sauté with garlic and olive oil.

• Shred daikon and toss with carrots and apple for a slaw.

• Add sliced or shredded radishes to potato salads.

• Stir finely chopped radish into plain low-fat yogurt and use as a sauce for fish.

• Garnish cold soups with sliced radishes.

• Toss sliced radishes in a lemony vinaigrette.

• Add radishes to stir-fries.

• Serve raw radishes with a soy-ginger dipping sauce.

DAIKON / 1 cup slices	
Calories	16
Protein (g)	1
Carbohydrate (g)	4
Dietary fiber (g)	1.4
Total fat (g)	0.1
Saturated fat (g)	0
Monounsaturated fat (g)	0
Polyunsaturated fat (g)	0
Cholesterol (mg)	0
Potassium (mg)	200
Sodium (mg)	19

KEY NUTRIENTS (%RDA/AI*)

Vitamin C	19 mg (22%)

For more detailed information on RDA and AI, see page 88.

raisins

The first raisins were probably grapes that had dried naturally on the vine, but more than 3,000 years ago people were picking grapes and laying them out in the sun to dry—a process that has remained virtually unchanged. (Today, most raisins are still sun-dried, though some are dried in ovens.) Raisins were a precious trade item in the ancient Near East and also highly valued in ancient Rome (where two jars of raisins could be exchanged for a slave). Spanish missionaries brought grapes to California in the 18th century, where the raisin industry began booming in the 1870s after a heat wave dried the grape crop on the vine. Today California's San Joaquin Valley produces nearly all the commercially grown raisins in the United States (and about 50 percent of the world's supply).

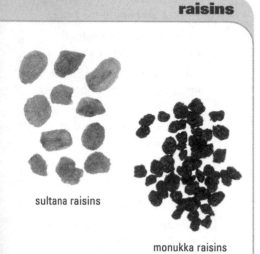

raisins

sultana raisins

monukka raisins

nutritional profile

Similar to all dried fruit, raisins are a concentrated source of nutrients, calories, and sugar, but they also provide good amounts of iron and potassium. To derive the most benefit from the type of iron in raisins ("nonheme"), eat raisins with vitamin C–rich foods, such as fresh citrus fruits or juices. Healthy amounts of both soluble and insoluble fiber are present in raisins as well.

in the market

Most raisins produced in the United States are made from five different types of grapes: Thompson Seedless (which are also the most popular green grapes for fresh consumption), Flame Seedless, Muscat, Sultana, and Black Corinth. It takes about 4½ pounds of fresh grapes to make 1 pound of raisins.

Currants Made from small Black Corinth grapes, currant raisins are seedless, tart, and tangy, and very dark in color. The tiny raisins (about one-fourth the size of Thompson Seedless raisins) are sometimes labeled "Zante Currants," referring to the Greek island where this type of grape first grew.

Flame Seedless raisins These come from the Flame Seedless red grape and are large, dark red, and extra sweet.

Golden Seedless raisins Like natural seedless raisins, these are also from Thompson Seedless grapes, but are oven-dried to avoid the darkening effect of sunlight. They are also treated with sulfur dioxide to preserve their light color.

Monukka raisins These large, dark, seedless raisins come from the black grapes of the same name. They're produced in limited quantities and are mostly available at health-food stores.

Muscat raisins Large, brown, and particularly fruity-tasting, these raisins are made from big, greenish-gold Muscat grapes. Since the grapes contain seeds, the raisins are seeded mechanically, or are sold with seeds. Muscats are considered a specialty item and are mostly used in baking.

RAISINS / ¼ cup	
Calories	107
Protein (g)	1
Carbohydrate (g)	29
Dietary fiber (g)	2.5
Total fat (g)	0.2
Saturated fat (g)	0.1
Monounsaturated fat (g)	0
Polyunsaturated fat (g)	0.1
Cholesterol (mg)	0
Potassium (mg)	299
Sodium (mg)	10

KEY NUTRIENTS (%RDA/AI*)	
Iron	0.9 mg (12%)

For more detailed information on RDA and AI, see page 88.

Natural seedless raisins These are sun-dried Thompson Seedless grapes. They account for almost all California raisins. The green grapes naturally develop a dark brown color as they dry in the sun, a process that takes from 2 to 3 weeks.

Sultanas These raisins, from the large, yellow-green Sultana grapes, are particularly tart and soft. They can be purchased in gourmet shops and health-food stores.

▶ Availability Boxes and bags of natural and golden raisins are available year round. Muscat raisins, preferred for holiday baking, are usually sold only in the autumn and winter months. Currants may only be found in specialty markets and larger supermarkets. Clusters of raisins still attached to the stem are sometimes displayed in specialty food stores.

choosing the best

When buying packaged raisins or currants, be sure that the box or bag is tightly sealed. Squeeze or shake the package to see if the fruit is soft—if the raisins rattle inside, they are dried out. When buying raisins in bulk at a gourmet shop or health-food store, choose moist-looking, clean fruit; don't buy raisins from uncovered bins.

▶ When you get home Unopened packages of raisins will keep almost indefinitely in the refrigerator. Once opened, reseal the package, excluding as much air as possible, or transfer the raisins to an airtight jar or bag. Proper storage will deter the fruit from drying out and will prevent its sugar from crystallizing on the surface. If refrigerated, the raisins will keep for up to a year; they will stay even longer in the freezer and will thaw quickly at room temperature.

preparing to use

If they've been correctly stored and are not dried out, raisins require no special preparation; however, you may wish to soften them by one of the following methods: To plump raisins for baking, cover them with hot liquid and let stand for 5 minutes. Or, let them soak overnight in the refrigerator. To conserve nutrients and flavor, use the least amount of liquid possible and then include the liquid in your recipe.

If raisins have dried out through improper storage, steam them over boiling water for 5 minutes. Or, sprinkle them with liquid, cover, and microwave for 1 minute, then let stand, covered, for 1 minute longer. Raisins that are stuck together in a hard clump will loosen up and separate if they are heated in a 300° oven for a few minutes.

When chopping raisins with a knife or chopper, coat the blade lightly with vegetable oil to keep the fruit from sticking to it. For easy grinding, freeze the raisins first, then use vegetable oil to coat the blades of your blender or food processor. When baking with raisins, dredge them in flour before adding them to batter to keep them from sinking to the bottom of the pan.

serving suggestions

• Add raisins to sautéed spinach.

• Add raisins to a meatball mixture.

• Add raisins to a spicy slaw.

• Make your own trail mix by combining raisins with popcorn, toasted pumpkin seeds, and grated Parmesan cheese.

• Soften raisins in fruit juice and puree. Use as you would prune butter.

• Add raisins to chicken salads.

• Add raisins to poultry stuffings.

facts & tips

In 1876 William Thompson, a Scottish immigrant living in the northern Sacramento Valley, introduced the Lady deCoverly seedless grape at the Marysville (California) District Fair. These grapes, which would become known as Thompson Seedless grapes, were thin-skinned, seedless, and sweet. Today, Thompson Seedless grapes account for nearly all of the California-grown raisins.

raspberries

These are the most expensive and most fragile berries, and their supply is extremely limited. A relative of the rose, and a bramble fruit like blackberries, raspberries have a delicate structure with a hollow core, so that they have to be handled very gently and eaten as soon as possible.

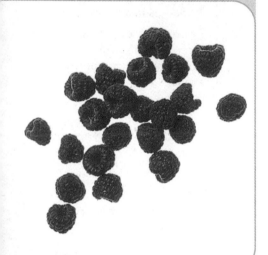

raspberries

RASPBERRIES / 1 cup	
Calories	60
Protein (g)	1
Carbohydrate (g)	14
Dietary fiber (g)	8.4
Total fat (g)	0.7
Saturated fat (g)	0
Monounsaturated fat (g)	0.1
Polyunsaturated fat (g)	0.4
Cholesterol (mg)	0
Potassium (mg)	187
Sodium (mg)	0

KEY NUTRIENTS (%RDA/AI*)

Vitamin C	31 mg (34%)

For more detailed information on RDA and AI, see page 88.

nutritional profile

Despite their apparent delicacy, these berries are packed with fiber (thanks in part to their tiny edible seeds); some of the fiber is soluble fiber in the form of pectin, which lowers cholesterol. Raspberries are also a good source of vitamin C.

in the market

Most cultivated raspberries are red, but there are also varieties in yellow, apricot, and amber, which are relatively similar in flavor and texture. Purple and black raspberries have a different, slightly sweeter, flavor.

Black raspberries Also called "blackcaps," these North American natives are blue-black, round, and small. They have a whitish "bloom" on the outside of the berry, which might be mistaken for mold, but it's a normal feature of the berry. Like the red raspberry, black raspberries are hollow, with no core.

Golden raspberries Described as tasting like a combination of apricots, bananas, and raspberries, these are deep gold in color and rich in flavor.

Purple raspberries These berries are hybrids of black and red raspberries. The fruits are purple with a white "bloom."

▶ Availability In the northeastern United States, local varieties are available at farmstands and farmers' markets from midsummer to late summer, but the bulk of our supply of this fresh fruit comes from the West Coast and is mainly available from June through October.

choosing the best

When raspberries are picked, the delicate cluster of fruits (each raspberry "seed" is actually an individual fruit) separate from the core, which gets left behind on the bush when the raspberries are picked. This makes the raspberries especially fragile, difficult to ship, and, naturally, expensive. Once raspberries reach market, they have a shelf-life of a day or two.

Choose berries very carefully; they are often packed in opaque boxes that may conceal inferior fruit beneath a display of perfect specimens on top. If the box is cellophane wrapped, your best bet is to examine the berries you can see, and check the box for dampness or stains, which indicate that the fruit below may be decaying. If the box is not wrapped, you can remove a few of the top berries and peek beneath.

Raspberries should be plump, dry, firm, well shaped and uniformly colored. Don't purchase berries that are withered or crushed.

▶ **When you get home** Raspberries can turn soft, mushy, and moldy within 24 hours. When you bring home a box of raspberries, turn it out and check the fruit. Remove soft, overripe berries for immediate consumption; discard any smashed or moldy berries and gently blot the remainder dry with a paper towel. Return the raspberries to the box or, better yet, spread them on a shallow plate or pan lined with paper towels. Raspberries should be used within a day or two of purchase.

Raspberries freeze beautifully, allowing you to enjoy them practically year round. You can buy prepackaged frozen berries, but these may have had sweetener added. Freezing berries yourself is simple. Spread them out in a single layer on a cookie sheet. Freeze the berries until they are solidly frozen, then transfer them to a heavy plastic bag.

preparing to use

Sort the raspberries again before serving, discarding any bad ones. Frozen berries need not be thawed before using them in recipes, but extra cooking time may be necessary.

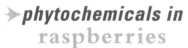

➤phytochemicals in raspberries

Similar to other berries, raspberries are rich in anthocyanin pigments, which give them their brilliant red hues. Anthocyanins are high in antioxidant capacity—and may prove to play a role in helping the body mop up free radicals, particles that can damage our cells and cause the onset of certain diseases.

serving suggestions

• Add raspberries to a seafood or chicken salad.

• Stir raspberries into a risotto or rice pilaf.

• Scatter raspberries over the top of a mozzarella and tomato salad.

• Fold raspberries into slightly sweetened ricotta cheese and use as a breakfast topping.

• Serve poached pears on a pool of raspberry puree.

• Combine raspberries with cooked lentils and cherry tomatoes for a cool summer salad.

• Fold raspberries and grated orange zest into vanilla frozen yogurt.

• Sprinkle on top of hot cereal.

rhubarb

Rhubarb, which looks like a pink celery stalk, is botanically a vegetable, but it is used as a fruit, largely in sauces and pies. (In some areas, it is referred to as "pie plant.") The ancient Chinese cultivated the plant for its roots, which were reputed to have medicinal properties, but rhubarb didn't gain acceptance as a food in the United States until the late 1700s.

While the stalks are delicious, the roots and leaves should not be eaten; indeed, the leaves are highly poisonous. At one time, the toxicity was attributed to their exceedingly high levels of oxalic acid, a substance that can interfere with iron and calcium absorption. However, the exact source of the leaf toxin has yet to be determined, since rhubarb stalks also contain significant amounts of oxalic acid (as do a few other foods, such as spinach and Swiss chard).

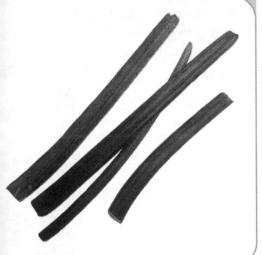

rhubarb

nutritional profile

Because the stalks have an extremely tart flavor, they require sweetening to make them appetizing, which, of course, increases their calorie content considerably. For example, half a cup of frozen, cooked, sweetened rhubarb has 139 calories compared with 29 calories in the same amount of unsweetened cooked rhubarb. Still, rhubarb can be combined with sweet fruits instead of sugar or honey to cut calories.

Two cups of fresh, diced rhubarb (which cooks down to about 1 cup) supplies over 20 percent of the daily requirement of vitamin C, potassium, and manganese. Good amounts of dietary fiber are present in rhubarb as well. If you're prone to kidney stones, your doctor may advise you to avoid rhubarb because it is high in compounds called oxalates, which may fuel stone formation in susceptible people. Oxalates interfere with the body's absorption of the calcium from rhubarb, even though the vegetable appears to be quite high in this mineral.

in the market

Rhubarb comes in many varieties, most of which fall into two basic groups:

Field-grown This group includes varieties that have dark red stalks and green leaves; field-grown rhubarb has a pronounced tart flavor.

Hothouse-grown These varieties have pink to pale red stalks and yellow-green leaves. It is milder than field-grown and less stringy.

▶ Availability Field-grown rhubarb appears in the market from April through June or July. Hothouse-grown rhubarb is mainly harvested from January through June, but some supermarkets carry it year round. Rhubarb is also available frozen.

RHUBARB / 2 cups raw	
Calories	51
Protein (g)	2
Carbohydrate (g)	11
Dietary fiber (g)	4.4
Total fat (g)	0.5
Saturated fat (g)	0.1
Monounsaturated fat (g)	0.1
Polyunsaturated fat (g)	0.2
Cholesterol (mg)	0
Potassium (mg)	702
Sodium (mg)	5

KEY NUTRIENTS (%RDA/AI*)	
Vitamin C	20 mg (22%)
Calcium	210 mg (18%)

*For more detailed information on RDA and AI, see page 88.

choosing the best

Rhubarb is sold loose and in 1-pound plastic bags, like celery. Whichever type is available, choose well-colored, good-sized, straight, firm stalks. If the leaves are attached, they should look fresh and crisp; small leaves usually indicate younger, more tender stalks.

▶ **When you get home** If you buy rhubarb stalks with the leaves still attached, cut off the leaves as soon as you get home. Never eat the leaves, raw or cooked. Place the stalks in plastic bags and store them in the refrigerator crisper, where they will keep for about a week.

You can freeze rhubarb raw or you can parboil it for about 30 seconds before freezing (which helps retain its color). Freeze whole stalks or cut the rhubarb into pieces. You can also freeze rhubarb puree. The rhubarb will keep in the freezer for a few months.

preparing to use

Hothouse rhubarb is ready to cook after it is rinsed and the tops and bottoms of the stalks are trimmed. For stewing or sauce-making, cut the stalks into 1- to 2-inch lengths. Mature field-grown rhubarb may need to have its stringy fibers removed: As you cut the stalks, peel the coarse fibers from the back of each piece with a paring knife.

---

serving suggestions

• Cook rhubarb with pears or apples for a different spin on applesauce. Add sugar to taste.

• Briefly blanch diced rhubarb and treat it as you would tomatoes for a salsa. Serve with meat, fish, or poultry.

• Cook rhubarb with pineapple juice, sweeten with a bit of honey, and use to top frozen yogurt.

• Sauté diced rhubarb and garlic in a mixture of olive oil and broth. Add mustard and use as a sauce for pork.

---

stewed rhubarb

Rhubarb tastes sweeter after it's cooked, so stew it first, then add sugar to taste. You may want to use less sweetener than your recipe calls for (or initially try about ½ cup of sugar per pound of rhubarb). Stewing rhubarb in orange juice rather than water both sweetens it and complements its flavor. Or, you can cook rhubarb in pineapple juice or with pineapple chunks.

Place the cut-up rhubarb in a saucepan (don't use aluminum or cast iron) with just enough water or juice to come a third of the way up the rhubarb (add some lemon or orange zest, if desired). Cover and bring to a boil, then reduce the heat and simmer gently until tender. After cooking, add more sugar to taste and cook for another 5 minutes to dissolve it.

If you're serving the stewed rhubarb cold, taste it again just before serving and add more sweetener, if necessary (sweetness is generally less intense when food is chilled).

rice

To Americans, rice is the most familiar food eaten in grain form. It is commonly served as a side dish in American households, but elsewhere in the world it forms the basis for most meals. In fact, half the world's people eat rice as their staple food. In some languages, the verb for "eat" means "eat rice."

Though rice is grown on every continent except Antarctica, China produces more than 90 percent of the world's rice crop.

Rice was first grown in the American colonies in the late 17th century. Today, the major rice-growing states are Arkansas, Louisiana, Mississippi, Missouri, Texas, and California (where rice was first introduced to feed the thousands of Chinese immigrants in the California territory in the mid 19th century).

Rice thrives in warm climates with abundant supplies of fresh water. The type of rice grown in the United States and some other parts of the world is called paddy rice. It is cultivated in fields that are surrounded by levees or dikes, which allow the fields to be flooded with water for most of the growing season. The purpose of the flooding is to subdue weed growth. The fields are drained before the rice is harvested (by machine, in industrialized countries; by hand, in less-developed ones). Another type of rice, upland rice, can be grown in wet soil and doesn't require flooding.

nutritional profile

Wholesome and nutritious, low in calories and fat, sodium-free, rich in complex carbohydrates, vitamins, minerals, and fiber—it's no wonder that rice is a staple food for a large segment of the world's population. Although rice is lower in protein than other cereal grains, its protein quality is good because it contains relatively high levels of the essential amino acid lysine.

When white rice is refined, it is milled and polished, a process that removes the bran and germ as well as valuable nutrients. In the United States, however, most white rice is enriched with thiamin, niacin, folate, and iron. Enriched white rice is a good source of these nutrients, as well as fiber and selenium.

Brown rice, which has only the outer hull removed, retains—along with its bran layer—thiamin, niacin, and vitamin B_6. And because the bran is not milled away, brown rice is a better source of fiber than white rice, supplying 3.5 grams of fiber per 1-cup serving, which is more than five times greater than white rice.

in the market

Rice can be classified according to size: long-grain, medium-grain, and short-grain. *Long-grain rice* accounts for about 75 percent of the domestic crop. The

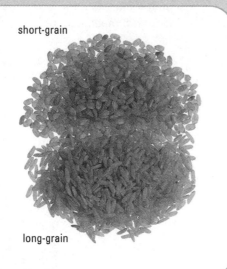

brown rice

short-grain

long-grain

BROWN RICE 1 cup cooked	
Calories	216
Protein (g)	5
Carbohydrate (g)	45
Dietary fiber (g)	3.5
Total fat (g)	1.8
Saturated fat (g)	0.4
Monounsaturated fat (g)	0.6
Polyunsaturated fat (g)	0.6
Cholesterol (mg)	0
Potassium (mg)	84
Sodium (mg)	10

KEY NUTRIENTS (%RDA/AI*)	
Thiamin	0.2 mg (16%)
Niacin	3.0 mg (19%)
Vitamin B_6	0.3 mg (17%)
Iron	0.8 mg (10%)
Magnesium	84 mg (20%)
Selenium	19 mcg (35%)
Zinc	1.2 mg (11%)

*For more detailed information on RDA and AI, see page 88.

slender grains are four to five times longer than they are wide. If properly cooked, they will be fluffy and dry, with separate grains. *Medium-grain rice* is about twice as long as it is wide and cooks up moister and more tender than long-grain. It is popular in some Asian and Latin American cultures, and is the type of rice most commonly processed to make cold cereals. *Short-grain rice* may be almost oval or round in shape. Of the three types of rice, it has the highest percentage of amylopectin, the starch that makes rice sticky, so the grains clump together when cooked. Easy to eat with chopsticks, it is ideal for dishes like sushi.

Brown rice This rice has had only its husk removed during milling. It is therefore naturally high in B vitamins and minerals, though with enrichment white rice actually ends up with higher levels of thiamin and iron. Because brown rice has its germ, it also has some vitamin E. It has a richer flavor and a chewier texture than white rice, and takes longer to cook, though *quick-cooking* and *instant* forms are available.

White rice (milled rice) The most popular form of rice, white rice has been completely milled to remove the husk, bran, and most of the germ. There are several types of white rice:

Enriched white rice is milled rice that has had thiamin, niacin, folate, and iron added after milling to replace some of the nutrients lost when the bran layer is removed. As a result, it is higher in these nutrients than brown rice.

Parboiled rice (converted rice) has been soaked and steamed under pressure before milling, which forces some of the nutrients into the remaining portion of the grain so that they are not totally lost in the processing.

Enriched parboiled rice is similar to regular white rice in terms of nutrition. The term "parboiled" is slightly misleading; the rice is not precooked and is actually somewhat harder than regular rice. As a consequence, it takes a little longer to cook than regular white rice, but the grains will be very fluffy and separate after they have been cooked.

Instant white rice is a quick-cooking rice that takes about 5 minutes to prepare. It has been milled and polished, fully cooked, and then dehydrated. It is usually enriched and only slightly less nutritious than regular enriched white rice, but it lacks the satisfying texture of regular rice.

specialty rices

Arborio This starchy white rice, with an almost round grain, is grown mainly in the Po Valley of Italy. Traditionally used for cooking the Italian dish risotto, it also works well for paella and rice pudding. Arborio absorbs up to five times its weight in liquid as it cooks, which results in grains of a creamy consistency.

> ➤ *phytochemicals in* rice

Whole grains, such as brown rice, are more nutritious than refined grains, since they retain the bran and the germ, which are not only rich in vitamins, minerals, and fiber, but also in beneficial phytochemicals. For example, research is exploring the potential benefits of oryzanol, a phytochemical that may help to guard against cardiovascular disease. Oryzanol is found in the outer layer of brown rice.

ENRICHED WHITE RICE
1 cup cooked

Calories	205
Protein (g)	4
Carbohydrate (g)	45
Dietary fiber (g)	0.6
Total fat (g)	0.4
Saturated fat (g)	0.1
Monounsaturated fat (g)	0.1
Polyunsaturated fat (g)	0.1
Cholesterol (mg)	0
Potassium (mg)	55
Sodium (mg)	12

KEY NUTRIENTS (%RDA/AI*)

Thiamin	0.3 mg (21%)
Niacin	2.3 mg (15%)
Folate	92 mcg (23%)
Iron	1.9 mg (24%)
Selenium	12 mcg (22%)

For more detailed information on RDA and AI, see page 88.

Aromatic rice This is an umbrella term for rices that have a toasty, nutty fragrance and a flavor reminiscent of popcorn or roasted nuts. They are primarily long-grain varieties.

Basmati Perhaps the most famous aromatic rice, basmati is grown in India and Pakistan. It has a nutlike fragrance while cooking and a delicate, almost buttery flavor. Unlike other types of rice, the grains elongate much more than they plump as they cook. Lower in starch than other long-grain types, basmati grains turn out fluffy and separate. Although it is most commonly used in Indian cooking, basmati can also be substituted for regular rice in any favorite recipe. Both *brown* and *white* basmati rices are available.

Bhutanese red This is a short-grain rice that is a staple in the small Himalyan kingdom of Bhutan. It has a nutty flavor and is slightly chewy.

Black Forbidden This black short-grain rice turns indigo when cooked. Use it as a substitute for regular rice in paella or for an intriguing risotto.

Black Japonica This fragrant rice is a blend of a Japanese short-grain black rice and a mahogany-colored medium-grain rice. It is slightly spicy and sweet.

Bomba From Spain, bomba is considered one of the two premier rice varieties for paella. This short-grain rice can absorb up to one-third more liquid than other rices while still retaining its integrity.

Della This aromatic long-grain rice, popular in the South, is similar in flavor to basmati rice.

Glutinous rice (sweet rice, sticky rice) Popular in Japan and other Asian countries, this very starchy rice is sticky and resilient, and turns translu-

rice bran

Like oat bran, rice bran is enjoying a reputation as a cholesterol-fighter. Researchers at the USDA have found that rice bran lowers blood cholesterol in animals just as much as oat bran. But scientists are interested in more than the fiber content of the rice.

Because of the composition of the rice kernel and the way it is milled, the processed bran ends up containing rice germ, which is rich in oil. Scientists in Japan and India have found that this highly unsaturated oil also has a substantial cholesterol-lowering effect. Although brown rice is exceedingly nutritious, it is not a concentrated source of fiber or oil.

Rice bran has been available in health-food stores for some time without arousing much enthusiasm: In its natural state, it tastes like sawdust and has a short shelf-life. But a range of products containing rice bran is now available—including rice cakes and cereals—that not only taste better, but have also been heat-stabilized to reduce spoilage.

Rice bran is also available packaged like wheat germ. An ounce of one brand contains 8 grams of dietary fiber—of which 2 grams are soluble—and 6 grams of fat. It also has 100 calories, 4 grams of protein, and generous amounts of thiamin, niacin, magnesium, and iron. Rice bran can be used just like wheat germ: Sprinkle it on cereal, salad, and yogurt or add it to baked goods. Unlike oat bran, rice bran doesn't turn gummy when cooked.

cent when cooked. Glutinous rice comes both short- and long-grain. It can be *white, brown,* or *black.*

Himalayan red Similar to long-grain brown rice, it has red rather than brown bran.

Jasmine This long-grain rice has a soft texture and is similar in flavor to basmati rice. It is available in both *white* and *brown* forms.

Kalijira (baby basmati) These miniature rice grains are similar in flavor to basmati rice and hail from Bangladesh. Because of its tiny grains, this rice cooks relatively quickly.

Sollana rice Like bomba rice, this short-grain Spanish rice can absorb lots of liquid while still retaining its shape. It is generally used to make paella.

Sticky rice See Glutinous rice (*opposite page*).

Thai black sticky rice (Thai purple rice) This long-grain, black glutinous rice turns a deep purple when cooked.

other rice products

Cream of rice This is very finely ground rice. Although store-bought versions are convenient, you can make your own cream of rice (or, even better, cream of brown rice) by grinding rice in a food processor.

Pinipig In the Philippines, glutinous rice grains are rolled (like oats) and used to make desserts and drinks.

Puffed rice This is an Indian ingredient similar to American crisped rice cereal, but it is not a brand-name cereal.

Rice bran See "Rice Bran" (*opposite page*).

Rice flour See Flour, Nonwheat (*page 326*).

Rice milk See "Other Milks," (*page 398*).

choosing the best

Whether buying rice in bulk or in packages, look for grains that are whole, not cracked or broken. Shop in a store that does a brisk business. Many varieties will be available in the supermarket, but for others you may need to shop in a specialty food store.

▶ **When you get home** Store rice in a closed container away from the heat. Because of the oil in its bran, brown rice has a more limited shelf-life than white rice. To preserve it, store it in the refrigerator.

trade-name rices

Certain aromatic rices that have been developed in this country are sold only under a trade name, including:

Christmas rice Red, with a slightly nutty, almost roasted flavor, this short-grain rice is not sticky when cooked and remains slightly crunchy.

Jasmati This is an American version of jasmine rice.

Kasmati This is similar to basmati.

Texmati This basmati-type rice was developed to withstand the hot Texas climate. It comes as a brown rice, as well as light brown and white.

Wehani Developed in California, this rice has an unusual rust-colored bran that makes it turn mahogany when cooked.

Wild pecan (popcorn rice) This tan rice (so-called because not all of the bran is removed) is a basmati hybrid, with a pecanlike flavor and a firm texture.

roots & tubers

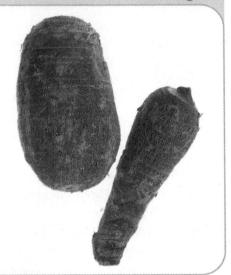

Hearty and nourishing, roots and tubers have been an important food category for thousands of years. Known as nature's buried treasures, roots and tubers are geophytes, a botanical term for plants with their growing point beneath the soil.

Roots are parts of a plant that usually grow downward, anchoring the plant into the ground, where they absorb moisture and nutrients. Examples of root vegetables include beets, carrots, celeriac, parsnips, sweet potatoes, and turnips.

Tubers form at the base of roots and are the swollen tips of stems that grow underground. They store energy in the form of starch to support new stem growth. Examples of tubers include potatoes, Jerusalem artichokes, jícama, and yams.

Rhizomes—such as arrowroot—look like roots, but they are actually swollen underground stems that can generate both new roots and stems.

With wildly varying characteristics, and flavors ranging from earthy to sweet, roots and tubers are arguably the most nutritious, economical, and versatile foods.

nutritional profile

Because these vegetables are so diverse, their nutritional make-up will be highly varied. As a result, no nutritional profiles accompany these entries; rather, information on the more commonly consumed roots and tubers, such as carrots and potatoes, will be found in the individual entries.

in the market

The more common roots and tubers are covered in their own entries. These include: Beets (*page 192*), Carrots (*page 216*), Horseradish (*page 363*), Parsnips (*page 440*), Potatoes (*page 488*), Radishes (*page 500*), Sweet Potatoes (*page 557*), and Turnips & Rutabagas (*page 583*).

Arrowroot (arrowhead, fung quat) Also called a Chinese potato, this underwater rhizome can be as small as a small onion (which it resembles) or as large as a coconut. Once cooked, it is like a slightly mealy potato. It needs to be peeled before using. This is the plant used to make arrowroot flour (*see Flour, Nonwheat, page 326*).

Batata See Sweet Potatoes (*page 558*).

Boniato See Sweet Potatoes (*page 558*).

Burdock This root vegetable is brown-skinned, with white flesh that darkens quickly when cut. Popular in Japan (where it's called *gobo*), burdock can be found in Asian grocery stores and some health-food stores. It also grows wild in North America; the plant can be recognized by its very large leaves and spiny burrs (the "cockleburs" that stick to your clothes when you walk through a meadow). Many people who eat burdock compare it to celery and artichoke, and consider the taste to be earthy and mildly sweet. Uncooked wild American burdock tastes very bitter, though cooking removes the bitterness. In the market, look for firm burdock roots. Don't be put off if the outside is dirty or muddy; just wash the root well.

Burdock is good source of magnesium, potassium, and folate; it is also high in inulin, a sugar that can sometimes cause flatulence.

Cassava See Yuca (*page 516*).

Celeriac Closely related to celery, this plant develops a knobby baseball-sized root with a crisp texture and intense celery flavor. (The stalks and leaves can be used to flavor soups and stews.) Although not very popular in the United States, celeriac is a favorite vegetable in France and Italy, where it is eaten both raw and cooked. Cooked celeriac and potato complement one another, and the two vegetables are often combined in one dish. Like celery, this fall and winter vegetable can also be used as a flavoring. Look for smallish, heavy, firm celeriac roots; although the outside may be dirty, it should be free of deep dents, cuts, or soft spots. If the stems and leaves are attached, they should be fresh and green. No matter how you're cooking celeriac, it needs to be scrubbed well. It can be baked in its skin, then peeled; for other cooking methods the thick skin should be pared off first. Slice or dice celeriac and braise or boil it until tender, or grate it or cut it into thin sticks for serving raw (in salads or as a crudité, with a creamy yogurt dressing or dip).

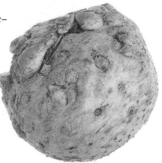

celeriac

Celeriac, like celery, is low in calories; vitamin C and potassium are its key nutrients.

Crosne (Chinese artichoke) These look like little, beige-skinned spiraled seashells. They are similar to Jerusalem artichokes in taste and texture.

Cushcush This is a species of tropical yam from the Caribbean with a variety of names: In Puerto Rico it's called *mapuey*; in Cuba it's an *aja*; in Jamaica it's *yampi*.

Jerusalem artichoke (sunchoke) This native American tuber resembles a small nubby potato or a piece of ginger. Jerusalem artichoke has been its common name since the 17th century, but it is also available in the market under the name "sunchoke," which is certainly more appropriate. The plant has no connection to either Jerusalem or artichokes, but is, in fact, a type of sunflower. So why is it called Jerusalem artichoke? One conjecture is that the French explorer Champlain sampled the vegetable in the early 1600s in Massachusetts, where it was cultivated by

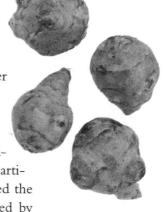

jerusalem artichokes

Native Americans, and he likened its taste to that of an artichoke. Some years later, after the "chokes" had been introduced to Europe, the English added Jerusalem—perhaps a corruption of *girasole* (an Italian word that means "turning to the sun," and is also the word for sunflower) or the mispronunciation of Terneuzen, a Dutch town that may have supplied the English with some of its first samples.

Like potatoes and other tubers, the Jerusalem artichoke stores carbohydrates, but most of them are in the form of inulin, a sugar that can sometimes cause flatulence. (If you have never sampled a sunchoke, you should eat it in small amounts until you are able to determine how your body will react to it.) The vegetable is also an incomparable source of iron, almost on a par with meat, yet without any fat content.

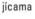

jícama

Jícama The growing popularity of Mexican food has popularized this root vegetable in the United States. Jícama is a white-fleshed tuber that can weigh from half a pound to 5 pounds or more. Shaped like a turnip, it has a thin brown skin and crisp, juicy flesh rather like a fine-textured apple. Its bland flavor enables jícama to be used in a variety of ways. You can serve raw slices or sticks sprinkled with lime juice and chili powder, or add it to salsa or salads; include slivers in stir-fries (a good substitute for water chestnuts); or boil or bake jícama like a potato. Look for hard, unblemished jícama roots that are heavy for their size. Peel the papery skin with a paring knife; store cut pieces of jícama in a container of cold water.

Although jícama can be used in some of the same ways as a potato, it is less starchy and lower in calories (a cup of sliced jícama has about 50 calories). The vegetable is a good source of vitamin C, and also contains some potassium, iron, and calcium.

Kumara See Sweet Potatoes (*page 558*).

Malanga A starchy tropical tuber with a nutlike flavor, malanga is called *yautia* by Puerto Ricans (*malanga* is the Colombian name). It is typically used as a bland foil for spicy side dishes or condiments. Sold in the Latin food section of some supermarkets and in Latin American grocery stores, malanga can be recognized by its yamlike shape (although it may weigh 2 pounds or more) and its rough, fuzzy brown skin, which reveals patches of yellowish or pinkish flesh beneath. Choose a firm, heavy root free of soft spots, and store it at cool room temperature for a day or two, or in the refrigerator crisper for up to a week. Peel malanga and boil, steam, or bake it until tender. Like potatoes, malanga can be served sliced, in chunks, or mashed, with a well-seasoned sauce or as a companion to a flavorful stew.

Name yam (tropical yam) The word *name* is the African word for yam. Name has a rough, dark skin and light-colored flesh. It is starchy and dry-fleshed and only slightly sweet. Use it as you would potatoes or sweet potatoes.

Parsley root This beige-colored vegetable is a subspecies of parsley that is grown for its roots. It tastes somewhat like celeriac and can be used in a very similar fashion. The tops can be used like regular leaf parsley.

Salsify "Oyster plant" is an old-fashioned name for this parsniplike root vegetable, as some people find the flavor reminiscent of oysters. The long, 1-inch-thick roots have tan skin and white flesh. (*Scorzonera,* a similar root, has brownish-black skin and cream-colored flesh.) Although it is not very common, you'll find this vegetable in some markets in the fall and winter; look for firm, plump, unblemished roots and store them in the refrigerator. After scraping or peeling the roots, place them in acidulated water to keep them from darkening. Like other root vegetables, salsify's starch turns to sugar during cold storage; it is also sometimes left in the ground over the winter to sweeten (like parsnips).

A single cup of cooked salsify has about 90 calories and provides riboflavin, vitamin B_6, and potassium.

Sunchoke See Jerusalem artichoke (*page 513*).

Taro The word taro (as well as dasheen, malanga, and other names) is applied to quite a number of starchy tropical tubers—all high-carbohydrate foods that are staples in the Pacific islands, Asia, the Caribbean, Africa, and parts of South America. Taro root's most familiar use is in poi, a sticky taro paste eaten in Hawaii. One of the more common forms of taro is a roughly cylindrical, brown-skinned root with white or pale purple flesh. You may find it in Spanish or Asian markets, and it may be cut open to display its quality. Choose a firm taro root with no shriveled or soft spots; store it in a cool, dry place or in the refrigerator crisper for no longer than 1 week. Taro resembles potatoes in flavor and uses: Boil, bake, or steam it (peeling it before or after cooking) and serve it with a flavorful sauce. Be sure to serve it hot, as it becomes very sticky as it cools.

Water chestnuts Anyone who has eaten in a Chinese restaurant is probably familiar with water chestnuts: Their crisp white flesh has a mildly sweet flavor and a crunchy texture that is actually closer to apples than to any kind of nut. In their fresh form, they do look like chestnuts, but they are not nuts (and have hardly any fat). Some sources classify this vegetable as a tuber, but it is technically a corm—the swollen tip of an underground stem that, like a tuber, stores carbohydrates for the plant's growth. The water chestnut grows underwater in mud. It has brown or black scalelike leaves and closely resembles a small, muddy tulip bulb.

water chestnuts

Since nearly all of the water chestnuts marketed in the United States come in canned form, most people have only seen the water chestnut with its scaly outer covering removed. Although fresh ones need to be peeled and cleaned, it is well worth the effort, since they are tastier than canned chestnuts and hold up especially well under cooking, gaining in sweetness while losing none of their crunch. When you buy fresh water chestnuts (primarily from Asian food markets), they should look sooty (they should not have been washed), but should be smooth, except for a few leaf scales. In addition, they should be rock hard and completely free of soft spots.

Yam Americans have appropriated the term yam and use it to mean orange-fleshed (as opposed to white- or yellow-fleshed) sweet potatoes. But in fact yams come from an entirely different, and large, botanical group of vegetables of the genus *Dioscorea*. (Sweet potatoes are all varieties of a plant classified as *Ipomoea batatas*.) Not only is the yam family large—there are some 600 species—but individual members of the family have attained record-breaking weights. An African species called elephant's foot produces a yam that can weigh up to 700 pounds. There are a handful of yams that eventually make it to the American market, by way of local African, Asian, or Caribbean populations: cushcush, name yam, Japanese yam, yama root, yamiamo. The names of these yams frequently translate simply as "yam."

Yamiamo This yam comes from Japan. It looks more like a severely elongated, cylindrical white potato than a yam. It has beige skin and white flesh, and it is fairly glutinous, with a texture similar to taro.

Yuca Also called manioc or cassava, this starchy tuber is cultivated in South America (where it originated), as well as in Africa, the Caribbean, the South Pacific, and Florida. Yuca is shaped like an elongated potato; it's about a foot long, weighs up to 3 pounds or so, and is covered with a hairy, brown, barklike skin enclosing soft, dense white flesh. Cooking it not only makes it palatable, but also eliminates a toxic substance that can form in varying amounts in the raw vegetable. Shop for yuca in Latin American markets, looking for dry, hard, clean roots with perfectly white flesh (grocers often cut them to show the inside). Yuca doesn't keep well, but it may stay fresh for a few days in the refrigerator or in a cool, dry place. To prepare the vegetable, cut it into thick slabs and peel them one at a time with a sharp paring knife. Yuca can also be dried and ground into flour; it is sold as tapioca flour (*see Flour, Nonwheat, page 326*). Tapioca pudding is made from beads of tapioca flour.

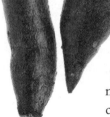

cassava

rye

Closely related and very similar in appearance to wheat (except for the bluish-gray color of the grain itself), rye probably originated in Asia and spread westward as a weed, infesting fields of wheat and barley. It was eventually recognized as a food plant and was first cultivated in eastern Europe during the 4th century B.C. Rye thrives where it is too wet and cold for other grains, and so has been widely consumed in Scandinavia, eastern Europe, and Russia for hundreds of years. In the United States, rye was introduced by British and Dutch settlers and became a staple in colonial New England. For years, New Englanders ate rye as a cereal grain, like rice or barley.

During the 20th century, rye production decreased considerably both here and abroad. Although still favored for breadmaking in Scandinavia and parts of eastern Europe, today the grain ranks eighth among cereal crops in world production. In the United States, only a quarter of the annual crop is set aside for human food (most Americans have never eaten rye except in commercial bread and crackers); the rest is used for the production of rye whiskey and other spirits, and for animal feed.

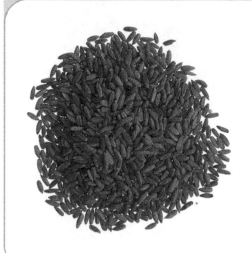

rye berries

nutritional profile

In addition to its hearty taste, rye is highly nutritious and provides protein, lots of fiber, B vitamins, and high amounts of the antioxidant mineral selenium.

in the market

The nutrient content of the whole-rye products listed below is far better than that of refined rye-flour products.

Cracked rye This type cooks more quickly than whole rye kernels. It can be added to soups, or cooked and eaten as a pilaf or hot cereal.

Flakes These resemble rolled oats and are made by the same process: The berries are heated and then pressed with steel rollers. Like oatmeal, rye flakes can be cooked as a hot breakfast cereal or mixed into yeast bread, quick bread, and muffin recipes.

Flour See Flour, Nonwheat (*page 326*).

Whole rye berries Also called whole kernels or groats, rye berries resemble wheat berries, and can be cooked just like them.

WHOLE-GRAIN RYE ¼ cup raw	
Calories	142
Protein (g)	6
Carbohydrate (g)	30
Dietary fiber (g)	6.2
Total fat (g)	1.1
Saturated fat (g)	0.1
Monounsaturated fat (g)	0.1
Polyunsaturated fat (g)	0.5
Cholesterol (mg)	0
Potassium (mg)	112
Sodium (mg)	3

KEY NUTRIENTS (%RDA/AI*)	
Thiamin	0.1 mg (11%)
Niacin	1.8 mg (11%)
Iron	1.1 mg (14%)
Magnesium	51 mg (12%)
Selenium	15 mcg (27%)
Zinc	1.6 mg (14%)

*For more detailed information on RDA and AI, see page 88.

salmon

Succulent, delicious, and nutritious, salmon is one of America's most popular fish. Salmon live in the ocean except during the spawning season, when they return to the coastal rivers and streams where they were born. Some types of salmon travel thousands of miles between the time they leave the rivers as juveniles until they return as adults. Farmed salmon are raised in salt water, though their flesh doesn't have the same rich nuances in flavor and texture as that of their wild ocean-roaming counterparts.

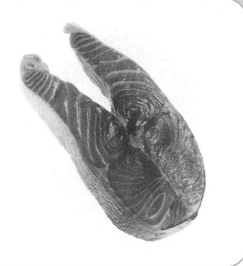

salmon steak

nutritional profile

The tender, rich meat of salmon provides substantial benefits, including protein, thiamin, niacin, vitamin B_6, vitamin D, potassium, selenium, and an impressive amount of vitamin B_{12}. Canned salmon containing the soft edible bones will also provide a respectable amount of calcium. Furthermore, though salmon contains cholesterol, it is low in saturated fat, which is more of a health risk than dietary cholesterol.

One of salmon's principal nutritional attributes, however, is its valuable omega-3 fatty acids. In fact, salmon is one of the top sources of these healthy fats. The American Heart Association revised its dietary guidelines to advise eating at least two servings of fish a week. It emphasized fatty fish such as salmon, since this is one instance where fat may help protect the heart. The rich oils in salmon contain polyunsaturated fatty acids called omega-3s, notably eicosapentaenoic acid (EPA) and docosahexaenoic acid (DHA). These omega-3s make platelets in the blood less likely to stick together and may reduce inflammatory processes in blood vessels (and elsewhere). Thus they reduce blood clotting, thereby lessening the chance of a fatal heart attack. Omega-3s can reduce triglycerides, the major type of fat that circulates in the blood. They may also make the heart less susceptible to dangerous, sometimes fatal, rhythm abnormalities. In addition, there's promising research showing that fish oil may help relieve inflammatory symptoms of autoimmune diseases such as rheumatoid arthritis or psoriasis.

And if you are wondering if farm-raised fish also contain these healthy fats, the answer is "yes." Studies have found that farmed fish are sometimes higher in omega-3s than wild fish, sometimes lower, depending on the species and other factors. Farmed fish do tend to have a higher total fat content. That would suggest that they contain more of the heart-healthy omega-3s (though as a proportion of the total fat content, the omega-3s may be lower). For instance, 3 ounces of cooked wild coho salmon has about 4 grams of fat (and 118 calories), while the farmed has 7 grams (and 151 calories).

FARMED ATLANTIC SALMON 3 ounces cooked	
Calories	175
Protein (g)	19
Carbohydrate (g)	0
Dietary fiber (g)	0
Total fat (g)	11
Saturated fat (g)	2.1
Monounsaturated fat (g)	3.8
Polyunsaturated fat (g)	3.8
Cholesterol (mg)	57
Potassium (mg)	327
Sodium (mg)	52

KEY NUTRIENTS (%RDA/AI*)	
Thiamin	0.3 mg (24%)
Niacin	6.9 mg (43%)
Vitamin B_6	0.6 mg (32%)
Vitamin B_{12}	2.4 mcg (99%)

*For more detailed information on RDA and AI, see page 88.

in the market

Several types of salmon are sold commercially, but the most important are: chinook, sockeye, coho, and pink. The pinkness of the flesh of salmon is directly related to their diet. Fish that eat lots of shrimp tend to have the pinkest flesh. Depending on the size of the fish, fresh salmon is sold whole, in fillets, and in steaks. Flash-freezing on fishing boats and deliveries by air bring most salmon varieties fresh to markets around the country. Most varieties, except coho, are available canned.

Atlantic salmon This is the only salmon native to the Atlantic. The population of wild Atlantic salmon has decreased over the years, but farmed Atlantic salmon accounts for more than 80 percent of the world's farmed salmon (Atlantic salmon is also farmed in the Pacific). They are similar to chinooks in oil content, but their flesh is a deeper orange in color. Much of the smoked salmon sold in this country comes from Atlantic salmon.

Chinook (king, spring) Caught in the icy waters of the North Pacific, the chinook is the largest, fattiest salmon variety and has firm, deep-red flesh. There is also a white-fleshed chinook salmon. Chinook is sold fresh, frozen, and smoked.

Coho (silver, medium-red) Found in the coastal waters of Alaska, the coho is less fatty than sockeye. The flesh is medium-red and very flavorful.

Chum (keta, chub, dog) Males develop caninelike teeth during spawning, thus the nickname dog salmon. Leaner than sockeye with firm, coarse, pale flesh, chums are not farmed. They make it to supermarkets as fresh fish in the fall.

Pink (humpback, humpie) Males develop large humps on their backs during spawning, thus the nickname. The smallest, leanest salmon, caught in the Pacific, it has soft, bland, pink flesh. It is the type most commonly used for canned salmon.

Sockeye (red, blueback) Second to the chinook in fat content, the sockeye salmon also has dark red flesh. It is the finest type of canned salmon, but it is also sold fresh.

FARMED COHO SALMON 3 ounces cooked	
Calories	151
Protein (g)	21
Carbohydrate (g)	0
Dietary fiber (g)	0
Total fat (g)	7.0
Saturated fat (g)	1.7
Monounsaturated fat (g)	3.1
Polyunsaturated fat (g)	1.7
Cholesterol (mg)	54
Potassium (mg)	391
Sodium (mg)	44

KEY NUTRIENTS (%RDA/AI*)	
Niacin	6.3 mg (39%)
Vitamin B_6	0.5 mg (28%)
Vitamin B_{12}	2.7 mcg (12%)
Selenium	12 mcg (22%)

*For more detailed information on RDA and AI, see page 88.

choosing the best

Fresh salmon does not keep well, so buy it the day you want to eat it, or at most, the day before. Do all other shopping first before buying fish, and get it into a refrigerator as soon as possible after buying it. On hot days, have the salmon packed in ice to keep it chilled in transit.

Look for flesh that is firm (it should spring back when touched), translucent, and moist, but with no liquid pooling around it. The smell should be sweet, not fishy. Ask if the fish has been frozen and thawed, so you will know if you can freeze it at home. Avoid buying salmon at bargain prices; they often indicate the store's effort to get rid of fish that's less than fresh.

Canned salmon, a pantry staple, is available everywhere. Look for the fattiest variety, because it's the tastiest.

Smoked salmon is best when purchased at a counter where it is freshly cut. Vacuum-sealed packs of smoked salmon are good if they have been properly stored in transit, so buy from reputable shops. Pick prewrapped salmon only in stores with a very high daily turnover.

▶ **When you get home** Salmon should be stored like all fresh fish (*see page 320*) and cooked the same day it is bought, or at most, the day after. Whole fish will keep better than steaks or fillets. As soon as you get salmon home, rinse it, place it on paper towels, seal it in a clean plastic bag, and store in the coldest part of the refrigerator or in a pan of ice.

To freeze fresh salmon, you need a freezer set at 0° or colder. Be sure to thaw frozen salmon in the refrigerator, not at room temperature. Cut large pieces (2 pounds or more) into steaks or fillets so they will freeze quickly. Rinse and pat dry, then tightly wrap individual pieces in heavy-duty freezer paper. Overwrap with foil or a freezer bag. Frozen salmon keeps about 3 months.

Smoked salmon keeps for up to 3 days wrapped tightly in the refrigerator. (For vacuum-packed smoked salmon, check the label for storage instructions.)

preparing to use

Before cooking, rinse fresh salmon and pat dry. Never leave fresh fish at room temperature. If marinating is called for, do it in the refrigerator.

CANNED SOCKEYE SALMON
3 ounces

Calories	130
Protein (g)	17
Carbohydrate (g)	0
Dietary fiber (g)	0
Total fat (g)	6.2
Saturated fat (g)	1.4
Monounsaturated fat (g)	2.7
Polyunsaturated fat (g)	1.6
Cholesterol (mg)	37
Potassium (mg)	321
Sodium (mg)	458

KEY NUTRIENTS (%RDA/AI*)

Riboflavin	0.2 mg (13%)
Niacin	4.7 mg (29%)
Vitamin B$_6$	0.3 mg (15%)
Vitamin B$_{12}$	0.3 mcg (11%)
Vitamin D	191 IU (48%)
Calcium	203 mg (17%)
Iron	0.9 mg (11%)
Selenium	30 mcg (55%)

*For more detailed information on RDA and AI, see page 88.

serving suggestions

• Add chunks of salmon to pasta sauces or chilis.

• Combine smoked salmon and reduced-fat cream cheese (Neufchâtel) in a food processor and blend to make a spread.

• Use canned or fresh salmon to make salmon cakes or burgers.

• Substitute salmon in a tuna salad and use as a stuffing for hollowed-out tomatoes.

• Make a salad: Combine chunks of cooked fresh salmon, cubes of cooked potato, pieces of fresh fennel, and diced red onion. Toss with a vinaigrette of olive oil, orange juice, and white wine vinegar.

• Brush fresh salmon steaks with balsamic vinegar and grill. Serve with a white bean and arugula salad.

• Poach salmon and serve it at room temperature or cold with a green sauce made with parsley, basil, spinach, lemon juice, and olive oil pureed in a blender.

scallops

The scallop is named for the handsome, fluted fan-shaped shells that surround the nuggets of tender-firm meat inside. Many people who aren't particularly fond of fish or shellfish enjoy the mild, sweet flavor of this bivalve mollusk.

Because scallops cannot close their shells tightly and tend to lose body moisture quickly, they die soon after being harvested. To preserve freshness, scallops are nearly always shucked and trimmed aboard fishing boats or on shore shortly after harvesting. For this reason, they are an easy type of shellfish to prepare and cook.

nutritional profile

The pale, creamy flesh of the scallop is low in cholesterol and supplies protein, vitamin B_{12}, vitamin E, potassium, and magnesium, as well as small amounts of omega-3 fatty acids.

in the market

There are two basic types of scallops available in fish markets—tiny bay scallops and much larger sea scallops. Calico scallops, a tiny variety of sea scallop sometimes sold as bay scallops, can also be found.

Bay scallops Ivory-colored, with a golden tinge, bay scallops are harvested from protected bays and shallow waters from New England to North Carolina, though they are most abundant from Cape Cod to Long Island. The shell grows to about 2 to 4 inches across, but the edible adductor muscle, or "eye" (what we call the scallop), is only about ½ inch in diameter. Bay scallops have a firm texture and very sweet, delicate flavor. There are about 100 bay scallops to the pound.

Calico scallops These small sea scallops (about ½ inch in diameter) are taken mainly from the Gulf of Mexico off of Florida. They're darker in color, less sweet, and not as firm as bay scallops, and are consequently considered inferior by many scallop fanciers. Because the shells must be steamed to open them, these scallops reach the consumer in a partially cooked state.

Sea scallops Translucent, ivory-colored sea scallops, harvested from deeper waters mainly along the Atlantic coast (but also from the Pacific) are much larger than bay scallops, with shells reaching 8 inches and the scallop itself measuring up to 2 inches in diameter. Chewier, with a less delicate flavor than bay scallops, they are often halved or quartered for use in recipes that call for the more expensive bay scallops. You get about 15 to 20 sea scallops to the pound.

▶ Availability The peak season for fresh bay scallops and sea scallops is October through March, although sea scallops can be found year round. Calico scallops are available fresh from December through May. Both bay scallops

sea scallops

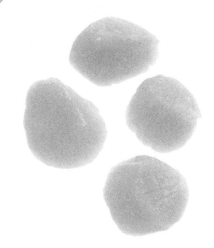

SCALLOPS 3 ounces cooked	
Calories	113
Protein (g)	18
Carbohydrate (g)	3
Dietary fiber (g)	0
Total fat (g)	3.4
Saturated fat (g)	0.6
Monounsaturated fat (g)	1.2
Polyunsaturated fat (g)	1.1
Cholesterol (mg)	34
Potassium (mg)	331
Sodium (mg)	435

KEY NUTRIENTS (%RDA/AI*)	
Vitamin B_{12}	1.5 mcg (62%)
Vitamin E	1.4 mg (10%)
Magnesium	58 mg (14%)

*For more detailed information on RDA and AI, see page 88.

and sea scallops can be purchased fresh-frozen or precooked and frozen, either breaded or plain.

choosing the best

Look for glossy firm scallops with a sweet smell; those with a strong odor of iodine or sulfur aren't fresh. Avoid unusually bright white scallops bulging at the sides and melting together; this may be a sign that they have been soaked in water to increase their weight or soaked with phosphates to keep them fresh longer.

Some unscrupulous markets have been known to cut out tiny "bay scallops" from the larger, less-tender sea scallops, or even substitute shark meat for scallops. If all the scallops seem uniform in size and shape, this could be a signal that they're not what they seem.

▶ When you get home Like all shellfish, it is important to keep scallops cold until you are ready to cook them to prevent bacterial contamination. Uncooked scallops should be stored like fresh fish (*see page 320*) and used the same day you purchase them.

You can freeze raw scallops, but they are better when they are cooked before freezing. Poach them, then freeze them in airtight containers or tightly sealed heavy-duty freezer bags. They should keep for 2 months if the freezer is set at 0° or colder. Be sure to thaw frozen scallops in the refrigerator, not at room temperature.

preparing to use

Some purists suggest cutting away the tough connective tissue known as the foot before cooking scallops, but if you're in a rush, this isn't necessary, since it is edible. Sea scallops are often halved crosswise to make them a more uniform size; they can also be quartered for use in place of bay scallops. Frozen scallops should be thawed in the refrigerator and can then be prepared just like fresh ones (drain any liquid and pat dry).

facts & tips

Because we do not eat the scallop animal itself but merely the adductor muscle (which holds the two halves of the shell together), there is less chance of contamination by pollutants. Other bivalves, such as clams and mussels for example, filter any pollutants in their environment through their organs, which is included in what we eat.

Nonetheless, people in high-risk health categories should not eat scallops raw. For more on shellfish safety, see pages 119–122.

serving suggestions

- Bake scallops in parchment along with sliced vegetables.
- Add bay scallops to pasta sauces.
- Skewer sea scallops, top with barbecue sauce, and grill.
- Add scallops to a seafood chowder or stew.
- Toss scallops with bread crumbs and grated Parmesan, drizzle with olive oil, and broil.
- Add scallops to vegetable stir-fries at the very end of cooking.
- Poach scallops and toss in a citrus dressing.
- Substitute scallops for shrimp in scampi, shrimp marinara, or other shrimp dishes.
- Add scallops to chicken and rice for a take-off on "paella."

seeds

Seeds are the means by which most plants propagate. Hence they contain a dense concentration of nutrients and essential oils that will be used by the new plants when and if the seeds get the opportunity to germinate. Although there are many foods we eat that are technically seeds—beans, peas, most nuts, and all grains—some seeds fall into a separate category defined more by their culinary use than anything else. These are loosely called edible seeds—not a semantic distinction, to be sure, just a cook's distinction. These seeds tend to be smaller (think of a sesame seed compared with a kidney bean) and have a higher proportion of fat. In fact, many seeds are used primarily for their oils. Though they are small, edible seeds can offer a substantial amount of flavor, texture, and nutritional benefits. On these pages are the seeds that we use one way or another as food, but there is a whole subset of edible seeds that we use as spices, such as caraway, cardamom, dill seed, and fennel (see "Herbs & Spices," page 614).

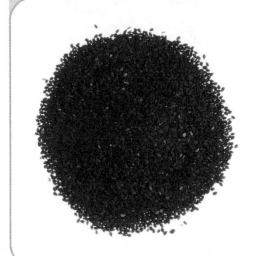

black sesame seeds

nutritional profile

Seeds offer a rich reservoir of nutrients such as iron, and phosphorus. And there is a moderate amount of protein in seeds, though the protein is incomplete. Seeds are used to make oils (see Fats & Oils, page 297), with sunflower, safflower, and sesame oils some of the more common examples.

Because of their fat content, seeds should be eaten in moderation, though it is noteworthy that the type of fats in seeds is primarily healthful polyunsaturated fats, some of which provide essential fatty acids. For example, flaxseed (see page 322) provide a beneficial type of fat called alpha-linolenic acid (ALA), which is linked to a reduced risk of heart disease. ALA is one of the essential fatty acids—that is, it's essential for life, and we must consume it in foods, because our bodies cannot manufacture it. The other commonly consumed seeds, such as sunflower seeds and pumpkin seeds, also provide important nutrients, such as vitamin E and iron.

HULLED SESAME SEEDS 1 tablespoon	
Calories	55
Protein (g)	3
Carbohydrate (g)	1
Dietary fiber (g)	1.1
Total fat (g)	5.1
Saturated fat (g)	0.7
Monounsaturated fat (g)	1.9
Polyunsaturated fat (g)	2.3
Cholesterol (mg)	0
Potassium (mg)	38
Sodium (mg)	4

in the market

Chia seeds Remember chia pets? Remember that when you mixed chia seeds with water they formed a gelatinous paste? Like flaxseed, chia seeds form a natural mucilage (a type of soluble fiber) when wet. In cooking, this translates to a good, nonfat thickener (add the gel to smoothies, soups, or pasta sauces). Used by Aztec warriors as a source of energy on long marches, chia seeds are high in protein (with all essential amino acids), alpha-linolenic acid, and fiber. Don't try eating the seeds that come with chia pets, though, unless you know that they don't treat their seeds with chemicals. A better source is a health-food store.

Egusi seeds In West Africa, egusi melons are a subspecies of the watermelon. Their seeds have a high oil content, and West Africans grind the seeds into a meal, which they use to thicken and flavor stews. Like pumpkin seeds, egusi seeds are generally sold in their hulls.

Flaxseed See Flaxseed (*page 322*).

Hemp seeds Hemp seeds (and the oil pressed from them) are high in unsaturated fats, including heart-healthy alpha-linolenic acid (ALA), an omega-3 fatty acid. Hemp is the same plant as *Cannabis sativa,* from which marijuana is made. But certain species can be bred and grown for seeds and oil, rather than for the psychoactive ingredient tetrahydrocannabinol (THC). Hemp seeds have traces of THC, but not enough to produce a high. Still, hemp is an illegal crop in the United States and can be grown in Canada and Europe only if the strains planted have minimal THC content. But hemp seeds and oil are a legal import here, provided the seeds have been heat-treated to prevent germination. Roasted hemp seeds make a nice snack.

Jackfruit seeds The seeds of the immense jackfruit (*see Exotic Fruits, page 287*) are huge: ¾ to 1½ inches long and ½ to ¾ inch thick. There may be from 100 to 500 seeds in a single jackfruit. The seeds have a starchy flesh not unlike chestnuts and must be boiled first and then roasted. They are often sold sweetened and canned (again, like chestnuts).

Lotus seeds The small, round white seeds of the lotus plant are most often sold as a canned, sweetened paste in Chinese markets. The paste is one of the classic fillings for Chinese moon cakes.

Papaya seeds Most people scoop out the papaya seeds and discard them, but they are edible. These glossy black seeds resemble peppercorns and have a spicy, pepperlike flavor that's been compared to nasturtium, watercress, and pepper. Rinse the seeds well and use them as a garnish; or dry them and grind them in a blender or food processor to the consistency of coarse ground pepper for use as a seasoning.

Poppy seeds The poppy's botanical name, *Papaver somniferum*, hints at the plant's unfortunate narcotic associations, but the milky sap that produces opium is long gone by the time the plant produces tiny seeds (each flower has about 30,000 of them). In addition to the plant's history as a drug, its nutty tasting, blue-black seeds have a long-standing culinary history, too. In fact, the Romans made something similar to halvah (*see sesame seeds, opposite page*) by roasting the seeds, mixing them with honey, and forming them into "candy" bars. And in Middle European cultures, poppy seeds were—and still are—ground and sweetened and used as a pastry filling called *mohn* (which actually just means poppy in German). In Indian markets you can find *white poppy seeds,* which Indian cooks use as a thickener. Use poppy seeds on top of baked goods (or kneaded into bread dough as Greek cooks do) or grind them with other spices to make a rich curry powder.

Pumpkin seeds See Pumpkin Seeds (*page 496*).

POPPY SEEDS / 1 tablespoon	
Calories	47
Protein (g)	2
Carbohydrate (g)	2
Dietary fiber (g)	0.9
Total fat (g)	3.9
Saturated fat (g)	0.4
Monounsaturated fat (g)	0.6
Polyunsaturated fat (g)	2.7
Cholesterol (mg)	0
Potassium (mg)	62
Sodium (mg)	2

KEY NUTRIENTS (%RDA/AI*)	
Calcium	127 mg (11%)
Iron	0.8 mg (10%)

For more detailed information on RDA and AI, see page 88.

Sesame seeds These tiny oval seeds, which grow on a tall annual plant, are basic to many of the world's cuisines, including those of Africa, India, and China. Dark sesame oil is a staple cooking ingredient in Asia. And tahini, a spread similar to peanut butter, is known as the "butter of the Middle East." Sesame seeds are also ground, mixed with honey, and formed into huge blocks for a Middle Eastern candy called halvah (although this term, which just means "candy," is also applied to similar mixtures made with various grains and nuts instead of sesame seeds). Sesame seeds were brought to America with the slave trade, and are still used in several popular Southern recipes (they are called benne seeds in the South). Their most familiar use in this country is as a topping on breads, buns, and rolls. You can buy *hulled* or *unhulled* sesame seeds; the unhulled, which are darker in color, have the bran intact and are an excellent source of iron and phosphorus. There are also *black sesame seeds*, but they are smaller and somewhat more bitter.

Squash seeds In addition to pumpkin seeds, other squash (and even melons) have seeds that are extremely tasty. Squash grown specifically for their seeds are often different from the plants grown for their vegetables. Growers reduce the space between the plants because the size of the fruit is of secondary concern.

Sunflower seeds See Sunflower Seeds (*page 555*).

Watermelon seeds Watermelon seeds are a favorite in China and the Middle East where they're eaten like sunflower seeds or pumpkin seeds. These seeds come from melons grown specifically for their seeds and are much larger than the seeds you find in watermelon cultivated to be eaten as a fruit.

choosing the best

Since most seeds are high in fat and subject to rancidity, buy seeds that are stored out of direct sunlight and away from other sources of heat. If buying in bulk, be sure that you are shopping at a store that does a brisk turnover.

▶ **When you get home** The high fat content of seeds makes them prone to rancidity; heat, light, and humidity will speed spoilage. Although seeds will keep for several months at room temperature in a cool, dry place, it's really best to keep them in the refrigerator. Better still, keep them in the freezer, where they will last a year or more.

preparing to use

Most seeds taste better if they are toasted before you eat or cook with them. Seeds can be toasted on the stovetop or in the oven; the cooking time will depend on the type of seeds and their fat content.

serving suggestions

• Top a salad with a sprinkling of toasted seeds.

• Stir toasted seeds and minced chives into yogurt cheese for a bagel or sandwich spread.

• Combine sesame seeds with bread crumbs and use as a coating for baked fish or poultry.

• Stir a spoonful of sesame butter (tahini) into a vegetable soup to enrich and thicken it.

• Knead poppy seeds into homemade pasta dough.

shellfish

Shellfish is a broad term for aquatic animals that have a shell or shell-like exoskeleton. Although you're likely to encounter far more types of fish than shellfish in a seafood store or on a restaurant menu, shellfish nevertheless exist in many varieties. Their flavors range from sweet to briny and their textures from "meaty" to soft and delicate. Many people who aren't fish eaters will happily consume lobster, shrimp, or scallops—foods that are as distinct from one another as they are from fish with fins.

There are two general categories of edible shellfish—crustaceans and mollusks. Crabs, crayfish, lobster, and shrimp are all crustaceans, whose segmented bodies are covered with armorlike sections of thick or thin shell. Mollusks include two-shelled bivalves (clams, oysters, mussels, and scallops) as well as univalves, such as abalone, periwinkles and other snails, conch, and whelk, which have a single shell covering a soft body. Another class of mollusks are the cephalopods, whose pliable body consists of a beaked head, an internal shell in some species, and tentacles sprouting directly from the head (cephalopod is derived from the Greek meaning "headed foot"). Squid and octopus are the most popular edible cephalopods.

nutritional profile

A healthy alternative to meat, shellfish provide high-quality protein and an array of important vitamins and minerals, as well as heart-healthy omega-3 fatty acids. Shellfish are naturally low in calories, but how you prepare them can have a significant effect upon their calorie content. For example, a 3-ounce serving of boiled or steamed shrimp has only 84 calories and derives only 10 percent of those calories from fat; an equivalent portion of breaded, deep-fried shrimp, on the other hand, packs about 240 calories—more than 45 percent of them from fat. In the case of clams, the calories go from 126 (12 percent from fat) for steamed clams to 202 (50 percent from fat) for fried clams.

Shellfish are also low in saturated fat, but depending upon the type of shellfish, they can have moderate to high amounts of cholesterol, which in the past, excluded them from low-cholesterol diets. However, research now indicates that dietary cholesterol is less of a health risk than saturated fat because it doesn't raise blood cholesterol as much as saturated fat does. Indeed, many types of shellfish (crabs, scallops, mussels, clams, and lobster, among them) are actually slightly lower in cholesterol than chicken or beef. In addition, research suggests that the cholesterol in shellfish may not be as well absorbed by the body as that in other foods.

in the market

The list that follows comprises a representative sampling of the more popular shellfish species in North America. The shellfish are identified by their most common names, although you will find that many varieties have local designations as well.

Abalone This mollusk grows wild in waters along the California coast, but because commercial fishing of abalone is prohibited, wild abalone must be captured by divers and is rarely found in the market. Farm-raised red abalone from California are widely available, however, and are often found in Asian markets. Red abalone average about 3 inches in shell length (you get about 6 abalone meats to the pound). Abalone can be purchased fresh, frozen, or dried, and is also available by mail order from growers in California.

Clams See Clams (*page 253*).

Conch Harvested from southern waters, and particularly popular in Florida and the Caribbean, the white meat of the conch is encased in a beautiful, brightly colored spiral shell. As with abalone and whelk, it is the conch's footlike muscle that is eaten, either raw or cooked. Conch can be purchased fresh or frozen in specialty seafood stores and is often found in Chinese or Italian markets. Conch is sometimes mistakenly referred to as whelk, which (though related) is an entirely different species.

Crab See Crab (*page 263*).

Crayfish (crawfish) See Lobster & Crayfish (*page 383*).

Lobster See Lobster & Crayfish (*page 383*).

Mussels See Mussels (*page 409*).

Octopus Possibly the strangest-looking sea creature used as food, the purplish-black octopus is caught primarily on the Pacific coast and is also imported. It is usually sold frozen (or thawed) and already dressed (cleaned). Octopus provides an extraordinary amount of vitamin B_{12}.

OCTOPUS / 3 ounces cooked	
Calories	140
Protein (g)	25
Carbohydrate (g)	4
Dietary fiber (g)	0
Total fat (g)	1.8
Saturated fat (g)	0.4
Monounsaturated fat (g)	0.3
Polyunsaturated fat (g)	0.4
Cholesterol (mg)	82
Potassium (mg)	536
Sodium (mg)	391

KEY NUTRIENTS (%RDA/AI*)	
Niacin	3.2 mg (20%)
Vitamin B_6	0.6 mg (32%)
Vitamin B_{12}	31 mcg (1,276%)
Vitamin E	2.0 mg (13%)
Iron	8.1 mg (101%)
Magnesium	51 mg (12%)
Selenium	76 mcg (139%)
Zinc	2.9 mg (26%)

For more detailed information on RDA and AI, see page 88.

COMPARING SHELLFISH 3 ounces cooked

As a general rule of thumb, 4 ounces of raw shellfish will yield 3 ounces of cooked. The ounce measurement of raw is for shucked or shelled meat.

	Calories	Fat (g)	% Calories from Fat	Saturated Fat (g)	Cholesterol (mg)	Omega-3s (g)
Abalone	179	1.3	6	0.2	145	--
Clams	126	1.7	12	0.2	57	0.3
Conch/Whelk	234	0.7	3	0.1	111	0
Crab	87	1.5	15	0.2	85	0.4
Crayfish	74	1.1	13	0.2	117	0.2
Lobster	83	0.5	5	0.1	61	0.1
Mussels	146	3.8	23	0.7	48	0.7
Octopus	140	1.8	12	0.4	82	0.3
Oysters	67	1.8	24	0.6	32	0.4
Scallops	113	3.4	27	0.6	34	0.8
Shrimp	84	0.9	10	0.3	166	0.3
Squid	117	4.0	31	0.9	239	--

Oysters See Oysters (*page 435*).

Periwinkles There are more than 300 species of this conical, spiral-shelled univalve (also known as winkles or sea snails). The most common edible varieties are the *Edible Periwinkle, Gulf Periwinkle,* and *Southern Periwinkle.* They can be purchased in specialty seafood stores and Asian markets and are also easily harvested by hand. Edible Periwinkles grow to only about 1 inch in size, so you'll need plenty to make a meal. The snails must be simmered briefly before the meat can be picked out with a toothpick.

Scallops See Scallops (*page 521*).

Shrimp See Shrimp (*page 530*).

Squid More streamlined than its relative, the octopus, this 10-armed cephalopod is netted on both coasts and is sometimes marketed as *calamari,* its Italian name. Squid has a firm, chewy texture and a mild flavor. It is sold both whole and dressed, and is available fresh or frozen. The squid's hollow body (also called the mantle or tube) is perfect for stuffing or may be cut crosswise into rings. The tentacles can be chopped into pieces and eaten as well. Squid contain a sac of brownish-black ink (used as protective camouflage in its ocean habitat); some recipes call for the ink, which is also sold in many markets, to be used in cooking the squid.

Whelk Harvested from cold waters from Maine to the Gulf of Mexico, the common northern whelk *(Buccinum undatum),* notable for its thick spiral shell, is the species most often found in the market. As with abalone and conch, it is the footlike muscle that's eaten. The flavorful meat is blotchy white, streaked with black. Whelk are mainly sold in Asian and Italian markets.

choosing the best

Shop for shellfish as you would for fish. Choose a reputable purveyor and follow your senses. Be sure fresh shellfish really smells fresh. If you are buying octopus or squid whole, the eyes should be bright, not cloudy. Fresh abalone should be alive and in the shell when purchased. Prod the abalone gently: The exposed muscle should move when touched. When buying frozen shellfish, select only tightly sealed packages with no ice crystals or any sign of refreezing. Always ask when cooked shellfish was cooked.

Make sure to purchase shellfish only when you can get home quickly to refrigerate it. In warm weather, or when you may be delayed on the trip home, have the shellfish packed in ice.

▶ **When you get home** Possibly the most perishable of all foodstuffs, any type of shellfish is highly susceptible to bacterial contamination and

---

a caution about raw shellfish

You may be aware that eating raw shellfish (such as oysters and clams) from contaminated waters can make you sick. But did you know that eating raw shellfish from waters that are certified clean also carries considerable heath risks? This is because the regulation of the shellfish industry is irregular at best, and agents charged with overseeing some 10 million acres of approved shellfish beds cannot keep up.

It's true, of course, that many people do eat raw shellfish without getting sick. If you decide to do so, make sure to buy the shellfish only from reputable markets or aquafarms. Also ask the dealer to show you the tag certifying that the shellfish were harvested from state-approved waters. If you gather your own shellfish, you should also exercise caution; check with local authorities about the safety of any waters where you intend to harvest. For more information on shellfish safety, see pages 119–122.

growth once it dies or gets too warm. Therefore, when you buy shellfish, it is imperative to keep it alive—and/or cold—until you are ready to cook and serve it (generally within a day or two of purchase). Live bivalves—such as clams, mussels, and oysters—can be kept refrigerated for 4 to 7 days.

Freeze all cooked shellfish in airtight containers or tightly sealed heavy-duty freezer bags. Most types of frozen raw or cooked shellfish will keep for 2 months if the freezer is set at 0° or colder. Be sure to thaw frozen shellfish in the refrigerator, not at room temperature.

preparing to use

Many popular types of shellfish, including shrimp, clams, mussels, and oysters, can be difficult to clean and prepare. Consult your fish seller for the best methods, or see the preparation information found in the individual entries in this book.

Abalone Because fresh abalone is purchased alive and in the shell, you will need to remove it before cooking. You can have your fish seller do this for you, or to easily separate the abalone meat from the shell yourself, simply drop it into boiling water for 10 seconds, remove immediately, and cut away the meat. Opinion varies on pounding fresh abalone to tenderize it. If you decide to do so, first cut the meat into thin steaks by slicing it horizontally across the muscle, or by slicing it vertically with the grain. Pound each slice with a light steady motion, using a wooden mallet or rolling pin. When properly pounded, abalone will feel soft and velvety. If the abalone has been frozen, the freezing process itself tenderizes the meat.

Conch and **whelk** Like abalone, conch and whelk can be bought live and in the shell. The method of extracting the animals, however, is quite difficult. So look for them already shelled, or have the fish seller shell them for you. Conch and whelk meat is often pounded to tenderize it, but freezing the meat before cooking also makes it tender.

Periwinkles Before cooking be sure to remove the hard, protective operculum from the end of each snail's foot or you'll have a crunchy meal.

Squid and **octopus** Both are commonly sold dressed and ready to cook. Wash them thoroughly before cooking. Some cooks feel that octopus must be pounded with a mallet to tenderize it before cooking; others find that cooking alone is sufficient.

sea urchins

These tiny creatures in spiny hard shells are members of a large group of marine animals called *Echinodermata,* which also includes starfish and sand dollars. Live sea urchins can be purchased at quality seafood purveyors or Asian markets: The spines should move when touched. To get to the edible roe (*uni* to sushi fans), which clings to the top inside part of the shell, you cut a circle in the bottom of the shell with scissors and scoop it out with a small spoon (be sure to wear gloves when doing so). Sea urchin roe is also packed and sold in trays for the retail market. Look for firm roe that is bright yellow or orange, not too dark or discolored. Because it is highly perishable, you may want to ask for a taste before buying.

shrimp

This crustacean ranks second to tuna as Americans' favorite seafood. Like chicken, its dense white meat has a fresh, mild flavor that marries well with a variety of ingredients. Unlike its close relatives, lobsters and crayfish, shrimp are primarily swimmers (rather than crawlers). They swim forward by paddling the legs (swimmerets) on their abdomens, but they can move backward quickly by using their fanlike tails. Shrimp are found in warm coastal water from Virginia on south, but the largest shrimp-fishing area is the Gulf of Mexico. The shrimp that are caught (in large baglike nets) are usually frozen right on the boat, or sometimes packed in ice for shipping "fresh."

Some 300 species of shrimp are sold worldwide, and are generally designated as warm-water or cold-water species. For the most part, the colder the water, the smaller and more succulent the shrimp. Though wild shrimp are caught in coastal waters of all continents, a number of shrimp farms also provide quantities of these delicious crustaceans.

Warm-water shrimp are caught in tropical waters. Much of the U. S. catch is harvested in the Atlantic and the Gulf of Mexico, but Latin America and Asia supply warm-water shrimp for import.

nutritional profile

A nutritious alternative to meat, shrimp are low in calories and saturated fat, and they supply protein, niacin, vitamin B_{12}, vitamin D, iron, selenium, and zinc.

Once considered a potentially unhealthy food, shrimp have suffered from an undeserved bad reputation. Health-conscious people sometimes still tend to shy away from shrimp, because they mistakenly assume that shrimp can cause high cholesterol. The truth is that although shrimp have about twice as much cholesterol as meat, they contain much less fat than meat, and their fat is largely unsaturated and includes heart-healthy omega-3 fatty acids.

Research suggests that dietary cholesterol is less of a health danger than saturated fat, which raises blood cholesterol more than dietary cholesterol does. A nourishing food that can be part of a heart-healthy diet, shrimp has emerged as a healthy food choice—just watch out for how shrimp is prepared. For example, in a typical serving of breaded shrimp, half of its weight may be the oil-soaked breading.

in the market

The commonest type of shrimp in the market is warm-water shrimp, a species that is classified by shell color—white, pink, and brown—though the differences in appearance and flavor are hard to detect. Fresh shrimp are sold in the shell and shelled and deveined. They are also sold cooked. Fresh-frozen

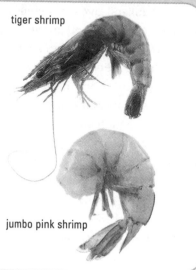

shrimp

tiger shrimp

jumbo pink shrimp

SHRIMP / 3 ounces cooked	
Calories	84
Protein (g)	18
Carbohydrate (g)	0
Dietary fiber (g)	0
Total fat (g)	0.9
Saturated fat (g)	0.3
Monounsaturated fat (g)	0.2
Polyunsaturated fat (g)	0.4
Cholesterol (mg)	166
Potassium (mg)	155
Sodium (mg)	191

KEY NUTRIENTS (%RDA/AI*)	
Niacin	2.2 mg (14%)
Vitamin B_{12}	1.3 mcg (53%)
Vitamin D	122 IU (30%)
Iron	2.6 mg (33%)
Selenium	34 mcg (61%)
Zinc	1.3 mg (12%)

*For more detailed information on RDA and AI, see page 88.

shrimp are sold in bulk: whole, shelled, and shelled and deveined, and either raw or cooked. You can also buy smaller quantities of cooked shrimp in cans or frozen in packages.

Brown shrimp These have a stronger, more pronounced iodine flavor than white shrimp. Their shells are reddish-brown.

Cold-water shrimp These are caught in the North Atlantic and northern Pacific, and have a firm texture and sweet flavor; they are usually sold cooked and peeled, but you can occasionally find them fresh. A popular type hails from Maine.

Pink shrimp Wild or farm-raised with light brown to reddish-pink shells, these shrimp are mild and sweet.

Rock shrimp So-named because of their rock-hard shells, their flavor is often compared to lobster.

Tiger shrimp Easily identified by their dark-striped shells, most of these shrimp are in the size range between Large and Jumbo, with 15 to 25 per pound. Because they are grown in warm, tropical waters, they grow quickly, making them the most widely distributed and marketed shrimp in the world. They have firm-textured meat and a mild flavor. Available frozen and raw, they are sometimes found in the market with their heads still on.

White shrimp These are wild or farm-raised and are harvested in waters from South Carolina to the Gulf of Mexico. White shrimp have firm flesh and a mild, sweet flavor.

choosing the best

Fresh shrimp should have a clean smell, with no trace of ammonia. If sold still frozen, shrimp should be solidly encased in ice. Cooked shrimp should be purchased the same day they were cooked (the same is true of cooked crab or

sizing shrimp

Shrimp come in a wide range of sizes; the larger the shrimp, the higher the price. In some areas of the country, very large shrimp may be called prawns, a term used in many other countries to refer to shrimp of any size. But in the United States, shrimp is the standard name for all types and sizes.

Size classifications range from Tiny (150 to 180 shrimp per pound) through Colossal (10 shrimp or less per pound). The usual sizes in the market are Medium (31 to 35 per pound), Large (21 to 30 per pound), and Jumbo (11 to 15 per pound).

Larger shrimp may cost more per pound, but this doesn't necessarily mean they taste any better than their smaller counterparts. However, buying larger shrimp will make the deveining and shelling task easier: Chances are you'll be buying the shrimp by the pound, not the piece; so you'll have fewer shrimp to shell.

lobster). If cooked in the shell, shrimp should be pinkish-orange, with opaque rather than translucent flesh. Fresh-cooked seafood shouldn't be displayed near raw fish or shellfish, as bacteria can migrate from the raw to the cooked.

▶ **When you get home** Uncooked shrimp should be stored like fish (*see page 320*) and used the same day you buy them. Do not freeze raw shrimp (since "fresh" shrimp have already been frozen once, and then thawed): Cook them first. Or, better still, buy frozen shrimp and be sure they are still solidly frozen when they reach your home freezer. Cooked, shelled, and deveined shrimp can be frozen in airtight packaging. Most types of frozen (raw or cooked) shrimp will keep for 2 months if the freezer is set at 0° or colder.

preparing to use

Shrimp purchased shelled and deveined are ready to be cooked, though this makes the shrimp more expensive. The less expensive option is to shell and devein them yourself. It's not difficult to do once you know how. You can shell the shrimp before cooking, or cook them with the shells on, which some people feel adds flavor to the dish.

To prepare uncooked shrimp, use a pair of scissors to cut through the shell down the back (outer curved side) of each shrimp, then pull off the shell and legs. (Remove the tail portion of the shell, or leave it on for decoration.) Use a knife tip or a metal skewer to pick out the black intestinal vein at the back; working under cold running water will help free the vein. Or use one of the special sheller/deveiner tools designed for this task.

For cooked shrimp, remove shells by peeling off the shell with your fingers. Devein as described above.

Always thaw frozen shrimp (in the refrigerator) before cooking it.

serving suggestions

• Cook shrimp and serve with a grapefruit and avocado salad.

• Use chopped cooked shrimp as an omelet filling.

• Add shrimp to a spicy tomato sauce and use as a pasta sauce.

• Use shrimp instead of clams in a chowder recipe.

• Stir chopped cooked shrimp into stiff mashed potatoes (leftover mashed potatoes work really well). Shape the mixture into cakes and sauté until golden brown.

• Combine chopped cooked shrimp with rice and use as a stuffing for flounder or another fish.

soyfoods

Extremely versatile and highly nutritious, soyfoods—soymilk, tofu, miso, and tempeh, to name just a few—are all derived from the soybean, a legume that was first cultivated in northern China in the 11th century B.C. The Chinese honored soybeans as one of the five sacred grains essential to the existence of civilization (the others were rice, barley, wheat, and millet), considering it to be both a food and a medicine.

While soybeans were widely eaten in many parts of the world, it wasn't until 1765 that they were first planted in the United States. They served primarily as animal feed until the 1920s, at which point they also began to be commercially crushed for their oil.

Soybean production greatly expanded in the United States during and after World War II. It was only then that the bean came to be recognized as the remarkable source of high-quality protein and other healthful nutrients that it remains today.

nutritional profile

Soybeans and their derivative soyfoods are well known for their superior nutritional and health benefits. Soybeans themselves are a rich source of B vitamins (thiamin, riboflavin, B_6, and folate), iron, potassium, magnesium, and cholesterol-lowering plant sterols. The nutritional value and make-up of any given soyfood depends on the individual method of processing. All soyfoods, regardless of processing, are low in saturated fat and contain no cholesterol. Two other potentially notable substances in soyfoods are its isoflavones (see *phytochemicals box, page 534*).

It is its high-quality protein, however, that distinguishes the soybean and its derivatives from other legumes. For some time it has been known that soy protein, when substituted for animal protein in the diet, lowers total and LDL ("bad") cholesterol and triglycerides without lowering HDL ("good") cholesterol, though no one knows why. Recently, the FDA authorized a nutrition label claiming that at least 25 grams of soy protein a day, as part of a low-fat diet, can lower blood cholesterol levels in people who have high cholesterol. Soy products containing at least 6.25 grams of soy protein per serving are allowed to bear the FDA-approved health claim label.

Despite this, researchers still disagree about whether it's the protein or some other substance in soy that provides these heart-healthy benefits. It is possible that it's the soy isoflavones, possibly acting as antioxidants, that are responsible. In addition, scientists are also looking at other cardioprotective components of soy, such as fiber.

There is no doubt that the health benefits of soy will continue to be studied for many years to come. Meanwhile, you are certainly better off eating cholesterol-free soyfoods instead of foods that are high in saturated fats.

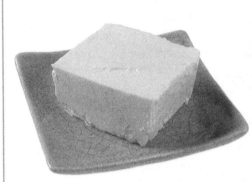

tofu

SOYBEANS / ½ cup cooked	
Calories	149
Protein (g)	14
Carbohydrate (g)	9
Dietary fiber (g)	5.2
Total fat (g)	7.7
Saturated fat (g)	1.1
Monounsaturated fat (g)	1.7
Polyunsaturated fat (g)	4.4
Cholesterol (mg)	0
Potassium (mg)	443
Sodium (mg)	1

KEY NUTRIENTS (%RDA/AI*)	
Thiamin	0.1 mg (11%)
Riboflavin	0.3 mg (19%)
Vitamin B_6	0.2 mg (12%)
Vitamin E	1.7 mg (11%)
Folate	46 mcg (12%)
Iron	4.4 mg (55%)
Magnesium	74 mg (18%)
Selenium	6 mcg (11%)

*For more detailed information on RDA and AI, see page 88.

in the market

No longer the exclusive darlings of health-food stores, soyfoods have gone mainstream and many products are now available at supermarkets in the United States. Just as the texture and taste of these products vary widely, so can their nutritional content. Therefore, be sure to read labels carefully. Listed below are some of the more common soyfoods found in the market today:

Edamame See Beans, Fresh (*page 184*).

Meat alternatives (meat analogs) Generally, soy alternatives to meat contain soy protein or tofu and other ingredients mixed together to simulate various kinds of meat, such as soy hot dogs and soy bacon. The products are sold frozen, canned, or dried, and can generally be used the same way as the foods they replace.

Miso A pungent, salty seasoning paste that originated in Japan, miso is made from a combination of soybeans and a grain such as rice or barley. It is fermented with salt, and sometimes a special mold is injected to produce its distinct, complex flavor. Miso comes in a range of different colors—white, yellow, red, and brown—and the darker the color, the deeper, and stronger, the flavor. Miso makes a flavorful soup base or seasoning, but should be used in moderation because its sodium content can exceed 900 milligrams per tablespoon.

Natto This fermented soyfood is produced by adding the bacterium *Bacillus natto* to lightly steamed soybeans. After fermenting for 15 to 24 hours, the soybeans develop a brown color, a sticky viscous coating, and a distinctive fermented odor and taste with ammonia overtones. Natto has been described by some as the Roquefort of soyfoods. Because the fermentation process breaks down the bean's proteins, natto is more easily digested than whole soybeans. Requiring no additional cooking, it is traditionally served as a topping for rice or noodles, in miso soups, or in salads. Natto can be found in Asian markets and health-food stores.

Soybeans See Beans, Dried (*page 181*) and Beans, Fresh (*page 184*).

Soybean sprouts See Sprouts (*page 543*).

Soy cheese This is a cholesterol-free cheese (although occasionally dairy products are added) that comes both firm and soft. Soft soy cheese is a good alternative to sour cream or cream cheese, while the firmer cheese can be used as you would dairy cheeses, though it does not melt the way dairy cheeses do. Firm soy cheese is often colored and/or flavored to resemble particular dairy cheeses, such as mozzarella or Cheddar. Check the label carefully as some brands of soy cheese may also contain dairy proteins, such as whey or

---

➤ phytochemicals in soyfoods

Soy contains a complex mix of phytochemicals, including isoflavones, some of which may act as estrogens or anti-estrogens. Soy isoflavones may also act as antioxidants and have other beneficial effects on blood vessels, the heart, blood cholesterol levels, and the brain.

• A diet rich in soy may help protect against several cancers, and again, it may be the isoflavones that are protective.

• Soy has also been heavily promoted as a remedy for such menopausal symptoms as hot flashes. However, its effectiveness in this respect is far from certain.

• Finally, soy isoflavones are under investigation for their role in building bone and delaying the onset of osteoporosis.

• The isoflavone content in a soyfood varies from high to low, depending on how the food is processed. For a comparison, see "Isoflavone Content of Soyfoods" (*opposite page*).

casein (caseinates), which some people may prefer to avoid due to allergies or diet preferences. Like regular cheese, soy cheese can be high in sodium and fat (although nonfat varieties are now sold).

Soy flour See Flour, Nonwheat (*page 325*).

Soy grits and **soy flakes** Soy grits are toasted, cracked soybeans that are usually the size of very coarse cornmeal. Soy flakes are made by running lightly dry-roasted whole soybeans through rollers (like rolled oats). Grits are high in protein and may be used the way you might use cracked wheat, as a side dish or cooked with other grains, such as rice, for example. Soy flakes are used the way you would rolled oats, usually cooked and served as a hot cereal.

Soymilk This is the liquid filtered from soybeans that have been soaked, finely ground, cooked, and strained. Because it is free of the milk-sugar lactose, soymilk is often substituted for cow's milk by people who have food allergies or who are lactose intolerant. It is also used by vegans who eat no animal products.

Plain, unfortified soymilk is an excellent source of high-quality protein, B vitamins, and iron. However, because soymilk contains a negligible amount of calcium, some brands are fortified with additional calcium and as well as vitamin D. Others are sweetened and/or flavored. Plain, unsweetened soymilk is approximately equivalent in calories to fat-free milk, but has about 10 times the fat content. Soymilk is most commonly found in aseptic (nonrefrigerated) cartons, but is also sold refrigerated. With the growing interest in lower-fat products, nonfat and "lite" soymilks are now appearing on the market. Unopened, aseptically packaged soymilk can be stored at room temperature for several months. Once opened, the soymilk must be refrigerated. It will

ISOFLAVONE CONTENT OF SOYFOODS

The USDA in collaboration with Iowa State University has compiled a listing of the isoflavone content of soyfoods. The values are expressed in milligrams per single serving of the food. The foods are organized from the most isoflavones to the least.

	Calories	Fat (g)	Isoflavones (mg)
Soybeans, dried, cooked (1 cup)	298	15	95
Soybean sprouts (¼ cup)	171	9.4	57
Soynuts (¼ cup)	194	9.3	55
Natto (½ cup)	186	9.6	52
Tempeh (4 ounces)	226	8.7	50
Soy flour, full-fat (⅓ cup)	121	5.7	49
Tofu, firm (4 ounces)	164	9.9	28
Soymilk (1 cup)	81	4.7	24
Edamame, cooked (4 ounces)	160	7.3	16
Miso (2 tablespoons)	71	2.1	15

about tofu

A versatile cooking ingredient, tofu (also known as soybean curd or bean curd) is a creamy white soy product sold in small blocks. It is made by coagulating the protein of soybeans, in somewhat the same way as cheese is produced. The soybeans are ground with water to produce soymilk, and an ingredient is added to form the soy protein into curds. If the coagulant is calcium sulfate (magnesium sulfate is another common coagulant), the resulting product has a high calcium content.

Tofu is also sometimes called "the cheese of Asia," and some types are similar in appearance to a block of farmer cheese; however, unlike cheese, tofu is very bland. In fact, tofu's greatest assets as an ingredient are that it can be cooked in many ways, and that it absorbs other flavors. Tofu can be stir-fried, broiled, grilled, sautéed, or baked (if marinated first in a spicy sauce, it will have a meaty taste). It can also be pureed to make dips, spreads, salad dressings—even thick shakes and cheesecakes. When mashed, it can be substituted for cottage cheese, ricotta, or even ground beef.

With only about 164 calories per 4 ounces of firm tofu, this soy product is a good, high-protein substitute for meat and whole-milk products. But it is also high in fat, with almost 10 grams per 4 ounces, though the fat is mostly unsaturated.

There are two basic types of tofu:

Silken Resembling custard, this type of tofu is always packaged and can be purchased soft, firm, or extra-firm. In addition, you may also find lower-fat or "lite" silken tofu (with less than 1 gram of fat per 4-ounce serving) in each of the three consistencies. Silken tofu can be used in desserts, spreads, sauces, and pie fillings. Pureed soft silken tofu is a good substitute for light cream or milk, while the firmer version can take the place of sour cream or yogurt.

Regular This type of tofu is more granular than silken tofu and also comes soft, firm, and extra-firm. Chinese-style tofu is often sold in a pillow-shaped block; Japanese-style tofu, which is less compressed, is sold in square-sided blocks. In Asian markets, tofu is often sold in bulk—the blocks floating in tubs of water. Individual water-packed plastic containers can be found in the produce section of many supermarkets. You can use this more textured tofu in stews, soups, or salads, or just slice it and eat as is.

If you buy tofu from an open tub (which is not recommended because of the potential for bacterial growth), shop at a store that has a good turnover and sniff the tofu to be sure it does not smell sour. Packaged tofu should have a "sell by" date stamped on its wrapping to guide you. With either type, rinse the tofu when you get it home, place it in a container of fresh cold water, and store it in the refrigerator, changing the water daily, and keep for no more than a week. You can also buy vacuum-packed tofu that does not need refrigeration until it is opened. Tofu freezes well. Be aware, however, that freezing changes the tofu's texture, making it slightly chewier.

If you or anybody in your household is in poor health, be sure to cook your tofu to 160°, even if it is packaged. This will prevent even the slightest chance of food poisoning.

FIRM REGULAR TOFU / 4 ounces

Calories	164
Protein (g)	18
Carbohydrate (g)	5
Dietary fiber (g)	2.6
Total fat (g)	9.9
Saturated fat (g)	1.4
Monounsaturated fat (g)	2.2
Polyunsaturated fat (g)	5.6
Cholesterol (mg)	0
Potassium (mg)	269
Sodium (mg)	16

KEY NUTRIENTS (%RDA/AI*)

Thiamin	0.2 mg (15%)
Calcium	775 mg (65%)
Iron	12 mg (149%)
Magnesium	66 mg (16%)
Selenium	20 mcg (36%)
Zinc	1.8 mg (16%)

*For more detailed information on RDA and AI, see page 88.

stay fresh for about 5 days. Soymilk is also sold as a powder, to be mixed with water. Soymilk powder should be stored in the refrigerator or freezer.

Soy sauce A piquant, dark brown, salty condiment that is popular throughout the world, soy sauce is derived from fermented soybeans that are mixed with roasted grain (wheat, barley, or rice are common), injected with a special yeast mold, and flavored with salt. The flavor, color, and consistency of soy sauce depends upon how it is processed. Different types of soy sauce include light, dark, mushroom, shoyu, and tamari. *Light soy sauce* (not to be confused with low-sodium, reduced-sodium, or "lite" soy sauce) is, in spite of its name, saltier than the darker varieties. *Dark soy sauce* is thicker, richer, and more pungent in flavor. *Mushroom soy sauce* has Chinese straw mushrooms added to it and has a pleasant, rich flavor. *Shoyu*, which is made in Japan, is a blend of soybeans and wheat. *Tamari,* also of Japanese origin, comes only from soybeans. It is thicker than Chinese-style soy sauce and has a strong, robust flavor that is retained after cooking. (Note, however, that though the strict definition of tamari is soybeans only, some brands also contain wheat.) Low-sodium and reduced-sodium soy sauces are available in most varieties. Use soy sauce to season dishes, sauces, and marinades. Even reduced-sodium soy sauce is relatively high in sodium, so be sure to use it in small amounts if you are salt sensitive.

> ## kecap manis
>
> Kecap (pronounced ket-jap) manis is a type of thick, sweet soy sauce used in Malaysian and Indonesian cooking. Kecap translates as "sauce added to food to enhance flavor" and if you're thinking that the word sounds a lot like ketchup, you're right—that's where our tomato condiment got its name. Kecap manis is made by flavoring a dark soy sauce with palm sugar, star anise, and garlic. It's used both in cooking and as a table condiment. Look for it in Asian grocery stores.

Soynut butter Made from roasted whole soynuts, which are then crushed into spreadable form and blended with soy oil and other ingredients, soynut butter has a slightly nutty taste and significantly less fat than peanut butter.

Soynuts (roasted soybeans) These are soybeans that have been soaked in water and then baked or roasted until lightly browned. They are sold whole or cracked in half and are similar in texture and flavor to peanuts.

Soy protein, textured Textured soy protein (TSP) usually refers to products made from defatted and dehydrated soy flour, although the term can also be applied to textured soy protein concentrates and spun soy fiber. When hydrated, TSP absorbs flavors well and has a chewy, meatlike texture. It is available in powder form as well as chunks, slices, and granules. It is often added to sauces, casseroles, and stews instead of ground beef. Dehydrated TSP has a long shelf-life, and may be stored in an airtight container at room temperature for up to 3 months. Once it is rehydrated, it should be refrigerated and used within a few days. *Textured vegetable protein (TVP)* is a brand name for a particular type of TSP, but many people simply refer to TSP as TVP.

Soy protein powder Popular with body builders who are trying to pump-up on protein, soy protein powder comes as either *soy protein concentrate* (from defatted soy flakes, containing about 70 percent protein and most of the bean's dietary fiber) or as *soy protein isolate* (a further refinement of defatted flakes resulting in a product that's 92 percent protein). Soy protein powder is a better source of protein than other soyfoods. Depending on the brand, one scoop (about 2 heaping tablespoons) can have about 20 to 28 grams of protein. By contrast, a 4-ounce serving of firm tofu has about 18 grams of protein and an 8-ounce glass of soymilk has only 6 grams of protein. It is important to note that soy protein powder may or may not contain nutritionally significant amounts of isoflavones depending on how the product is made. Soy protein isolate contains less than soy flour and tofu, but still has significant amounts.

Soy yogurt Made from soymilk, this product has the texture and consistency of dairy yogurt. Soy yogurt is available in different flavors with and without active cultures. It is an excellent substitute for sour cream.

Tempeh This soyfood, a useful meat substitute, originated in Indonesia. To make it, soybeans are cooked (usually with grains like rice or millet) and then aged with a special culture that breaks the cooked beans down and binds the mixture into a firm substance that can be sliced. Tempeh contains even more protein than tofu, and is a bit more flavorful (some find it smoky or nutty, others say it tastes like chicken). You'll find tempeh and prepared foods based on it in health-food stores, either refrigerated or frozen.

Tofu See "About Tofu" (*page 536*).

Yuba Yuba is made by lifting and drying the thin layer formed on the surface of heated soymilk once it has cooled. It has a high protein content and is most commonly found as brittle, brown sheets that must be reconstituted before use. Once softened, it can be added to stocks, soups, stews, and the like.

---

easy homemade soymilk

Traditionally soymilk is made from whole soybeans, but it can easily be made using soy flour instead. Keep in mind that soymilk made at home has a "bean-ier" flavor than the packaged soymilk available at most supermarkets. Here's how to do it:

Bring 3 cups of water to a boil, then slowly add 1 cup of soy flour (do not use toasted soy flour), stirring constantly with a whisk to prevent lumps. Reduce the heat and simmer for 20 minutes, stirring occasionally.

Line a colander with a double layer of dampened cheesecloth and place the colander over a large bowl. Strain the soy-flour mixture through the lined colander. Stir in a favorite flavoring, if you like, and refrigerate until chilled.

---

serving suggestions

• Marinate thick slices of extra-firm tofu in a teriyaki sauce and grill.

• Use textured soy protein in chili, spaghetti sauce, sloppy joes, enchiladas, or veggie burgers.

• Fill manicotti with a mixture of chopped cooked spinach and mashed tofu.

• Slice tempeh, dip it in lightly beaten egg whites and flour, and sauté until crisp. Serve on a roll with barbecue sauce.

• Substitute soymilk for cow's milk in cheese sauces and soups.

• Add soy flour to bread and pizza doughs.

• Make a healthful smoothie with soynut butter, "lite" soymilk, soy protein powder, honey, and banana slices.

• Use soynuts in muffins, cookies, or brownies. Or combine them with cereal and dried fruit in a trail mix.

spinach

A fleshy-leafed member of the *Cheopdiaceae* (goosefoot) family, which also includes Swiss chard and beets, spinach has a rich, hearty flavor that is delicious both raw in salads or cooked. Its broad, tender leaves as well as the tiny, more tender stems are both edible. Due to advances in breeding, spinach can now be purchased both crinkly or flat-leafed, and with leaves that are a vivid red at the center.

Believed to have originated in Asia, spinach was a relative latecomer to Europe, arriving sometime during the Middle Ages. It gained popularity rapidly, and was particularly appreciated by the French and Italians.

No one knows when the vegetable was first cultivated in the United States, but by the early 19th century, seed catalogues offered three varieties, and spinach was an established part of the national cuisine—though not necessarily a favorite dish, since cooks customarily boiled it to a flavorless, gray-green mush. Fortunately more appealing ways of preparing spinach have made this vegetable widely appreciated today.

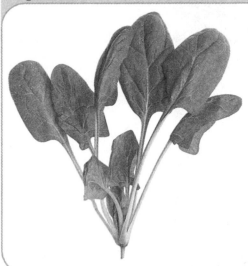

spinach

nutritional profile

Just 1 cup of cooked spinach offers an impressive array of vitamins and minerals, including riboflavin, vitamin B_6, folate, and magnesium. Furthermore, spinach is exceptionally rich in the carotenoids beta carotene, lutein, and zeaxanthin, which are masked by the abundant green pigment chlorophyll. To enhance the availability of these fat-soluble carotenoids, and to get the full benefit from this leafy green, it's best to eat spinach cooked with a small amount of fat, such as olive oil.

It's important to note that while spinach does provide iron—and also calcium—these minerals cannot be completely used by the body because the vegetable also contains a compound called oxalic acid, which limits their absorption. In short, spinach's value really rests in its other nutrients.

in the market

The commonest spinach in the market is a type called Savoy. Other, more unusual, spinaches can be found at specialty grocers and in some farmers' markets.

Baby spoon Rich-green, baby spoon spinach is similar to Savoy, but as its name suggests, is smaller in size. Crispy and coarse, it is sweeter than the larger variety. The tender small stems are edible, too.

Flat or **smooth-leaf** This type has unwrinkled, spade-shaped leaves that are easier to clean than the crinkly leaved varieties. It is the type generally used for canned and frozen spinach, as well as in soups, baby foods, and other processed foods.

SPINACH / 2 cups raw	
Calories	13
Protein (g)	2
Carbohydrate (g)	2
Dietary fiber (g)	1.6
Total fat (g)	0.2
Saturated fat (g)	0
Monounsaturated fat (g)	0
Polyunsaturated fat (g)	0.1
Cholesterol (mg)	0
Potassium (mg)	335
Sodium (mg)	47

KEY NUTRIENTS (%RDA/AI*)	
Beta carotene	2.4 mg (22%)
Vitamin C	17 mg (19%)
Folate	116 mcg (29%)
Iron	1.6 mg (20%)
Magnesium	47 mg (11%)

*For more detailed information on RDA and AI, see page 88.

Red spinach Growing in popularity, striking red spinach leaves are round, thick, and rich-green with an attractive red center. Tender and very tasty, the flavor of this lovely variety is deliciously sweet and succulent.

Savoy With crinkly, curly leaves and a dark green color, this is the type of spinach sold fresh in bunches at most supermarkets. Springy and crisp, it's particularly good in salads.

Semi-Savoy The slightly crinkled leaves of semi-Savoy offer some of the texture of Savoy but are not as difficult to clean. It is cultivated for both the fresh market and for processing.

choosing the best

Fresh spinach is sold both loose and in bags, which usually hold about 10 ounces. Loose spinach is easier to evaluate for quality, since you can examine each leaf individually.

Select small spinach leaves with good green color and a crisp, springy texture; reject wilted, crushed, or bruised leaves, and those with yellow spots or insect damage. Look for stems that are fairly thin; coarse, thick ones indicate overgrown spinach, which may be leathery and bitter. Fresh spinach should smell sweet, never sour or musty.

If only bagged spinach is available where you shop, check for yellowed leaves and squeeze the bag to see whether the contents seem resilient.

▶ When you get home Don't wash spinach before storing it: After a day or so, it will begin to wilt and decay. Instead, leave packaged spinach in its cellophane bag, or wrap loose spinach in paper towels, place the wrapped spinach in a large plastic bag, and store in the refrigerator crisper. Fresh spinach will keep for 3 to 4 days.

spinach that's not spinach

There are a number of vegetables in the market today masquerading under the name spinach. While some of these actually look like spinach, others have little resemblance. Moreover, all are members of different botanical families. Keep an eye out for these ringers:

Chinese spinach (Indian spinach) This is just another name for amaranth (*see page 158*).

Malabar spinach While this green tastes like spinach, it's from quite another family and grows as a vine. *(For more on this odd green, see page 354.)*

New Zealand spinach This tender green has fleshy stems and leaves that resemble spinach, but a less astringent taste. Because it grows well in hot summer temperatures and with little watering, it is popular with home gardeners. Like spinach, New Zealand spinach contains oxalic acid, which makes its calcium and iron less available for absorption by the body.

Water spinach (*ong choy*) This green vegetable looks like watercress (not spinach) and like that plant, thrives in a watery environment (it's also called swamp spinach). However, it probably gets its name from its mild spinach flavor. It is a common ingredient in Chinese cooking and is available mostly in Chinese markets.

preparing to use

Your first priority is to get rid of the grit. Fresh spinach—especially the crinkly Savoy type—often has sand trapped in the leaves and stems, and therefore requires careful washing. Trim off any roots, then separate the leaves and drop them into a large bowl of lukewarm water; agitate the leaves gently with your hands. Lift out the leaves, letting the sand and grit settle, then empty and refill the bowl and repeat the process until the leaves are clean. Keep in mind that even though bagged spinach is often labeled "prewashed," it should still be rinsed to clean away any sand and grit.

Loose spinach usually has more stem on it than bagged spinach, but both need to be stemmed if the stems are not very thin and tender. Pinch off the stems and also the midribs (the part of the stem that extends into the leaf), if they are thick and tough. You can easily stem spinach by folding each leaf in half, vein-side out, and pulling up on the stem as you hold the folded leaf closed.

To crisp spinach for salad, wash the leaves, then dry them in a salad spinner or shake them dry in a colander. Wrap the spinach in paper towels, place in a plastic bag, and refrigerate for no longer than a few hours before using.

Spinach that is to be cooked doesn't have to be dried; in fact, there is usually just enough water clinging to freshly washed leaves so that they can be steamed without additional cooking liquid.

SPINACH / 1 cup cooked	
Calories	41
Protein (g)	5
Carbohydrate (g)	7
Dietary fiber (g)	4.3
Total fat (g)	0.5
Saturated fat (g)	0.1
Monounsaturated fat (g)	0
Polyunsaturated fat (g)	0.2
Cholesterol (mg)	0
Potassium (mg)	839
Sodium (mg)	126

KEY NUTRIENTS (%RDA/AI*)	
Beta carotene	8.9 mg (80%)
Thiamin	0.2 mg (14%)
Riboflavin	0.4 mg (33%)
Vitamin B_6	0.4 mg (26%)
Vitamin C	18 mg (20%)
Vitamin E	1.7 mg (11%)
Folate	263 mcg (66%)
Calcium	245 mg (20%)
Iron	6.4 mg (80%)
Magnesium	157 mg (37%)
Zinc	1.4 mg (12%)

*For more detailed information on RDA and AI, see page 88.

serving suggestions

• Stuff chicken breasts with a mixture of spinach, mint, and feta cheese and bake.

• Puree steamed fresh spinach with buttermilk and fresh basil for a cold summer soup.

• Blanch large spinach leaves and use as wrappers for soft, light fillings, such as sautéed mushrooms and cooked rice.

• Top baked potatoes with sautéed chopped spinach and grated Parmesan cheese.

• Stir yogurt into chopped or pureed cooked spinach for a low-fat version of "creamed" spinach.

• Steam spinach, drain well, and toss with a dressing made of soy sauce, dark sesame oil, and a pinch of sugar. Sprinkle with toasted sesame seeds.

• Add chopped raw spinach to macaroni and cheese or lasagna before baking.

• Add shredded spinach leaves to soups just before serving.

sprouts

Sprouts are plant seedlings that are harvested shortly after germination. Tender and crisp, these succulent shoots are no longer the exclusive domain of Chinese cuisine or health-food stores. In fact, sprouts have become a common sight at salad bars and in the produce sections of many supermarkets. Their culinary appeal lies in the refined crunchiness they add to dishes, backed up by a delicate flavor that can be enjoyed whether the sprouts are cooked or eaten raw. And because they are young—just a few days from the seed stage—sprouts always taste tender and sweet. They have another distinctive feature: You can grow them yourself at any time of the year *(see "Grow Your Own Sprouts," opposite page)*.

It is important to note, however, that since 1995 raw sprouts have emerged as what the FDA calls "an important cause of foodborne illness." Indeed, over the years both salmonella and *E. coli* bacteria in raw sprouts have made thousands of people sick worldwide. The problem can arise with any type of sprouts and has nothing to do with whether they are organically or conventionally grown. It occurs because sprouts are soaked in water and grown in warm, humid conditions—the perfect environment for fostering the growth of harmful bacteria. And it's not just during sprouting that the problem occurs; the seeds can become contaminated during harvesting and storage as well.

In recent years, growers and the FDA have begun working to eliminate any unsanitary conditions in harvesting and sprouting, and raw sprouts continue to be sold widely. In fact, if you are in good health, you may prefer to continue eating raw sprouts, since cooking them does eliminate the crisp texture. However, if you have a serious illness, an impaired immune system, or are elderly, you may not want to take the risk of getting sick from contaminated sprouts. Also, very young children should not be given sprouts.

nutritional profile

While there are many different sprouts available, the more popular ones—alfalfa, mung bean, broccoli, and radish to name a few—provide a number of vitamins and minerals and hardly any calories or fat. Sprouts from nutrient-dense seeds like lentils, mung beans, or soybeans offer the broadest range of nutrients. Broccoli sprouts also provide the phytochemical sulforaphane *(see "Phytochemicals in Broccoli Sprouts," opposite page)*.

in the market

Today there are dozens of types of sprouts available through supermarkets, specialty food stores, health-food stores, and even at some farmers' markets. In addition to the popular types listed below, you may also find *wheat sprouts, lentil sprouts, pea sprouts,* and *red bean sprouts*—as well as those from *basil,*

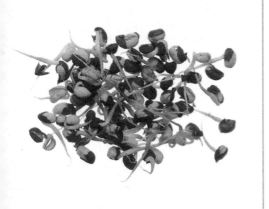

red bean sprouts

MUNG BEAN SPROUTS 2 cups	
Calories	62
Protein (g)	6
Carbohydrate (g)	12
Dietary fiber (g)	3.7
Total fat (g)	0.4
Saturated fat (g)	0.1
Monounsaturated fat (g)	0.1
Polyunsaturated fat (g)	0.1
Cholesterol (mg)	0
Potassium (mg)	310
Sodium (mg)	13

KEY NUTRIENTS (%RDA/AI*)	
Thiamin	0.2 mg (15%)
Riboflavin	0.3 mg (20%)
Niacin	1.6 mg (10%)
Vitamin B$_6$	0.2 mg (11%)
Vitamin C	28 mg (31%)
Folate	127 mcg (32%)
Iron	2.0 mg (24%)
Magnesium	44 mg (10%)

*For more detailed information on RDA and AI, see page 88.

caraway, dill, fennel, mustard, or *coriander seeds.* Spicy sprout mixtures that contain radish sprouts in combination with clover or another milder sprout are also available. Because each type of sprout has its own shape, taste, and texture, you'll probably want to experiment with different ones to see which appeal to you the most.

Adzuki bean These very sweet, lentil-shaped beans form fine, grasslike sprouts that have a nutty taste.

Alfalfa Notable for their mild, nutty flavor and crunchy texture, these white sprouts have yellow to dark green leaves. They are too delicate too cook, but are excellent in salads or sandwiches.

Broccoli These delicate green sprouts, with tiny white stems, have a pleasant, mildly spicy and refreshing taste that's reminiscent of radishes (they don't taste at all like broccoli).

Clover An alfalfa sprout look-alike, most clover sprouts are produced from red clover; the tiny seeds resemble poppy seeds.

Daikon radish (*kaiware*) These sprouts have silky stems, leafy tops, and a peppery-hot taste.

Mung bean Larger and crunchier than alfalfa, with a blander flavor, these thick white sprouts are a staple in Asian dishes. Unlike more delicate sprouts, they hold up well in stir-fries. Canned mung bean sprouts are a poor substitute for fresh.

Soybean More strongly flavored than mung bean sprouts, soy sprouts are a rich source of protein. They do, however, contain small amounts of toxins that can be harmful when the sprouts are eaten in large quantities. To prevent complications, cook soybean sprouts for at least 5 minutes. If you consume them infrequently, there's no need to cook them.

> ### ▶ *phytochemicals in* broccoli sprouts
>
> Broccoli sprouts are a particularly concentrated source of sulforaphane, a substance that has been shown to mobilize the body's natural cancer-fighting resources and reduce the risk of developing cancer. While all cruciferous vegetables (including broccoli, Brussels sprouts, kale, and cauliflower) contain this substance, broccoli sprouts appear to be the richest source of it.

grow your own sprouts

Growing sprouts is not difficult, and almost any seed, bean, or grain can be sprouted. To reduce the risk of bacterial contamination you should first soak the seeds in a chlorine bleach solution (1 tablespoon of bleach to ¼ cup of water per tablespoon of seeds) for 10 minutes before sprouting. Afterward, rinse the seeds in water. Keep in mind that while this process reduces the risk of pathogenic bacteria, it doesn't eliminate the risk entirely.

1. After rinsing the beans, seeds, or grains thoroughly, place them in a clean quart-sized glass jar. (A quart jar is large enough to accommodate the sprouts from ⅓ cup of most seeds, beans, or grains.) Fill the jar three-quarters full with tepid water. Cover the mouth of the jar with cheesecloth and secure with a heavy rubber band. Soak, unrefrigerated, overnight.

2. Next morning, drain the beans, seeds, or grains well and rinse with fresh water. Drain well once again, and place the jar on its side in a dark area.

3. Rinse and drain the seeds, beans, or grains twice a day, returning the jar to the dark place after each rinsing. Sprouting times vary, but most are ready in 2 to 3 days. To turn the sprouts green, place them in indirect sunlight on the last growing day.

Sunflower Mildly flavored, like alfalfa sprouts, sunflower sprouts are sweeter and much crunchier.

▶ Availability Since sprouts grow indoors hydroponically—that is, in water—they are generally available year round, although some are less likely to show up in the hot summer months because of their susceptibility to heat.

choosing the best

The best way to get ultrafresh sprouts is to grow your own. It's not difficult, however, to tell whether those you find in the market are in prime condition. Sprouts are sold loose (sometimes immersed in water), in plastic bags, or in clear plastic boxes (often containing the pad of absorbent material on which the seeds were sprouted). In each case, you can clearly see and evaluate the quality of the sprouts. They should be moist and crisp, and should look and smell clean; look out for sliminess, discoloration, mold, or a sour smell.

Mung bean sprouts may have their split seed cases still attached; these will wash away when you rinse the sprouts. If you buy mung bean sprouts from an open, water-filled container (as they are displayed in many Asian markets), be sure that a serving implement is provided and that the sprouts are not scooped out by hand.

▶ When you get home Refrigerate sprouts in their container or loosely packed in plastic bags (tightly packed, sprouts will be crushed and begin to decay quickly). Do not wash sprouts before storing, and plan to keep bagged sprouts for no more than 3 days. Boxed sprouts will keep for 4 to 5 days. Snip the sprouts as needed, leaving the tangle of roots in the box. Check your stored sprouts frequently and be sure to remove any that have become slimy or discolored.

Mung bean sprouts can be frozen for several months if they are to be used in cooking; the texture will not be as crunchy, however.

preparing to use

Sprouts sealed in plastic bags or boxes are sold clean and need no additional washing. Those that are available in bulk, however, may need to be rinsed before using. Any that seem slightly wilted can be revived by a 10-minute soaking in ice water; pat them dry with paper towels before using. Rinse mung bean sprouts in a bowl of water, stirring them gently with your hand, and discard the seed casings, which will float to the top.

squash, summer

Squash are gourds—fleshy vegetables protected by a rind—that belong to the *Cucurbitaceae* family, which also includes melons and cucumbers. Although some grow on vines and others on bushes, all are commonly divided into one of two main groups, summer squash and winter squash (*see Squash, Winter, page 549*). This nomenclature sprang from the fact that summer squash were once only available in the summer, whereas winter squash, a hardier group, could "winter over" and were available in the winter months. The more accurate distinction between the two is that summer squash, with their soft shells and tender, light-colored flesh, are picked while immature; winter squash, with their hard shells and darker, tougher flesh and seeds, are not harvested until maturity.

Like corn and beans, squash is a notably American food. It sustained Native Americans for some 5,000 years and then helped nourish the early European settlers, who quickly made the vegetable a mainstay of their diet. New England colonists adapted the word squash from several Native American names for the vegetable, all of which meant "something eaten raw" (presumably referring to summer squash, though both Native Americans and colonists also ate squash cooked).

yellow squash

straightneck

crookneck

nutritional profile

Summer squash are more than 95 percent water, and so offer only a modest amount of nutrients. The high water content, however, means that they are very low in calories (about 19 per cup of raw sliced squash).

In spite of its low nutritional profile, summer squash are not completely without merit. They have good amounts of vitamin C (more in raw squash than cooked), fiber, potassium, and magnesium. In addition, because summer squash skin is edible, you get the benefits of its carotenoid pigments. In fact, green-skinned zucchini is a leading source of lutein and zeaxanthin, carotenoid pigments that team up to help protect us against cataracts and age-related macular degeneration.

in the market

The most popular summer squash in the United States is the familiar and prolific green zucchini—entire cookbooks have been devoted to it. But it is only one among several common types of summer squash, which vary mainly in shape and color. All are similar enough in flavor and texture to be interchangeable in recipes.

YELLOW SQUASH 1 cup cooked	
Calories	36
Protein (g)	2
Carbohydrate (g)	8
Dietary fiber (g)	2.5
Total fat (g)	0.6
Saturated fat (g)	0.1
Monounsaturated fat (g)	0
Polyunsaturated fat (g)	0.2
Cholesterol (mg)	0
Potassium (mg)	346
Sodium (mg)	2

KEY NUTRIENTS (%RDA/AI*)	
Vitamin C	10 mg (11%)
Magnesium	43 mg (10%)

For more detailed information on RDA and AI, see page 88.

Baby acorn squash This is the familiar winter squash, it's picked young, when the whole vegetable is edible, skin and all.

Chayote Although best known in the South and Southwest, chayote (chy-o-tay, to rhyme with coyote) is becoming increasingly popular throughout the country. This pale or dark green (or white) pear-shaped summer squash is also called mirliton, vegetable pear, and christophene. Unlike other summer squash, it has a large central seed and a fairly thick, deeply ridged skin. It also requires a longer cooking time. Mexican cooks savor the central seed, which has faint almond overtones.

chayote

Cucuzza squash (bottle gourd) This mild-flavored Italian squash has pale green skin and white flesh. Though it can grow up to 3 feet long, it is usually harvested at shorter lengths, when it has the shape of a bowling pin.

Globe squash These round squash look like zucchini molded into a round shape.

Golden zucchini This is the gold version of your garden variety zucchini. It's about the same size and shape, but has a deep golden-yellow skin and a dark green stem. Its flavor is sweeter than that of green zucchini.

Pattypan (cymling, scallop) This greenish-white, disk-shaped squash is convex at both its top and bottom, with a scalloped edge. Its flesh is white and quite succulent. Yellow pattypan squash (such as Sunburst) is similar but more cup-shaped. Pattypan squash are also available as miniatures.

Scallopini squash This looks like pattypan squash, but it's larger and a dark, glossy green.

Yellow crookneck This squash tapers from a bulbous blossom end to a curved, narrow stem end. Its pale yellow skin has a slightly pebbled texture and its flesh is yellow.

Yellow straightneck Almost a twin of crookneck, this squash forms a tapering cylinder without a curved neck. Its skin may be pebbled like crookneck's, or smooth, while the flesh is paler. Along with its crookneck cousin,

squash blossoms

Yellow-orange flowers appear first on the vines that produce squash. These blossoms are not only edible but are considered a delicacy by many. They are also extremely low in calories and are a good source of vitamin C, potassium and the carotenoid beta carotene.

Although the flowers of any type of squash can be eaten (their flavor faintly resembles that of squash), the most frequently consumed are zucchini blossoms. Unfortunately, they are usually served battered and deep-fried, which adds fat and calories. More healthful ways of preparing them include: sautéed in a small amount of oil; stuffed with a low-fat filling and then briefly sautéed; or lightly steamed.

these are the classic summer squash, which some markets simply label "summer squash."

Zucchini The shape of a zucchini resembles that of a lightly ridged cucumber; its skin is medium to deep green, with paler flecks or stripes. Zucchini also comes in a miniature, baby version.

choosing the best

Summer squash can grow quite large (home gardeners often discover baseball-bat-sized zucchini hidden under the plant's large leaves), but these overgrown specimens have coarse, stringy flesh and large seeds. Summer squash taste best when small- to medium-sized—not more than 7 inches long (pattypan squash should be no more than 4 inches across). Choose squash that are also firm and fairly heavy for their size; otherwise, they may be dry and

chinese squash

This is an extremely confusing category for Americans, because many Chinese squash are called melons, even though they are not at all sweet and are cooked like vegetables. The fact that squash and melon are in the same botanical family is responsible for the taxonomic overlap.

Bitter melon (bitter cucumber) This Asian squash looks like a warty cucumber, and true to its name, it is bitter (though the younger the melon, the milder its flavor). The yellow seed core is usually removed before cooking.

Fuzzy melon (mo qua, hairy melon) This fleshy, mild squash tastes like cucumber. When picked young, it's covered with tiny white bristles (not unlike a cucumber).

Luffa (Chinese okra) Ridges run the length of this squash, which is probably what earned it the name Chinese okra. Its interior is soft and spongy (like an overgrown zuc-chini) and it has a mild flavor when young. Older squash (which can grow to 9 feet) are bitter and have a strong laxative effect. The gourd that is grown to produce loofah sponges is a different species in spite of the similar name.

Opo squash This is the Asian version of the Italian cucuzza squash (*see opposite page*).

Winter melon This enormous squash (it grows to 100 pounds) is used not only in China, but also in Japan, India, and Thailand. Outwardly, winter melon resembles a big round watermelon. A typical example weighs about 12 pounds and is often sold cut up into manageable pieces. Its skin is greenish with a whitish blush. The white flesh has the texture of watermelon. Like other summer squash (the winter in its name is a misnomer), winter melon is about 95 percent water and has a very subtle—some would say bland—taste.

cottony within. Farmers' markets and greengrocers sometimes offer baby summer squash, just 1 to 2 inches long; these are particularly tender and sweet.

The skin of summer squash is thin and fragile—delicate enough to puncture with a fingernail. Unfortunately, some shoppers do just this—they prick the skin to test for tenderness, leaving the squash susceptible to decay. Look for squash with sound, glossy exteriors; avoid those with skins showing nicks, pits, bruises, or soft spots. The squash should be plump (not shriveled), the stem ends fresh and green. The color should be uniform and bright.

▶ **When you get home** Unlike winter squash, which does well at room temperature, summer squash is more fragile and should be refrigerated.

preparing to use

Wash summer squash well and trim the ends. Summer squash need not be peeled or seeded unless it is oversized and has a thick skin or large seeds. There are some exceptions to this: Luffa should have its ridges and skin peeled. And chayote, unless it is very small, has quite tough skin, which should be peeled. When peeled, chayote exudes a sticky liquid that may burn or even numb the skin, so peel the vegetable under cold running water. Halve the chayote and remove the seed; it can be cooked with the squash, as it has a pleasant almondlike flavor. If you are cooking chayote whole, you can slip off the skin after cooking.

Because summer squash is mostly water, it will exude a lot of liquid during cooking. If you want to prevent a cooked dish containing the vegetable from becoming "waterlogged," salt the squash before heating it. Follow the procedure given for salting eggplant on page 277, making sure to rinse and drain the squash well after salting.

ZUCCHINI 1 cup cooked	
Calories	25
Protein (g)	2
Carbohydrate (g)	5
Dietary fiber (g)	2.2
Total fat (g)	0.3
Saturated fat (g)	0.1
Monounsaturated fat (g)	0
Polyunsaturated fat (g)	0.1
Cholesterol (mg)	0
Potassium (mg)	446
Sodium (mg)	5

KEY NUTRIENTS (%RDA/AI*)	
Vitamin C	14 mg (15%)

*For more detailed information on RDA and AI, see page 88.

serving suggestions

• Cut summer squash into ½-inch-thick lengthwise slabs. Brush with some olive oil and grill.

• Puree cooked chayote with toasted cumin and nonfat sour cream. Sprinkle with toasted almonds and serve as a vegetable side dish.

• Throw cubes of any summer squash into soups at the last minute. Cook until just heated through.

• Cook shredded summer squash with some salt and vinegar. Drain and use as a sandwich relish.

• Make a summer squash slaw: Shred zucchini or yellow squash (you don't have to peel it). Toss with a little lemon juice or vinegar and set aside. Make a dressing of low-fat yogurt, black pepper, and minced dill. Drain the squash and toss with the dressing. Serve at room temperature.

squash, winter

Winter squash are hard-skinned edible members of the gourd family. In contrast to tender, young summer squash, winter squash are harvested at a mature stage, when their skins have grown hard. Because of these protective skins, winter squash have a much longer storage life than their summer counterparts—some can keep for several months at home, or longer in a commercial facility. Harvested in the fall, for example, they can be stored throughout the winter in a cool, dry place. However, winter squash are no longer bound to a particular season. Today, the term simply refers to hard-skinned varieties that keep well (as compared to summer squash, such as zucchini, that do not).

Unlike their summer counterparts (*see Squash, Summer, page 545*), which tend to be rather similar in taste, winter squash have very distinctive flavors. They also come in a variety of colors—white, yellow, orange, green-brown, gray, and even light blue, to name a few. Winter squash are almost always cooked. The seeds, which are high in protein and fat, are usually discarded (although some, such as pumpkin seeds, can be eaten if toasted and husked). Winter squash blossoms are also edible (*see "Squash Blossoms," page 546*).

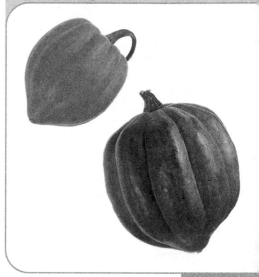

acorn squash

nutritional profile

The deep yellow to deep orange flesh of winter squash is darker than that of summer varieties, and it is more nutritious, richer in complex carbohydrates, and in many cases, beta carotene. Pumpkin and butternut squash offer outstanding amounts of this healthful yellow-orange pigment: 1 cup of pumpkin contains 7.8 milligrams of beta carotene and 1 cup of cooked butternut squash supplies 10 milligrams. Additional carotenoid pigments, alpha carotene and lutein, lend vivid autumn color to winter squash and help to defend the body's cells against disease-causing free radicals.

Dietary fiber and a wealth of nutrients are also plentiful in winter squash. Ample amounts of both soluble and insoluble fiber in squash may help to regulate cholesterol levels and to relieve constipation. Winter squash offers appreciable amounts of the B vitamins thiamin and vitamin B_6, as well as of vitamin C, magnesium, potassium, and iron. Winter squash is also one of a handful of good low-fat sources of vitamin E.

in the market

Winter squash vary greatly in size—from small acorn squash and sweet dumplings to pumpkins that can reach 200 pounds. Though they exhibit a

ACORN SQUASH 1 cup baked, mashed	
Calories	137
Protein (g)	3
Carbohydrate (g)	36
Dietary fiber (g)	11
Total fat (g)	0.3
Saturated fat (g)	0.1
Monounsaturated fat (g)	0
Polyunsaturated fat (g)	0.1
Cholesterol (mg)	0
Potassium (mg)	1,071
Sodium (mg)	10

KEY NUTRIENTS (%RDA/AI*)	
Thiamin	0.4 mg (34%)
Niacin	2.2 mg (13%)
Vitamin B_6	0.5 mg (28%)
Vitamin C	27 mg (29%)
Vitamin E	1.6 mg (11%)
Folate	46 mcg (11%)
Iron	2.3 mg (28%)
Magnesium	105 mg (25%)

For more detailed information on RDA and AI, see page 88.

range of flavors, most varieties can be substituted for one another in recipes. The one exception is spaghetti squash, which has uniquely textured flesh that pulls apart to form slender strands.

Although hundreds of varieties of winter squash are grown, the three most commonly found in the supermarket are acorn, butternut, and Hubbard. Most of the others mentioned below are available at specialty food stores or farmers' markets.

Acorn Excellent for baking, this acorn-shaped squash, which tapers at one end, measures about 6 inches long. Its deeply ridged skin is dark green with orange markings. One variety, known as *Golden Acorn,* is a glowing pumpkin color; another variety, sometimes called *Table Queen,* is white. All have deep yellow flesh. The biggest drawback to this variety is that the skin is quite hard, and therefore difficult to cut.

Australian blue (Queensland blue) This large squash with a gray-blue exterior has an orange, pumpkin-flavored flesh that can be used in place of pumpkin in recipes.

Banana This large cylindrical squash (one type weighs up to 30 pounds) has thick skin, which ranges in color from pale yellow to ivory, and a finely textured yellow-orange flesh. It is generally cut into smaller portions for sale.

Buttercup With a drumlike shape and a turbanlike cap on its blossom end, this squat squash generally weighs from 2 to 6 pounds. Orange and green varieties are available. The deep orange flesh is very sweet and mild, with a flavor similar to butternut squash.

Butternut Weighing 2 to 5 pounds, with deep orange, mildly sweet flesh, this long-necked bell-shaped squash has a smooth, tan skin that is softer and easier to cut than that of the acorn or Hubbard. The most widely grown winter squash, it has a small seed cavity and provides a lot of flesh for its size.

Calabaza (calabasa) Generally, this large squash is bright orange, but it can be found with green, yellow, or cream-colored skin and orange striations. Sweet and moist when cooked, with a flavor similar to that of butternut squash, it's most often sold in portions, frequently in Hispanic markets.

Carnival This pretty yellow, orange, and green squash can grow to the size of a medium-sized pumpkin. It has a sweet squash flavor and a smooth, moist texture.

Delicata (bohemian) The 1- to 2-pound oblong delicata has cream-colored skin with stripes that vary in color from green to orange. Its flesh is orange-yellow and extremely sweet, rich, and moist.

Golden Nugget This orange, hard-skinned, pleasantly sweet-tasting buttery squash looks like a miniature pumpkin. With only enough flesh for one serving, it tastes best when baked, like acorn squash.

Hubbard Members of an old, extensive group of squash, Hubbards are usually plump in the middle and more tapered at the neck. Their bumpy, hard skin varies in color from dark-green to blue-gray. Over the years, the popularity of Hubbards has diminished because they are so big—the smallest

BUTTERNUT SQUASH 1 cup baked, mashed	
Calories	98
Protein (g)	2
Carbohydrate (g)	26
Dietary fiber (g)	6.9
Total fat (g)	0.2
Saturated fat (g)	0.1
Monounsaturated fat (g)	0
Polyunsaturated fat (g)	0.1
Cholesterol (mg)	0
Potassium (mg)	696
Sodium (mg)	10

KEY NUTRIENTS (%RDA/AI*)	
Beta carotene	10 mg (93%)
Thiamin	0.2 mg (15%)
Niacin	2.4 mg (15%)
Vitamin B$_6$	0.3 mg (18%)
Vitamin C	27 mg (41%)
Vitamin E	1.6 mg (11%)
Folate	47 mcg (12%)
Iron	1.5 mg (18%)
Magnesium	71 mg (17%)

*For more detailed information on RDA and AI, see page 88.

weigh 5 pounds, the largest more than 15 pounds. In the supermarket, they are often sold precut.

Kabocha This orange-fleshed, turban-shaped squash has a rough shell with deep green and pale green stripes. Averaging 2 to 3 pounds, its deep yellow-orange flesh is sweeter, less fibrous, and somewhat dried than other winter squash and tastes a little like sweet potato or pumpkin.

Pumpkin See Pumpkin (*page 494*).

Spaghetti squash (calabash, vegetable spaghetti) When cooked, the flesh of this unique squash forms spaghetti-like strands that can be pulled out with a fork. It has a mild taste and crisp texture, but requires more time and care to prepare than other squash (*see "How to Prepare Spaghetti Squash," page 552*).

Sugar loaf (orange delicata) Smaller and shorter than the common delicata, the sugar loaf has orange or tan skin and green stripes. It is moist and creamy with a sweet, buttered-corn flavor.

Sweet dumpling Like the Golden Nugget, this small squash (it's about the size of an apple) has only enough flesh to serve one person, and can be cooked halved or whole. The skin is light-colored, usually with dark green or orange stripes. The flesh is sweeter than that of many winter squash varieties.

Turban An orange base and bright stripes in several colors distinguish this turban-shaped squash, which is capped with a knob similar to that on buttercup squash. It is typically 4 to 5 inches long and 6 to 8 inches wide. The finely textured orange flesh is usually quite sweet and dry. This pretty squash is often used as a table decoration or soup tureen.

serving suggestions

- Stuff manicotti with a blend of pureed winter squash and nonfat cottage cheese.

- Substitute mashed winter squash for pumpkin in pies, quick breads, and muffins.

- Add chunks of peeled winter squash to soups, stews, and chilis.

- Halve and seed acorn squash, stuff with a flavorful rice mixture, and bake.

- Puree roasted winter squash soup with broth and seasonings to make a soup. Garnish with toasted squash seeds.

- Cut rings of acorn squash (no need to peel), drizzle with maple syrup, and bake.

- Mash cooked squash with sautéed onions or garlic and herbs.

- Combine chunks of cooked squash with cooked corn, tomatoes, and bell peppers.

- Use whole small steamed or baked squash (or even small pumpkins) as serving bowls for soups or stews: Scoop out the flesh after baking and use it in the soup, or mash it and reserve for another use.

choosing the best

The size you buy will depend on your needs. There is no such thing as an "overgrown" winter squash; the longer the squash grows, the sweeter it will be. However, after picking, squash may be damaged by poor storage. Clues to good quality are a smooth, dry skin, free of cracks or soft spots. Moreover, the skin should be dull; a shiny skin indicates that the squash was picked too early and will not have the full sweetness of a mature squash.

Deep color is also a sign of a good winter squash. Green acorn squash may have splashes of orange, but avoid any that have orange on more than half the surface; butternut squash should be uniformly tan, with no tinge of green. A winter squash should feel heavy for its size. If possible, choose squash with their stems attached, as these are also indicators of quality: The stems should be rounded and dry, not collapsed, blackened, or moist.

Some very large squash, such as calabaza, banana, or Hubbard, are sold cut into quarters or chunks and wrapped in plastic. When buying cut squash, look for a good interior color.

▶ **When you get home** Winter squash is one of the best-keeping vegetables. Uncut squash should last for 3 months or longer in a cool, dry place. Storage below 50° (as in the refrigerator) will cause squash to deteriorate more quickly, but refrigerator storage is acceptable for a week or two. Cut squash will keep for up to a week if tightly wrapped and refrigerated.

preparing to use

Rinse off any dirt before using. The hard skin of some types of winter squash can prove challenging to cut: Use a heavy chef's knife or a cleaver, especially for larger squash. First, make a shallow cut in the skin to use as a guide to prevent the knife blade from slipping. Then place the blade in the cut and tap the base of the knife (near the handle) with your fist (or, if necessary, with a mallet or hammer) until the squash is cut through. Scoop out the seeds and fibers and cut the squash into smaller chunks, if desired. Small, very hard-skinned squash, such as Golden Nugget, may be impossible to split before cooking; bake or steam them whole.

If peeled chunks of squash are required, cut the squash into pieces, then peel them with a sturdy, sharp paring knife. Very hard-skinned squash is much easier to peel after cooking.

how to prepare spaghetti squash

Unique among winter squash, spaghetti squash requires a little extra work after cooking to remove its spaghettilike flesh. Here are some tips on preparing it:

• To bake spaghetti squash whole, pierce the shell in several places with a fork, then put the squash in a baking pan. Bake in a 350° oven for 1 hour to 1 hour and 45 minutes, or until the squash gives when squeezed (protect your hand with a potholder).

• To cook squash halves (a time-saver), cut the raw squash lengthwise (not crosswise) through the middle; this will allow you to get the full spaghettilike length of the strands when you scoop them out. Place the halves, cut-side up, in a pot (or pots, if large) and add 2 inches of boiling water. Cover and simmer until tender, adding more water, if necessary. This method is, in effect, steaming—the water should remain below the cut edge of the squash, so that the flesh cooks by steam.

• When cool enough to handle, cut the squash in half lengthwise if it was cooked whole. Scoop out the seeds and fibers. Then take a fork and begin to scrape at the squash flesh. As you tease it apart, the flesh will separate into strands. Continue scraping down to the shell, transferring the forkfuls of strands to a pot to keep them warm as you remove them.

• Serve spaghetti squash with your favorite pasta sauce or chill the crunchy strands and toss them with a light vinaigrette dressing, fresh herbs, and perhaps chunks of fresh tomato to make a dish similar to a light pasta salad.

strawberries

The strawberry, as we know it today, is the product of horticultural fiddling around, beginning with a wild strawberry plant from Virginia that was introduced to Europe in the 16th century. Several hundred years later, this original North American plant was crossbred with a plant from South America to produce the ancestor of just about every commercial breed of strawberry grown in the world today. Further horticultural fiddling in the United States has produced strawberries suited to the climate of each of the states (and it's all 50 of them) that grows strawberries.

nutritional profile

These plump, sweet, rubylike berries are nutritional jewels: They're rich in dietary fiber and offering good amounts of vitamin C (more than any other berry).

in the market

Some 70 varieties are produced commercially, mostly in California and Florida. Two of the dominant California varieties are the *Pajaro* and the *Chandler*.

Day neutrals The "day neutral" varieties, such as *Tristar*, are a type of strawberry that produces fruit all summer long. However, they are usually grown on a smaller scale because of their labor-intensive cultivation. The fruits are smaller than other berries, but good and sweet.

Wild strawberries Also called *fraises des bois* (strawberries of the woods), wild strawberries are now cultivated to a small extent in California. These thumbnail-sized berries are prized for their intense flavor. If you're a good forager, you may find an overlooked patch of these tiny strawberries growing in a pasture or meadow in midsummer.

choosing the best

For best flavor, buy strawberries when they're in season where you live; they'll undoubtedly be riper and tastier than berries that have been transported in from distant regions. Also, the closer the berries are to the market, the less damage they're likely to suffer in transit.

Choose strawberries very carefully; they are often packed in opaque boxes that may conceal inferior fruit beneath a display of perfect specimens. If the box is cellophane wrapped, your best bet is to examine the berries you can see, and check the box for dampness or stains, which indicate that the fruit below may be decaying. If the box is not wrapped, you can remove a few of the top berries and peek beneath.

Strawberries should be plump, dry, firm, well shaped and uniformly colored. Don't purchase berries that are withered or crushed. The berries them-

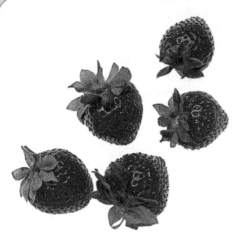

strawberries

STRAWBERRIES / 1 cup	
Calories	46
Protein (g)	1
Carbohydrate (g)	11
Dietary fiber (g)	3.5
Total fat (g)	0.6
Saturated fat (g)	0
Monounsaturated fat (g)	0.1
Polyunsaturated fat (g)	0.3
Cholesterol (mg)	0
Potassium (mg)	252
Sodium (mg)	2

KEY NUTRIENTS (%RDA/AI*)

Vitamin C	86 mg (96%)

*For more detailed information on RDA and AI, see page 88.

selves should be a true, rich red (although the shade of red differs among varieties). Pale, greenish, or yellowish fruit is unripe and will be hard and sour. The leafy caps should look fresh and green.

▶ **When you get home** Strawberries are highly perishable; they can turn soft, mushy, and moldy within 24 hours. When you bring home a box of berries, turn it out and check the fruit. Remove any soft, overripe strawberries for immediate consumption; discard any smashed or moldy berries and gently blot the remainder dry with a paper towel. Place the berries in a shallow refrigerator container lined with paper towels.

preparing to use

Keep the caps of strawberries intact until after they're rinsed and drained, as the opening left by the removal of the cap will allow the berries to absorb water. Rinse the fruit, drain, and gently pat dry. Use a paring knife, or a pincerlike strawberry huller to take off the caps and the hard white core of flesh directly beneath the cap.

Strawberries freeze well, allowing you to enjoy them practically year round. You can buy prepackaged frozen berries, but these may have had sweetener added, which can double their calorie content. Freezing strawberries yourself is simple. Pick over the berries, but do not wash them; then spread them out in a single layer on a baking sheet. Place the berries in the freezer until they are solidly frozen, and then transfer them to a freezer container. They'll keep for 10 months to a year.

Frozen berries need not be thawed before using them in recipes, but extra cooking time may be necessary. Commercially frozen berries do not require washing, but home-frozen berries should be quickly rinsed under cold water.

sunflower seeds

Sunflower seeds come from the center of the magnificent, daisylike flower of the familiar North American sunflower plant. Named because its flowers resemble the sun, and because they twist on their stems to follow the sun throughout the day, this imposing plant can grow as tall as 10 feet.

Native Americans use the seeds of this wild plant in a variety of ways: They ate the seeds for a snack and possibly squeezed them for their oil. The seeds were also pounded into a meal, which was then combined with other vegetables, or cooked up as a mash, or used to make bread.

Around 1500, Spanish explorers took the indigenous North American sunflower to Europe, where it was considered an exotic curiosity and was used for ornamental purposes. By the 18th century, someone had discovered that the tightly packed flowerheads contained seeds that were valuable at the very least for their oil. In Russia, sunflower seeds took off in a big way, and were prized for their oil as well as their kernels. By the late 19th century, the seeds had made their way back to the United States as a commercial food product imported from Russia. Only recently has the sunflower become a cultivated crop in the United States.

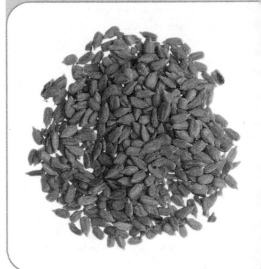

sunflower seeds

nutritional profile

Sunflower seeds are an outstanding source of the antioxidant vitamin E, and they also supply good amounts of folate, iron, manganese, selenium, vitamin B_6, zinc, protein, and fiber, as well as essential linoleic acid. Though they are a nutrient-dense food with a concentrated array of vitamins and minerals, sunflower seeds nonetheless are rather high in calories, so include them in your diet in moderation.

in the market

While the majority of the sunflower seed crop is destined to be processed for oil, the rest of the seeds are for consumption and are of a different type: Oil seeds are generally small and black; the delicately flavored seeds that we eat are "confectionery" seeds.

The plump, nutlike kernels of the "confection sunflower" grow in teardrop-shaped, gray-and-white shells. The seeds are allowed to dry on the flower (covered so the birds can't get them). The dried seeds are then removed and processed into a variety of forms:

HULLED SUNFLOWER SEEDS 1 ounce	
Calories	162
Protein (g)	6
Carbohydrate (g)	5
Dietary fiber (g)	3.0
Total fat (g)	14
Saturated fat (g)	1.5
Monounsaturated fat (g)	2.7
Polyunsaturated fat (g)	9.3
Cholesterol (mg)	0
Potassium (mg)	195
Sodium (mg)	1

KEY NUTRIENTS (%RDA/AI*)	
Thiamin	0.7 mg (54%)
Vitamin B$_6$	0.2 mg (13%)
Vitamin E	14 mg (95%)
Folate	64 mcg (16%)
Iron	1.9 mg (24%)
Magnesium	100 mg (24%)
Selenium	17 mcg (31%)
Zinc	1.4 mg (13%)

*For more detailed information on RDA and AI, see page 88.

Kernels Sunflower seeds are hulled and the kernels are either packaged *unroasted, dry-roasted* (in a slow oven), or *oil-roasted.* The roasted kernels are usually also salted.

Oil See Fats & Oils (*page 298*).

Whole unhulled The seeds of sunflowers are dried on the flower and then removed, but not hulled. The whole unhulled seeds are then brined.

choosing the best

When buying whole in-shell sunflower seeds in bulk, check to see that they have clean, unbroken shells. Sample a few to be sure that they're crisp and fresh, not limp, rubbery, or off-tasting. There shouldn't be a lot of dust and debris in the bin. Because they are high in fat, sunflower seeds are susceptible to rancidity; shop at a store where there is a rapid turnover in bulk products.

▶ When you get home Because of their high fat content, sunflower seeds that you won't be using within a few days should be kept in a cool, dry place in a tightly closed container. Better still, keep them in the refrigerator or freezer. If they are properly wrapped, freezing will not significantly affect their flavor or texture.

preparing to use

If sunflower seeds are hulled, you can use them as they are. To heighten their flavor or to crisp them if they've gotten soggy, raw (unroasted) sunflower seeds can be either oven-toasted or toasted in a dry skillet on top of the stove.

serving suggestions

• Grind sunflower seeds and substitute for some of the flour in a pie crust.

• Substitute sunflower seeds for pine nuts in pesto.

• Make sunflower seed butter by grinding the seeds in a food processor until pasty. Use as you would peanut butter.

• Sprinkle toasted sunflower seeds over salads.

• Sauté vegetables and top with toasted sunflower seeds.

• Add sunflower seeds to muffin, quick bread, and cookie recipes.

• Add roasted sunflower seeds to rice puddings.

sweet potatoes

Sweet potatoes are edible roots, not tubers like potatoes. In fact, sweet potatoes aren't even related to potatoes. They are members of an entirely different family, the morning glory family. The resemblance to other members of the vining morning glory family is evident in the leafy vines that can be grown from sweet potato cuttings.

Native to the New World, the sweet potato plant (*Ipomoea batatas*) was introduced to Europe by Columbus (and to Asia by other explorers). A valued food for Native Americans, and widely cultivated in Colonial America, where it often provided the chief means of sustenance for early homesteaders and for soldiers during the Revolutionary War, the sweet potato was considered a fundamental staple food. As one Colonial physician put it, the sweet potato was the "vegetable indispensable."

Sweet potatoes have a rich natural sweetness, which is produced by an enzyme in the potato that converts most of its starches to sugars as the potato matures. This sweetness continues to increase during storage, and when the potato is cooked.

In spite of their appealing flavor and spectacular nutrition profile (they are among the most nutritious foods in the vegetable kingdom), many people eat sweet potatoes only on Thanksgiving. In fact, in the past 20 years, the per capita consumption of sweet potatoes has gone down instead of up.

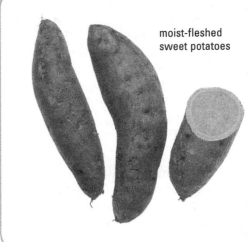

sweet potatoes

moist-fleshed sweet potatoes

nutritional profile

High in fiber and rich in vitamins and minerals, sweet potatoes provide a dynamic assortment of nutritional benefits. They are low in calories (about 143 calories per average-sized sweet potato), and they also supply handsome amounts of vitamin B_6, vitamin C, iron, and potassium. Also well worth noting is the sweet potato's vitamin E content: One potato provides over 25 percent of the RDA, almost unheard of in a low-fat food. And the orange color of sweet potato flesh indicates the presence of carotenoids. In fact, one orange-fleshed sweet potato supplies over 100 percent of the daily requirement for beta carotene. The darker the flesh of a sweet potato, the more beta carotene. (Chances are the tropical white-fleshed varieties have little to no beta carotene.)

Though many people assume that sweet potato skin is inedible, it is in fact every bit as edible as white potato skin. This is important, because the skin boosts the amount of important nutrients in this delicious root vegetable.

in the market

There are two main types of sweet potato: *dry-fleshed* and *moist-fleshed* (these are descriptives, not market terms). The starchier, dry-fleshed types have a tan skin and light-colored flesh ranging from almost white to a light yellow. Their texture is much more akin to baking potatoes. The moist-fleshed sweet potatoes have a dark, red-brown skin with orange to deep-orange flesh. This latter type dominates the market, perhaps because they are sweeter. There is rarely any distinction in the market among sweet potatoes, except for the following:

Batata This dry-fleshed sweet potato is rounder than American sweet potato types and has a mottled red-purple skin. The batata's name is taken from the species name for all sweet potatoes: *Ipomoea batatas*. It is a favorite in Puerto Rican and other Latin American cuisines.

Boniato (Cuban sweet potato) A boniato is a white sweet potato similar to a batata. Boniatos can be found in Hispanic markets, especially in Cuban neighborhoods; they are now being grown in Florida.

Jersey sweets There are a number of varieties of dry-fleshed sweet potato that include Jersey in their varietal name (for example, Big Stem Jersey and Little Stem Jersey) and some markets will identify any dry-fleshed sweet potato as a Jersey or Jersey sweet.

Kumara Another tropical sweet potato, kumara is what the sweet potato is called in New Zealand. The traditional variety of sweet potato grown there is called the Owairaka Red, which is a direct descendant of an American sweet potato introduced to New Zealand in the 1850s by an American whaling ship. The kumara has red skin and white flesh.

White sweet potato This is a generic term used to identify what are loosely called tropical sweet potatoes. Their flesh is lighter in color than orange-fleshed sweet potatoes. Although it all started with a North American plant, the sweet potato has been adapted to many tropical regions around the world. Depending on where the sweet potato comes from it may be called batata, kumara, camote, or boniato, to name a few.

Yam Moist-fleshed sweet potatoes are often called "yams," but this is a misnomer: The true yam (botanical family *Dioscoreaceae*) is a large (up to 100 pounds) root vegetable grown in Africa, South America, and the Caribbean (*see Roots & Tubers, page 516*). However, common usage has made the term "yam" acceptable when referring to sweet potatoes. (Although the USDA requires that the label "yam" always be accompanied by the term "sweet potato," this is rarely respected in the market.)

choosing the best

Select sweet potatoes that are heavy for their size, and buy similar-sized potatoes of the same variety (don't mix dry- and moist-fleshed types) if you plan to cook them whole; this will keep the cooking time uniform. Choose potatoes that are smooth, hard, and free of bruises or decay, which may appear as

SWEET POTATO / 1 medium (4 ounces) baked, with skin	
Calories	143
Protein (g)	3
Carbohydrate (g)	34
Dietary fiber (g)	3.7
Total fat (g)	0.1
Saturated fat (g)	0
Monounsaturated fat (g)	0
Polyunsaturated fat (g)	0.1
Cholesterol (mg)	0
Potassium (mg)	458
Sodium (mg)	11

KEY NUTRIENTS (%RDA/AI*)	
Beta carotene	12 mg (107%)
Riboflavin	0.1 mg (11%)
Vitamin B$_6$	0.4 mg (22%)
Vitamin C	26 mg (28%)
Vitamin E	4.1 mg (27%)
Iron	2.2 mg (27%)

*For more detailed information on RDA and AI, see page 88.

shriveled or sunken areas or black spots. Even if cut away, a decayed spot may have already imparted an unpleasant flavor to the entire potato.

▶ **When you get home** Despite their rugged appearance, sweet potatoes have a thin skin that is easily damaged, and they are subject to rapid spoilage. To help preserve them, growers cure them—that is, they store them at a high temperature and humidity for about 10 days before sending them to market. This process also enhances the vegetable's natural sweetness.

After purchase, sweet potatoes should be kept in a cool (55° to 60°), dry place, such as a cellar, pantry, or garage—never in the refrigerator, where they may develop a hard core and an "off" taste. In fact, when sweet potatoes are stored at low temperatures, their natural sugars turn to starch, which does nothing to enhance their flavor.

Sweet potatoes will keep for a month or longer if stored at 55°; if kept at normal room temperature, they should be used within a week.

preparing to use

Sweet potatoes may be somewhat dirty, especially if bought at a farmstand or a farmers' market. You should brush off any excess dirt before storing, but don't wash the potatoes until you are ready to cook them, as the moisture will hasten spoilage.

Moist- and dry-fleshed sweet potatoes are interchangeable in recipes (although the cooking times may vary). Try not to combine the two types in a single dish, however, as their differing textures and cooking times may affect the outcome of the recipe. (Moist-fleshed varieties take longer to cook than dry-fleshed. The exception to this is in the microwave, where the higher water content of the moist-fleshed sweet potatoes makes them cook faster.)

Scrub the potatoes under cold running water before cooking. When cutting sweet potatoes, always use a stainless steel knife so that the flesh will not discolor.

serving suggestions

• Use batata or boniato in place of white potatoes in a potato pancake recipe.

• Make a multi-potato salad with sweet potatoes, blue potatoes, and boniatos. Make a dressing with yogurt, mashed roasted garlic, chipotle peppers, and a little olive oil.

• Add shredded raw sweet potato to hamburger, meatloaf, and meatball mixtures.

• Toss chunks of cooked sweet potato, diced tomato, minced scallion, toasted cumin, and lime together for a nonfat salad.

• Stir cubes of sweet potato into chili.

• Add tropical sweet potato to regular mashed potatoes.

• Toss cubes of batata or boniato with cut-up asparagus, sun-dried tomatoes, some olive oil, and crushed fennel seed. Roast in a 450° oven until cooked through.

• Stir mashed sweet potatoes into tomato-based pasta sauces.

• Combine mashed sweet potato with some Parmesan and use as a ravioli stuffing.

sweeteners

Starting at a very early age, humans seem to have a "sweet tooth." This instinctive desire for sweet tastes may be part of an evolutionary design that encourages infants to accept life-sustaining milk with its slight sweetness (human breast milk is quite sweet). And though this childhood tendency changes as we get older and begin to seek out other basic tastes (such as salty, bitter, and sour), many adults still retain their sweet tooth.

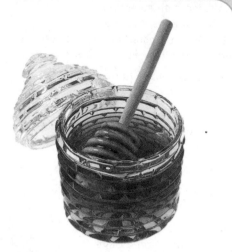

honey

Not only does sugar add sweetness to foods and beverages, it has culinary applications as well, adding tenderness to dough, stability to baking mixtures, and contributing to the preservation of some foods. However, the problem with eating too many sugary foods is that they tend to leave little room for more nutritious foods. Much of the sugar we consume is added to processed foods, such as sodas, cookies, and candy. These added sugars are the main reason why sugar now accounts for 16 percent of all calories consumed by Americans; 20 years ago, it supplied 11 percent. (Soda alone is responsible for about one-third of all the sugar calories consumed.)

nutritional profile

All sugars are simple carbohydrates: glucose and fructose from fruits, honey, and some vegetables; lactose from milk; sucrose from cane or beet sugar. All of these sugars offer minimal nutritional value, except for blackstrap molasses, which contains small amounts of such minerals as calcium, iron, magnesium, and potassium. Beyond that, the sugars all provide comparable calories: around 50 per tablespoon for most. Those sugars that are fine and powdery have fewer calories per tablespoon (about 30), because a tablespoon of these weighs less than the same volume of other sugars. Very dense, low-moisture syrups, such as honey, contain more calories per tablespoon (about 64). Of course, sugar substitutes are essentially calorie-free.

in the market

granulated sugars

What most people would call sugar in this country is granulated highly refined cane sugar and is the most common form both for table use and for cooking. Not only are there many forms of cane sugar, but also sugars from other plant sources.

Beet sugar Sugar beets are sliced, then the liquid is extracted, partially evaporated, and boiled off. The resulting sugar crystals are white and can be used like granulated sugar.

Brown sugar This moist sugar is granulated cane sugar that has molasses added to it. It comes in both light and dark forms. *Dark brown sugar* has more molasses than the light and has a stronger flavor. *Light brown sugar* has less molasses and less of a molasses flavor; it is also a little less moist. They can be used interchangeably. Dry, *granulated brown sugar* is also available.

Cane sugar Sugar is made from sugarcane that is chopped, has some water added, and is then heated, clarified with the addition of lime, and evaporated. The resulting syrup is then centrifuged to extract the sugar crystals. The liquid by-product of this process is called molasses. The two main categories of cane sugar are white refined sugar and brown sugar.

Date sugar Made from ground, dehydrated dates, this very sweet sugar does not dissolve when added to liquids.

Demerara sugar This "raw," pale brown, coarse-textured cane sugar is from Demerara, an area in Guyana where the cane grows in rich, volcanic soil. It is often used as coffee sugar.

Fructose Fruit sugar, twice as sweet as refined cane sugar, provides moisture in baked goods. It's sold in both a granular and liquid form. Commercial fructose is not extracted from fruits, but is created by treating glucose with enzymes.

Fruit sweetener Made from grape juice concentrate blended with rice syrup, this sweetener is about 80 percent as sweet as white sugar. It is sold in both granular and liquid form.

Jaggery (palm sugar, gur) Made from the reduced sap of either the sugar palm or the palmyra palm, this sugar is dark brown and crumbly. The two most common forms of jaggery are the solid cake form (the reduced sap

sugar myths

Sugar seems to perpetually be the object of misperception and myth.

Myth: Sugar is the leading cause of obesity.

Fact: Eating more calories than you burn adds pounds to the body—and for most people the lion's share of excess calories comes from eating too much fat, not sugar. Many "sweets" (cakes, ice cream, cookies) actually get most of their calories from fat, not sugar. Thus, many a "sweet tooth" is a "fat tooth."

Myth: Only refined sugar causes cavities.

Fact: Refined sugar remains the leading dietary cause of tooth decay, but sugars such as fructose in fruit and lactose in milk may promote decay, as may some foods high in fermentable carbohydrates, such as bread and rice.

Myth: Artificial sweeteners will help you lose weight.

Fact: Studies have failed to show that artificial sweeteners keep people from gaining weight, much less help them lose significant amounts.

Myth: Sugar makes children hyperactive.

Fact: Though for years parents have been blaming a high sugar intake for their children's uncontrollable behavior, studies have found no evidence for this.

Myth: You can become addicted to sugar.

Fact: There's no scientific evidence for this.

Myth: Sugar in fruit is good, sugar in candy is bad.

Fact: The sugar in most fruit is primarily fructose, which has few, if any, advantages over sucrose.

Myth: Honey and brown sugar are healthier than sucrose.

Fact: Sugar is sugar, and no type offers significant nutritional advantages over the others.

is traditionally dried in coconut shells) and a soft type with a spreadable texture. Sometimes the syrup is smoked, giving the jaggery a black color and smoky flavor. It is generally found in East Indian markets. It is available in both granular and liquid form.

Maple sugar This is maple syrup with all the liquid evaporated, leaving behind a dry sugar. It comes both in pressed cakes as well as in a granulated form. Except for the fact that it is very expensive, this is a good substitute for refined sugar because the mouth perceives it as much sweeter than white sugar and it has fewer calories.

Muscovado (Barbados) sugar This "raw" cane sugar is similar to brown sugar, but with a richer, more complex flavor. It comes both light and dark.

Palm sugar See Jaggery (*page 561*).

Piloncillo (panela, panocha) Raw sugarcane is crushed to extract the juice, then boiled to evaporate the liquid. It is poured into cone-shaped molds and sold in cone shapes in Hispanic markets.

Raw sugar True raw, unrefined sugar is not allowed to be sold in the United States because of the presence of dirt, insect fragments, and other unknown particles. Sugar sold as "raw" in this country has actually gone through at least 50 percent of the refining steps. Examples of "raw" sugar are: Demerara, Muscovado, and Turbinado.

Rock sugar (Chinese rock sugar) This lightly caramelized cane sugar is amber in color and not quite as sweet as regular granulated sugar. It is used in many Chinese dishes.

Sucanat Juice from organically grown sugar cane is turned into granular sugar by a process that does not involve any chemical additives. It is light brown and has a mild molasses taste.

Turbinado sugar Raw cane sugar crystals, derived from the first pressing of sugarcane, are steam-cleaned, but not bleached, to produce a blond, delicate, molasses-flavored sugar that is similar to Demerara, but with smaller crystals.

White refined sugar (granulated sugar, table sugar, sucrose) Made primarily from sugarcane, but also from sugar beets, this highly refined, free-flowing sugar is the type most Americans know as sugar. In addition to the typical granulated sugar, this comes in a number of other granulations, from coarse to fine. *Coarse sugar* is large crystals of granulated sugar, used for decorating baked goods. *Superfine sugar* is finer than granulated sugar and dissolves instantly. It is therefore often used in drinks and may be referred to as bar sugar. In England it is known as castor sugar. *Confectioners' sugar (10X sugar, icing sugar)* is granulated sugar that has been crushed to a very fine powder. It often has a small amount of cornstarch added to prevent clumping. This is used in baking and to make frostings.

stevia

An herbal extract from a member of the chrysanthemum family, stevia is widely used as a calorie-free sweetener in South America and Japan. Under the Dietary Supplement Act of 1994, stevia, like other herbal products, can be sold as a "dietary supplement." It still can't be used as a food additive, so stevia isn't used in any commercial products.

liquid sweeteners

Barley malt syrup Roasted, sprouted whole barley is combined with water and cooked down to produce this brown liquid. It has a flavor similar to light molasses.

Corn syrup Corn syrup is made by converting the starches in corn to sugar. *Light corn syrup* is clarified, removing any particles. *Dark corn syrup* has caramel coloring added and has a stronger flavor than light.

Honey This thick, sweet liquid is made by bees from flower nectar. The honey's color and flavor come from the source of the nectar. There are hundreds of different honeys and, in general, the darker the honey, the stronger the flavor. In addition to the standard liquid honey, it comes in a few other forms: In *comb honey*, the liquid honey is sold still in the chewy, edible comb. *Chunk-style honey* has bits of chewy honeycomb included in the jar along with the honey. *Whipped honey* is honey that has been processed by controlled crystallization to give it a thick, smooth, spreadable consistency. It is sometimes called *honey butter* or *creamed honey*.

Malt syrup (malt extract) This natural sweetener is made from a mash of evaporated ground corn and sprouted barley. It has an earthy flavor and is less sweet than honey.

Maple syrup In Colonial America, Native Americans taught the early settlers how to tap the sugar-maple tree for its sap and how to boil the sap down to evaporate the water and produce the thick, sweet syrup the Indians called "sweetwater." Because the processing of maple syrup is time consuming and labor intensive, it is rather expensive. Maple syrup is available graded according to color and flavor. Fancy or Grade AA is light amber and mild in flavor. Grade A, which comes in both medium and dark amber, is mellow with a delicate maple flavor. Grade B is dark and full-bodied with deep maple flavor, and Grade C is very dark with a molasseslike flavor. Maple syrup is also boiled further to produce thicker products: *Maple honey* is maple syrup that's been boiled until it achieves the consistency of honey. *Maple cream (maple butter)* is boiled longer still and is thick and spreadable. At the far end of the spectrum is maple sugar (*see opposite page*). There are also maple-syruplike products called *pancake syrups*, which are corn syrups mixed with varying amounts of real maple syrup. Some pancake syrups have no maple syrup at all, and are flavored with artificial maple extract.

Molasses When granulated sugar is extracted from sugarcane, the remaining brownish-black liquid is called molasses. The type of molasses depends on what part of the sugar-refining process produces it. *Light molasses* comes from the first boiling of the sugar syrup in the sugar-making process.

honey facts

Our attraction to honey goes back to antiquity. In fact, references to honey can be traced back to 9,000 years ago in the form of cave paintings. And so prized was honey that the ancient Romans used it instead of gold to pay their taxes.

Though some preliminary studies show that honey does contain antioxidants, most people don't eat large enough amounts of honey to reap any of the benefits; a tablespoon of honey is not a significant source of anything, except calories.

This flavorful sweetener comes with one important caveat: Honey should never be fed to infants under the age of 12 months. Because their digestive systems are immature, babies less than 1 year of age are susceptible to infant botulism, an illness that can originate from spores (microorganisms) in honey that have no effect on adults (older children and adults have sufficient amounts of stomach acids to kill the bacterium quickly).

Dark molasses is the by-product of the second boiling of the sugar syrup. *Blackstrap molasses,* the strongest and most bitter of the three, comes from the third boiling. Molasses also comes in either sulfured or unsulfured. Unsulfured molasses, made from the juice of sun-ripened sugarcane, is the lightest and most delicately flavored. Sulfured molasses is made from green, immature sugarcane that's been treated with sulfur during the sugar extracting process. It has a stronger flavor than unsulfured molasses.

Rice syrup This thick amber syrup is made from a combination of sprouted barley and cooked brown rice that is fermented to convert the starches to sugar.

Sorghum molasses (sorghum syrup) The juice from stalks of sorghum (a cereal grass) is boiled down to produce this thick, mild-flavored syrup, which is similar to light molasses.

Treacle This is what the British call molasses.

sugar substitutes

Artificial sweeteners are now usually called sugar substitutes or low-calorie or noncaloric sweeteners, largely because the word "artificial" makes many people uncomfortable. In addition, the distinction between artificial and natural is sometimes impossible to draw. While several new sugar substitutes are waiting for FDA approval, there are currently only a few used in the United States.

Acesulfame-K (acesulfame potassium) This sugar substitute was approved by the FDA in 1989 and is used in soft drinks (sometimes combined with aspartame), candy, baked goods, and other foods. More than 90 studies have given it a clean bill of health, though some consumer groups still worry about it. Acesulfame-K passes through the body unchanged and is thus noncaloric. It contains only a small amount of potassium per serving. It does not break down when heated and can be used in baked goods and other cooked foods.

Aspartame Approved by the FDA in the early 1980s, aspartame is made from two amino acids (the building blocks of proteins) and has almost no calories. It's used in countless foods and beverages, but can't be used in most baked goods. Aspartame has been more intensively studied than almost any other food additive. Leading authorities, including the FDA, American Medican Association, and the World Health Organization, have concluded that it is safe. Aspartame's only proven danger is for people with phenylketonuria, an uncommon genetic disorder—the labels warn about this.

Sorbitol This occurs naturally in some fruits and berries. It is not quite as sweet as sucrose, and in addition to being used as an artificial sweetener, it is also used as a thickener and stabilizer in candy and numerous food products.

storing sugar

Most granulated sugar will keep for a long time without any special storage (sugar is used as a preservative, after all). To keep brown sugar moist, make sure the package is tightly sealed. Once opened, seal the package tightly and keep it in a dry cabinet. If brown sugar has hardened, cut an apple and place the apple in a container with the hardened sugar: The sugar will get soft within a day or two and stay soft as long as the apple is in the container.

Honey can crystallize, but this doesn't affect its flavor. If it has crystallized, place the closed jar in a pan of simmering water and heat until the honey has softened and no crystals remain.

facts & tips

There are some sugar substitutes—such as sorbitol and other forms of reduced-calorie sugar alcohols—that provide the sweet taste found in many sugar-free candies, cookies, and chewing gums. Foods made with sugar alcohols affect blood glucose levels less dramatically than sugar and therefore require little or no insulin for metabolism. Thus, sugar alcohols are often used in foods for people with diabetes.

swiss chard

Swiss chard (also known simply as chard) is a cruciferous vegetable and member of the beet family. Unlike other beets, it's grown for its stems and leaves, not its root; its distinctive flavor is akin to (but milder than) that of beet greens. The plant's dark green leaves are wider and flatter than beet greens, and they have a full-bodied texture similar to spinach (for which chard is a good substitute). The fleshy, delicately flavored, celerylike stalks of Swiss chard are edible; in fact, in Europe, they are considered the best part of the plant.

nutritional profile

A rich source of beta carotene and potassium, Swiss chard also supplies fiber, vitamin C, and magnesium. The vegetable is also a superb low-fat source of the antioxidant vitamin E, which is usually found in high-fat foods. In addition, Swiss chard supplies a tremendous amount of vitamin K, which is needed to make a protein that's essential for bone formation. Though it contains iron, Swiss chard also contains a compound called oxalic acid, which may limit the mineral's absorption by the body.

in the market

The fleshy stalks and ribs of Swiss chard are most commonly either white or red. There are thin-stemmed and thick-stemmed chard varieties. If you prefer the leaves to the stalks, choose a thin-stemmed variety; if you enjoy the crunchy stalks, go for a thick-stemmed type. Most red chard is thin-stemmed.

Bright Lights This variety comes in a rainbow of colors. The stalks and veins range in color from white to gold to orange to pink to purple. Occasionally the green leaves have bronze or copper hues. This newly developed chard is tender and sweet, and each color tastes slightly different.

Bright Yellow A yellow-stemmed variety, this chard's flavor is a bit earthier than white chard and less so than red.

Fordhook Giant Probably the most widely available variety, it has large, thick, white stalks and crinkled leaves.

Rhubarb chard (ruby red) With dark green, crinkled leaves and thin, tender red stalks, this chard has a sweet, earthy flavor that is a little stronger than that of the white variety.

choosing the best

Swiss chard should be displayed in a chilled case to preserve its crispness and sweetness. Look for a fresh green color. The leaves should not be yellowed or

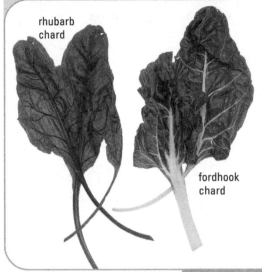

swiss chard

rhubarb chard

fordhook chard

SWISS CHARD	
1 cup cooked	
Calories	35
Protein (g)	3
Carbohydrate (g)	7
Dietary fiber (g)	3.7
Total fat (g)	0.1
Saturated fat (g)	0
Monounsaturated fat (g)	0
Polyunsaturated fat (g)	0.1
Cholesterol (mg)	0
Potassium (mg)	961
Sodium (mg)	313

KEY NUTRIENTS (%RDA/AI*)	
Beta carotene	3.3 mg (30%)
Riboflavin	0.2 mg (12%)
Vitamin C	32 mg (35%)
Vitamin E	3.3 mg (22%)
Iron	4.0 mg (49%)
Magnesium	150 mg (36%)

*For more detailed information on RDA and AI, see page 88.

browned; they should be moist, crisp, and unwilted, and unblemished by any tiny holes, which usually indicate insect damage. Be sure that the stems are juicy and crisp.

preparing to use

Unless the chard is young, the stalks should be separated from the leaves and given a little extra cooking time. Wash chard leaves and stems before using, as they are likely to have sand or dirt clinging to them. Separate the leaves from the stems if the chard is large, and swish the leaves around in a large bowl of cool water. Lift the leaves out, letting the sand and grit settle; repeat if necessary. Slice or chop as your recipe directs. Don't heat Swiss chard in an aluminum pot; the chard contains oxalates that will cause the pot to discolor. Start cooking the stems a few minutes before adding the leaves.

serving suggestions

• Steam chard, garlic, and green peas. Puree in a food processor with lemon juice, broth (enough to make a soup consistency), and nonfat sour cream. Reheat very gently for a nonfat cream of vegetable soup.

• Chop stems and leaves, sauté in olive oil, and use as a filling for a frittata or omelet.

• Wrap whole fish or fillets in chard leaves and bake or steam.

• Sauté both stalks and leaves with raisins and pine nuts.

• Use raw tender baby chard (preferably in a range of colors) to perk up a salad.

• Stuff large chard leaves as you would cabbage, using the chopped stems as part of the filling.

• Add shredded chard to vegetable soups and stews.

• Use chard in an Italian dessert based on savory greens, called crostata di verdure.

• Use chard instead of spinach in a Greek spinach pie recipe.

tea

Our love affair with tea goes back thousands of years. The Chinese were cultivating the tea plant about 4,000 years ago and sometime in the 8th century A.D. the Japanese discovered it. During the 17th century, Europeans were introduced to tea for the first time by the Dutch and the Portuguese, who had picked it up in their travels to Asia. Tea soon became an important item of trade. The British took up tea drinking with a passion unequaled by any other European people. Tea soon became England's national drink, with that country importing about 40,000 pounds of tea in 1699, and as much as 240,000 pounds in 1708. Dutch and English colonists brought tea to the New World, and early settlers in America soon embraced this soothing new beverage.

In the world at large, the countries with the highest consumption of tea are India and China, who together are responsible for producing 80 percent of the world's tea. Though America as a nation consumes quite a few metric tons of tea a year, the per capita consumption is quite low: only ½ cup daily.

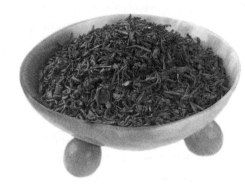

green tea

nutritional profile

The fluoride in black, green, or oolong tea may help to strengthen tooth enamel, fight cavities, and prevent dental plaque. However, apart from fluoride, tea contains only a little potassium and folate, and traces of other minerals. Unless you add sugar or honey, tea has just 2 calories per cup.

in the market

There are over 3,000 varieties of tea grown worldwide, and all of them come from the same type of plant, a small shrub (*Camellia sinensis*). Each type of tea has certain flavor characteristics associated not only with the variety but also with the soil and climate in which it is grown (much like wine grapes). But beyond the subtle flavor differences from tea to tea, there are three main categories of tea—black, oolong, and green—that are a function of how the tea leaves are processed.

The majority of teas are processed this way: The freshly picked tea leaves (usually the tender leaves from the top of the plant) are dried slightly, then crushed (to bring out the essential oils), and finally "fermented." Though this final stage is called fermentation, it is not the result of an introduced organism (as yeast is in winemaking), but rather is oxidation caused by a natural enzyme in the tea leaves themselves. This "fermentation" brings out the tannins and oils (wherein lies the caffeine), and changes the color of the tea leaves to brown.

In addition to the broad categories based on fermentation, teas are also identified by a leaf-grading system. For black teas, the grades are: souchong,

> ### facts & tips
> It's fine to use milk in tea, if you like it. You may have heard that milk "binds" some of the beneficial polyphenols in tea, but this has not been proven to be the case.

➤ phytochemicals in
tea

Green tea is a likely choice these days for people looking for health benefits from their beverages. But current research indicates that all tea is good for you, as long as it comes from the leaf of *Camellia sinensis*—as do all green, black, and oolong (red) teas.

The chemicals that make tea a potential protector of health are called polyphenols. Though green tea was once thought to have the most polyphenols, it turns out that black tea has a similar amount. The most potent polyphenol in tea is a substance called EGCG (epigallocatechin gallate), which belongs to a group of flavonoid phytochemicals called catechins.

The polyphenols in tea seem to operate in a variety of ways: For example, halting the damage that free radicals do to cells, neutralizing enzymes essential for tumor growth, and deactivating cancer promoters.

Yet studies of these and other antioxidants have yielded contradictory results. These substances can certainly protect against oxidation in a test tube, but in the human body they can have the opposite effect—acting as pro-oxidants as well as antioxidants. Or they may have no effect at all.

While tea may have health benefits, it clearly is no panacea. Stomach cancer, for example, remains a major killer in China and Japan, where the highest amounts of green tea are consumed. But the evidence keeps mounting that tea has health benefits. Think of it as an adjunct to other good health habits—not as a miraculous potion that will keep you well by itself.

orange pekoe, and pekoe. For green teas, the leaf grades are: gunpowder and young hyson. There are several other identifiers for types of tea, including classic blends (such as Earl Grey) and districts (such as Darjeeling).

black teas

Black teas are fully fermented, and because of this, they are also the highest in caffeine. They are also the most popular type of tea in this country.

Assam This is a robust, large-leafed tea from India.

Ceylon This Sri Lankan black tea has a floral aroma.

Darjeeling From the Darjeeling region of India, this is a favorite of tea connoisseurs, and is probably the world's most expensive tea. Because it is so costly, many "Darjeelings" are actually blends (though the packaging should say if the tea is 100 percent Darjeeling). Darjeeling also comes as an oolong.

Keemun One of the best Chinese black teas, it has a rich bouquet and good flavor.

Lapsang souchong This distinctive Chinese black tea has a smoky flavor.

Ti kuan yin A sought-after tea, this is available as both a black tea and an oolong. Its name translates as "iron goddess of mercy."

Yunnan From southwest China, this is similar to Ceylon.

oolong (red) teas

This is the type of tea found in most Chinese restaurants in this country. Like black tea, it is fermented, but for shorter periods of time. Within this category, there are some that are more fermented than others.

Black dragon The word "oolong" translates into English as black dragon.

Cantonese oolongs These oolong teas from Canton are very lightly fermented.

Formosa oolongs These teas are fermented for almost as long as black teas and are the most caffeinated of the oolongs.

Jade oolong This lightly fermented tea has overtones of green tea and a delicate flavor.

Jasmine This is an oolong that has had night-blooming jasmine blossoms added to it for a floral scent. It is most often made with pouchong oolong.

Pouchong This medium oolong is rarely exported to the United States, except in a form scented with jasmine, gardenia, or lychee.

green teas

Green teas are completely unfermented. The fresh leaves are air-dried and then roasted (or steam-dried). This heating process halts the natural enzymatic action that is involved in fermentation. Green teas have almost no caffeine. There are dozens of green teas from China, Japan (where green tea is the tea of choice), and Korea. There are also teas from areas that do not by tradition produce green teas; for example, Sri Lanka and India are now making unfermented versions of their classics, such as Darjeeling green. One of the most famous green teas is Gunpowder from China, named because the loose tea leaves are rolled into gunpowder-colored pellets.

tea blends

Some of the better-known teas (at least to Westerners) are tea blends, many of them created by British tea companies in honor of members of the royal family, or as private blends for wealthy customers. Though there are hundreds of such blends, a handful have gained worldwide popularity.

Earl Grey No strict formula defines this—it's usually a blend of Darjeeling, Ceylon, and Chinese black teas—but it is always flavored with the oil of bergamot (a sour, inedible orange cultivated for its aromatic oils).

English Breakfast This is not so much a specific blend as a category of blend, which suggests a mixture of several strong Chinese black teas.

Irish Breakfast This is a mix of strong black teas.

Lady Londonderry This tea was created by a famous tea company in London for one of its customers. It is a blend of black teas from India, Sri Lanka, and Formosa.

Prince of Wales This is a proprietary blend created by the Twinings tea company and is a blend of black teas from south China.

choosing the best

Tea lovers would probably unite in recommending loose tea over tea bags, which are most often made from a grade of tea leaf called fannings or dust—fragments of tea leaf broken off from the larger leaves. These leaf fragments are used in tea bags because they have a greater surface area and brew really quickly. This same increased exposure to air is what makes tea-bag tea less-fragrant than loose tea. In addition, tea-bag teas are often middle-of-the-road teas with no special character.

▶ **When you get home** Because air and light can diminish the flavor of tea, it should be stored in opaque, airtight containers.

teatime

Though tea is an important Asian tradition, for Westerners the culture of tea is quintessentially British. In England, tea (and teatime) has been elevated to a national institution. As teatime rapidly became a common practice in England, it also evolved into two different customs, created loosely along class lines: Low Tea (afternoon tea) was for the aristocrats and the wealthy, who enjoyed an array of biscuits, little cakes, sweets, and other desserts along with their pots of tea at 4 P.M. High Tea, on the other hand, was usually had by the middle and lower classes, and was served at 5 or 6 P.M.; more of an early dinner, it featured substantial foods like meat and vegetables, along with the tea.

teff

Native to North Africa, teff is the minuscule seed of a wild grass. It takes 150 grains of teff to match the weight of one grain of wheat, and one grain of teff is about twice the size of the period at the end of this sentence. The word "teff" is thought to originate from the Ethiopian word *teffa,* which means lost, because if you drop it, you won't find it. Teff is cultivated by the Ethiopians, who use its flour to make a type of fermented (think sourdough) pancakelike bread called *injera.* Teff is also grown in this country, and while its acceptance has not exactly been meteoric, it is gradually garnering some interest. Teff has a mild, sweet, and nutlike flavor.

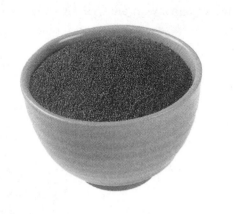

teff

nutritional profile

Teff has a good supply of thiamin and an exceptional amount of fiber and iron.

in the market

Teff can be found in health-food stores and specialty food shops. Whole-grain teff is available in three colors and the rule of thumb seems to be the darker the color the more earthy the flavor.

Brown teff Brown teff is earthy and robust with a nutty flavor. The darkest brown is reminiscent of hazelnuts.

Red teff Like brown teff, red teff is full-flavored and robust.

White teff This is the most delicate and mild teff, with an almost chestnutlike flavor.

Teff flour See Flour, Nonwheat (*page 326*).

preparing to use

You can cook teff grains as they are, or toast them in a dry skillet (or in a little olive oil) before using.

TEFF / ¼ cup raw	
Calories	204
Protein (g)	7
Carbohydrate (g)	41
Dietary fiber (g)	7.7
Total fat (g)	1.5
Saturated fat (g)	--
Monounsaturated fat (g)	--
Polyunsaturated fat (g)	--
Cholesterol (mg)	0
Potassium (mg)	282
Sodium (mg)	10

KEY NUTRIENTS (%RDA/AI*)	
Thiamin	0.2 mg (18%)
Iron	4.2 mg (52%)

For more detailed information on RDA and AI, see page 88.

serving suggestions

• Substitute teff flour for part of the flour in biscuits.

• Add cooked, cooled whole-grain teff to homemade pizza dough.

• Substitute raw teff for some of the poppy seeds in a poppyseed cake.

• Use teff as a thickener for soups and stews.

• Add raw teff to pancake, waffle, quick bread, and muffin recipes.

• Cook whole-grain teff like a breakfast cereal.

tomatoes

Although botanically a fruit—specifically, a berry—the tomato is prepared and served as a vegetable. (As a result of a tariff dispute, it was officially proclaimed a vegetable in 1893 by the Supreme Court of the United States.) A member of the nightshade family (which includes deadly nightshade as well as potatoes, bell peppers, and eggplant), the tomato is a native South American plant that was brought to Europe by Spanish explorers in the 16th century. Europeans, however, believed it to be poisonous and used it only as an ornamental houseplant. Not until the 19th century was the tomato widely accepted as a food, and even then it was customarily cooked for hours to neutralize its "poisons." Only in the second half of that century were raw or lightly cooked tomatoes consumed by Europeans and Americans.

nutritional profile

Extremely popular and highly versatile, tomatoes provide dietary fiber, some B vitamins, iron, potassium, and a good amount of vitamin C. Cherry tomatoes and fresh plum tomatoes are a decent low-fat source of the antioxidant vitamin E. And iron and potassium are found in ample amounts in canned tomatoes and also in sun-dried tomatoes, which are another good source of fiber. However, one of the key nutritional bonuses derived from tomatoes is a carotenoid that makes tomatoes red: lycopene. Research shows that this plant pigment may help to prevent prostate cancer and possibly heart disease (*see "Lycopene in Tomatoes," page 573*). While a few other foods contain lycopene, tomatoes are the major dietary source of this important carotenoid.

in the market

There are thousands of tomato varieties, but most fall into one of the following categories:

Beefsteak tomatoes These generally large (up to 6 inches in diameter), elliptical tomatoes are extremely "meaty." In other words, they have a high flesh-to-seed ratio. Prized by home gardeners, beefsteaks are only seasonally available. A distinguishing characteristic of some beefsteaks is an odd puckering or scarring at the blossom end known as "cat facing."

Cherry tomatoes Round and bite-sized, these tomatoes are often served in salads and as garnishes. Their skin may be red or yellow. Varieties of "heirloom" cherry tomatoes are sometimes available at specialty food markets.

Currant tomatoes The tiniest of the species, these tomatoes grow in clusters and measure only about ¾ inch in diameter. They are available in both red and yellow varieties and have a sweet, crisp flesh.

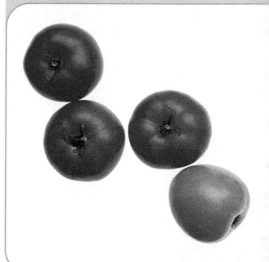

tomatoes

TOMATO / 1 medium	
Calories	48
Protein (g)	2
Carbohydrate (g)	11
Dietary fiber (g)	2.5
Total fat (g)	0.8
Saturated fat (g)	0.1
Monounsaturated fat (g)	0.1
Polyunsaturated fat (g)	0.3
Cholesterol (mg)	0
Potassium (mg)	504
Sodium (mg)	20

KEY NUTRIENTS (%RDA/AI*)	
Thiamin	0.1 mg (10%)
Vitamin B$_6$	0.2 mg (11%)
Vitamin C	59 mg (66%)
Iron	1.0 mg (13%)

*For more detailed information on RDA and AI, see page 88.

Grape tomatoes Now widely available in supermarkets, these sweet, firm-textured, grape-shaped tomatoes are slightly more elongated than cherry tomatoes. Because they don't have as much juice as cherry tomatoes do, "squirting" accidents are minimized.

Heirloom tomatoes About 25 years ago some dedicated individuals began saving what they could of the remaining open-pollinated (without human intervention) seed varieties, and these have become known as "heirloom seeds." An increasing number of growers are now using these seeds to produce an extensive array of heirloom tomatoes. Notable for their intriguing coloration (ranging from white to black, and yellow- or pink-striped to variegated), as well as their often amusing names (Mortgage Lifter, Box Car Willie, White Wonder, to name a few), these tomatoes are also prized for their excellent flavor. Because they are thin-skinned and fragile, they don't ship well and are therefore not available in most supermarkets. Look for them at specialty food stores and farmers' markets during tomato season and use them soon after purchase for the best flavor.

> ➤ **phytochemicals in tomatoes**
>
> A number of phytochemicals in tomatoes are under review for their disease-fighting properties. Most notably, the antioxidant quercetin is linked to a reduced risk of certain types of cancer and is being studied for its potential to protect against clogged arteries and degenerative eye disease.

Pear tomatoes (teardrop) These small, pear-shaped tomatoes (about the size of cherry tomatoes) have an intense, sweet-tomato flavor. There are red and yellow versions available.

Plum tomatoes (Italian, Roma) These egg-shaped tomatoes are meatier and less juicy than slicing tomatoes, and are therefore ideal for making sauces and adding to other cooked foods. They are also the type most commonly used for making sun-dried tomatoes and canned whole tomatoes.

Slicing (round) tomatoes This is an umbrella term for medium-to-large tomatoes, including the globe varieties usually found in supermarkets.

Yellow or **orange tomatoes** These are sometimes advertised as "low-acid" tomatoes. They are, in fact, not lower in acid than other tomatoes, but higher in sugar, which produces a very mild, sweet flavor. Like red tomatoes, these have plenty of vitamin C and potassium, but they don't have lycopene.

▶ **Availability** Over the last hundred years, tomatoes have been bred for hardiness in a variety of climates, and today commercial crops are cultivated in every state. Local growers supply tomatoes to every region of the country in season, mainly summer to fall. Out of season, most U.S.-grown tomatoes are either hothouse varieties or varieties shipped from Florida or California. Of course, many of the tomatoes Americans eat are home grown. (The tomato is the number-one vegetable favored by backyard gardeners.)

choosing the best

As a rule, never buy tomatoes from a refrigerated case; the cold damages them (*see "Those Pale Winter Tomatoes," page 574*). Tomatoes displayed loose are easier to evaluate than those packed in boxes. Look for plump, heavy tomatoes with smooth skins. They should be free of bruises, blemishes, or deep cracks, although fine cracks at the stem ends of ripe tomatoes do not affect flavor. Make sure the leaves of greenhouse tomatoes are fresh and green.

Ripe tomatoes are fragrant, but even mature green ones should have a mild fragrance that promises future ripeness. If they have no aroma at all, the tomatoes were probably picked when immature, and will never ripen. Fully ripe tomatoes are soft and yield to the touch; buy them only if you plan to use them immediately. Overripe tomatoes, provided they are not moldy or rotting, are perfect for making sauce, and even briefly cooking fresh tomatoes releases their lycopene. Choose whatever size tomatoes are appropriate for your intended use; size has no bearing on flavor, texture, or quality.

▶ **When you get home** Room temperature (above 55°) is best for storing tomatoes; don't refrigerate them. Place less-than-ripe tomatoes in a paper bag

lycopene in tomatoes

Recent research has shown that the carotenoid lycopene may be an even more potent antioxidant than beta carotene, and that it may help prevent cancer, notably of the prostate, as well as cardiovascular disease. Here are some lycopene facts:

• Population studies suggest that people who consume lots of lycopene-rich foods have a lower risk of not only prostate cancer but also cancer of the cervix, skin, bladder, breast, lung, and digestive tract.

• Lycopene may reduce the risk of cancer in several ways. For instance, it seems to stimulate the immune system to battle cancer cells. As an antioxidant, it helps block the destructive effects of free radicals in the body, especially when there's enough vitamin E around. It also interferes with "growth factors" that stimulate cancer.

• It may help protect LDL ("bad") cholesterol from oxidation, and thus may lower the risk of coronary artery disease.

• Lycopene is fat-soluble, so you absorb more of it when you eat a little fat in the same meal with your tomato—perhaps a little olive oil or cheese.

• Deep red tomatoes have more lycopene than pale ones or yellow-green ones. Vine-ripened tomatoes have more than those that are picked green and allowed to ripen later. And those grown outdoors in the summer have more than greenhouse tomatoes.

• Ounce for ounce, processed tomato products (sauce, puree, juice, even ketchup) or cooked tomatoes contain two to eight times as much available lycopene as raw tomatoes. Processing makes lycopene more available and more easily absorbed by the body. These products are also more concentrated sources of lycopene because of the water lost in processing.

The chart below shows the best tomato sources of lycopene, according to the USDA. Other key sources include red and pink grapefruit (about 2 milligrams per ½ cup), watermelon (about 6 milligrams per ¾ cup), and guava (about 5 milligrams for 1 fruit).

Food	Lycopene
Tomato juice (1 cup)	20 mg
Vegetable juice cocktail (1 cup)	20 mg
Pasta sauce (½ cup)	19 mg
Tomato puree (½ cup)	18 mg
Tomato sauce (½ cup)	17 mg
Lasagna* (6 ounces)	13 mg
Tomato soup (1 cup)	12 mg
Tomatoes, canned (½ cup)	11 mg
Tomato paste (2 tablespoons)	8 mg
Ketchup (2 tablespoons)	5 mg
Tomato, fresh (medium, 4 ounces)	4 mg
Pizza (3-ounce slice)	4 mg
Minestrone soup (1 cup)	2 mg

*Depends on the amount of tomato sauce, of course, not the type of pasta.

those pale
winter tomatoes

The tomatoes that are available in the winter months often bear little resemblance to their in-season counterparts: They may be pale red or streaky greenish-pink in color, rock hard, and taste much blander. Year-round demand has led growers and breeders to develop thicker-skinned hardy varieties that can withstand the rigors of shipping long distances. Because of this, and because of the way these tomatoes are handled on their way to the market, their taste, texture, and juiciness often suffer in comparison to tomatoes available in peak season. Still, it's possible to get a winter tomato with a decent flavor in the off-season if a few key criteria have been met during growing and shipping.

The picking stage

To increase their durability, tomatoes are picked when they are still green—a stage referred to as "mature green"—or just when they begin to show a spot of pink at the blossom end, a stage known as "breaker." Tomatoes at either stage are fully developed, they just haven't begun the ripening process.

To speed along the ripening process of mature green and breaker-stage tomatoes, growers and shippers often spray them with ethylene gas. Though it sounds like a synthetic creation, ethylene is the same organic compound (actually a ripening hormone) produced naturally by many fruits—oranges, bananas, honeydew melons—as well as by tomatoes. Left on the vine, a tomato will produce its own ethylene, but the external application of ethylene gas is used to initiate and promote the ripening process.

Since not all tomatoes in a crop develop at the same rate, it is inevitable that some will be picked too early, and you may occasionally get a tomato that, although it turns completely red, never develops a palatable flavor or texture. But if handled properly these tomatoes have the potential to develop good flavor and juicy texture. A study by the USDA has found that artificial exposure to ethylene has little if any effect on a tomato's nutritional value. Another study at the University of Georgia, which compared tomatoes left on the vine to ripen to those treated with ethylene, found that the treated tomatoes have the same "sensory attributes and post-harvest quality" and only minor differences in taste and texture.

Are "vine ripened" better?

The term "vine ripe" has no standard definition and can be misleading, as it covers a wide range of ripening stages. It usually refers to tomatoes that have been picked at the breaker stage, but tomatoes picked at any time can carry the label. Generally, tomatoes shipped to nearby markets are picked at a greater degree of ripeness than tomatoes shipped across the country. And since most greenhouse tomatoes are grown close to their market, they are also likely to be left on the vine a bit longer. However, as long as a tomato is handled properly, where it ripens should make little difference in ultimate flavor and texture.

Temperature: the crucial factor

To help ensure that the tomatoes you buy will at least taste adequate, don't buy any that have been refrigerated. Exposure to temperatures under 55° during growth or after harvest prevents a tomato from ripening satisfactorily. Unfortunately, shippers and retailers sometimes keep tomatoes with other vegetables, like lettuce or broccoli, under refrigeration, destroying their ripening potential. It's difficult to identify a tomato damaged by the cold until you get it home and slice it—the skin pulls away easily from the flesh, and the tomato will be mealy and virtually tasteless. Ask the produce manager of the supermarket under what conditions the tomatoes were shipped and stored. Another key to flavor is to buy tomatoes slightly under-ripe, and then let them ripen at room temperature for a few days (put them in a paper bag with an apple or a banana).

with an apple or banana; the ethylene gas given off by the fruit will hasten the ripening process. Keep the tomatoes out of sunlight—they will overheat and ripen unevenly—and arrange them, stem-side up, to prevent bruising. Once the tomatoes are red and yield to the touch, they will keep for a day or two at room temperature.

preparing to use

Wash tomatoes gently in cold water before serving them. To cut tomato slices, stand the tomato upright and cut from top to bottom—the slices will retain their juices better than those cut from side to side. Add sliced tomatoes to salads or sandwiches at the last minute because they begin to release their juices as soon as they are cut; contact with salty condiments or dressings will draw out more juice.

To remove excessive seeds or juice, cut the tomato in half crosswise, then hold each half, cut-side down, and squeeze it gently (you can sieve the juice and drink it, if you like). If you need very well drained tomato halves (for a stuffed tomato recipe, for instance), salt them lightly, then place them, with the cut side down, on several layers of paper towel.

When a recipe calls for peeled tomatoes, drop them into boiling water and blanch for 15 to 30 seconds (the harder the tomato, the longer it requires).

CANNED NO-SALT-ADDED TOMATOES / 1 cup	
Calories	46
Protein (g)	2
Carbohydrate (g)	11
Dietary fiber (g)	2.4
Total fat (g)	0.3
Saturated fat (g)	0.1
Monounsaturated fat (g)	0.1
Polyunsaturated fat (g)	0.1
Cholesterol (mg)	0
Potassium (mg)	545
Sodium (mg)	24

KEY NUTRIENTS (%RDA/AI*)	
Niacin	1.8 mg (11%)
Vitamin B$_6$	0.2 mg (13%)
Vitamin C	34 mg (38%)
Iron	1.3 mg (17%)

*For more detailed information on RDA and AI, see page 88.

serving suggestions

• Bake or broil halved tomatoes.

• Sauté cherry tomatoes with garlic and herbs and use as a topping for pasta or fish.

• Puree tomatoes with roasted peppers and fresh basil for a summer soup.

• Halve plum tomatoes, drizzle with olive oil, and slow-bake for 2 to 3 hours in a 250° oven, until very tender and sweet. Serve warm or at room temperature.

• Puree fresh tomatoes and add vinegar and herbs for a low-fat salad dressing.

• For a flavorful salsa, mix coarsely chopped ripe tomatoes with some minced onion, garlic, and chopped fresh cilantro or parsley. Add lime juice and chopped hot peppers (or a few drops of hot pepper sauce)

to taste. Let the mixture stand for a few minutes and serve at room temperature.

• Toss chunks of cooked sweet potato and fresh tomato with cumin, salt, and lime juice for a side salad.

• Hollow out large fresh tomatoes (save the pulp) and fill the tomatoes with a mixture of cooked couscous, chopped mint, grated carrot, the chopped tomato pulp, and finely diced red onion. Season with salt and pepper or fresh lemon juice.

• Stir chopped tomatoes into green peas and season with chili powder.

• Puree reconstituted sun-dried tomatoes and add to store-bought low-fat mayonnaise. Use as a sandwich spread.

Remove the tomatoes with a slotted spoon and cool briefly under running water. The skin can then be rubbed off easily. You can also spear tomatoes individually on a cooking fork and turn them slowly over a gas flame until the skin splits and can be pulled off. Or, you can loosen the peel in a microwave by heating the tomato for 15 seconds on high power.

tomato products

Tomatoes are sold in myriad forms other than fresh. It used to be that fresh was always better than canned. Well, not when it comes to tomatoes. Compared with fresh tomatoes, canned and processed tomato products are more concentrated and so can have up to five times the lycopene. What's more, processed tomatoes are cooked, which makes it easier for the body to absorb the lycopene. Today tomato products are sold in vacuum-packed boxes as well as cans and jars.

In general, canned tomatoes may be designated "solid pack," which means no liquid has been added, or they may be packed in tomato juice, puree, or paste; the label will indicate the packing medium. Salt or other flavorings, such as bay leaf or basil, may also be included.

Since canned tomatoes with added salt may have twelve times the sodium of unsalted, be sure to check the ingredients list on the label to see if salt has been added (many salt-free brands don't necessarily have the words "no salt added" prominently displayed). The following are the tomato products most commonly found in the market:

Whole tomatoes Often the plum or Roma variety, these are mature whole tomatoes that have been cooked, peeled, and cored.

Diced tomatoes These tomatoes are excellent for stews and chunky pasta sauces.

Crushed tomatoes Use these tomatoes to make a quick soup or tomato sauce.

Stewed tomatoes Tomatoes are labeled stewed when other vegetables (onion, green pepper, celery, for example) and/or seasonings (such as oregano, thyme, sage) are mixed in.

Tomato puree A concentrated form of tomato juice and tomato pulp, puree has the consistency of a thick tomato sauce, and may contain salt.

Tomato sauce This product is the same as tomato puree, except that the sauce has been seasoned. Be sure to read the labels; some brands have whopping amounts of sodium added. There are also a huge variety of tomato-based **pasta sauces** on the market, and the added fat and sodium levels in some brands can be sky-high. One popular brand of marinara sauce gets 40 percent of its calories from fat and contains nearly 800 milligrams of sodium per ½-cup serving. Brands with added cheese or meat can be even higher in fat and sodium.

Tomato paste This very concentrated form of tomatoes is sold in cans or in tubes. By law, tomato paste must be concentrated to more than 24 percent solids (compared with 8 to 24 percent for tomato puree).

Sun-dried tomatoes These are plum tomatoes that have been dehydrated to preserve them and intensify their flavor. They are sold packed in oil or dry. The tomatoes that are not packed in oil are usually reconstituted by soaking in hot water before being used in cooking.

triticale

Unlike many other grains, nutty-sweet triticale (pronounced tri-ti-KAY-lee) does not have a history that covers several millennia. It was developed in 1875, when a Scottish botanist crossed wheat with rye in hopes of creating a food grain with the good baking qualities and high yield of wheat and the robust growing habit and protein content of rye. The few seeds he was able to germinate from the hybrid were sterile, but in 1937, a French researcher succeeded in producing a fertile cross of wheat and rye.

Subsequent research beginning in the 1950s led to great improvements in the new grain, called triticale after the Latin genus names for wheat (*Triticum*) and rye (*Secale*). Triticale is not grown in great quantities in the United States, and therefore is more likely to be found in health-food stores or through mail-order sources.

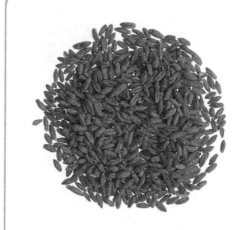

triticale

nutritional profile

Triticale is a specialized high-fiber, high-protein grain that is also a good source of thiamin and minerals.

in the market

Triticale comes in the same forms as wheat or rye. All of the forms can be found in health-food stores.

Cracked This has a shorter cooking time than the whole berries. You can make your own cracked triticale by processing the whole berries in a blender until they are coarsely chopped.

Flakes (rolled triticale) Like rolled oats, these are triticale berries that have been steamed and flattened.

Flour See Flour, Nonwheat (*page 327*).

Triticale berries Like wheat berries, whole triticale berries have not been stripped of their nutritious bran and germ. They are twice the size of wheat berries and need to be soaked overnight in the refrigerator before cooking.

choosing the best

As with any grain product, buy triticale in well-wrapped packages. If purchasing in bulk, buy from a store with good turnover. Buy what you'll need for a couple of months and store it in the freezer.

▶ When you get home To prevent bug infestation, store triticale in a tightly sealed container. In the summer months, if you have room, store the container in the refrigerator or freezer.

TRITICALE / ¼ cup raw	
Calories	161
Protein (g)	6
Carbohydrate (g)	35
Dietary fiber (g)	8.7
Total fat (g)	1.0
Saturated fat (g)	0.2
Monounsaturated fat (g)	0.1
Polyunsaturated fat (g)	0.4
Cholesterol (mg)	0
Potassium (mg)	172
Sodium (mg)	2

KEY NUTRIENTS (%RDA/AI*)	
Thiamin	0.2 mg (17%)
Iron	1.2 mg (15%)
Magnesium	62 mg (15%)
Zinc	1.7 mg (15%)

For more detailed information on RDA and AI, see page 88.

tuna

Americans eat more tuna than any other fish (or shellfish), though about 95 percent of it is consumed in canned form. A member of the mackerel family, tuna is a large saltwater fish, which may weigh up to 1,500 pounds, depending on the species.

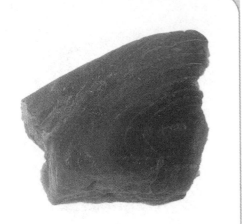

tuna steak

nutritional profile

All species are good sources of high-quality protein with very little saturated fat. Rich in beneficial long-chain omega-3 fatty acids, tuna is also an excellent reservoir of B vitamins such as thiamin, niacin, and vitamin B6. It is also an exceptional source of the antioxidant mineral selenium. Canned tuna is also a rich source of nutrients, though it's best to buy water-packed tuna, which has less fat and sodium than tuna in oil.

in the market

There are only a half dozen or so species of tuna that are of commercial importance. Albacore and blackfin tuna are used to make "white meat" canned tuna; yellowfin and skipjack are the "light meat" tunas.

Albacore This is the most commercially important tuna—in its canned form. Because most albacore ends up in a can, it is rare to find it fresh in the market.

Bluefin This is the largest of the tunas. Young bluefins have lighter flesh and are not too strongly flavored; older bluefins have dark red flesh and a more pronounced flavor.

Skipjack This is a lighter-fleshed, milder-flavored tuna similar to yellowfin. It's often used for sushi or sashimi.

Yellowfin This tuna is one of the more common tuna types available as fresh steaks in fish markets. Its flesh is darker than albacore, but still light enough to qualify for the "light meat" designation in cans.

choosing the best

Fresh tuna is most commonly sold in steaks (which are usually about one-fourth of a whole cross-section slice of the fish). As a general rule of thumb for fresh tuna, the darker the flesh, the stronger the flavor. Indeed, tuna's deep red almost "beefy" color is darker than that of other types of fish. Like good beef, fresh tuna should be reddish, not brown, when you buy it.

▶ **When you get home** It's best to use fresh tuna within a day of buying it, although it can be kept an extra day or two if it is of very high quality and was very fresh when purchased. Place it, still in the wrapper from the market, in a glass or enameled pan in the coldest part of the refrigerator. Fill a plastic bag with crushed ice and place it on top of the fish. Check the fish daily and pour off any liquid that may have accumulated in the bottom of the pan.

YELLOWFIN TUNA 3 ounces cooked	
Calories	118
Protein (g)	26
Carbohydrate (g)	0
Dietary fiber (g)	0
Total fat (g)	1.0
Saturated fat (g)	0.3
Monounsaturated fat (g)	0.2
Polyunsaturated fat (g)	0.3
Cholesterol (mg)	49
Potassium (mg)	484
Sodium (mg)	40

KEY NUTRIENTS (%RDA/AI*)	
Thiamin	0.4 mg (36%)
Niacin	10 mg (63%)
Vitamin B6	0.9 mg (52%)
Vitamin B12	0.5 mcg (21%)
Iron	0.8 mg (10%)
Magnesium	54 mg (13%)
Selenium	40 mcg (72%)

*For more detailed information on RDA and AI, see page 88.

turkey

Turkeys roamed the Americas thousands of years ago, and the Pilgrims, landing in Massachusetts in 1620, found them a valuable game bird. Four wild turkeys were served as part of the first Thanksgiving feast in 1621, starting a tradition that has endured to this day. Benjamin Franklin regarded the turkey so highly that he proposed naming it the official bird of the United States instead of the bald eagle, declaring that ". . . the Turkey is a much more respectable Bird, and withal a true native of America."

In the past, turkey was regarded as a once-a-year treat at Thanksgiving or Christmas—90 percent of all turkeys were sold during November and December—and many cooks felt that whole birds entailed too much work to serve at other times of the year. But today more people are making turkey a part of their regular diet. Turkey breast is the leanest of all meats, supplying just 115 calories and less than a gram of fat per 3-ounce serving (skinned). In addition, turkeys are now produced in greater numbers and are available in many forms, in contrast to a decade ago when turkeys were mostly available whole. Consumers can select the parts they prefer, such as whole or half breasts, cutlets, drumsticks, thighs, wings, and tenderloins; these cook much faster than a whole bird. Convenience and nutritional awareness have contributed to a 230 percent increase in turkey consumption since 1970.

nutritional profile

As with chicken, almost all of the fat in turkey is found in the skin. However, turkey meat is so low in fat that eating 3 ounces of roasted breast meat with skin would furnish only 130 calories, 19 percent of them coming from fat. The dark meat is higher in fat than the light meat, but it is still relatively lean if eaten without the skin.

Turkey is high in the nutrients for which meat is known. It is not only an excellent source of protein, but also of riboflavin, niacin, vitamin B_6, vitamin B_{12}, selenium, iron, and zinc.

in the market

The wild turkeys of yesteryear have largely been replaced—at least for food—by domestic turkeys, which are farm-raised birds bred for their broad breasts and juicy, flavorful flesh. Domestic turkeys weigh 6 to 24 pounds and have large breasts in relation to their legs and wings—they are so out of proportion, in fact, that domestic turkeys cannot fly more than a few feet at a time.

Most of the turkeys found on the market are young and will have tender meat. The most common types of turkey are:

Fryer/roasters The youngest and most tender turkeys available, fryer/roasters are under 16 weeks old at slaughter. Their small size—5 to 9

TURKEY BREAST 3 ounces cooked, skinless	
Calories	115
Protein (g)	26
Carbohydrate (g)	0
Dietary fiber (g)	0
Total fat (g)	0.6
Saturated fat (g)	0.2
Monounsaturated fat (g)	0.1
Polyunsaturated fat (g)	0.2
Cholesterol (mg)	71
Potassium (mg)	248
Sodium (mg)	44

KEY NUTRIENTS (%RDA/AI*)	
Niacin	6.4 mg (40%)
Vitamin B_6	0.5 mg (28%)
Vitamin B_{12}	0.3 mcg (14%)
Iron	1.3 mg (16%)
Selenium	26 mcg (47%)
Zinc	1.5 mg (13%)

*For more detailed information on RDA and AI, see page 88.

TURKEY DARK MEAT 3 ounces cooked, skinless	
Calories	138
Protein (g)	25
Carbohydrate (g)	0
Dietary fiber (g)	0
Total fat (g)	3.7
Saturated fat (g)	1.2
Monounsaturated fat (g)	0.8
Polyunsaturated fat (g)	1.1
Cholesterol (mg)	95
Potassium (mg)	209
Sodium (mg)	67

KEY NUTRIENTS (%RDA/AI*)	
Riboflavin	0.2 mg (16%)
Niacin	3.0 mg (18%)
Vitamin B_6	0.3 mg (19%)
Vitamin B_{12}	0.3 mcg (14%)
Iron	2.1 mg (26%)
Selenium	32 mcg (58%)
Zinc	3.5 mg (32%)

*For more detailed information on RDA and AI, see page 88.

pounds—makes them good choices for small families. They can be roasted, broiled, or grilled.

Hens These female turkeys, 5 to 7 months old, weigh between 8 to 18 pounds. Some cooks believe that hens have a larger proportion of white to dark meat. Hens can be roasted, broiled, or grilled.

Toms There are those cooks who believe that the only relevant difference between a tom and a hen is size—tom turkeys weigh up to 24 pounds. Others insist that toms have tastier meat. Like hens, toms can be roasted, broiled, or grilled.

Mature hens or toms These are older turkeys and are not often found on the market. They are best stewed or poached.

Turkey parts All-white-meat *breasts* come in whole or half form, with the bone in or boneless. *Breast steaks* are crosswise cuts ½ to 1 inch thick; breast steaks that are ¼ to ⅜ inch thick are called *cutlets. Tenderloins* are the whole muscles on the inside of the turkey breast. Tenderloins are also sliced lengthwise into ½-inch-thick steaks, called *tenderloin steaks. Thighs* and *drumsticks* are all-dark-meat sections sold separately or together as hindquarters. *Wings* are white-meat sections sold with the bone in.

Ground turkey Provided that it's made from mostly breast meat, ground turkey can be a leaner substitute for ground beef. Packaged ground turkey often contains skin and dark meat, however, and may derive 54 percent of its calories from fat. But some processors do sell turkey ground from breast meat only (check the ingredient label). You can be sure of very lean ground meat if you buy fresh turkey parts—breast cutlets or tenderloins, for example—and have the butcher grind them for you, or grind them yourself.

COMPARING TURKEY **3 ounces cooked**

As a general rule of thumb, 4 ounces of raw boneless turkey will yield 3 ounces of cooked. For 3 ounces of cooked turkey from a bone-in piece, start with about 8 ounces of raw. Before cooking, you should trim any visible fat. The turkey cuts are listed by percentage of calories from fat. Ground turkey is often labeled by the percentage of lean meat (by weight), rather than the fat percentage, though it can vary.

	Calories	Fat (g)	% Calories from Fat	Saturated Fat (g)	Cholesterol (mg)
Ground (87% lean)	200	11	50	2.9	87
Ground (93% lean)	170	8	42	2.5	80
Dark meat, with skin	155	6.0	35	1.8	100
Dark meat, skinless	138	3.7	24	1.2	95
Breast, with skin	130	2.7	19	0.7	77
Breast, skinless	115	0.6	5	0.2	71

choosing the best

Like chicken, turkey is graded by the USDA if the processors request and pay for it. The graded turkey sold in supermarkets is Grade A, which means that it is well shaped, free of feathers, and has a layer of fat. Check that the skin is unbroken, free of cuts, tears, bruises, or blemishes. When buying turkey parts, choose those which are moist and pink. The skin, if any, should be creamy-white, not bluish.

The "sell by" date on fresh turkey is 7 days after the bird has been processed. The turkey is fresh until then, and for a day or two afterward. Don't buy fresh turkey—whole or parts—unless you plan to cook it within that time period.

Frozen turkeys should be rock hard and stored well below the freezer line in the freezer case. Make sure the package is tightly sealed and the turkey is free of freezer burn and ice crystals. Avoid packages that have a lot of frozen liquid in them; the fluid indicates that the turkey was defrosted and refrozen. If frozen turkey is properly handled at the store and at home, there should be no difference in quality between fresh and frozen birds.

When buying a whole bird, make sure to select one that will fit into your oven. The number of people you plan to feed will determine the size of bird you buy. Allow ¾ pound per person (1 pound per person if you want leftovers). If the bird is over 12 pounds, you should allow ½ pound per person, since larger birds have a greater proportion of meat to bone.

► **When you get home** As soon as you get whole fresh turkey home from the store, place it in the coldest part of the refrigerator. If the bird comes with giblets, remove them and store in a separate container; they should be used or frozen within 24 hours. Rewrap the turkey in butcher paper or heavy-duty aluminum foil. Above all, see that the package does not leak juices onto other foods; overwrap the turkey or place it on a platter in the refrigerator.

If you've bought a whole turkey and find you cannot use it within one or two days of purchase, freeze it. However, home freezers are not cold enough (or perhaps large enough) to quick-freeze a whole bird so as to eliminate the risk of salmonella. It is therefore essential that the turkey be cut into parts first. Rinse the turkey parts in cold water and dry them with paper towels, then wrap them in heavy-duty aluminum foil or freezer paper, and seal the package tightly.

preparing to use

Keep turkey refrigerated until you plan to use it. Rinse it under cold running water and pluck out any stray pinfeathers with your fingers or a pair of tweezers. (If you're preparing a whole bird that has previously been frozen,

serving suggestions

• Use lean ground turkey to replace some of the beef in hamburgers, chili, meatballs, meat-based pasta sauces, and meatloaf.

• When making turkey burgers, be sure to include ingredients that will help the burger retain juices (turkey breast meat can get quite dry). For each 4-ounce burger mix in about ⅓ cup of such ingredients as: minced mushrooms, fresh bread crumbs, grated apple, grated carrot, softened bulgur, or crushed cracker crumbs.

• Use turkey cutlets in place of veal scallops in recipes.

• Use turkey legs (which are generally cheaper than other parts) to make homemade turkey stock (*follow directions for the stock in "Chicken Soup," page 241*).

remove the giblets and the neck before rinsing.) Be sure to wash the counter top, sink, utensils, and your hands with hot, soapy water after handling raw turkey.

Never thaw a frozen turkey at room temperature. The turkey will thaw from the outside in, leaving the surface prone to bacterial growth before the inside has fully thawed. The safest way to thaw a frozen turkey is in the refrigerator. The length of time it takes will depend on the size of the bird. Place the turkey in a shallow baking pan or on a tray to catch the moisture as the bird defrosts.

Defrosting a turkey in cold water takes a shorter time, but requires some vigilance. Check the wrapping to make sure there are no tears, then place the wrapped bird in the sink or a large container and cover the turkey with cold water. (If the package is torn, place the turkey in a tightly sealed plastic bag.) Change the water every 30 minutes to keep it cold. This method significantly reduces thawing time.

You can thaw turkey parts in your microwave. Plan to cook the turkey immediately after thawing.

Whether you're preparing a whole bird or turkey parts, leave the skin on during cooking. The skin will help keep the meat moist and juicy, and won't increase the fat content of the turkey as long as it is removed before eating.

stuffing story

Starchy stuffings—such as those made with bread or rice—are especially prone to bacterial contamination; the bacteria in the raw poultry can get into the stuffing and multiply. Consider cooking the stuffing separately from the turkey; it will save you time and work. An unstuffed turkey cooks faster than a stuffed one. Before roasting, simply flavor the cavity with some chopped onion, celery, apple, and herbs. Add a clove or two of garlic if you like.

If you do decide to stuff the bird, do so just before you're ready to cook it. Stuff the bird loosely (tightly packed stuffing cooks more slowly, and stuffing expands as it cooks). Fold the neck skin over the back of the turkey and secure with skewers or toothpicks. Tie the legs together with clean string, or use metal (or plastic) "hocklocks," if they're provided. Once the turkey is cooked, check the internal temperature of the stuffing with a meat thermometer; it is done at 165°. Never let a stuffed turkey sit at room temperature for any length of time. Remove the cooked stuffing from the turkey immediately and serve it separately; keep the remaining stuffing in a warm oven (200°) or refrigerate it in a tightly closed container.

turnips & rutabagas

Like cabbage, to which it is related, the turnip has long been thought of as "plain folks" food. It is economical; it grows well in poor soil; it keeps well; and it supplies complex carbohydrates. One of the cruciferous vegetables in the *Brassica* genus, the turnip can be cultivated for its root—which is a good source of complex carbohydrates—as well as for its greens, which are rich in vitamins and minerals. Rutabagas look similar to turnips (and have a similar sweet-earthy taste), but are a separate botanical species that probably evolved from a cross between a turnip and a wild cabbage.

Of the two, turnips (*Brassica rapa*) have a much older history. They were eaten by the Romans as well as by the people of Europe during the Middle Ages; eventually, they were brought to America by both French and English colonists. They are especially appreciated in the South. Rutabagas (*Brassica napus*) are comparatively new—the first record of them is from the 17th century, when they were used as both food and animal fodder in southern Europe. In England, they were referred to as "turnip-rooted cabbages," and their popularity in Scandinavia eventually earned them the name of Swedish turnips, or "swedes" (rutabaga comes from the Swedish word *rotabagge*, meaning "round root"). Americans were growing rutabagas as early as 1806. Warm temperatures (above 75°) can damage rutabagas and, as a result, they are planted chiefly in northern states and in Canada, while turnips are found in every state.

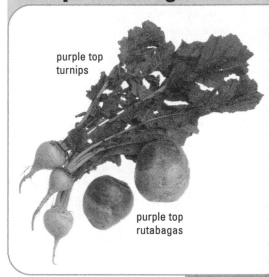

turnips & rutabagas

purple top turnips

purple top rutabagas

nutritional profile

Turnips and rutabagas are rich in complex carbohydrates, with good amounts of both insoluble and cholesterol-lowering soluble fiber. The sweet, crisp flesh of these vegetables also contains modest amounts of protein and a surprisingly high concentration of vitamin C: One cup of fresh rutabaga cubes provides over 35 percent of the daily requirement of this vitamin and 1 cup of turnip cubes meets about 20 percent of our daily needs. In addition, rutabagas supply some B vitamins, iron, and a sizable amount of potassium.

Yellow-fleshed rutabagas also contain some beta carotene, while white-fleshed turnips have none.

in the market

Turnips come in an astonishing range of shapes and sizes, depending on the age and variety. More or less smoothly spherical or top-shaped, the most

TURNIPS	
1 cup cubes, cooked	
Calories	33
Protein (g)	1
Carbohydrate (g)	8
Dietary fiber (g)	3.1
Total fat (g)	0.1
Saturated fat (g)	0
Monounsaturated fat (g)	0
Polyunsaturated fat (g)	0.1
Cholesterol (mg)	0
Potassium (mg)	211
Sodium (mg)	78

KEY NUTRIENTS (%RDA/AI*)

Vitamin C	18 mg (20%)

For more detailed information on RDA and AI, see page 88.

common varieties have a creamy-white skin that shades to purple or reddish-pink or green at the top. (The top of the root develops above the ground, and exposure to sunlight causes it to become pigmented while the lower part, buried in earth, does not.)

Rutabagas are considerably larger than most turnips. Their skin is tan, with a dark purple band at the crown, and they have an irregular shape. They have firm yellow flesh, and a strong, sweet flavor.

You may be able to find turnips or rutabagas by one of the varietal names listed here in a farmers' market, but supermarkets are unlikely to label these root vegetables anything other than "turnips" and "rutabagas."

turnips

Amber globe Unlike typical top-shaped turnips, this type is round and has yellow skin. It has sweet, pale yellow flesh.

Baby bunch turnips These small marble-sized turnips are white with firm white flesh. Their flavor is like a combination of apple and radish.

Golden ball (orange jelly) This variety has sweet, bright-orange flesh and is occasionally available in farmers' markets.

Purple top This is the most common turnip available and the one that most people are used to seeing in the supermarket. They have white skin and a bright purple crown and mild white flesh.

White globe These round turnips are completely white, without the typical purple top of other turnips. The flesh is sweet and mild.

rutabagas

American purple top This is the most common rutabaga. It is (as its name suggests) purple at the crown and yellow below.

Ruta-Bits This small variety of rutabaga comes to the market unwaxed. They are thin-skinned and don't need to be peeled.

choosing the best

Newly harvested turnips are sometimes sold in bunches with their leaves, which should be crisp and green. If in good condition, the leaves can be cooked and eaten (*see Greens, Cooking, page 355*). Topped turnips (with the greens cut off) are frequently sold in plastic bags. Leaf scars at the stem end of topped turnips should be few. The turnips themselves should always be firm and heavy for their size, with a minimum of fibrous root hairs at the bottom. Their surface should be smooth, not shriveled or bruised. Smaller turnips are sweeter and more tender than large ones, which may be bitter and pithy. Bunched turnips are usually about 2 inches in diameter; topped turnips about 3 inches.

Rutabagas are almost always trimmed of their taproots and tops, and are often coated with a thick layer of clear wax to prevent moisture loss. The skin that's visible through the wax should be free of major scars and bruises. Watch

RUTABAGA	
1 cup cubes, cooked	
Calories	66
Protein (g)	2
Carbohydrate (g)	15
Dietary fiber (g)	3.1
Total fat (g)	0.4
Saturated fat (g)	0.1
Monounsaturated fat (g)	0.1
Polyunsaturated fat (g)	0.2
Cholesterol (mg)	0
Potassium (mg)	554
Sodium (mg)	34

KEY NUTRIENTS (%RDA/AI*)	
Thiamin	0.1 mg (12%)
Vitamin B$_6$	0.2 mg (10%)
Vitamin C	32 mg (36%)
Iron	0.9 mg (11%)

*For more detailed information on RDA and AI, see page 88.

out for mold on the surface of the wax. Rutabagas should feel firm and solid, never spongy. For the sweetest flavor, choose smallish rutabagas, about 4 inches in diameter.

▶ **When you get home** Both turnips and rutabagas keep well. Cut off turnip greens and bag them separately for storage (they keep for just a few days).

preparing to use

Both turnips and rutabagas can be eaten raw, but large ones may be strongly flavored. Avoid cooking turnips in aluminum or iron pots, as their flesh may darken. However, this discoloration isn't a problem with rutabagas, which have more stable pigments.

Turnips are usually peeled before cooking (or using raw), although very young, fresh turnips need not be. A vegetable peeler will remove the thinnest possible layer of skin. First, trim a slice from the top and bottom of each turnip and halve the vegetable around the "equator." Then peel and slice, dice, or cut into julienne strips, as required.

The wax applied to rutabagas must be peeled (along with the skin) before cooking. It's easier to peel rutabagas if you quarter them first. Use a sharp paring knife for peeling; it will be easier than a vegetable peeler.

facts & tips

Like other cruciferous vegetables, turnips and rutabagas can become more strongly flavored when cooked. However, the odors from both vegetables are quite mild compared to, say, Brussels sprouts and cabbage. You will find that when turnips and rutabagas are well prepared, their sweet, somewhat peppery flesh makes them an excellent side dish as well as a tasty addition to salads, soups, and stews.

serving suggestions

· Add sliced rutabagas to potatoes as they cook for mashed potatoes.

· Add grated turnip or rutabaga to potato pancakes.

· Add chunks of rutabaga or turnips to soups and stews.

· Shred baby turnips and serve raw in a lemony dressing.

· Serve thin slices of rutabaga as part of a crudité platter.

· Make a slaw with shredded raw turnips and apples.

· Sauté shredded turnips, carrots, and parsnips with olive oil and carrot juice for a side dish.

· Serve baby turnips sautéed with their greens still attached.

· Quarter well-scrubbed turnips and roast them with garlic and olive oil.

walnuts

Walnut trees grow in temperate zones throughout the world. Because they are used in so many dishes and are so popular, walnuts represent an important commercial crop. In the 18th century, while establishing Spanish missions there, Franciscan monks planted the Persian (English) walnut in California, where a mild climate and deep fertile soil provided ideal growing conditions. California now provides 99 percent of this country's supply of English walnuts, and two-thirds of the world's supply.

nutritional profile

In the past, nuts were considered nutritional villains. However, research reveals them to be a healthy food choice. What distinguishes walnuts from other nuts is that they (and their oil) contain alpha-linolenic acid (a heart-healthy omega-3 fatty acid), which research suggests may help prevent heart attacks. Not many foods are rich in alpha-linolenic acid (ALA): In addition to walnuts, only canola oil, flaxseed oil, and soybean oil are high in ALA. The monounsaturated fats and polyunsaturated fats in walnuts can also lower blood cholesterol, especially when substituted for saturated fat in the diet. In addition, walnuts contain cardioprotective plant sterols, which are naturally occurring plant compounds that block the absorption of cholesterol into the bloodstream.

in the market

Walnuts are available shelled (in halves and pieces) and unshelled. Walnuts are also pressed for their oil (*see Nut Oils, page 300*).

Black walnuts These walnuts have very tough, dark outer hulls and inner shells that are thicker than those of English walnuts. The shells have to be cracked under so much pressure that the nutmeats are usually crushed as a result. Black walnuts have a rather distinctive, "cheese-y" flavor that's not to everyone's taste, but aficionados of these walnuts will nevertheless go to great lengths to get their hands on them.

Butternuts Also called "white walnuts," the nutmeats looks like the letter U, or a life-preserver vest.

English walnuts Also called Persian walnuts, these are the walnuts that most people are familiar with. They are native to Asia and Europe; California is now the major world producer.

Heartnuts This Japanese walnut variety has a shell that looks like a flattened heart. It easily splits in two, releasing the whole nutmeat. Heartnuts are available on an extremely limited, and mostly local, commercial scale.

▶ Availability Because black walnuts, butternuts, and heartnuts are marketed on a very small scale, you may find them only in farmers' markets and some specialty food stores during the fall and early winter.

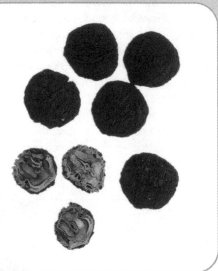

black walnuts

ENGLISH WALNUTS 1 ounce	
Calories	182
Protein (g)	4
Carbohydrate (g)	5
Dietary fiber (g)	1.4
Total fat (g)	18
Saturated fat (g)	1.6
Monounsaturated fat (g)	4.0
Polyunsaturated fat (g)	11
Cholesterol (mg)	0
Potassium (mg)	142
Sodium (mg)	3

KEY NUTRIENTS (%RDA/AI*)

Magnesium	48 mg (11%)

*For more detailed information on RDA and AI, see page 88.

choosing the best

When buying walnuts in the shell, look for undamaged shells with no tiny wormholes. Shake the nuts. Those that rattle or feel extra light may be withered or dried out inside.

When buying shelled walnuts, look for a freshness date on the jar, can, or bag. If visible, the nuts should be plump and uniform in size.

Buy nuts in bulk only if you are sure the store has a rapid turnover of their stock to ensure freshness. Check to see that the nuts are crisp. Don't buy them if they are limp or rubbery, or smell musty or rancid; their high oil content makes them susceptible to spoilage.

▶ **When you get home** Walnuts are more perishable than other nuts because of their high polyunsaturated fat content, but keep well if properly stored. Heat, humidity, and light will speed spoilage.

In their shells, walnuts will keep for 6 months to a year if stored in a cool, dry place. For longer storage, keep them in the refrigerator or freezer.

Keep shelled walnuts in their original package until you are ready to use them. Store in a cupboard or other cool, dry place. They will stay fresh until the date marked on the package. If there is no date, count on them lasting for 3 to 4 months.

Once the package is opened, wrap the nuts well and store them in the refrigerator or freezer. The nuts will stay fresh for 6 months in the refrigerator and for a year in the freezer.

If shelled walnuts seem a little soft (but do not smell rancid), freshen them by spreading them on a baking sheet and heating them in a very low oven (150°) for a few minutes.

preparing to use

English walnut shells split readily with the squeeze of a nutcracker, allowing the removal of whole nutmeats. Nut picks can be helpful, however, in teasing them out. Black walnuts, on the other hand, have very tough, dark outer hulls, and the shells are rock hard. They usually have to be broken with a very hard hammer blow or in a vise. (Some people even resort to running over black walnuts with their car.) Because so much force must be used to break the shell, halves are virtually impossible to rescue and the meats have to be picked out in pieces with a nut pick.

Chop walnuts by hand with a sturdy chef's knife. Chopping walnuts in a blender or food processor is hard to do without turning them into butter, so process a small amount at a time and pulse the machine on and off only once or twice. If you're finely grinding them for a cake, process them with a small amount of the flour and proceed with the recipe.

Peeling Occasionally a recipe will direct you to remove the bitter walnut skin. To do this, drop shelled walnuts into boiling water and blanch for 1 minute. Drain, rinse under cold water, and rub the skin off. Place the nuts on a cookie sheet and bake at 350° for 10 minutes or until crisp.

watercress

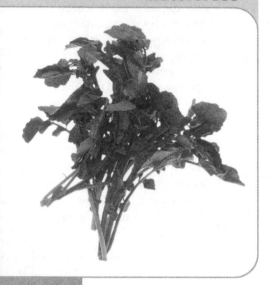

watercress

A member of the *Cruciferae* (mustard) family, which includes broccoli, kale, and mustard greens, watercress has small, crisp, dark green leaves and a pungent, slightly bitter, peppery flavor. It grows wild in streambeds and in the wet soil along pond margins. For the commercial market, however, watercress seedlings are started in dry soil, then placed in special pools of flowing clean, cool water.

Like many members of the mustard family, the nourishing leafy sprigs of watercress have long been touted for their medicinal properties, and over the centuries the plant has been employed as a diuretic, expectorant, purgative, stimulant, and antiscorbutic (to prevent scurvy), among many other uses. Hippocrates, the renowned Greek father of medicine, purportedly selected the location for his first hospital because of its proximity to a stream where watercress grew. It wasn't until the mid-1800s, however, that watercress was introduced to the United States by European immigrants, and today Florida is the major commercial supplier to the U.S. market.

Watercress is considered by many in the culinary world to be a highly underrated and underused vegetable. Not only can it add zest to salads, sandwiches, soups, and sauces, but like other cruciferous vegetables, it has great nutritional value as well.

nutritional profile

Watercress provides generous amounts of the carotenoid beta carotene, which has potent antioxidant properties that may help to defend against heart disease and certain forms of cancer. Our bodies convert substantial amounts of beta carotene to vitamin A in a safe, carefully regulated process that prevents toxic levels of vitamin A from accumulating.

Watercress also offers fiber, potassium, and, most notably, vitamin C. Just 2 cups of raw, chopped watercress supplies an impressive one-third of the daily requirement for this indispensable vitamin.

in the market

While watercress *(Nasturtium officinale)* can easily be found in most markets, there are two other less well-known watercress relatives that are also occasionally available, usually in specialty food stores or farmers' markets.

Garden cress (curly cress, pepper cress) Like watercress, garden cress *(Lepidium sativum)* has a pungent, peppery flavor and can be used instead of watercress in recipes. Some types have curly leaves. A similar species, *wild peppergrass (L. virginicum)* is not cultivated, but can be picked for salads.

WATERCRESS / 2 cups	
Calories	8
Protein (g)	2
Carbohydrate (g)	1
Dietary fiber (g)	1.0
Total fat (g)	0.1
Saturated fat (g)	0
Monounsaturated fat (g)	0
Polyunsaturated fat (g)	0
Cholesterol (mg)	0
Potassium (mg)	224
Sodium (mg)	28

KEY NUTRIENTS (%RDA/AI*)	
Beta carotene	1.9 mg (17%)
Vitamin C	29 mg (32%)

*For more detailed information on RDA and AI, see page 88.

Upland cress (winter cress, broadleaf cress, creasy greens) Resembling watercress in both form and flavor, upland cress *(Barbarea verna)* produces very small, almost square, green leaves that have a slight notching on the leaf margins. The stems can grow 6 to 8 inches long.

choosing the best

Choose watercress with bright green, unwilted leaves and crisp, moist stems. There should be no sign of yellowing or wilting.

▶ **When you get home** You can place a bunch of watercress, stems down, in a container of water like a bouquet of flowers. Cover it loosely with a plastic bag and refrigerate; it will keep for 2 or 3 days. Don't put watercress in the vegetable crisper, where it's likely to get bruised and crushed.

preparing to use

Wash watercress just before using: Trim the bottom inch or so off the stems, then cut the band or string that holds the bunch and drop the watercress into a basin of water. Swish the watercress in the water, then lift it out, leaving any dirt behind in the basin. Repeat the process, if necessary.

➤phytochemicals in watercress

Watercress and its cruciferous cousins are known to be excellent sources of a family of cancer-fighting phytochemicals called isothiocyanates. Promising experimental research suggests a certain type of isothiocyanate in watercress, called phenyl ethyl isothiocyanate (PEITC), may detoxify carcinogens linked to lung cancer.

facts & tips

The poisonous marshwort or "fool's cress" *(Apium nodiflorum)* is often mistaken for watercress, alongside which it is sometimes found growing. Fool's cress may readily be distinguished by its hemlock-like white flowers, and when out of flower, by its finely toothed and somewhat pointed leaves, which are much longer than those of watercress and of a paler green color.

serving suggestions

· Sprinkle chopped watercress over scrambled eggs.

· Make a salad dressing by blending watercress with lemon juice, salt, pepper, and some olive oil.

· Stir cooked, pureed watercress into mashed potatoes. Thin down the mixture with some broth or milk to make a soup.

· Toss watercress with chunks of kiwifruit, orange, and grapefruit, and serve alongside roasted meat or poultry.

· Stir chopped watercress into a potato salad.

· Blend chopped watercress with reduced-fat cream cheese (Neufchâtel) or yogurt cheese for a sandwich spread.

· Quickly steam or stir-fry watercress as you would spinach and eat it as a side dish.

watermelon

The watermelon is so thoroughly associated with America and backyard barbecues, that most people would probably be surprised to discover how global this fruit is, not to mention the fact that China is the top watermelon producer in the world. Watermelon is a member of the gourd family and is thought to have originated in Africa. Depicted in Egyptian hieroglyphics (hard to imagine), watermelons also were sometimes placed in the burial tombs of kings to nourish them in the afterlife.

Because the flesh of this fruit is over 90 percent water, the watermelon was a valuable and portable source of nourishment and water for explorers, desert nomads, and dwellers living in arid regions where natural water was scarce or contaminated. Over the years, watermelons spread from the Mediterranean to China, and eventually through much of the world via trade routes, finally landing in America with the slave trade.

nutritional profile

This all-American favorite offers ample amounts of lycopene, a nourishing carotenoid that has been receiving lots of attention for its potential to protect against certain cancers, including prostate cancer. According to the USDA, 4 ounces of watermelon (about ¾ cup diced) supplies an impressive 6 milligrams of lycopene.

in the market

There are more than 50 varieties of watermelon. Generally, they are divided into *"picnic"* and *"ice-box"* varieties. Picnic types usually weigh 12 to 50 pounds and are round, oblong, or oval. Ice-box varieties—designed to fit into a refrigerator—weigh 5 to 10 pounds and are round or oval. Most watermelons have the familiar red flesh, but there are white-fleshed, yellow-fleshed, and orange-fleshed varieties, too. There is no appreciable taste difference among them. There are also seedless varieties (which have been in existence for over 60 years). Note, though, that seedless does not really mean that there are no seeds; it just means that the seeds that exist are small in number and very soft; thus the watermelon qualifies as seedless. No varietal names get associated with watermelons in the marketplace, though there are some colorful ones: New Dragon, Sugar Baby (a completely round, unstriped green picnic watermelon), Yellow Doll (yellow-fleshed), King of Hearts (seedless red), and Black Boy.

▶ Availability Watermelons are theoretically available all year, but some markets only stock them in the warm summer months, when they expect their peak sales.

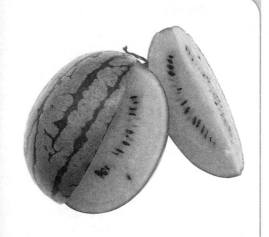

yellow watermelon

WATERMELON 1 cup cubes	
Calories	49
Protein (g)	1
Carbohydrate (g)	11
Dietary fiber (g)	0.8
Total fat (g)	0.7
Saturated fat (g)	0.1
Monounsaturated fat (g)	0.2
Polyunsaturated fat (g)	0.2
Cholesterol (mg)	0
Potassium (mg)	176
Sodium (mg)	3

KEY NUTRIENTS (%RDA/AI*)	
Thiamin	0.1 mg (10%)
Vitamin B$_6$	0.2 mg (13%)
Vitamin C	15 mg (16%)

*For more detailed information on RDA and AI, see page 88.

choosing the best

Watermelons are sold whole, or cut into halves, quarters, or smaller pieces. Skin color ranges from deep green to gray, solid to streaked or dappled; look for a melon with a rind that is neither very shiny nor very dull, but shows a waxy "bloom." The underside should have a creamy-white spot (where it sat on the ground as it ripened in the sun). This so-called "ground spot" changes from pale white to a creamy-yellow at proper harvest maturity. If the stem is still attached, it should look dry and brown; if the stem is green, the melon was picked too soon, and if it has fallen off, the fruit may be overripe.

Of course, if your market sells cut melons, the fruit should be perfect for immediate consumption, as it will not improve once it is cut. With cut melons, you can check the color and texture of the flesh, and usually smell the delectable fragrance of a ripe melon even through the plastic wrapping.

Cut watermelon should have dense, firm flesh that is well colored for its type, with dark seeds. White seeds are a sign of immaturity (seedless varieties may contain a few small white seeds). If the piece of melon has seeds that have begun to separate from the flesh, white streaks, or large cracks in the flesh, don't buy it.

▶ **When you get home** An uncut watermelon can, if necessary, be stored at room temperature for up to a week, but in summer, when room temperatures can be quite high, the fruit should be refrigerated or kept on ice. It takes 8 to 12 hours to chill a whole watermelon thoroughly. Cut watermelon should be wrapped and refrigerated.

preparing to use

To cut a watermelon into wedges for eating, halve the watermelon lengthwise, then halve each piece lengthwise again to give you four quarters. Cut each quarter-piece crosswise into wedge-shaped slices.

For salads, halve the watermelon lengthwise and use a melon baller to scoop out the flesh.

serving suggestions

- Puree watermelon, pour into ice cube trays, and freeze. Use to chill summer drinks.

- Cube watermelon and combine with cubes of cucumber, diced red onion, and toasted pumpkin seeds. Toss with a sherry vinegar dressing for a summer salad.

- Cube watermelon and freeze. Add the frozen melon to smoothies instead of ice cubes.

- Puree watermelon, strawberries, and fresh mint for a refreshing summer soup. Serve topped with grated lime zest and a dollop of nonfat sour cream.

- Blend watermelon, basil, parsley, and red onion. Strain and mix with olive oil, rice wine vinegar, and black pepper for a vinaigrette.

- Very finely mince watermelon and drain slightly. Stir into reduced-fat sour cream along with minced chives. Serve as a sweet-savory sandwich spread.

facts & tips

Leave it to the Japanese to figure out how to grow watermelons that take up less space in the refrigerator. Farmers in the southern Japanese town of Zentsuji force watermelons to grow inside glass cubes, creating a box-shaped watermelon that fits conveniently on refrigerator shelves. However, this convenience has a hefty price tag: over $80 per watermelon.

wheat

Wheat is one of the oldest harvested grains. Probably descended from a wild grass that was harvested as early as 10,000 B.C., domestic wheat was first cultivated in western Asia 6,000 years ago. Wheat was milled into flour for bread in ancient Egypt and was the grain of choice during the Roman Empire. Wheat fell behind barley, rye, and potatoes as a staple food in Europe during the Middle Ages, but it reemerged as the preeminent grain in the 19th century. It was brought to the New World by European settlers in the 1700s, and by the mid-19th century was established in what would later be America's wheat belt.

As the most important cereal crop in the world, wheat—mainly in the form of bread and noodles—nourishes more people than any other grain. Unlike many other grains, such as oats, corn, sorghum, and millet, wheat is not typically used as animal feed, but is processed directly into human food (although wheat bran and germ, the nutrient-dense by-products of flour refining, are given to livestock). The bulk of the wheat grown is milled into flour—usually white flour. But there are forms of wheat, with their bran and germ intact, that can be eaten as a main or side dish.

The United States ranks among the top five wheat-growing nations in the world, exporting half of the annual wheat crop to other nations.

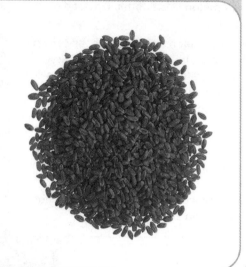

wheat berries

nutritional profile

A highly nutritious food source, wheat is low in fat and provides complex carbohydrates, insoluble and soluble fiber, and an assortment of vitamins and minerals. Though its protein is incomplete, when combined with other cereal grains, animal proteins, or legumes, it becomes complete.

The nutritional value of wheat is determined by how it is processed: Whole wheat retains its natural bran and germ, and thus retains a full range of nutrients. Highly nutritious, it offers a good supply of protein, B vitamins, and minerals, including iron and magnesium, and plays a role in a heart-healthy, anti-cancer diet. Refined wheat has been stripped of its bran and germ, and thus most of its fiber and many nutrients. Although refined-wheat foods are usually enriched with a few vitamins and minerals (sometimes even with fiber), not all of the nutrients that existed in the whole grain are replaced.

A nutrient-dense food, wheat germ is the germ or "heart" of the wheat kernel, and is packed with folate, thiamin, magnesium, and vitamin B_6, iron, selenium, vitamin E, zinc, and fiber. Wheat bran is the outer layer of the wheat kernel, and it also makes a nutritious addition to baked goods, offering fiber, B vitamins, protein, and iron.

BULGUR / 1 cup cooked	
Calories	151
Protein (g)	6
Carbohydrate (g)	34
Dietary fiber (g)	8.2
Total fat (g)	0.4
Saturated fat (g)	0.1
Monounsaturated fat (g)	0.1
Polyunsaturated fat (g)	0.2
Cholesterol (mg)	0
Potassium (mg)	124
Sodium (mg)	9

KEY NUTRIENTS (%RDA/AI*)	
Niacin	1.8 mg (11%)
Iron	1.8 mg (22%)
Magnesium	58 mg (14%)

*For more detailed information on RDA and AI, see page 88.

To find a whole-wheat product without spending hours inspecting labels, look for the word "whole" before "wheat." If the first ingredient is whole-wheat flour, you're getting what you need. Do not be fooled by the following words: Enriched, unbleached, bromated, stone ground, granulated, 100% wheat, rye, pumpernickel, multi-grain, 7-grain, semolina, or organic. These products may contain little or no whole grains. And "hearty wheat," "stoned wheat," or "multi-grain" crackers are made from refined (white) wheat flour.

While wheat foods can be highly nutritious, people who have celiac disease or gluten sensitivity (*see "Gluten Sensitivity," page 596*) and are allergic to wheat and wheat products should read food labels carefully to check to see if a product contains wheat.

➤ *phytochemicals in* wheat

The nutritious bran and germ layers of whole wheat are rich in beneficial phytochemicals called flavonoids, lignans, and saponins that may help to reduce the risk of cancer and heart disease. Whole-wheat foods—such as wheat berries, bulgur, cracked wheat, and whole-wheat flour—are made from the whole grain, which preserves the disease-fighting substances from these layers.

in the market

The thousands of known varieties of wheat all fall into one of six classes, determined by the planting season, hardness of the grain, and the color of the kernel. Hard Red Winter, Hard Red Spring, Soft Red Winter, Hard White, Soft White, and Durum wheat are the major classes. *Winter wheats* are planted in the fall; they lie dormant during the winter, revive to grow again in the spring, and are harvested early in the summer. *Spring wheats* are

new products from ancient grains

There are over 30,000 varieties of wheat, all of which developed from one common ancestor called wild einkorn. The wheats most commonly grown today are different genetically from this original wheat, but two ancient strains are now being marketed, mostly in health-food stores. Called kamut and spelt (or farro), these were among the wheats found growing when humans first walked the earth.

Similar nutritionally to modern wheats, kamut and spelt are available in the form of whole grains, flours, and pastas. Even though they are botanically considered forms of wheat, they may be labeled "wheat-free"—presumably to attract the attention of those with wheat sensitivities. One packaged spelt product says it is an "alternative to wheat" and its product-information flyer states that it is "perfect for wheat-sensitive people." But whether or not spelt or kamut can be tolerated by individuals with wheat allergies or gluten sensitivity has yet to be established by scientific research, and those with such allergies should consult their doctors before experimenting with these grains.

planted in the spring and harvested late in the summer. The hard wheats have a higher protein-to-starch ratio than the soft wheats. *Durum*, the hardest wheat of all, is processed into semolina and used to make pasta. *Hard Red Winter* and *Hard Red Spring* wheats are milled into bread flour and all-purpose flour, as are *Hard White* wheats. *Soft Red Winter* and *Soft White* wheats produce flours that are well-suited for making cakes, crackers, cookies, and pastries.

Bulgur A processed form of cracked wheat (*below*), but with a more pronounced flavor, bulgur is produced by a method similar to that used for converted rice: The whole-wheat kernels are steam-cooked and dried, then the grain is cracked into three different granulations. Traditionally, the coarsest grain is used for pilaf; the medium, for cereal; and the finest, for tabbouleh. Bulgur requires less cooking time than cracked wheat. It can also be "cooked" by soaking, without heat.

Cracked wheat This product is made from wheat berries that have been ground into coarse, medium, and fine granulations for faster cooking. Cracked wheat has an agreeably wheaty flavor and can replace rice or other grains in most recipes; it cooks in about 15 minutes and retains a slight crunchiness afterward. It's possible to make cracked wheat at home by processing wheat berries in a heavy-duty blender. Process 2 cups of wheat at a time on high speed for about 4 minutes.

Farina Also sold as Cream of Wheat, farina is made from the endosperm of the grain, which is milled to a fine granular consistency and then sifted. Although the bran and most of the germ are removed, this cereal is sometimes enriched with B vitamins and iron. Farina is most often served as a breakfast cereal, but can also be cooked like polenta.

Farro See Spelt (*opposite page*).

Flour See Flour, Wheat (*page 328*).

WHEAT GERM 2 tablespoons	
Calories	52
Protein (g)	3
Carbohydrate (g)	7
Dietary fiber (g)	1.9
Total fat (g)	1.4
Saturated fat (g)	0.2
Monounsaturated fat (g)	0.2
Polyunsaturated fat (g)	0.9
Cholesterol (mg)	0
Potassium (mg)	128
Sodium (mg)	2

KEY NUTRIENTS (%RDA/AI*)	
Thiamin	0.3 mg (23%)
Vitamin B$_6$	0.2 mg (11%)
Vitamin E	3.9 mg (26%)
Folate	40 mcg (10%)
Iron	0.9 mg (11%)
Selenium	11 mcg (21%)
Zinc	1.8 mg (16%)

For more detailed information on RDA and AI, see page 88.

serving suggestions

- Add spelt (farro) to a minestrone instead of pasta.

- Cook wheat berries and toss with a lemon vinaigrette, dried fruit, and shredded grilled chicken.

- Add wheat germ to pancake, waffle, and bread recipes in place of some of the flour.

- Make risotto using wheat berries, spelt, or kamut instead of rice.

- Replace some of the meat in a chili with soaked and drained medium-grain bulgur.

- Substitute cooked cracked wheat for bread in a poultry stuffing.

- Cook rolled wheat flakes as you would oatmeal.

- Add wheat flakes or cracked wheat to casseroles or stews.

- Substitute seitan for chicken in a stew or add it to a soup or stir-fry.

- Lighten meatball, meatloaf, or hamburger mixtures by replacing some of the meat with soaked and drained bulgur.

Kamut An ancient relative of modern-day wheat, this high-protein grain has a buttery, nutty flavor. It is generally available both in whole grains and in processed forms, such as pasta and puffed cereal.

Pasta See Pasta, Wheat (*page 445*).

Rolled wheat (wheat flakes) These are wheat berries that have been flattened between rollers and are not to be confused with ready-to-eat wheat-flake breakfast cereals. Rolled wheat flakes resemble rolled oats, but are thicker and firmer.

Seitan (wheat meat) This vegetarian stand-in for meat is derived from high-gluten wheat flour. Chewy and dense, seitan is a flavor-sponge that absorbs sauces and seasonings very well.

Spelt (farro, dinkle) High in fiber, protein, and B vitamins, this ancient wheat relative has a nutty flavor and a slightly crisp texture.

Triticale See Triticale (*page 577*).

Wheat berries Also called groats, these are wheat kernels that have not been milled, polished, or heat treated. Wheat berries are brown and nearly round in appearance; they take over an hour to cook, but the time can be reduced if they are presoaked. Wheat berries have a robust, nutlike flavor that goes well with other hearty foods. They can be used for grain-based main dishes, served as a side dish, or added to soups and yeast-bread doughs.

Wheat bran The rough outer covering of the wheat kernel, wheat bran is very high in insoluble fiber.

WHEAT BRAN 2 tablespoons	
Calories	16
Protein (g)	1
Carbohydrate (g)	5
Dietary fiber (g)	3.1
Total fat (g)	0.3
Saturated fat (g)	0.1
Monounsaturated fat (g)	0.1
Polyunsaturated fat (g)	0.1
Cholesterol (mg)	0
Potassium (mg)	86
Sodium (mg)	0

KEY NUTRIENTS (%RDA/AI*)	
Iron	0.8 mg (10%)
Magnesium	44 mg (11%)
Selenium	6 mcg (10%)

For more detailed information on RDA and AI, see page 88.

wheat germ vs. wheat bran

For years people have been buying wheat germ to sprinkle on breakfast cereals, yogurt, and salads, as well as to add to baked goods and casseroles. Now, with nutritionists emphasizing the importance of fiber, wheat germ has been joined on supermarket shelves by wheat bran. What are the nutritional differences between the two?

Wheat germ contains a fair amount of polyunsaturated fat, deriving almost 25 percent of its calories from fat. It is an especially good source of thiamin, vitamin E, and selenium. Two tablespoons supply 3 grams of protein and 2 grams of dietary fiber. Defatted wheat germ is available, but it's lower in vitamin E; unlike regular wheat germ, it doesn't have to be stored in the refrigerator.

Wheat bran is also a nutritional storehouse; it offers magnesium, iron, and selenium. Two tablespoons contain 1 gram of protein, less than a half gram of fat, and 3 grams of dietary fiber.

If you eat whole-wheat cereals and baked goods, then you're already getting the germ and the bran. Otherwise, try adding some packaged wheat germ and bran to your diet; you'll be enhancing the nutrient value of the foods, as well as their flavor and texture.

Wheat germ oil See Fats & Oils (*page 298*).

Wheatena This is the trade name for a very finely cracked wheat product sold for use as a hot cereal. It has a pleasant, nutlike flavor and is among the most nutritious of hot cereals.

Wheat germ The embryo of the wheat berry, wheat germ is packed full of vitamins, minerals, and protein. It has a nutty flavor and is used to add nutrients and flavor to many dishes.

choosing the best

When buying whole grains, they should be whole, not cracked, and with little or no chaff. Purchase wheat products from a store that has a brisk turnover and keeps the grains out of the heat.

▶ **When you get home** Store in a cool dry place for 2 months; freeze for longer storage.

preparing to use

Whole grains bought in bulk should be picked over and washed to remove dust or debris before cooking.

gluten sensitivity

Gluten is a component of wheat: It makes flour elastic and smooth. Other cereal grains, such as rye and barley, have a related compound. Gluten contains a protein called gliadin. A small percentage of people are born with an intolerance to gliadin. It produces an immune reaction in them, with such symptoms as diarrhea, weight loss, and skin rashes. Eventually, damage to the small intestine may result. This condition is known as GSE (gluten sensitive enteropathy), celiac disease, or nontropical sprue.

GSE is essentially a genetic ailment, though other factors, such as infection, may trigger the condition. It is more common in people of European descent than in others. Estimates of the number of Americans and Canadians who have GSE vary markedly: Some experts say it is as many as 1 in 150. Sometimes children born with gluten sensitivity have mild symptoms or none, and go undiagnosed until adulthood. Only a physician can diagnose GSE; the treatment is usually a lifelong gluten-free diet.

Many people troubled by indigestion, fatigue, or other symptoms conclude they are allergic to wheat or gluten and decide to change their diets. While it's true that wheat, along with peanuts and shellfish, is one of the foods most likely to cause allergic reactions, true food allergies are rare.

Self-diagnosis is never a good idea. If you have chronic indigestion or always feel exhausted, you should get medical advice to pinpoint the cause. If you prove to be gluten-sensitive, you'll need help to plan your diet. For example, you'll find lots of products labeled "gluten-free" and/or "wheat-free "in the supermarket. This can be confusing: A wheat-free product can still contain gluten and would not be suitable for a person with GSE. Corn and rice products are fine—they contain no gliadin.

wild rice

Wild rice is not really a true rice, but the seed of an aquatic grass from a completely different botanical family. Archaeological findings indicate that wild rice has been a native North American food for at least 1,000 years. And ever since the Native Americans first introduced wild rice to the early explorers, settlers, and fur traders, this grain has been much sought after.

Wild rice is grown in shallow areas in lakes, tidal rivers, and bays in fresh water between 2 and 4 feet deep. The "rice" is located in the head of stalks that can grow to be 9 feet tall. Until modern methods for mechanical harvesting were established, wild rice was harvested by hand: Native Americans would bend the stalks into their canoes so that they could strike the seeds from the heads with their paddles or wooden sticks. They then sun-dried or parched the seeds over a fire to crack the hulls, allowing the grain to be released.

Domestication of wild rice began relatively late compared with other grains and cereals. Commercial crops of this nutritious grain—which is sometimes referred to as the "caviar of grains"—are now grown in man-made paddies or shallow lakes. After harvesting, the large seeds are steamed, dried, dehulled, and cleaned to produce the delicious dark brown grain. Once exclusively the province of regional Native American tribes (who by law were the only ones allowed to harvest it in this country), wild rice is now cultivated on a broader scale. Interestingly, this broader cultivation includes Australia, which has been growing wild rice since the early 1990s.

Wild rice has a complex, nutlike flavor, and its slender grains (when properly cooked and not overcooked) are pleasantly chewy; they can be used in poultry stuffing and salads as well as in side dishes. While its high price may deter you from making it a regular part of your diet, you will find that a little goes a long way. Wild rice blends well with other rices or can be served on its own: 1 cup dry cooks up to 3 or 4 cups, which is enough for six servings.

nutritional profile

Wild rice has more protein than other rices, and just under 10 percent of the RDA for a number of B vitamins, including niacin and D_6.

choosing the best

Connoisseurs of wild rice claim that truly "wild" wild rice has more flavor than the cultivated variety. However, this information is not required on labels, so you may not be able to choose wild rice based on this criterion.

preparing to use

Wild rice is usually rinsed before cooking.

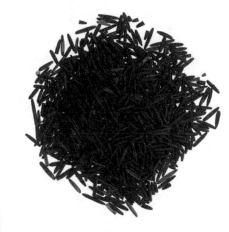

wild rice

WILD RICE / ½ cup cooked	
Calories	82
Protein (g)	3
Carbohydrate (g)	17
Dietary fiber (g)	1.5
Total fat (g)	0.3
Saturated fat (g)	0
Monounsaturated fat (g)	0
Polyunsaturated fat (g)	0.2
Cholesterol (mg)	0
Potassium (mg)	82
Sodium (mg)	3

KEY NUTRIENTS (%RDA/AI*)	
Zinc	1.1 mg (10%)

For more detailed information on RDA and AI, see page 88.

yogurt

Not so long ago most Americans considered yogurt a product for health-food faddists. At that time, relatively few people were aware that yogurt had been a staple in certain parts of Asia, the Middle East, and Eastern Europe for centuries. Yogurt has been commercially produced in the United States since the early 1940s, but didn't become popular until the 1970s. In its various manifestations, yogurt has emerged from the health-food store into the mainstream supermarket in a big way, with consumption in this country soaring (even if a lot of it is in the form of frozen yogurt).

Commercially produced yogurt is made by curdling cow's milk with purified cultures of special "friendly" bacteria that cause the milk sugar (lactose) to turn into lactic acid. The milk is then warmed in an incubator for several hours, during which time the yogurt thickens and develops its creamy-texture and distinctively tart, yet subtle, flavor.

nutritional profile

Possibly because it was an exotic food in this country until about 30 years ago, yogurt retains a certain mysterious quality. Most people classify it as a healthy food—which it certainly is, as long as you avoid the high-fat, sugar-laden varieties.

Cup for cup, low-fat yogurt has about 150 milligrams more calcium than low-fat milk, and provides more than one-third of your daily needs. It's also a good source of protein; yogurt supplies 50 percent more protein than milk, since it is usually thickened with nonfat milk solids. It also has good amounts of B vitamins (especially vitamin B_{12}) and minerals.

Low-fat yogurt (or better yet fat-free yogurt) is a good thing to keep around if you're watching your calorie and fat intake. Both are low in calories, considering the nutrients they provide, and can substitute for high-fat items like mayonnaise and sour cream.

In order to thicken or stabilize yogurt and increase its shelf-life, some brands have added gelatin, starches, pectin, or gums. These additives are not harmful, but they sometimes give the yogurt a slightly "unnatural" stiffness or thickness.

Fruit yogurts are less nutritious than plain, since the fruit takes up space in the cup—thus you get less yogurt, fewer vitamins and minerals, and much more sugar. If the fruit is from preserves, which it often is, the yogurt supplies even fewer nutrients. Choose plain yogurt, because it has the fewest calories—you can add your own fruit or sweeteners if you like.

Some yogurts contain artificial flavors or colors, as well as sweeteners (natural and artificial), such as sugar, honey, molasses, corn syrup, fructose, or aspartame. A cup of regular sweetened vanilla, lemon, or coffee yogurt contains the equivalent of 3½ teaspoons of sugar; fruit flavors may have as much

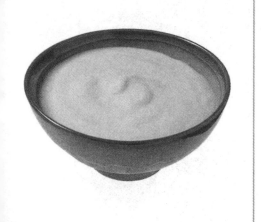

yogurt

PLAIN LOW-FAT YOGURT 1 cup	
Calories	154
Protein (g)	13
Carbohydrate (g)	17
Dietary fiber (g)	0
Total fat (g)	3.8
Saturated fat (g)	2.5
Monounsaturated fat (g)	1.0
Polyunsaturated fat (g)	0.1
Cholesterol (mg)	15
Potassium (mg)	573
Sodium (mg)	172

KEY NUTRIENTS (%RDA/AI*)	
Riboflavin	0.5 mg (40%)
Vitamin B_{12}	1.4 mcg (57%)
Calcium	448 mg (37%)
Magnesium	43 mg (10%)
Selenium	8 mcg (15%)
Zinc	2.2 mg (20%)

*For more detailed information on RDA and AI, see page 88.

as 7 teaspoons per cup. Some extra-rich yogurts have egg yolks added.

A number of health benefits are attributed to the active bacterial cultures in yogurt. One benefit for which there is good evidence applies to people with lactose intolerance—that is, they have trouble digesting the lactose (milk sugar) in dairy products. These people can eat yogurt with live cultures since the bacteria help in digesting lactose.

The bacteria in yogurt are also promoted as "probiotics," which help replace intestinal flora destroyed by illness or when antibiotics are taken. In fact, though, among the hundreds of strains of bacteria identified by scientists, only a very few strains appear able to "colonize" the large intestine to produce such a benefit. And there is no evidence that any of the living bacteria in commercial yogurts act in this way. Instead, the bacteria in yogurt are digested before reaching the large intestine.

If you still want to purchase yogurt with live cultures, look for products that say "contains active cultures" or "contains live cultures" on the container. Note that "made with active cultures" is not enough; all yogurts are made with active cultures, but the bacteria may be killed off if the yogurt is pasteurized or heated after it is fermented (this does not reduce the calcium or the vitamin content). Just keep in mind that, unless you are lactose intolerant, there is no evidence that those live cultures are going to do much of anything for you.

In the market

Plain, or unflavored, yogurt is the original and most versatile of yogurts. It contains from 100 to 160 calories per cup. All yogurts, from fat-free to whole-milk, come in a variety of flavors, ranging from simple vanilla with added sugar to fruit-flavored. The fruit-flavored yogurts fall into two categories: Sundae-style yogurts, in which

yogurt drinks

Once upon a time, when yogurt was exotic, no one would have considered buying a drinkable yogurt. But now that yogurt is firmly mainstream, yogurt drinks, too, have become commonplace. Yogurt drinks are really just thinner, pourable versions of the spoonable yogurts and come in the same range of flavors. There are also a couple of slightly different drinks available:

Kefir A close cousin of yogurt, kefir also has its roots in Eastern Europe. It was originally a beverage made from mare's milk, fermented with a cultured "starter"—akin to a sourdough starter—until it developed a low alcohol content. A modern nonalcoholic version sold in the United States is made in much the same way as yogurt but using different cultures. It tends to be somewhat less tart than plain yogurt. Kefir can be made from whole or low-fat milk, and is sold plain and fruit-flavored.

Lassi This Indian yogurt drink can occasionally be found in East Indian markets, but it is more often homemade. It is made by thinning yogurt with a little water and adding either savory spices (such as cumin) or sweet fruit juices (like mango).

COMPARING YOGURT 1 cup							
	Calories	Fat (g)	% Calories from Fat	Saturated Fat (g)	Cholesterol (mg)	Calcium (mg)	% RDA for Calcium
Fat-free, plain	137	0	0	0	5	488	41
Low-fat, plain	154	4.0	23	2.5	15	448	37
Whole-milk, plain	149	8.0	48	5.1	32	296	25
Low-fat, with fruit	238	3.2	12	2.1	14	384	32

the fruit is at the bottom of the container and must be stirred in; and blended, custardlike, Swiss- or French-style yogurts, in which the fruit is distributed throughout the yogurt. In addition, custard-style yogurts are usually made with egg yolks.

plain yogurt

Whole-milk The richest of the plain yogurts, whole-milk yogurt has from 6 to 8 grams of fat per 8-ounce serving. Some brands of whole-milk yogurt (called farm-style) come with a layer of yogurt cream on top. To reduce the fat content, lift this off and discard it rather than stirring it in.

Low-fat Low-fat yogurt may contain anywhere from 2 to 5 grams of fat per 8-ounce serving (0.5 to 2 percent milk fat by weight).

Fat-free Fat-free yogurt contains less than 0.5 percent milkfat by weight. It is less tangy than either low-fat or whole-milk yogurt and makes a good stand-in for sour cream.

yogurt cheese

Yogurt thickens when the whey is drained from it. The resulting mildly tart yogurt "cheese," or curd, can be substituted for sour cream or cream cheese in recipes, depending on how long you let the yogurt drain. You can buy an inexpensive yogurt cheese "funnel" or make your own out of common kitchen items. Use any type of plain low-fat or whole-milk yogurt that does not contain gelatin, as gelatin keeps the whey from draining off. Fruit yogurts will not work well, but flavored yogurts that do not have solids in them (such as vanilla, coffee, or lemon) can be made into tasty dessert cheeses by this method.

To make yogurt cheese, line a strainer or colander with dampened cheesecloth, a clean white cloth napkin or towel, or paper towels; place the strainer over a bowl. (You can also use a simple funnel-shaped drip coffee filter—the type that sits atop the cup or pot—lined with a paper filter.) Stir the yogurt, then spoon it into the strainer. Cover the strainer with plastic wrap and place the strainer and bowl in the refrigerator.

The thickness of the resulting product will depend on the type of yogurt you use and how long it drains. As a rule of thumb, an hour or two will yield a yogurt "sour cream"; 6 to 8 hours, or overnight draining, will produce a yogurt "cream cheese."

For appetizer dips and/or sandwich spreads Try flavoring yogurt "cream cheese" or "sour cream" with herbs, spices, or chopped vegetables. For instance, add minced garlic and fresh or dried herbs such as basil, thyme, dill, or oregano. Or flavor the dip or spread with chili or curry powder, chopped scallions or chives, pureed roasted bell peppers, capers, anchovies, or mustard. Add shredded carrots, chopped cooked spinach, or pureed artichoke hearts.

For dessert Consider sweetening the "cream cheese" or "sour cream" with honey, brown sugar, or frozen fruit juice concentrate, and/or flavoring it with vanilla or almond extract, nutmeg, cardamom, or ginger. You can fold in grated citrus zest or chopped dried fruit, if desired. Serve it with fresh fruit (it's especially good with bananas or berries) or plain cookies. You can make a chocolate cheese spread for fruit slices (or a simple frosting for cake or cookies) by adding cocoa powder to sweetened "cream cheese."

Yogurt "sour cream" can be used instead of mayonnaise in tuna or chicken salad. When heating yogurt "sour cream" (as part of a sauce or creamy soup, for example), take the same precautions you would with regular yogurt to keep it from curdling or breaking.

other yogurts

Goat's milk yogurt Like sheep's milk yogurt, this is a full-flavored yogurt with a slightly more pronounced gamy flavor. If you're a fan of goat cheese, you'll enjoy goat's milk yogurt.

Labneh (labne) This thick Middle Eastern yogurt "cheese" is smooth and creamy like sour cream. It is often eaten with a drizzle of olive oil and chopped mint, and served with pita bread.

Sheep's milk yogurt This is a rich and creamy full-flavored yogurt with a slightly gamy flavor.

Soy yogurt See Soyfoods (*page 538*).

choosing the best

All commercial yogurts are freshness dated. Be sure to check the date, and select the latest-dated carton you find on the shelf. If you prefer fruited yogurt, select one made with fresh fruit rather than preserves.

▶ **When you get home** Keep yogurt in its original container in the refrigerator. An unopened container of yogurt with live cultures should keep for about 10 days past the "sell by" date; pasteurized yogurt will keep even longer. However, check to see that the yogurt looks and smells fresh when you open it.

facts & tips

In the 1970s there was an advertising campaign to promote interest in yogurt. The ads featured vigorous 100-year-old denizens of the Georgian steppes who attributed their longevity to yogurt. It turned out that these yogurt-eaters were not as old as they claimed: They had falsified their birth records to avoid being conscripted into the army.

serving suggestions

- Stir toasted cumin, minced pickled jalapeños, and chopped roasted pumpkin seeds into yogurt, and use as a topping for chili.

- Use yogurt as a part of a marinade for chicken.

- Use low-fat yogurt instead of sour cream in baking.

- Mash potatoes with plain low-fat yogurt instead of butter or sour cream.

- Make a smoothie with sliced bananas, strawberries, yogurt, and a couple of ice cubes.

- Stir diced cucumber, minced cilantro, and sliced scallions into yogurt for a refreshing accompaniment to curries.

- Make your own fruit yogurt by stirring an all-fruit spread into plain yogurt.

- Stir herbs and spices into yogurt and use as a dip for crudités.

- Finely chop garlic and stir it into yogurt along with a little olive oil, and use as a sauce for pasta.

- Use yogurt to lighten a potato salad dressing.

how to
read a food label

Foods that are sold in fresh form usually don't come with any nutritional information—which is why the food entries in this book are accompanied by nutrition charts. Most packaged foods sold in the United States carry food labels, however, and these offer a convenient source of information about nutritional content once you understand what the figures on them mean. The information on food labels appears in a standard panel under the heading "Nutrition Facts"—a format mandated by the Food and Drug Administration (FDA) in 1994, when it revamped regulations concerning food labeling and required that the Nutrition Facts panel be carried on practically all packaged foods.

You will find the panel on foods from milk and juice to pasta, cereal and bread, cookies and crackers, and canned or frozen produce. While the panel is not required on raw meats, most supermarkets provide this information on the packaging. Labeling is also not required on fresh produce, but some types of produce sold in packages, such as carrots or celery, do carry a Nutrition Facts panel.

For every food product, manufacturers must provide nutritional data for specific nutrients—notably total calories, total fat, saturated fat, cholesterol, sodium, vitamin A, vitamin C, calcium, and iron—and they have the option of providing even more information. For each type of food (say, frozen vegetables), the data must be given for a standard serving size. The use of standard serving sizes allows consumers to compare calorie and nutrient content between similar products.

understanding "daily values"

You will notice that in this book the nutrition charts with each food entry show a food's vitamin and mineral content based on Recommended Dietary Allowances, or RDAs. The RDAs, established by the National Academy of Sciences, are the most authoritative guidelines for recommended intakes of specific nutrients in a person's daily diet (see page 88). You won't see RDAs on food labels. Instead, the Nutrition Facts panel uses another set of numbers called Daily Values, or DVs, for a person's daily recommended intake—and lists the "% Daily Value" that each nutrient in a serving contributes for someone consuming 2,000 calories a day.

The DVs actually comprise two sets of numbers. Those for macronutrients, such as fat, protein, and carbohydrates, are known as Daily Reference Values (DRVs); the values for micronutrients—the vitamins and minerals—are termed Reference Daily Intakes (RDIs). But for simplicity's sake, on labels both sets of numbers are referred to as DVs.

In contrast to the RDAs, which vary for men and women and by age group, the DV for each vitamin and mineral is a single number that is set high enough to provide sufficient intakes for everyone. Certainly this simplifies reading a label. However, the DVs are based on recommendations—RDAs, actually—that were established in 1968. Confusingly, although the RDAs themselves were most recently updated between 1997 and 2002, the DVs were not. The Food and Drug Administration (FDA) intends to update DVs in the future to reflect current RDAs, but it will take some years to establish, and then implement, the updated values.

In the meantime, there is no reason to get caught up in struggling with either set of numbers, since there aren't major differences between the DVs and the RDAs. When buying packaged foods, you can certainly use the DVs as a guide for assessing your nutrient intake.

additional information

A limited number of health claims can also appear on food labels. The claims must be scientifically established and approved by the FDA.

Nutrition Facts

Serving Size: ½ cup
Servings Per Container: 4

Amount Per Serving
Calories 260 Calories from Fat 120

	% Daily Value*
Total Fat 13g	20%
Saturated Fat 5g	25%
Cholesterol 30mg	10%
Sodium 660mg	28%
Total Carbohydrate 31g	11%
Dietary Fiber 0g	0%
Sugars 5g	
Protein 5g	

Vitamin A 4%	•	Calcium 15%	
Vitamin C 2%	•	Iron 4%	

* Percents (%) of a Daily Value are based on a 2,000 calorie diet. Your Daily Values may vary higher or lower depending on your calorie needs:

Nutrient		2,000 Calories	2,500 Calories
Total Fat	Less than	65g	80g
Sat. Fat	Less than	20g	25g
Cholesterol	Less than	300mg	300mg
Sodium	Less than	2,400mg	2,400mg
Total Carbohydrate		300g	375g
Fiber		25g	30g

Calories per gram:
Fat 9 • Carbohydrate 4 • Protein 4

The Nutrition Facts panel must display information for the key nutrients shown in the top half. If space allows, the lower portion of the panel can also indicate the Daily Values for fat, cholesterol, sodium, total carbohydrate, and dietary fiber. In this example, the amount of fat in a serving is 13 grams, or 20% of the 65-gram limit that represents the Daily Value for fat in a 2,000 calorie-per-day diet.

For instance, products that are low in sodium may indicate on their label that "diets low in sodium may reduce the risk of high blood pressure, a disease associated with many factors." Some other established claims concerning nutrient/disease relationships are: calcium and osteoporosis; fat and cancer; saturated fat and cholesterol and coronary heart disease; fiber and cancer; soluble fiber and coronary heart disease; folate and neural tube birth defects; and soy protein and risk of coronary heart disease. Loose and unsubstantiated terms such as "heart-smart" or "health-wise" are no longer allowed.

There are also rules governing which products can be labeled as organic. Organic products must originate from farms that are certified by a state or private agency accredited by the United States Department of Agriculture (USDA), meaning that they follow farming practices that qualify for the organic label. The labeling indicates whether products are made from ingredients that are 100 percent organic, or whether the product contains a lesser amount of organic ingredients. For instance, products that contain less than 70 percent of organic ingredients can use the word "organic" on the ingredient list, and can list what percentage of the product is organic, but cannot use the USDA seal or other certifying logo

putting the "facts" together

While regulations governing food labels may seem confusing, the information itself actually serves to help consumers make informed decisions when comparison shopping. Learning how to read a Nutrition Facts panel and understand the percent DVs will also help you plan a balanced diet. The sample label at left lists all of the nutrients a manufacturer is required to cover.

Some DVs, such as those for total fat, saturated fat, and cholesterol, are amounts you should try not to exceed. Other values, such as those for vitamins, minerals, and fiber, are amounts you should aim to achieve.

The information below will help you put these and other label terms into perspective.

Serving size Serving sizes are standardized by product type and reflect the amounts people tend to eat. (Previously, the serving size was up to the manufacturer.) What qualifies as a serving depends on the type of food. For example, the reference serving size for cookies is 30 grams (a little more than 1 ounce) and the serving is for the number of cookies that comes closest to weighing 30 grams.

Total fat and saturated fat Total fat is defined as the sum of all fatty acids (saturated, polyunsaturated, and monounsaturated) plus triglycerides. The manufacturer is also required to provide the number of grams of saturated fat per serving, and has the option of listing figures for polyunsaturated and monounsaturated fats.

Keep in mind that the percentages shown are not percentages of total calories that come from fat, but rather the percentages a serving contributes towards the Daily Values in a 2,000 calorie-per-day diet. The DVs for total fat and saturated fat represent the upper limits considered acceptable—65 grams and 20 grams, respectively—for a 2,000 calorie diet.

At some point, food labels will also include a figure for trans fatty acids—unsaturated fats that have become more saturated (and therefore more unhealthy) during processing for use in margarines, crackers, cookies, and other snack foods (*for more information on trans fatty acids, see "Trans Fats," page 298*).

Cholesterol The DV for cholesterol represents the recommended maximum daily cholesterol intake, which is 300 milligrams. The "% DV" on the Nutrition Facts panel tells you the percentage of cholesterol the individual food contributes to this amount. (Note that while many snack foods are cholesterol-free, they may still be high in total fat, saturated fat—which can raise blood cholesterol levels—and calories.)

Sodium Again, the DV for sodium is considered the maximum suggested amount (2,400 milligrams per day). Many processed foods, including soups, frozen vegetables with special sauces, and even some cereals, contain high amounts of sodium in a single serving. Some reduced-fat foods also contain high amounts of sodium. (Fresh whole foods, by contrast, provide very little sodium.) If you are buying processed or canned foods, shop for low-sodium versions. To reduce the sodium in canned vegetables, tuna, and beans, rinse them in water.

Total carbohydrate The total carbohydrate content is given in grams, as are the amounts of dietary fiber and sugars. The manufacturer may also break down the fiber values into soluble and insoluble fiber. The value for sugars includes naturally occurring sugars, such as lactose in yogurt or milk and fructose in fruit juice, in addition to added sugars like corn syrup.

If you are buying packaged breads or other grains, note the dietary fiber content on the label. Look for foods that provide at least 3 grams of fiber per serving to help you meet the recommended 25 to 30 grams of fiber daily. People with diabetes who are on a restricted diet will want to pay attention to the total carbohydrate value.

Vitamins and minerals Manufacturers are required to list the percentage of the daily value of vitamin A, vitamin C, calcium, and iron supplied by a serving of a food. Listing of other vitamins and minerals is voluntary, unless a claim has been made about the nutrient, or they are added to supplement the food (as in breakfast cereals that supply 100 percent of your daily need of various vitamins and minerals). If a food supplies less than 2 percent of the DV for the required four nutrients, the value does not have to be listed on the label.

food label glossary

Food labeling regulations now spell out which nutrient content claims are allowed, and under what circumstances they can be used. Here are the core terms and their definitions:

Free, as in "fat-free," means that a product is either absolutely free of that nutrient or contains an insignificant amount:
• Less than 0.5 grams per serving of fat, saturated fat, or sugar
• Less than 2 milligrams of cholesterol
• Less than 5 milligrams of sodium
• Less than 5 calories

Fortified, enriched, added, or **more** are all claims that mean a food must have at least 10 percent more of the DV for a particular nutrient (say, dietary fiber, potassium, or an essential vitamin or mineral) that was not originally in the food, or was present in smaller amounts.

Healthy can be used on a label if a food is low in fat and saturated fat, and a serving does not contain more than 480 mg of sodium or more than 60 mg of cholesterol. In addition, foods must provide at least 10 percent of one or more of the following: vitamins A or C, iron, calcium, protein, or fiber. Certain foods, like frozen dinners, are required to contain at least two of these nutrients.

High and **good source** focus on nutrients for which higher levels are desirable—for example, fiber or calcium. "High" must equal 20 percent or more of the DV for that nutrient in a serving. (The FDA has also approved "rich in" or "excellent source" as synonyms.) "Good source" means a serving contains 10 to 19 percent of a nutrient's DV.

Lean and **extra lean** can be used to describe the fat content of meat, poultry, seafood, and game. "Lean" foods have less than 10 grams of fat, 4 grams of saturated fat, and 95 milligrams of cholesterol per serving. "Extra lean" means less than 5 grams of fat and 2 grams of saturated fat.

Light or **lite,** when applied to a nutritionally altered food product, means that it contains one-third fewer calories or half the fat of the food from which it was derived. In addition, the term "light in sodium" can indicate that the sodium content of a low-calorie, low-fat food has been reduced by 50 percent. "Light" can also refer to taste, color, and texture, provided qualifying information is included.

Low can refer to total fat, saturated fat, cholesterol, sodium, and calories. It means that a relatively large amount of a food can be eaten without exceeding the DV for the "low" nutrient.
• "Low-fat" foods contain less than 3 grams of fat per serving.
• "Low-saturated fat" foods provide less than 1 gram of saturated fat per serving.
• "Low-sodium" can be used for foods that contain less than 140 milligrams of sodium. (A claim of "very low" can also be made, in which case the food provides 35 milligrams or less per serving.)
• "Low-cholesterol" is allowed on foods that have less than 20 milligrams of cholesterol and less than 2 grams of saturated fat.
• "Low-calorie" foods have less than 40 calories per serving.

Reduced or **less** is a comparison claim applied to total fat, saturated fat, cholesterol, sugar, sodium, and total calories. To be labeled "reduced," a food must have 25 percent less of a nutrient (or calories) than the regular product. The comparison must also be shown on the label.

water

We can live for several weeks without the nutrients in foods, but without water we would die in a few days. Much of our weight is water: The average person totes 10 to 12 gallons of it. Blood is 83 percent water, muscles are 76 percent water, and even 22 percent of bone is water. It's an essential component of every body fluid, from saliva to urine. It's in your cells and around your cells. It enables you to digest food and excrete wastes. It cushions and lubricates brain and joint tissue. It is essential as a lubricant, and it is the major component of saliva, mucous secretions throughout the body, and the fluids that bathe the joints. Water helps move food through the digestive system. It also helps regulate a person's body temperature by distributing heat and cooling the body through perspiration.

Under average circumstances the body loses and needs to replace 2 to 3 quarts of water every day. Perspiring, sneezing, breathing, urinating, defecating, nursing a baby—all these functions and others deplete the body of water. Depending on how much exercising or physical work you do, and how hot or cold the air is, you may lose more. Loss of body fluids is called dehydration, which can decrease exercise performance and, in its extreme forms, can lead to muscle spasms, sharp drops in blood pressure, and other serious symptoms. Luckily, the human body is equipped with a very sensitive regulator for water balance. When your fluid supply needs replenishing, you feel thirsty and you drink. Replacing this water is part of the job of living.

However, thirst may not be a reliable indicator when you're exerting yourself physically. Especially when doing physical work or exercising over long periods, you need to drink even if you don't feel thirsty—before, during, and after exertion. Very dry environments such as airplane cabins may also dehydrate you. You'll be more comfortable if you drink extra fluids (nonalcoholic) when flying. Cold, dry winter air also depletes the body of water.

Age is also a factor that can affect fluid intake. The body's water balance regulator becomes less sensitive in older people, who often don't drink enough and so may become dehydrated.

wellness recommendation

On average, you need to consume the equivalent of eight 8-ounce glasses of water a day—more in extremes of climate or if you're exerting yourself. Not all this fluid needs to be plain water. Milk and other beverages consist almost entirely of water. Many foods are mainly water, particularly fruits, greens, and other vegetables. Soups are mostly water. Even meats contain some water.

Caffeinated beverages such as coffee, tea, or cola tend to promote urination, but they too count, in part, as fluid intake. You certainly don't end up with a water deficit from drinking a cup of coffee or tea. In other words, they don't dehydrate you. Concentrated alcoholic beverages, such as vodka or brandy, have a more pronounced dehydrating effect.

It's a good idea to drink a glass of water or juice on arising in the morning, since you've had no fluids for many hours. If you are constipated, increasing your fluid intake can help. If you are upping your fiber intake (fruits, vegetables, and especially grains), you need to increase your fluid intake at the same time, which may help prevent cramps or gas.

To replace fluids you lose during exercise, drink 4 to 8 ounces of water or other non-dehydrating fluid every 10 to 20 minutes. Drink at least another 8 ounces when you're finished.

In hot weather, drink plenty of water before, during, and after any exercise.

How do you know if you are consuming enough fluids? Notice the color of your urine. If you urinate regularly and your urine is light yellow, you're drinking enough. If it's dark yellow, increase your fluid intake.

bottled water

About half of Americans now drink bottled water, which has the fastest-growing sales of any beverage. But don't assume that bottled water is safer or more healthful than tap water. Some studies have found that tap water tends to have lower bacterial counts than bottled. This doesn't mean that the bottled waters contained enough bacteria to cause illness, but enough to raise a red flag. Some earlier studies had also found that bottled waters are often out of line with the standards set for U.S. tap water. Some bottled waters are, in fact, merely repackaged tap water.

If you have young children and they drink only bottled water, make sure they use fluoride toothpaste and/or a fluoride rinse, and consider fluoride treatments from a pediatric dentist as well. Many, if not most, bottled waters contain little or no fluoride. Since fluoride helps protect against tooth decay, it's doubly important that your kids get proper dental care if they drink only bottled water.

For adults, fluoridated water may also play a role in building strong bones and warding off osteoporosis. Studies have shown that women who live in areas with naturally fluoridated water suffer fewer osteoporotic fractures and have generally greater bone strength than those who drink nonfluoridated water.

If you care about conservation of resources, tap water is by far the best choice. Millions of tons of plastic are used every year to make water bottles; disposing of these bottles contributes to air pollution.

Bottom line: If your tap water comes from a municipal system, there is no reason to forsake that water for the bottled variety.

If you do buy bottled water, you're probably better off buying brands bottled by members of the International Bottled Water Association; their plants are inspected by the National Sanitation Foundation, an independent nonprofit organization that tests products and certifies they meet certain standards. Check the label.

cooking glossary

Cooking has a great effect on the flavor and texture of the foods we eat, and also on their nutritional value. With improved knowledge of the physical and chemical changes that cooking causes in food, and greater understanding of the value and conservation of vitamins, minerals, and other valuable constituents in food, cooking methods have undergone a minor revolution in recent decades.

Tastes have changed, too. During the first half of the 20th century, overcooking was the rule: To make foods more digestible, many were boiled or stewed for hours. Under such treatment, vegetables and fruits turned mushy, while meat and poultry were rendered stringy and flavorless—their flavors and nutritional value obliterated.

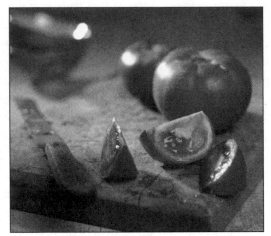

Today, the quality of "freshness" is appreciated, even in cooked foods. Both dry-heat methods (such as roasting and baking) and moist-heat techniques (such as blanching, steaming, and braising) are used by health-conscious cooks to produce crisp-tender vegetables, bright-colored fruits, and moist, flavorful meats and poultry. These techniques help conserve nutrients as well as taste and texture: The cook need only give some attention to details such as cooking time and temperature; how much liquid to add; whether or not to cover the pan; and the importance of serving certain cooked foods promptly. Even healthy frying (sautéing and stir-frying) is fine if broth or a small amount of olive or vegetable oil is used instead of large quantities of butter or other animal fat.

The glossary that follows presents the most common cooking techniques for the foods de-scribed in this book. A general understanding of how these processes work will help you choose techniques for cooking a wide range of foods with healthful, delicious results.

Baking This dry-heat method cooks food by surrounding it with heated air in an oven or covered barbecue grill. Vegetables, grains, legumes, meat, poultry, and fish (as well as casseroles and cakes) can be cooked by this method. Firm fruits, such as apples, pears, peaches, and plums, can be baked with spices and/or sweetener for a healthy dessert. The food may be covered to keep it moist: Consider wrapping chicken or fish in cabbage or lettuce leaves, or enclosing it in parchment (*opposite page*). Or it can be left uncovered to let the air circulate around the food and evaporate the moisture.

Among vegetables, potatoes are probably the most commonly baked. Other sturdy root vegetables (such as beets and rutabagas), as well as winter squash, also lend themselves to this method, as do onions and garlic (baking renders them sweet and mild). Place whole vegetables on a baking sheet or in a shallow baking dish, or wrap them in foil. Sprinkle halved or cut vegetables with a few tablespoons of liquid and cover them to keep them from drying out. Bake in a moderate oven (about 350°) until the vegetables are tender when pierced.

To bake grains, do so in a casserole or baking dish, just as you would simmer them on the stove-top: Stir in a measured amount of liquid and any seasonings or additional ingredients, then cover and bake in a 350° to 400° oven until the liquid is absorbed and the grain is tender. Baking should take the same amount of time as simmering, or slightly longer. The advantage of baking is that it requires little attention, and there is less chance of burning.

Dried beans and peas (legumes) are usually pre-cooked before baking. They are then typically slow-baked with other ingredients, such as onions, molasses, or tomato sauce, to flavor them.

Naturally, chicken parts, thick chops, whole fish, and fish steaks can be baked. And you can also bake both "fully-cooked" and "cook before eating" hams. To keep chicken, meat, or fish from drying out during baking, either marinate it beforehand, or cook it in a sauce or coating (a crumb crust, for instance), or cook some vegetables in the same pan. Covering the food with foil or a lid will help keep it moist. Use a shallow baking dish and turn the food occasionally for even cooking.

To bake fruits, core or pit the unpeeled fruit. Stuff the fruits, if desired, with chopped dried fruit or nuts, and place them in a baking dish with a small amount of liquid—water, fruit juice, or wine. Cover with foil and bake in a 325° oven until tender, basting occasionally with the liquid.

Baking in parchment Also called cooking *en papillote,* this method seals moisture into lean chicken breasts or fish fillets. You can use special cooking parchment (it's usually cut in a large heart shape for this purpose), but it's possible to obtain a similar result with aluminum foil. Cut large squares of foil, then place a boneless chicken breast or fish fillet on each square. For a one-dish meal, place the chicken or fish on a bed of cooked rice (or other grain) and top with thinly sliced vegetables, then season with your favorite herbs and spices. Fold the wrapping over the contents, crimp the edges together to seal the packet, and bake in a 400° to 425° oven until cooked through. Serve the dish directly from the parchment.

Blanching Also called parboiling, blanching means cooking food briefly in a large quantity of rapidly boiling water. It is typically used to quick-cook tender vegetables or to precook sturdier ones before finishing them with another technique such as braising or baking. A very brief blanching also loosens the skins of tomatoes, peaches, and plums, making them easier to peel. However, because immersing vegetables in lots of water can leach out water-soluble nutrients, many people prefer to steam them for the same purpose instead (*see page 613*).

To blanch vegetables, bring a large pot of water to a boil. Drop in the vegetables a few at a time, then cover and return the water to a boil. Cook just until the vegetables are bright-colored and barely crisp-tender. (You may want to use a timer, as blanching often takes a minute or less.) Drain the cooked vegetables in a colander and cool them under cold running water (or place the colander in a bowl of ice water). This stops the cooking and sets the bright color.

Boiling Though microwaving (*page 610*) and steaming (*page 613*) are preferred for cooking vegetables (because these methods help preserve nutrients), some vegetables cook more efficiently when they are boiled. Examples of vegetables that need to be boiled are dense vegetables such as dried beans, potatoes, or turnips. Cooking these vegetables in their skin helps protects against nutrient loss.

There is another method of boiling that is more accurately called steam-boiling. In this method, cut-up vegetables are started in a minimal amount of boiling water in a tightly covered pot. The water on the bottom of the pan converts to steam and steam-cooks the vegetables. A small amount of oil should be added to keep the vegetables from scorching. Here's how to steam-boil: Using about ½ cup of water per pound of vegetables, bring the cut-up vegetables, oil, and water to a boil in a tightly covered pan. Then adjust the heat to maintain a slow boil. Check during cooking to be sure the water does not boil away.

Braising This moist-heat method cooks meat, poultry, or vegetables slowly in their own juices plus a little added liquid. Slow-cooking in liquid softens the connective tissue of meat without hardening the protein, so this is one of the best methods for tenderizing and flavoring lean cuts of meat that would be tough and stringy if broiled or roasted. Pot roast is an example of braised meat.

Whether you're braising meat, poultry, or vegetables, you can use wine, broth, or juice (or a combination) instead of water. The liquid will cook down to a thick, savory sauce to serve with the food, thus preserving nutrients that might otherwise be lost. Vegetables are often braised along with meat and poultry; they add flavor as well as moisture.

Sometimes foods are precooked before braising: Fatty meats, such as short ribs, can also be blanched before braising to remove some of the fat. Meat and poultry may also be seared or browned before braising to intensify their flavors and produce better color.

To braise meat or poultry, start by browning the meat, if desired, in a lightly oiled nonstick pan—a deep skillet or Dutch oven works well. (Dredging the food in flour first helps brown it and thickens the cooking liquid.) Pour off any excess fat, then add a small amount of liquid—to a depth of not more than ½ inch. Adjust the heat so the liquid simmers, then cover the pan tightly and cook until the meat is very tender, adding more liquid if necessary. You can braise on the stovetop or in a low (300° to 325°) oven. Remove the meat when it is done and cook down the liquid on the stovetop until it forms a thick sauce. If possible, braise the meat the day before you plan to serve it; when refrigerated, the fat will congeal on the surface of the liquid and can then be easily removed.

To braise vegetables, place them in a heavy skillet with enough liquid to cover the bottom. Cover the pan and simmer over low heat until tender, basting occasionally.

Broiling and grilling Properly done, broiling and grilling (over gas or charcoal) yield meat, poultry, and fish that are crisp on the outside and juicy inside. These methods are also good alternatives to frying for vegetables such as eggplant, tomatoes, and summer squash. Oven broilers heat the food from the top, while barbecue grills heat it from the bottom. *(See also Panbroiling, opposite page)*.

These cooking methods work well for tender cuts of meat such as steaks or chops that are from 1 to 2 inches thick, kebabs, thick ground-meat patties, bone-in poultry parts, and thick fish steaks or whole fish (very lean meats and thin chicken or fish fillets can quickly toughen or overcook from the high heat). Marinating and basting help keep broiled or grilled foods moist and flavorful. Be careful with sugary barbecue sauces, however, as they can quickly scorch and burn.

For healthier broiled foods, use a pan with a rack that allows fat to drip off (this will also prevent flare-ups caused by burning fat). When grilling over coals, be sure to trim all visible fat. As a further precaution, push the hot coals to the sides of the barbecue and place a foil pan of water under the meat; any fat will then drip into the pan rather than onto the coals. Never broil or grill meat until it is blackened; if this occurs inadvertently, scrape or cut off the charred area.

Broil or grill meat about 4 inches from the heat source; chicken and turkey should be 6 to 8 inches from the heat. Start poultry pieces with the bone side toward the heat—bone-side up for broiling, bone-side down for grilling. Have the grill rack or broiler pan very hot—trying to grill or broil at a low temperature results in dried-out rather than juicy, well-browned food. Turn the food halfway through the cooking time, using tongs to avoid piercing the pieces and releasing juices. Be careful not to overcook and dry out meat or poultry when broiling or grilling.

Sturdy vegetables can be broiled or grilled, too. When broiling, place halved or thickly sliced vegetables (or whole baby vegetables) on the broiler pan. Brush them lightly with oil (or baste them during cooking with broth or juice) and broil about 4 inches from the heat. When the vegetables begin to brown, turn them and broil the other side. When grilling vegetables on the barbecue, it's best to use a grill topper rather than placing the food directly on the rack, where it is likely to stick, break apart, and fall into the fire.

Frying Cooking food in a deep or shallow pan of hot fat is obviously not a healthful method. However, two frying methods—sautéing/panfrying (*page 612*) and stir-frying (*page 613*)—can be modified so that little or no fat is required.

Microwaving This method of cooking is, for some foods (such as vegetables), the healthiest. It's undeniably fast, and little or no liquid is used. When microwaving vegetables, cover or wrap them to hold in moisture and help them cook more evenly. This includes hard-shelled squash, which should be halved for quicker cooking and to prevent them from exploding. You don't need to cover whole baking potatoes; but do pierce them several times before cooking. If you are microwaving more than one potato, arrange them in a circle and allow additional cooking time.

Meats and poultry don't do well in a microwave, because they are difficult to brown.

Fish, on the other hand, lends itself very nicely to microwaving: It doesn't require browning and it retains nearly all of its moisture when micro-waved, as though it had been perfectly poached or steamed.

Microwave cooking times vary with the quantity of food and the type of oven you use: The owner's manual is your best guide to finding the correct times. Test for doneness after the shortest cooking time, if a range of times is given. To ensure that food cooks evenly, it should be stirred several times, or the platter or dish it is on should be turned midway through the cooking time if the microwave doesn't have a rotating lazy susan.

Panbroiling (pangrilling) Steaks, chops, patties, and small whole fish can be cooked by this stovetop version of oven broiling. Special stovetop grilling pans with raised grids allow the fat to pool away from the food for healthier cooking. Use nonstick cooking spray or a little oil if necessary. (Fish will probably require some oil in the pan.) Heat a heavy, lightly oiled (preferably nonstick) grill pan until very hot. Place the meat or fish in the pan and cook, uncovered, until one side is browned, then turn and cook the other side. Cook thick cuts of meat slowly over medium heat, and thinner cuts of meat, patties, and whole fish over medium-high heat.

Poaching This method calls for cooking food in barely simmering water or other liquid on the stovetop. Eggs are the food most commonly poached, but poaching is also a gentle cooking technique for meat, poultry, and fish. Chicken breast is often poached for chicken salad; poached beef is good with a robust horseradish or mustard sauce. Fruit can also be poached, singly or in combination, for a dessert or main-dish accompaniment. For best flavor, poach food in well-seasoned broth, a combination of broth and wine, or fruit or vegetable juice, as appropriate.

When poaching meat, poultry, or fish, place the food in cold liquid and bring it to a bare simmer—never a rapid boil. Partially cover the pan, or use a round cut out from parchment paper that fits just inside the pan; this "lid" allows excess steam to escape while holding in the heat. When the food is cooked, you may strain the poaching liquid and cook it down (thickening it if necessary) to serve as a sauce. Or, reserve the poaching liquid and use it as a soup base.

To poach fruit, it's best to cook it in a small amount of barely simmering liquid, partially covered. You can cook the fruit in a sugar syrup to sweeten it, or poach in water, wine, or fruit juice (add whole or ground spices to the poaching liquid for more flavor). Turn the fruit occasionally, and baste it with the poaching liquid if it is not completely immersed.

Pressure cooking Long before the microwave arrived on the scene, the pressure cooker was the secret to quick cooking. It's also a healthful method, since this type of pot in effect steams the food, and does so in minutes. Follow the instructions that come with your pressure cooker for the correct cooking times and techniques.

Some foods require special procedures, especially if you're using an older pressure cooker. Grains must be rinsed before cooking to remove excess starch, which can block the steam valve during cooking. Foam clogging the valve can also be a problem with dried beans. With both beans and grains, adding a few teaspoons of oil will help prevent excessive foaming. Don't fill the pot more than one-third full, to allow plenty of space for the grains or beans to expand.

Roasting A standard cooking method for large cuts of meat and whole chickens, turkeys, and other poultry, roasting is not a demanding technique, but it does require temperature regulation and timing. A constant temperature (which can be from 350° to 450°, depending on the food and the recipe) causes less shrinkage and conserves more nutrients. It was once thought that initial high heat "sealed in" juices, but this is now known not to be true.

Traditionally, meat for roasting had a liberal layer of fat on it. Leaner cuts and lean poultry were "larded" or "barded," that is, strips of fatty pork or bacon were inserted through or wrapped around the food to keep it moist. Neither is a healthy option, but leaner roasts do benefit from marinating and/or basting (with broth, not fatty pan drippings). Rubbing the meat with a teaspoon of olive oil will also help without adding much fat. Poultry cooked in its skin—which can be removed before the bird is eaten—has a natural protective coating, but basting with broth, fruit juice, or cider will help keep a roasting bird moist. (It is best to baste chicken or turkey only at half-hour intervals to avoid lowering the oven temperature and increasing the cooking time.)

Cooking both meat roasts and poultry on a rack allows fat to drip off. Cooking vegetables or fruit with a roast also supplies moisture; however, if the potatoes, onions, carrots, or apples you place in the pan are sitting in drippings, they will not be a healthful addition to your meal. Place them on the rack or on top of the meat, or consider them simply as seasonings to be discarded.

To roast beef, lamb, or pork, prepare the meat and place it on a rack in an open roasting pan. Place the roast in a preheated oven and cook until a meat thermometer inserted in the thickest portion of the roast registers the correct temperature, according to the recipe. Remember that the size, shape, and cut of the roast, its temperature when placed in the oven, and the accuracy of your oven thermostat can affect cooking time. A good meat thermometer—and your own experience—are your best guides.

When cooking a chicken or turkey, place it breast-side up on a rack in a roasting pan. Roast, uncovered, until a thermometer inserted in the under part of the thigh registers the correct temperature, according to the recipe. If parts of the bird brown too quickly, protect them with a loose tent of foil.

Whether you're serving meat or poultry, allow the roasted food to stand for 15 to 20 minutes before carving; this lets it finish cooking (the internal temperature will go up about 5° as it sits) and also allows the juices to be reabsorbed evenly throughout so they are not lost during carving.

Vegetables can be roasted, too. Sturdy ones such as white and sweet potatoes, winter squash, eggplant, turnips, carrots, beets, cauliflower, onions, and garlic develop a rich, sweet flavor when roasted at a high temperature—in a 425° to 450° oven. Leave the vegetables whole, or halve or quarter large ones; roast them with the skin on. Brush the vegetables with a little oil so they do not dry out. Potatoes in their skins, corn on the cob in its husk, and other vegetables can be grilled, too, if convenient.

Sautéing/panfrying Food that is sautéed is cooked in a hot pan (usually a skillet) in a small amount of fat. The term comes from the French verb *sauter,* which means "jump," because the pan should be hot enough to make the food do that. You can sauté thin cuts of meat such as pork medallions, veal scallops, and boneless chicken breasts, as well as fish fillets and whole small fish. The food may be breaded or dusted with flour; chicken may be sautéed without the skin. Also, grains such as rice or kasha are sometimes sautéed before simmering to intensify their flavor. When cut-up foods are sautéed, they need to be moved around to cook them evenly, a method that closely resembles stir-frying.

Sautés traditionally call for butter and/or oil; if you use a nonstick pan, you can manage with very little fat. Alternatively, use a nonstick cooking spray or sauté in a small amount of broth or even water. (Such liquids do not get as hot as fat, so the cooking process changes slightly.) The pan should be big enough to hold the food without crowding, or it will steam rather than sauté.

Heat a skillet or sauté pan (with a tablespoon of fat or a few tablespoonfuls of broth) until hot but not smoking. Add the food and if whole pieces, cook until browned on one side, then turn and cook on the second side. When sautéing meat or poultry, turn it with tongs instead of a fork, so you do not pierce it and release the juices. To turn fish, use a spatula. Cut-up food should be stirred to keep it from sticking. If using broth or water, add more as the liquid evaporates.

Simmering Most Americans cook rice by this basic method, and it works equally well for other whole and cracked grains. By using a measured quantity of liquid (so none is poured off after cooking), you conserve most of the nutrients in the grain. You can simmer grains in water, broth, milk, or juice for added flavor (acidic juices will slow the cooking, so they should be added after the grain is partially cooked).

To simmer, bring a measured amount of liquid to a boil in a pot with a tight-fitting cover. Stir in the grain and re-cover the pot. When the liquid returns to a boil, reduce the heat so that it simmers and cook, covered, until the grain is tender and the liquid is absorbed. It's best not to uncover the pot during cooking, but you may want to check it once—quickly—toward the end of the cooking time to make sure that the liquid has not been absorbed prematurely, allowing the grain to scorch. Add more liquid, if necessary.

To simmer grains that have been precooked by sautéing (as for most pilafs), bring the measured amount of liquid to a boil in a separate pot, then stir the liquid into the grain. Cover tightly, reduce the heat, and simmer until fully cooked.

Cereal grains used for porridge, such as cream of wheat or oatmeal, are stirred into rapidly boiling water or milk and then stirred constantly for about a minute to keep them from lumping. They are then simmered, covered or uncovered, until thick. Stir occasionally to keep the cereal from sticking, and be sure to add more boiling liquid if necessary.

Steaming This is an ideal cooking method: Because the food is not immersed in water, most nutrients are retained. Almost any food that can be boiled or simmered can also be steamed. It works well for vegetables and can also be used for boneless chicken breasts, fish, and some grains. Use a metal steaming basket or a bamboo steamer, or improvise a steamer, if necessary, with a metal strainer or colander. Place the food in the steamer over boiling water, using a pot with a tight cover. A large steamer that leaves space for the steam to circulate around and through the food does the most efficient job. If the water threatens to boil away before the food is done, add more boiling water (adding cold water lengthens the cooking time).

Steeping Bulgur and other cracked grains, such as barley grits, can be cooked this way, and will be slightly chewier than if they were simmered. Place the grain in a heatproof bowl and pour in boiling water or broth to barely cover it. Cover and let stand for 15 to 30 minutes, or until most of the liquid has been absorbed; drain in a strainer if necessary, then fluff with a fork before serving.

Stewing Similar to braising (*page 609*), stewing is cooking food in liquid. But while braising uses a small amount of liquid, stewing usually involves enough liquid to immerse the food being cooked. The cooking liquid in stewing is most often retained and becomes part of the dish.

Stews are usually made with relatively small cubes of meat or cut-up poultry. Browning the meat before stewing makes a more flavorful dish; dredging the meat in flour first enhances the browning and helps thicken the stew. Pour off any accumulated fat after browning, then add enough boiling liquid (water, broth, or wine) to cover the meat. Cook, covered, until the meat or poultry is tender. Time the addition of vegetables so that they will be done at the same time as the meat. You'll want to add dense, firm vegetables such as carrots or turnips earlier than more delicate ones like mushrooms or peas. Stews often improve in flavor after standing for a day.

You can also stew whole chickens and large cuts of meat. Sometimes vegetables are added to the stewing liquid and the meat and vegetables are served together, with the broth on the side. Other times, the meat or poultry is cooked without any vegetables and the broth is discarded.

Stir-frying A stir-fry of mixed vegetables, or meat or poultry with vegetables, is a colorful, satisfying meal or side dish. If you use a wok or a heavy nonstick skillet, you can stir-fry with a minimum of oil (about a tablespoon). Or, you can stir-fry with broth.

Cut all of the ingredients into thin, uniform pieces. Heat the oil or broth in the pan until very hot but not smoking. Once the food has been added, toss it constantly, using a rubber, heatproof spatula, until the vegetables are crisp-tender.

If you are cooking more than one vegetable, start with the densest, then add more delicate vegetables toward the end; some require just seconds in the wok. Or, stir-fry each vegetable individually, transfer it to a dish when cooked, and stir-fry the next. When making a stir-fry that includes both meat or poultry and vegetables, cook the vegetables first, then remove them from the pan and set aside before cooking the meat or poultry.

herbs & spices

An excellent way to enhance the flavors of food when you're cutting back on fat is to use herbs and spices creatively. The following guide will help you choose appropriate seasonings for different foods. Fresh herbs are becoming more widely available all the time: Look for them in the produce department of your supermarket or at a specialty greengrocer. Buy fresh herbs as needed: Wrap them in damp paper towels, place in plastic bags, and refrigerate. If using fresh herbs in a cooked dish, add them toward the end of the cooking time so that their delicate flavors are not lost. (*See also Green Herbs, page 349.*)

Dried herbs (as well as spices) are available in supermarkets, specialty food stores, and many ethnic markets, as well as by mail order. If you prefer to grind your own spices, for use on their own or in blends, use a spice grinder or small coffee grinder dedicated to the purpose. It's best to grind small batches for maximum freshness. Store dried herbs and spices in airtight containers in a cool, dark place to conserve their flavors and aromas.

Achiote See Annatto *(at right).*

Adobo seasoning This all-purpose Mexican blend is spicy without being overly hot. It typically contains black pepper, cumin, Mexican oregano, onion, and garlic; however, certain brands may also include turmeric, salt, cayenne, lemon-pepper, or other spices. To make your own: Combine 3 tablespoons each of oregano and ground cumin with 1½ tablespoons each of garlic powder, onion powder, and black pepper. Makes about ½ cup.

Ajowan seed (ajwain, Bishop's weed, omum) Closely related to caraway and cumin, this seed is grown predominantly in India, Pakistan, Egypt, and Afghanistan. Though it looks like a large celery seed, it tastes very much like thyme. It is most often used in lentil and bean dishes. In India, a drink made of water and ajowan is used to cure an upset stomach, and some people believe it helps relieve intestinal gas. Use less than you think at first, because the flavor is intense.

Allspice This small, dry, dark-brown berry is native to the West Indies and Central and South America, though it is usually associated with Jamaica. So named because its flavor is said to be reminiscent of cinnamon, nutmeg, and cloves, allspice lends a warm, slightly sweet and spicy flavor to both savory and sweet dishes. It can be purchased whole or ground. Add a few whole berries when making chicken, beef, or fish stock. Or add ground allspice to pot roasts or beef stews. You can also combine ground allspice with other spices to make a rub for poultry or meat or use it to give a kick to homemade applesauce, poached pears, and fruit compotes, as well as cookies, cakes, and quick breads. It is also the primary ingredient in jerk seasoning (*see page 619*).

Amchoor Also known as mango powder, this spice is made from green, unripe mangoes that are sliced, sun-dried, and ground into a fine powder. It is used in northern Indian cooking, lending a tangy, sour fruit flavor to soups, curries, and vegetable dishes. It is also used to tenderize meat and poultry. You can add amchoor to stir-fries or to any dish to which you'd add a splash of lemon or vinegar. Look for it in Indian markets and specialty food shops.

Anise seed Anise belongs to the *Umbelliferae* family of herbs, which also includes parsley and dill. The seeds have a sweet, licoricelike flavor. Available whole or ground, anise seed is a favorite ingredient in spice cakes, cookies, and other desserts. It also goes well with pork and seafood, and a little of this spice can add an intriguing note to braised beef or cooked cabbage. Anise oil is made from the seeds and is used mainly in baking.

Annatto (achiote) These colorful, flavorful seeds come from the fruit of an evergreen tree native to Mexico, Latin America, and the Caribbean, and are widely used in these cuisines. Each fruit produces about 50 seeds, which contain a red pigment. The seeds themselves are inedible, but they are used to make a flavorful oil for cooking. The dried seeds are heated in oil to which they impart a rich red color and a musky flavor. Annatto oil is often used instead of saffron to color and flavor rice dishes, for frying chicken or fish, and for braising pork or beef for enchiladas. Look for annatto seeds in markets selling Latin American products or at specialty food stores. Choose those that are rusty-red; if they are brown, they are old and flavorless. To make annatto oil: Mix ½ cup of annatto seeds for every 1 cup of vegetable oil or light olive oil in a small saucepan. Simmer over very low heat for 10 minutes, strain out the seeds, and refrigerate the oil. Use a tablespoon or two as needed.

Asafoetida (devil's dung, stinking gum) This seasoning, derived from several species of giant fennel that grow mainly in Iran and India, takes its name from the Persian word *aza* (resin) and the Latin *fetida,* which means stinking. The name accurately describes asafoetida's most obvious attributes: a dry, resinlike texture and a strong, garlicky odor. A common ingredient in Indian cooking, it can be found in solid bricks or in powder form in Indian markets. Use it sparingly to lend an interesting flavor to fresh and salted fish, vegetables, and beans. Store asafoetida in a closed jar, or the aroma will permeate your entire house.

Basil See Green Herbs (*page 349*).

Bay leaf There are two varieties of bay leaves commonly available, Turkish and California. Considered the best in the world by many, Turkish bay leaves are dull-green and have more depth of flavor than the shiny bright-green aromatic California variety. They are usually sold dried, in whole leaf or powdered form. If using the whole leaves, be sure to add them at the start of cooking to give them time to release their flavor; remove them from the dish before serving. Add bay leaves to meat, poultry, and fish stocks; to soups, stews, and braised dishes; and to tomato and other sauces.

Bay seasoning Crumbled bay leaves, celery seed, ginger, cayenne, and mustard are just a few of the dozen or so spices in this blend, which is commercially sold as Old Bay Seasoning. Originally created in the Chesapeake Bay area to use in crab boils, bay seasoning is far more versatile today. Use

it to season liquids for poaching fish, shellfish, or chicken; in soups; in spaghetti and barbecue sauces; and in vegetable dishes. To make your own: In a spice grinder, combine 3 tablespoons each of celery seeds and black peppercorns, 1½ tablespoons of sweet Hungarian paprika, 1 tablespoon of yellow mustard seeds, 2 teaspoons of ground ginger, 1 teaspoon of cardamom seeds, 10 bay leaves, and 1 teaspoon of cloves. Makes about ½ cup.

Bouquet garni This classic French combination of herbs always includes a couple of sprigs of fresh parsley and thyme, and a bay leaf. Like a "bouquet," the herbs are traditionally tied together in a bundle (or in a piece of cheesecloth) so that they can be easily removed at the end of cooking or once the flavor has been imparted to the dish. A bouquet garni is frequently used to flavor soups, stocks, and stews. Dried bouquet garni herbs are also marketed, but are a far cry from fresh.

Caraway seed The seeds of a plant in the parsley family, caraway is most often associated with rye bread. However, the seeds are also used in main dishes and salads in German and other northern European cuisines. Try caraway seeds in potato or cucumber salad or coleslaw, in meatloaf, or sprinkled over cooked noodles. The ancient Greeks used caraway to calm an upset stomach and today the Germans make a caraway liqueur called Kummel to serve after a heavy meal.

Cardamom Native to India, this aromatic, sweet spice (reminiscent of lemon, mint, and pine with hints of pepper) is used in many cuisines, notably Indian, Middle Eastern, African, and Scandinavian. It lends an interesting note to both sweet and savory dishes. You can purchase whole cardamom pods (they come green, white, or black), the hulled seeds, or ground cardamom. Green cardamom is more flavorful than white; black cardamom has a somewhat smoky flavor. Commercial ground cardamom is the least flavorful form; it's best to grind your own from the seeds. Use cardamom in homemade curry powder, in meat and vegetable dishes, in rice pilafs, and in baked goods.

Cassia buds Occasionally available from specialty spice stores, these are the dried unripened flower buds of the same cassia tree that gives us cassia cinnamon (see *Cinnamon, at right*). While the buds closely resemble cloves in appearance, their flavor is more like that of cassia cinnamon, but sharper and more flowery. Use cassia buds as you would cloves in sweet and savory recipes, including fruit desserts, curries, pilafs, chilis, and meat dishes.

Cayenne This pungent seasoning, also known as hot red pepper, is made by grinding dried hot red cayenne chili peppers. It is commonly used in Mexican, Indian, Chinese, Cajun, and Tex-Mex dishes. Cayenne is also good in marinades and barbecue sauces for meat, poultry, and fish, or in any dish that needs a peppery kick. If you're sensitive to spicy food, use just a pinch to begin with, then taste and add more cayenne, if desired.

Celery seed Commercially available celery seed comes from a wild celery called lovage. It has a concentrated celery flavor and should be used sparingly in recipes. Add it to split-pea soup, fish chowders, salad dressings, dips, hot or cold potato dishes, and stuffings. It's also often used in pickling mixtures.

Charnushka See Nigella sativa (*page 620*).

Chervil The dried form of this slightly sweet, anise-flavored herb (a member of the parsley family) has a stronger flavor than its fresh counterpart. Dried chervil is a common ingredient in *fines herbes* (*page 618*). It is also often used in cold dishes, since heat quickly causes its flavor to dissipate. Try adding it to potato, chicken, or tuna salad, or to cold vegetable dishes. You can also sprinkle it on a soup at serving time.

Chili powder There are two categories of chili powder. One is a blend (commonly found in supermarkets) that includes not only chilies (usually Anaheim), but spices such as cumin, garlic powder, and salt as well. The other is pure chili powder, which contains nothing but ground chilies. Pure chili powder can be made from a single type of chili pepper (and should be so labeled), or it may be a combination of several different types of chili peppers. Each type of chili pepper has its own flavor and heat characteristics. Try buying several different kinds of chili powder, each made from a different single pepper, and make your own blend. Chili powder can be used as part of a rub for meat, poultry, or fish; be added to soups, stews, and chilis; or be mixed into savory bread, pizza, and pie doughs.

Chives See Green Herbs (*page 349*).

Chinese five-spice powder See Five-Spice Powder (*page 618*).

Cilantro See Green Herbs (*page 350*).

Cinnamon One of the oldest spices known, cinnamon comes from the inner bark of evergreen trees native to Asia. The variety found in supermarkets is usually cassia cinnamon (*Cinnamonium cassia*), also known as Chinese cinnamon, although it may not be indicated on the packaging. Cassia is a dark, reddish-brown color and has a robust, bittersweet flavor. It typically comes in rolled sticks and in ground form; it may also be purchased in small chunks from specialty stores. Cassia buds (*see page 615*) come from the same tree and are occasionally available. Another variety of cinnamon, Ceylon cinnamon (*Cinnamonium zeylanicum*), also known as "true cinnamon," has a sweeter more citrusy flavor. In addition to its familiar uses in desserts and fruit dishes, cinnamon is a traditional ingredient in Moroccan and Greek chicken and beef dishes and fruited rice pilafs. Use this spice to season winter squash, sweet potatoes, carrots, and parsnips. Serve whole cinnamon sticks as stirrers in hot cider or fruit juice.

Citric acid (sour salt) This white powder is usually extracted from the juice of acidic fruits such as lemons, limes, pineapples, and gooseberries. It has a strong, tart flavor and is used in sweet and sour dishes and beverages. Look for it in the supermarket, packed in small bottles labeled citric acid, citric salt, or sour salt. Because it is often used in Jewish cooking, it may sometimes be found in the kosher foods section.

Cloves The dried unopened nail-shaped buds of the tropical evergreen clove tree, reddish-brown cloves are sold both whole and ground. They are typically combined with other sweet spices in apple desserts, gingerbread, and pumpkin pie. Their pungency also enhances split pea and bean soups, as well as baked beans, chilis, and barbecue and tomato sauces. Try cloves with fresh pork and ham, lentil and chick-pea dishes, and winter squash or sweet potatoes.

Coriander seeds The tiny, round, yellow-tan seeds of the coriander plant have no flavor resemblance to the plant's leaves (which are commonly called cilantro; see Fresh Herbs, page 350). Coriander comes both as whole seeds and ground. Pungently spicy, yet sweet and slightly fruity (like an orange), coriander is a key component in curries and is often used in spice cakes and cookies. A touch of coriander also perks up savory soups, roast pork, and salad dressings.

Crab boil (shrimp spice) This is the generic name for a mixture of herbs and spices—typically allspice, mustard seed, cayenne, dill seed, bay leaf, coriander seed, thyme, pepper, and salt—that is added to a large pot of boiling water to flavor cooked crab and sometimes shrimp. The mixture of herbs and spices varies from manufacturer to manufacturer. To make your own: Combine 2 tablespoons each of black peppercorns, mustard seeds, and coriander seeds with 1 tablespoon each of cloves, allspice, dill seed, thyme, and red pepper flakes. Add 12 bay leaves. Makes about ¾ cup.

Cubeb (Java pepper, tailed pepper) This Indonesian member of the pepper (*Piperaceae*) family is similar in flavor to black pepper, but with a hint of allspice. The small, reddish-brown seeds may be difficult to find, but try looking in Indonesian markets. Use cubeb as you would black pepper in any dish, or in a recipe calling for both pepper and allspice.

Cumin The seed of a plant in the parsley family, nutty-flavored whole or ground cumin seeds are often a component of chili powder; indeed the spice is commonly used to flavor many Mexican and Tex-Mex dishes. Cumin is also a key component of curry powder. To bring out its flavor, lightly toast cumin before adding it to a dish. Combine it with ground coriander, oregano, salt, and a touch of sugar and rub it onto chicken, fish, beef, or lamb before grilling. Cumin also complements cooked carrots and cabbage, chick-peas, lentils, and other legumes. There is also a *black cumin*, which has a stronger, more exotic flavor than regular cumin. It's available in Indian markets

(where it will be labeled *kali jeera*). It is used by cooks in northern Indian and Pakistan to flavor meat and rice dishes. Because of its strong flavor, use it in small amounts.

Curry leaves (kari leaves) Sold both fresh and dried in Indian markets, curry leaves are a popular ingredient in Indian, Indonesian, Malaysian, and Thai cuisines. Although they bear the name curry, and have a strong curry fragrance, the leaves are not used in curry powder. Use the fresh or dried leaves to season rice or bean dishes, or gently heat the leaves in oil and use the oil in cooking. You can also grind the dried leaves with coconut and chili peppers and add the mixture to a chutney during cooking.

Curry powder This blend of spices can vary widely, but generally includes turmeric, cardamom, coriander, cumin, fenugreek, cinnamon, and white, black, and/or cayenne pepper. Commercial curry powder typically comes in two styles: sweet and hot. Because some supermarket blends are not marked either way, your best bet is to look at the ingredients list and see how many types of pepper are used in the blend and where they fall in the listing (if they're first, it's hot). Use curry powder in soups, stews, and vegetable dishes, or as part of a rub for meats, fish, or poultry. To make your own: In a small, dry skillet, heat 4 teaspoons each of cumin seeds, coriander seeds, and cardamom seeds, and 2 teaspoons of peppercorns, until lightly toasted. Transfer to a spice grinder and finely grind. Stir in 2 tablespoons of turmeric and ¾ teaspoon each of ground cinnamon and fenugreek. Makes about ½ cup.

Dill seed These seeds of the dill plant are stronger and more flavorful than the leaves of the plant. Dill seed is a traditional favorite in German and Scandinavian cuisine, where it is often used in pickling, salad dressings, cucumber and potato salads, and fish dishes. It can also be added to bread doughs, cole slaw, and seafood boils.

Dill See Green Herbs (*page 350*).

Epazote (Mexican tea, wormseed) This leaf of a wild Mexican herb has a slightly citrusy, bitter flavor. It is an essential ingredient in Mexican bean dishes (perhaps for its supposed ability to reduce flatulence). The flat, pointed leaves are available whole or ground in Latin markets. Try adding 1 tablespoon to a large pot of chili or to bean soups; or simmer epazote with beans before adding them to soups or stews.

Fennel seeds See Fennel (*page 303*).

Fenugreek Cultivated since ancient times, aromatic fenugreek has a bittersweet, savory flavor. It is used extensively in Middle Eastern, southern Indian, and North African cuisines, and is best known as an indispensable ingredient in most curry powders (most people smelling fenugreek would identify it as the typical smell of curry powder). Both the whole dried seeds as well as ground fenugreek are available. The spice is also used in chutneys, and can be added to vegetarian dishes, soups, and stews.

Filé powder (gumbo file) This seasoning (used in Cajun and Creole cooking as a thickener for soups, stews, and gumbos) is made from the ground dried leaves of the sassafras tree. It has a woodsy flavor, reminiscent of root beer. Always add filé powder to a dish just before it comes off the heat, or it may thicken too much.

Fines herbes A classic *fines herbes* mixture always consists of finely chopped chervil, chives, parsley, and tarragon. However, depending on the manufacturer, it may also contain sweet marjoram and savory, or other herbs. This light combination of herbs goes well with chicken, fish, or vegetable dishes.

Five-spice powder This blend of spices—which includes cinnamon, ground cloves, fennel seed, star anise or anise seed, and Szechuan peppercorns—is mainly used in Chinese cooking. Added to sauces, or combined with brown sugar and used as a rub for pork or chicken (Chinese-style or not), it lends a wonderful sweet and spicy flavor. To make your own: In a spice grinder, finely grind 2 tablespoons each of Szechuan peppercorns, star anise, and fennel seeds. Stir in 2 tablespoons each of ground cinnamon and ground cloves. Makes about ½ cup.

Galangal (laos powder) A close relative of ginger, galangal is an important ingredient in Indonesian and Southeast Asian cuisines (and Thai dishes in particular). Although chunks of dried galangal can be purchased, powdered galangal is easier to work with and more readily available. The flavor of galangal is similar to ginger, but more flowery and peppery. Use it as you would ginger. It is commonly combined with lemongrass in Thai cooking.

Garam masala *Garam* is the Indian word for "warm" or "hot" and *masala* means blend. This mixture of dry-roasted ground spices from the colder climes of northern India adds warmth to any dish it's used in. While variations abound, garam masala generally consists of a combination of coriander, black pepper, cardamom, cinnamon, cloves, ginger, and nutmeg, but also may include other spices such as nigella sativa, fennel, or fenugreek. Typically used in Indian dishes, it can also be added to Western stews and soups and be used as a rub for roasts. Try several brands to see which you prefer. To make your own: Remove cardamom seeds from 1 tablespoon of cardamom pods and toast in a dry skillet along with 2½ tablespoons each of cumin seeds and coriander seeds, 1½ tablespoons of peppercorns, 1 teaspoon of whole cloves, and 1 cinnamon stick. Toast over low heat, stirring frequently, until aromatic. Transfer to a bowl and cool before grinding in a spice grinder. Makes about ½ cup.

Ginger See Ginger (*page 338*).

Grains of paradise (melegueta pepper) This spice, a relative of cardamom, grows mainly in Ghana and is used in many West African dishes. The seed has a strong flavor that tastes like a combination of pepper, ginger, and cardamom. It can be used as a substitute for black pepper, or you can add some to your peppermill along with other peppercorns.

Herbes de Provence This blend of dried herbs is so named because it contains herbs that commonly grow in the south of France. The mix usually contains basil, rosemary, marjoram, fennel seeds, lavender, sage, summer savory, and thyme. Look for it in small packets or little clay crocks in your supermarket or specialty food stores. To make your own: Combine equal parts of all of the herbs listed above.

Horseradish See Horseradish (*page 363*).

Horseradish powder Made of ground, dried horseradish, the powder can be mixed with water to reconstitute it or can be stirred directly into tomato sauces, ketchup, sour cream, or yogurt.

Jerk seasoning This herb and spice blend from Jamaica is used in the preparation of grilled meat (usually pork), chicken, and fish. The spicy seasoning usually consists of a fair amount of allspice, along with thyme, cinnamon, ginger, cloves, and pepper. Both liquid and dry forms are available. To make your own: Combine 2 tablespoons each of ground allspice and thyme with 1 tablespoon each of ground black pepper, ground cinnamon, and ground ginger, and 1½ teaspoons of ground cloves. Makes about ½ cup. The dry mixture can be mixed with vinegar to make a wet marinade.

Juniper berries Perhaps most famous for lending a slightly medicinal flavor to gin, these blue-black berries from the juniper bush are also used in marinades for seasoning game such as rabbit, venison, and squab. Sold dried, the berries should be lightly crushed to release their flavor and can then be added to both wet and dry marinades, and to sauces and stuffings.

Kaffir lime leaves From the kaffir lime tree, which grows in Southeast Asia and Hawaii, these leaves are shiny dark-green when fresh and dull gray-green when dried. Both the fresh and dried leaves are available in Asian markets. Kaffir leaves have a pronounced floral aroma and impart a lemon flavor when added to soups and stews. The flavor marries well with hot chilies and the leaves are often added, along with coconut milk, to Thai curries and soups. Like bay leaves, use them whole and remove them from the dish before serving.

Kali jeera See Cumin (*page 617*).

Kokum powder The kokum tree, native to southern India, bears dark-purple to black fruit. It's the fruit's skins that are dried and ground into this powder. Kokum powder has a tangy, salty flavor and is used in Indian cooking to season curries, chutneys, pickles, vegetable dishes, and beans and lentils. Look for it in Indian grocery stores.

Laos powder See Galangal (*opposite page*).

Lavender Dried lavender flowers, often imported from Provence, are typically added to desserts to lend their sweet, flowery flavor. Try steeping lavender in milk for puddings (be sure to strain before using). You can also add it to spice rubs for lamb. Be wary about how much you use, however; the perfumey flavor can become overpowering.

Lemongrass (citronella, sereh) This fragrant grass has a long, somewhat tough stalk, a bulbous root, and a sweet, lemonlike flavor without any acidity. The dried bulb is available in small crosscut sections or in powder form. Lemongrass is an essential ingredient in Thai cooking, where it is used in soups, stews, curries, and sauces. It combines well with garlic and ginger and lends a mellow, lemony note to any dish it is used in.

Loomi In the Middle East, ripe limes are boiled in salted water, sun-dried until the interior blackens, and ground into a powder called loomi. The powder has a strong, tangy taste similar to lime zest. Try loomi in legume and meat dishes. It's available at Middle Eastern markets.

Mace The bright-red membrane that covers the nutmeg seed, mace becomes yellow-orange when dried. Both ground mace and whole mace (called mace "blades") are available. Mace has a flavor similar to nutmeg, but is slightly stronger. You can use mace in the same way as you would nutmeg—just use less of it. It is the classic spice for poundcake.

Mahlab The dried pit of a tree similar to the sour cherry, mahlab is available in both whole and ground form. Used extensively in the Middle East (especially in Turkey and Syria) it lends a slightly bitter almond flavor to baked goods and is also used to season vegetable, meat, poultry, and fish dishes. Although ground mahlab is sold, it's best to buy the seeds whole and grind them yourself just before using, because the spice's flavor dissipates quickly.

Marjoram (sweet marjoram) A member of the mint family, and a close relative of oregano (which can also be called wild marjoram), this gray-green herb has a more delicate flavor than oregano. Most often found dried, it's especially good in tomato sauces and other tomato-based dishes, and also adds flavor to lentils and beans. Try it with summer squash and potatoes, and with fish, lamb, and veal.

Mint See Green Herbs (*page 351*).

Mustard seed There are three types of mustard grown for their seed: white (*Brassica alba* or *Brassica hirta*), brown (*Brassica juncea*), and black (*Brassica nigra*). *White mustard seeds* (which are actually yellow) are the mildest and are the type commonly found in supermarkets. They are typically used in making ballpark mustard and as a pickling spice. Smaller *brown mustard seeds* (also known as Asian) are more pungent than white and are used in Asian and African cooking. *Black mustard seeds,* the most expensive and hardest to find because they are not produced much anymore, are the strongest-flavored of all. Mustard seeds are often briefly toasted in a dry skillet before being added to a dish; this gives them a nutty flavor. Use mustard seeds in sauces for meat, poultry, and fish; in marinades, salad dressings, relishes, and chutneys; and in pickle brines. Powdered mustard is finely ground mustard seeds.

Nigella sativa (charnushka, black onion seed, black caraway, kaloonji) These tiny, matte-black seeds have a smoky, peppery flavor that is also reminiscent of onions. They are often found atop Jewish rye breads or on the Indian bread called naan. They are also the seeds you find in Armenian string cheese. In India, nigella sativa is also used in braised meat dishes, with vegetables and legumes, in chutneys, and in some garam masala mixtures. To achieve the fullest flavor, gently toast the seeds in a dry skillet before using them.

Nutmeg The seed of the fruit of the nutmeg tree, native to the Spice Islands, nutmeg is sold whole and already ground. For maximum flavor, it's best to buy the whole nutmeg (the seeds keep indefinitely) and grate it yourself as you need it. This pungent, sweet spice is a favorite in fruit desserts and baked goods. A pinch of nutmeg also enhances braised or stewed meats and poultry, as well as spinach, broccoli, cauliflower, and carrots. It's also a key ingredient in béchamel (a classic white sauce).

Oregano A relative of mint, oregano is considered the quintessential Italian herb. However, it is also commonly used in Mediterranean and Mexican cooking. Indeed, the two types of dried oregano available are Mediterranean and Mexican. The Mediterranean variety, commonly found in supermarkets, is milder than the Mexican, which is generally used in spicy dishes, such as chili and salsa. Whichever type of oregano you choose, it should be added at the beginning of cooking so its flavor develops. Try oregano in tomato sauces and tomato-based soups, salad dressings, and marinades. Or use this aromatic herb to season grilled poultry, lamb, or shrimp, and mushrooms, green beans, and summer squash.

Paprika (pimentón) Paprika is made by drying and grinding mild to slightly hot peppers of the *Capsicum* genus. Most paprika comes from Spain or Hungary, and to a lesser extent California. *Spanish paprika* is either made from sun-dried or smoked peppers, depending upon the region it comes from. It is available in three varieties— dulce (sweet), agridulce (bittersweet), and picante (hot)—each made from a different type of pepper. Sweet Spanish paprika can be used in any dish calling for paprika; the bittersweet is good for more complex dishes; and the hot (which is hot without being too fiery) is fine for spicy dishes. Smoked Spanish paprika (also available sweet, bittersweet, and hot) adds a deep, smoky, full flavor to dishes. *Hungarian paprika,* which ranges in color from bright-red to rusty-brown, comes in eight different heat levels, from sweet to very hot. However, only three are available in the United States: sweet (labeled "Noble Rose"), medium-hot, and hot. The best Hungarian paprika is from the towns of Kalocsa and Szeged; the name should appear on the label of finer brands. *California paprika* is sweet and mild, with a deep red color. Don't use it in dishes requiring long cooking, because it tends to brown.

Parsley See Green Herbs (*page 351*).

Pepper Considered the world's most popular spice, pepper comes from the berry of the pepper plant (*Piper nigrum*), a climbing vine native to India and Indonesia. Interestingly green, white, and black peppercorns all come from the same plant, but are harvested at different stages of the pepper's growth. Green are the youngest, black are riper, and white are almost fully mature peppercorns. Two very popular types of *black peppercorns* are

Tellicherry and Malabar, which are not varieties of pepper but size designations. The peppercorns are harvested and then dried and sifted to separate the larger peppercorns (Tellicherry) from the smaller ones (Malabar). *White peppercorns* are peppercorns that have had the black outer shell removed. The method by which this is done determines the type of white pepper: Muntok pepper is the result of soaking the peppercorns in water until the shell loosens; Sarawak pepper is processed by running a constant stream of water over the shells. White pepper is preferred for pale-colored dishes because it doesn't show up as dark specks. Because *green peppercorns* are harvested before they are mature, they are usually sold fresh (typically packed in brine, vinegar, or water) rather than dried (though you can find them freeze-dried). Although pepper is available as whole peppercorns, as well as cracked and coarsely or finely ground, it's best to buy the whole peppercorns because pepper rapidly loses it's pungency once ground. Grind peppercorns yourself as needed (a simple peppermill is an inexpensive kitchen requisite). For an unusual dessert, sprinkle a little finely ground black pepper over vanilla ice milk or frozen yogurt.

There are also some spices called "pepper" that don't come from the pepper plant at all. These include *pink peppercorns*, which are from an unrelated weed, sometimes called Florida holly; Szechuan peppercorns (*page 622*); and melegueta pepper (*see Grains of paradise, page 618*).

Pickling spices This blend, used for pickling and canning, generally contains mustard seed, allspice, cracked cinnamon sticks, ginger, chili peppers, cloves, pepper, and cardamom—but the combination varies depending upon the manufacturer. To make your own: Combine 3 tablespoons of cracked cinnamon sticks with 2 tablespoons each of allspice berries, mustard seed, and coriander seed; 1 tablespoon each of cracked black peppercorns and crushed dried chili peppers; and 1 teaspoon each of whole cloves and cardamom seeds. Add 8 bay leaves, crumbled. Makes about ¾ cup.

Pomegranate seed The slightly sweet, dehydrated seeds of the pomegranate can be found in Indian, Middle Eastern, and specialty food stores. Their crunchy texture and sweet flavor add an interesting dimension anywhere they're used. A common ingredient in Indian lentil and pea dishes, pomegranate seeds also give a burst of flavor to chutneys, and rice and chicken dishes. Try some sprinkled on a salad of feta cheese and toasted walnuts or use them as a topping for frozen yogurt or ice cream.

Poppy seed See Seeds (*page 524*).

Poultry seasoning While this blend often contains rosemary, marjoram, and thyme, it *always* includes sage. Depending upon the manufacturer, it may also contain one or more of the following ingredients: pepper, dehydrated red and green peppers, savory, allspice, and/or dill. Use poultry seasoning to flavor stuffings; as part of a marinade for poultry or pork; in soups and stews; or as an ingredient in a salad dressing. To make your own: Combine 3 tablespoons of rubbed sage, 2 tablespoons each of rosemary (crumbled) and marjoram, and 1 tablespoon thyme. Makes about ½ cup.

Pumpkin pie spice This sweet and spicy mixture is what makes pumpkin pie so appealing. It generally contains cinnamon, allspice, nutmeg, ginger, and cloves. While pumpkin pie is the "signature dish" for which the blend is known, it also makes a great addition to butternut squash soup, pumpkin ravioli, sweet potatoes, cookies, cakes, quick breads, and sweet rolls. To make your own: Combine 4 tablespoons of ground cinnamon, 2 tablespoons of ground ginger, 1 tablespoon of ground allspice, 1½ teaspoons of ground nutmeg, and 1 teaspoon of ground cloves. Makes about ½ cup.

Ras el hanout This complex Moroccan spice blend with floral undertones can have anywhere from 12 to 50 ingredients. The name, which translates as "top (or head) of the shop," indicates that it's the spice merchant's finest blend. The mixture often contains black pepper, ginger, rose petals, cubeb, cardamom, nigella sativa, mace, nutmeg, cloves, lavender, cayenne, coriander, and cumin. In Morocco it is used to season couscous, vegetables, olive oil, and rice dishes.

Rosemary This herb comes from an evergreen shrub. Indeed, a branch of fresh rosemary looks like a small sprig of evergreen, and is just as fragrant. If you enjoy rosemary's assertive flavor, try using it to season chicken, lamb, pork, salmon and tuna; tomato sauces and soups; and potatoes, mushrooms, and peas. Be light-handed however, because a little goes a long way and too much rosemary can give a dish a distinctly forestlike flavor. When using fresh rosemary, it's necessary to remove the hard, needlelike leaves from the stem, then chop and crush them thoroughly. Even dried rosemary should be crushed or crumbled.

Saffron The most expensive of spices, saffron comes from a particular species of crocus (*Crocus sativus*). The spice is sold as "threads"—the whole stigmas of the flower—or powdered, often in small glass vials. Powdered saffron loses its flavor more readily than the stigmas. Just a pinch is needed to add a brilliant yellow color and an exotic, slightly medicinal taste to Spanish, Italian, and Indian rice dishes (such as paella, risotto, or pilaf); to seafood and poultry; and to sauces and soups. Saffron stigmas should be lightly toasted in a dry skillet, then crushed and dissolved in a small amount of warm water (just a teaspoon or so) before adding them to any dish.

Sage This native Mediterranean herb is most familiar as a seasoning for poultry stuffing. Sold as whole leaves (fresh or dried), rubbed (crumbled), and ground, sage has a bold, rather musty flavor and aroma. Try it with any type of poultry, or with pork, veal, or ham. Or use it in cheese sauces; in bean or vegetable soups and seafood chowders; or with cooked mushrooms, lima beans, peas, tomatoes, or eggplant.

Salam leaf (Indonesian bay leaf) Similar in size and shape to curry leaves (*see page 617*), these small green leaves turn brown once dried and impart a slightly sour, astringent flavor to a dish. Like bay leaves, they must be removed before serving.

Salt See Salt (*page 624*).

Sesame seeds See Seeds (*page 525*).

Star anise (Chinese anise) This star-shaped, dark-brown pod (from an evergreen native to China) has 5 to 10 points, each containing a pea-sized seed. Similar to anise seed, but from a different botanical family, it has a more pronounced, rather bitter licorice flavor. Because the flavor is so strong, the points are always broken off and only a few are used (along with their seeds) in a dish. Powdered star anise is also available and is one of the main ingredients in five-spice powder

(*see page 618*). Star anise can be used in braising liquids for meat and poultry; in fruit compotes; or in any dish where a strong licorice flavor is desired.

Sumac berries (sumaq) Available both whole and ground, these intense brick-red to dark-purple berries come from a bush that grows wild throughout the Middle East and in parts of Italy. Sumac is used extensively in Turkey, Syria, and Lebanon, where it is preferred over lemon for its mildly tart fruity flavor and aroma. It is often used in ground form to both spice up and give a slightly red hue to fish and shellfish dishes, rice and lentil recipes, and to yogurt toppings for kebabs. The whole berries may be soaked in hot water, then mashed to release their juice; the strained juice can then be used in marinades and salad dressings. Whole sumac berries can also be lightly toasted in a dry skillet and then ground for use in stews and soups.

Summer savory This slightly peppery herb goes particularly well in salad dressings and with vegetables such as peas, green beans, Brussels sprouts, and potatoes. It is also a delicious addition to bean, pea, and lentil dishes. In addition, summer savory enhances poultry, fish, lamb, and pork, and may even be used to perk up cooked fruit.

Szechuan peppercorns (Chinese pepper) Native to the Szechuan province of China, Szechuan peppercorns are not true pepper, but the dried berry of a deciduous prickly ash tree. The berry has a rough reddish-brown shell and a black seed. The black seed is bitter and not used; the shell is used whole or ground as a seasoning in savory dishes. Szechuan peppercorns have a warm, peppery flavor without being hot. If you purchase the whole shells, lightly toast them in a dry skillet before grinding them in a spice grinder. The toasting releases their fragrance and flavor. The ground peppercorns can be used as is or combined with salt to make an all-purpose seasoning mixture.

Tarragon Essential in French cooking, tarragon has a faint undertone of anise or licorice. Because it is so flavorful, the herb may overshadow other herbs, so use it with discretion. Tarragon is an excellent choice with shellfish, such as crab or shrimp, or with poached, baked, or broiled fish. It also complements poultry. Try it in a vinaigrette or other salad dressing, and with potatoes, peas, asparagus, carrots, mushrooms, or tomatoes.

Thyme This versatile herb, though quite strong in flavor, is compatible with many foods. It is also an essential ingredient in bouquet garni (*see page 615*). Thyme is available fresh and in dried leaf and ground form. Add a little to tomato sauces; vegetable soups and clam and other seafood chowders; beef stew or pot roast; poultry stuffings; and cooked vegetables, such as summer squash and green beans.

Turmeric Native to the Orient, but now cultivated in India and the Caribbean, turmeric (the ground dried rhizome of a gingerlike plant) is the ingredient that makes curry powder yellow. It is also what makes ballpark mustard bright yellow. Its flavor is warm with a slightly bitter undertone. Used extensively in Moroccan and East Indian cooking to add both color and flavor to dishes, it particularly complements lamb and vegetable curries. You can find it in powdered form in supermarkets.

Vanilla bean Long, thin vanilla beans are the dried fruits of a celadon-colored orchid (*Vanilla planifolia*), the only orchid to bear such fruit. Rich in aroma and sweet in flavor, vanilla beans are primarily used to flavor sweet dishes. The three most common types are *Bourbon-Madagascar, Mexican,* and *Tahitian.* Those from Madagascar are regarded as the most flavorful, with the vanilla beans from Mexico running a close second. The Tahitian beans, while intensely aromatic, are not as flavorful. To release the flavor of a vanilla bean, cut it lengthwise and scrape out the moist seeds into whatever dish you're preparing. Or, if you're flavoring a syrup, custard, or fruit dish, simply cut the bean and heat it along with the other ingredients. Once warmed, allow the bean to steep in the liquid for the fullest flavor. Once used, the bean can be rinsed, dried, and placed in your sugar canister where it lends its perfume to the sugar. You can also make your own vanilla extract by steeping the cut vanilla bean in a jar of grain alcohol or vodka. While vanilla is generally used in sweet dishes, it can lend a subtle note to some savory sauces as well. Whole ground vanilla beans are also made into vanilla powder, available at some specialty markets.

Zatar This popular Middle Eastern blend consists of thyme, sumac berries, sesame seed, and salt. It is typically mixed with olive oil and used to top breads such as pita, but it can also be sprinkled on yogurt or a soft cheese, such as goat cheese. Its flavor is slightly tart and earthy. Purchase zatar at Middle Eastern markets.

salt

The crystals we recognize as salt—its chemical name is sodium chloride, NaCl—are formed when water evaporates from a saline solution. While many types of salt do come from the sea (*see sea salt, below*), salt is also harvested from large inland bodies of water, such as the Great Salt Lake in Utah, and from subterranean deposits left by ancient oceans. The following are the most common types of salt:

Table salt This is the type of salt most of us use in cooking and as a condiment. It is actually finely ground, refined rock salt to which magnesium carbonate is added to keep it flowing freely. Iodized table salt also has potassium iodide added to help prevent thyroid disease. Low-sodium (or light) table salt is also available; it's good for people who need to restrict their sodium intake.

Kosher salt This is a large-grained, noniodized salt that's frequently used in koshering meats and pickling. Kosher salt is also good for topping breads, pretzels, and focaccias. Don't substitute kosher salt teaspoon for teaspoon for table salt; because the grains are larger, the measure will be off.

Crystal rock salt This is the same salt that's used on the highways to melt snow. In its unrefined form, rock salt is not eaten, but is often used in crank-style ice-cream makers and as a bed for raw and baked shellfish. Finely ground and refined, it's used for table salt.

Sea salt This salt comes in myriad varieties, tastes, and colors, depending on where it is harvested. The composition varies considerably according to the minerals and salts in the nearby land. Avoid the highly refined sea salt often sold in supermarkets; it is washed and boiled, which removes the minerals. Instead, look for unrefined, natural sea salt, available in specialty food markets, ethnic markets, and by mail order.

gourmet salt

The following salts can be expensive, but they are some of the best in the world.

Fleur de sel Called the "caviar of salt," this fragile gray-pink sea salt from the marshes of Guérande in Brittany is gathered from the surface crust on sel gris (*below*). It has a complex flavor that some say is reminiscent of violets. Its name, however (which in French means "salt flower"), comes from the floral filagree of its light and fluffy crystals.

Halen môn This Welsh sea salt is harvested from the Atlantic waters surrounding the Isle of Anglesey, or Ynys Môn (un-iss-mon) in Welsh. Its crystals are pure-white and very crunchy.

Hawaiian black It's the small amount of evaporated black lava that's added to this salt that gives it its color.

Hawaiian red These large, burnt-sienna crystals get their color from the iron oxide in the small amount of baked red clay (*alaea* in Hawaiian) that's added.

Indian black (kala namak, sanchal) More grayish-pink than black when ground, this salt comes large-grained (rock) or ground. It has a decidedly sulfurous flavor.

Jordanian pink From the Dead Sea, this coarse-grained salt is light-pink in color.

Maldon crystal This popular salt, produced by a small family business in Maldon, in Essex, England, has fine, pyramid-shaped crystals and a slightly sweet flavor.

Sel gris From Brittany and Normandy, this moist, large-grained light-gray sea salt gets its color from the clay that lines the basins in which it is dried. Fleur de sel (*above*) comes from the lightest, topmost crust of sel gris from Guérande. For every 80 pounds of sel gris produced, there is one pound of Fleur de sel.

Sicilian sea salt This black salt, produced along this island's western coast, becomes dusky-pink when ground; it has pungent, sulfurous notes.

vinegar

Vinegar has been used in one form or another for more than 10,000 years. It's been employed as a preservative, a beauty aid, a cleanser, a drink, a medicine, and a condiment, among other things. From the Latin *vinum* for wine and *acer* for sour, vinegar was once just that, sour wine. Today vinegar can be made from wine, fruit, rice, and other grains. Though the original vinegars were a happy accident with wine going sour naturally, commercially made vinegars involve a more complicated, two-step process: The first step is called alcoholic fermentation in which yeast converts the sugars in the juice (grape, fruit, or other) to alcohol; the second step is called acetic fermentation, in which bacteria convert the alcohol to acid.

The following list represents some of the more available vinegars:

Grain vinegar Though grains do not inherently have sugar, their starches can be converted to sugar, which are then processed into alcohol and from there into vinegar. *Distilled white vinegar* is made from the acid fermentation of dilute distilled alcohol. With its sharp bite, it is often used in pickling or preserving. *Malt vinegar* (the vinegar of choice for British fish and chips) comes from malted barley or sour unhopped beer.

Vinegar made from rice, which is used extensively in Asian cuisine, comes in several varieties. The mildest is *white rice vinegar*, made from glutinous rice. *Black vinegar*, generally produced from glutinous rice, water, and salt, may also be made from sorghum or millet instead of rice. The flavor, a pleasant balance between sweet and tangy, has a slightly smoky undertone. A third variety of rice vinegar, *red rice vinegar*, is not quite as dark as black rice vinegar, and is tangy and sweet but not smoky. *Brown rice vinegar* from Japan is a rich golden brown, and pleasantly sweet and tangy.

Wine vinegar These vinegars are made from a variety of wines. Some of the more common wine vinegars are: white wine, red wine, Champagne, sherry, brandy, and vin santo. There are also wine vinegars made from specific grape varietals and or regional wines, all with a slightly different flavor. Wine vinegars tend to be higher in acid than many other vinegars and are used as the base for infused vinegars.

Fruit vinegar Any fruit that has enough sugar can become a vinegar, though few are turned into commercial vinegars. The most common fruit vinegar, *apple cider vinegar*, has a mild, slightly sweet flavor. *Pineapple vinegar* is a Mexican ingredient, and is hard to find in this country.

One of the most famous and most popular fruit vinegars is sweet *balsamic vinegar*, which is made in Modena, Italy, from highly concentrated grape juice that never becomes wine, but is reduced by cooking and then aged in a succession of barrels, each from a different wood. Made predominantly from the Trebbiano grape, it comes in both a commercially made (*industriale*) and traditionally made (*tradizionale*) form. As you might surmise, the commercially made is manufactured in bulk, while the traditional is a much longer and more painstaking process. The commercial balsamic may or may not be aged, is sweet and tart, and is a perfect everyday vinegar. The traditional should be used sparingly as it is often thick and syrupy, it is also quite expensive.

Other vinegar *Coconut vinegar*, made from coconut water fortified with palm sugar, is a light-colored, low-acid vinegar available in Filipino grocery stores. *Cane vinegar* is made from sugar cane and has a slightly sweet flavor. *Honey vinegar* retains some of the finer characteristics of the honey from which it is made.

Infused vinegar Vinegars can be infused with flavors of any number of ingredients, including fruits, herbs, and spices. Raspberry, pear, cranberry, plum, blueberry, date, fig, cherry, orange, pomegranate, and key lime are just a few of the fruit vinegars available. Some of the more popular herb vinegars are tarragon, basil, and thyme. Other flavors may include chili peppers, citrus zest, garlic, cloves, or vanilla. There are also myriad combinations of fruit, herb, and spice infusions.